Modern Techniques in SPINE SURGERY

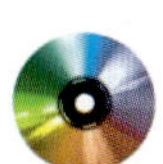

System requirement:

- Operating System – Windows XP or above
- Web Browser – Internet Explorer 8 or above, Google Chrome, Mozilla Firefox and Safari
- Essential plugins – Java and Flash player
  - Facing problems in viewing content – it may be your system does not have java enabled.
  - If Videos don't show up – it may be the system requires Flash player or need to manage flash setting
  - You can test java and flash by using the links from the troubleshoot section of the CD/DVD.
  - Learn more about flash setting from the link in the troubleshoot section.

Accompanying CD/DVD-ROM is playable only in Computer and not in DVD player.

CD/DVD has Autorun function – it may take few seconds to load on your computer. If it does not works for you then follow the steps below to access the contents manually:

- Click on my computer
- Select the CD/DVD drive and click open/explore – this will show list of files in the CD/DVD
- Find and double click file – "launch.html"

DVD Contents

1. Minimally Invasive Lumar Endoscopic Surgery
2. Minimally Invasive Surgery - Transforaminal Interbody Fusion
3. Anterior Endoscopic Cervical Microdecompression of Disc and Foramen
4. Transforaminal Approach

Modern Techniques in SPINE SURGERY

Arvind Bhave MS (Orth) IPTM FICOE FMISS
Professor, Department of Orthopedic Surgery
Bharati Vidyapeeth Medical College
Spine Surgeon, Deenanath Mangeshkar Hospital and Inlaks and Budhrani Hospital
Pune, Maharashtra, India

Forewords
Kuniyoshi Abumi
S Rajasekaran

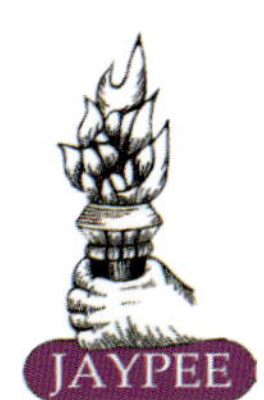

The Health Sciences Publisher
New Delhi | London | Philadelphia | Panama

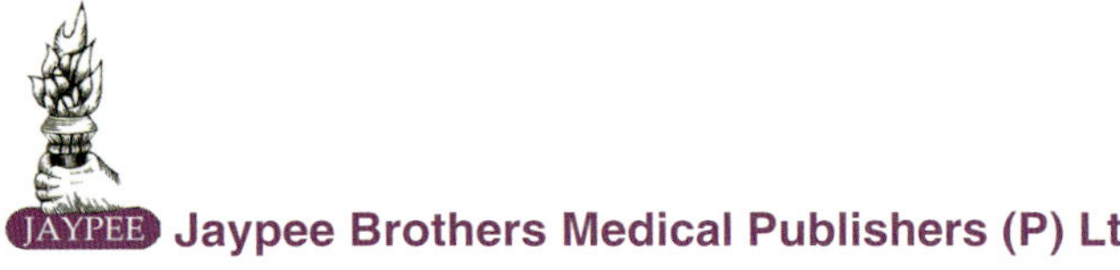

Jaypee Brothers Medical Publishers (P) Ltd

Headquarters

Jaypee Brothers Medical Publishers (P) Ltd
4838/24, Ansari Road, Daryaganj
New Delhi 110 002, India
Phone: +91-11-43574357
Fax: +91-11-43574314
Email: jaypee@jaypeebrothers.com

Overseas Offices

J.P. Medical Ltd
83, Victoria Street, London
SW1H 0HW (UK)
Phone: +44-2031708910
Fax: +44(0)20 3008 6180
Email: info@jpmedpub.com

Jaypee-Highlights Medical Publishers Inc
City of Knowledge, Bld. 237, Clayton
Panama City, Panama
Phone: +1 507-301-0496
Fax: +1 507-301-0499
Email: cservice@jphmedical.com

Jaypee Medical Inc
The Bourse
111 South Independence Mall East
Suite 835, Philadelphia, PA 19106, USA
Phone: +1 267-519-9789
Email: jpmed.us@gmail.com

Jaypee Brothers Medical Publishers (P) Ltd
17/1-B Babar Road, Block-B, Shaymali
Mohammadpur, Dhaka-1207
Bangladesh
Mobile: +08801912003485
Email: jaypeedhaka@gmail.com

Jaypee Brothers Medical Publishers (P) Ltd
Bhotahity, Kathmandu
Nepal
Phone: +977-9741283608
Email: kathmandu@jaypeebrothers.com

Website: www.jaypeebrothers.com
Website: www.jaypeedigital.com

Inquiries for bulk sales may be solicited at: jaypee@jaypeebrothers.com

Modern Techniques in Spine Surgery

First Edition: 2015

ISBN 978-93-5152-530-1

Printed at Replika Press Pvt. Ltd.

Dedicated to

My Guru, all my teachers
My parents & Family members
All my patients, friends & well wishers
Whose guidance and well wishes have made this possible

Contributors

A Mezentsev MD
Sytenko Institute of Spine and
Joint Pathology
Kharkiv, Ukraine

Abhilash N Dhruv
MS (Orth) (Bom) D Orth FCPS Diploma (SICOT)
Consultant Spine Surgeon
Chief, Mumbai Spine Scoliosis and
Disc Replacement Centre
Specialist in Minimal Access Spine Surgery
Bombay Hospital
Mumbai, India

Ajoy P Shetty MS DNB (Ortho)
Consultant Spine Surgeon
Department of Orthopedics and
Spine Surgery
Ganga Hospital
Coimbatore
Tamil Nadu, India

Ali M Maziad MD MChOrth
Orthopedic Surgery Specialist
Spine Surgery and Surgical Informatics Fellow
California Spine Institute – IPILAB
University of Southern California
CA, USA

Ameer S Theruvath
Indian Spinal Injuries Centre
New Delhi
India

Amer F Samdani MD
Orthopedic Surgeon
Shriners Hospital, North Broad Street Clinic
South Philadelphia, USA

Arvind Bhave MS (Orth) IPTM FICOE FMISS
Professor, Department of Orthopedic Surgery
Bharati Vidyapeeth Medical College
Spine Surgeon
Deenanath Mangeshkar Hospital and
Inlaks and Budhrani Hospital
Pune, Maharashtra, India

Arvind G Kulkarni
MS (Orth) (Bom) D Orth FCPS Diploma (SICOT)
Consultant Spine Surgeon
Chief, Mumbai Spine Scoliosis and
Disc Replacement Centre
Specialist in Minimal Access Spine Surgery
Bombay Hospital
Mumbai, India

Ashish S Ranade
Pediatric Orthopedic Surgeon
Deenanath Mangeshkar Hospital
Pune, India

Boissiere L MD PhD
Department of Spine Surgery
P Wertheimer Hospital
East Hospital Group
59 Boulevard Pinel, 69394 Lyon
France

Bong-Jin Lee MD PhD
Department of Orthopedic Surgery
Cheju Halla General Hospital Jeju
Korea
Department of Rehabilitation Medicine
Catholic University of Korea
College of Medicine
Seoul, Korea
Moon-Kim's Institute of Orthopedic Research,
Seoul, Korea

Cédric Barrey MD PhD
Department of Neurosurgery and Spine Surgery
Pierre Wertheimer Hospital
GHE, Claude Bernard Lyon 1 University
Hospices Civils de Lyon
Lyon, France

D Petrenko MD
Sytenko Institute of Spine and Joint Pathology
Kharkiv, Ukraine

D'acunzi G MD
Department of Spine Surgery
P Wertheimer Hospital
East Hospital Group, 59 Boulevard Pinel
69394 Lyon, France

Daniel Gastambide MD
International Intradiscal Therapy Society
(President–2010 and Member since 1994)
Founding Member
Ex-President and Current Treasurer of the GIEDA
Member of ISMISS, SICOT, SFCR
Paris, France

Darwono A Bambang MD
Division of Orthopedic and Spine
Gading-Pluit Hospital
Jakarta, Indonesia

Deduch N MD
Professor, Chief of Department of
Pathomorphology Sytenko Institute of Spine and
Joint Pathology
Kharkov, Ukraine

Eric O Klineberg MD
University of California Davis Medical Center
Department of Orthopedic Surgery
Sacramento
CA, USA

Fujio Ito MD
Aichi Spine Institute
Gouhigashi
Aichi, Japan

George Huang MD
Oita Orthopedic Hospital
Oita-shi, Japan

HS Chhabra MBBS MS (Orth)
Chief of Spine Service and Medical Director
Indian Spinal Injuries Centre
New Delhi, India
Chairman, Prevention Committee—ISCoS, Board
Member—IGASS
Executive Member—AO Spine
Joint Secretary—ASSI
Executive Member—ASCoN, Secretary— SCS

Hanlim Moon MD PhD
Spine Center, Department of Orthopedic Surgery
Cheju Halla General Hospital
Jeju, Korea
Department of Rehabilitation Medicine
Catholic University of Korea
Seoul, Korea
Moon-Kim's Institute of Orthopedic Research
Seoul, Korea

Hideki Ohta MD
Oita Orthopedic Hospital
Oita-shi, Japan

Hirotaka Kida MD
Oita Orthopedic Hospital
Oita-shi, Japan

Ho-Yeon Lee MD PhD
Department of Neurosurgery
Wooridul Spine Hospital
Seoul, Korea

Ioannis Avramis MD
University of California Davis Medical Centre
Sacramento, CA, USA

Jang-Cheol Sihn MD
Department of Orthopedic Surgery and Traumatology
Cheju Halla General Hospital
Jeju, Korea
Moon-Kim's Institute of Orthopedic Research
Seoul, Korea

Janusz Bonkowski
Neurosurgeon
St. Georges Hospital
Christchurch
New Zealand

Jeong-Lim Moon MD PhD
Department of Orthopedic Surgery
Cheju Halla General Hospital
Jeju, Korea
Department of Rehabilitation Medicine
Catholic University of Korea
College of Medicine, Seoul, Korea
Moon-Kim's Institute of Orthopedic Research
Seoul, Korea

Jin-Fu Lin MD
Consultant Spine Surgeon
Department of Orthopedic Surgery
Central Clinic Hospital
Taipei, Taiwan

Jiyoung Cho
Wooridul Spine Hospital
Seoul, Korea

John C Chiu MD DSc FRCS
Director, Neurospine Surgery
Department of Neurosurgery
California Spine Institute
Thousand Oaks
Carlifornia, USA

Kim-Soon Oh MBBS MSurg (Orth)
Consultant Surgeon
Island Hospital Spine Centre
Georgetown, Penang, Malaysia
Associate Professor
Department of Orthopedics
Allianze University College of Medical Sciences
Penang, Malaysia
Advisor, Faculty of Medicine and Health Sciences
Universiti Tunku Abdul Rahman
Kuala Lumpur
Malaysia

Koji Sato MD
Department of Orthopedic and Spine Surgery
Nagoya Daini Red Cross Hospital
Aichi, Japan

Lance K Mitsunaga MD
University of California
Davis Medical Center
Department of Orthopedic Surgery
California, USA

Malyshkina S MD
Deparment of Pathomorphology
Sytenko Institute of Spine and Joint Pathology
Kharkov, Ukraine

Manabu Ito MD PhD
Professor, Department of Advanced Medicine for Spine and Spinal Cord Disorders
Hokkaido University Graduate School of Medicine, Sapporo, Japan

Mehmet Zileli
Professor, Department of Neurosurgery
Ege University
Izmir, Turkey

Min Geun Yoon MD
Department of Orthopedic Surgery
Cheju Halla General Hospital
Jeju, Korea
Department of Rehabilitation Medicine,
Catholic University of Korea
Seoul, Korea

Minoru Yamada
Aichi Spine Institute
Aichi, Japan

Mohit Arora
Indian Spinal Injuries Centre
New Delhi, India

Motohide Shibayama
Aichi Spine Institute
Aichi, Japan

Munish Gupta MD
Professor, Davis Medical Center
Department of Orthopedic Surgery
University of California
California, USA

Myung-Sang Moon MD PhD FACS
Professor Emeritus
Catholic University of Korea
Seoul
Director, MKIOR
Seoul, Korea
President, International Society of Musculoskeletal Infection
President, International Society for Study of Soft Lumbar Spine Stabilization
Patron (Honorary), Neurospine Surgeon's Association – India.

Naresh Kumar MBBS MS (Orth) DNB (Orth) FRCS
Associate Professor
Department of Orthopedic Surgery
Yong Loo Lin School of Medicine
National University of Singapore
Senior Consultant
University Spine Centre
University Orthopedics,
Hand and Reconstructive Microsurgery Cluster
National University Health System
Singapore

Nicholas Pirnia MD
University of California Davis Medical Centre
Sacramento
CA, USA

Perrin G MD
Department of Spine Surgery
P Wertheimer Hospital
East Hospital Group
59 Boulevard Pinel
69394 Lyon, France

Petrenko D MD
Department of Minimal Invasive and Instrumented Spine Surgery
Kharkiv, Ukraine

Pil Sun Choi
Coordinator of the Minimally Invasive Spine Surgery Study Group
Institute of Orthopedics and Traumatology (IOT)
Hospital Das Clínicas (Hc)
School of Medicine of the University of São Paulo (FMUSP), Hospital Abreu Sodré (AACD)
Av. Pacaembu 1003
São Paulo, Brazil

Radchenko Vladimir A MD
Professor, Chief of Department of Minimal Invasive and Instrumented Spine Surgery
Vice-Director of the Institute
Sytenko Institute of Spine and Joint Pathology of Academia of Medical Science
Kharkiv, Ukraine

Rajat Mahajan
Indian Spinal Injuries Centre
New Delhi, India

Rishi M Kanna MS MRCS FNB Spine
Associate Consultant Spine Surgeon
Department of Orthopedics and Spine Surgery
Ganga Hospital, Coimbatore, Tamil Nadu, India

S Rajasekaran
MS DNB FRCS (Ed) MCh (Liv) FRCS (Eng) PhD
Professor and Head, Department of Orthopedics
Trauma and Spine Surgery
Ganga Hospital, Coimbatore
Tamil Nadu, India

Sambhav Shah MBBS MS (Orth)
Clinical Fellow
University Spine Center
University Orthopedics
Hand and Reconstructive Microsurgery Cluster
National University Hospital
Singapore

Sang-Ho Lee MD PhD
Department of Neurosurgery
Wooridul Spine Hospital
Seoul, Korea

Satishchandra Gore
Prime Surgical Centre
Off Law College Road
Damle Path
Next to Kanchan Galli
Near Film and Television Institute of India
Pune, Maharashtra, India

Seog In Moon
Department of Orthopedic Surgery
Cheju Halla General Hospital
Jeju, Korea
Department of Rehabilitation Medicine
Catholic University of Korea, College of Medicine
Seoul, Korea
Moon-Kim's Institute of Orthopedic Research
Seoul, Korea

Shipra Chaudhary
Indian Spinal Injuries Centre
New Delhi, India

Shoji Ikeda
Aichi Spine Institute
Aichi, Japan

Shu Nakamura
Aichi Spine Institute
Aichi, Japan

Siddharth Shah MBBS MS (Orth)
Clinical Fellow, Department of Orthopedic Surgery, National University Hospital
5 Lower Kent Ridge Road
Singapore

Suken A Shah MD
Division Chief, Spine and Scoliosis Center
Clinical Fellowship Director, Department of Orthopedics
Nemours/Alfred I duPont Hospital for Children
Associate Professor, Department of Orthopedic Surgery and Pediatrics
Jefferson Medical College, Thomas Jefferson University, USA

Sung-Sim Kim MD PhD
Spine Center, Department of Orthopedic Surgery
Cheju Halla General Hospital
Jeju, Korea
Department of Rehabilitation Medicine
Catholic University of Korea, Seoul, Korea
Moon-Kim's Institute of Orthopedic Research
Seoul, Korea

Sung-Soo Kim MD PhD
Department of Orthopedic Surgery
Cheju Halla General Hospital, Jeju, Korea
Department of Rehabilitation Medicine
Catholic University of Korea, College of Medicine
Seoul, Korea
Moon-Kim's Institute of Orthopedic Research
Seoul, Korea

Tomohiko Yamada
Aichi Spine Institute
Aichi, Japan

Tsubasa Sakai MD
Oita orthopedic hospital
Oita-shi, Japan

Vishnu Prasad MS DNB Orth
Fellow in Spine Surgery
Department of Orthopedics and Spine Surgery
Ganga Hospital
Coimbatore, Tamil Nadu, India

Yasushi Miura
Aichi Spine Institute
Aichi, Japan

Yoshiharu Takemitsu MD PhD
Oita Orthopedic Hospital
Oita-shi, Japan

Yoshiyuki Matsumoto MD
Oita Orthopedic Hospital
Oita-shi, Japan

Young-Wan Moon MD PhD
Department of Orthopedic Surgery
Sam-Sung Medical Center
Sungkyunkwan University
Seoul, Korea

Yuichirou Morishita MD PhD
Oita Orthopedic Hospital
Oita-shi, Japan

Foreword

Development of modern technology among various areas of the natural science had provided significant changes in the field of spinal surgery. Advent, qualitative progress and dissemination of magnetic resonance image brought major changes in strategy of diagnosis for spinal disorders. New optical technology advanced endoscopic surgery in both of the anterior and posterior spine surgeries. Innovative metallic and non-metallic materials provided some sort of changes for surgical treatment of spinal disorders from the craniocervical junction to the sacroiliac joint. Surgeons, engineers and industry interactively contributed their expertise to the advancement.

Modern Techniques in Spine Surgery was conceived as a convenient textbook covering the broad area of spinal disorders and whole spinal levels. Arvind Bhave as editor, however, selected authors focusing scientists who have originality in basic spinal science or diagnostic method and who have innovative procedures in spine surgeries. Therefore, the book accomplished presenting full of innovative matters in spinal science. Especially, it is impressive that chapters concerning surgical techniques contain anatomical explanation written from standpoint of practitioners of innovative surgical procedures. Some of the novel procedures will be a standardized and spread universally in the near future.

Readers will find this book to be derived from a broad base of background of basic sciences and more applied disciplines (e.g., mechanical/chemical engineering, orthopedics, neurosurgery, etc). Bhave and chapter authors should be congratulated for their contribution producing wonderfully organized textbook for spine surgeons.

Kuniyoshi Abumi MD
Director and Vice-President
Sapporo Orthopedic Hospital- Center for Spinal Disorders, Sapporo, Japan
Professor Emeritus, Hokkaido University, Sapporo, Japan

Foreword

Medical science and especially the field of Spine Surgery has progressed tremendously in the last one decade, making it difficult for any individual surgeon to stay current with all the advances. Improvements in techniques, newer instruments, new technologies and improved devices are evolving continuously from different parts of the world and it is important that one remains aware of these developments so that the best is available to one's patient. This textbook, very aptly termed as *Modern Techniques in Spine Surgery* has 38 Chapters covering the entire spectrum of spine surgery. I am really pleased to see experts from all over the world as authors of these very well written and illustrated chapters. I am confident that this will be a useful addition to every spine surgeon's collection.

S Rajasekaran
MS DNB FRCS (Ed) MCh (Liv) FRCS (Eng) PhD
Professor and Head
Department of Orthopedics, Trauma and Spine Surgery
Ganga Hospital, Coimbatore
Tamil Nadu, India

Preface

The book *Modern Techniques in Spine Surgery* is a unique collection of articles of new and old techniques in spine. The chapters are contributed by the world leaders and experienced spine surgeons who have given practical advice and tips to overcome common pitfalls. The standard techniques for common spine problems are discussed and what is new is added.

I feel this book can be used as a study guide and reference book for the spine community.

Arvind Bhave

Acknowledgments

I sincerely thank:

All the contributors of this book who have spent a lot of their time, energy and expertise to make this book.

Professor Abumi and Professor Rajasekaran for the Forewords of this book.

Shri Jitendar P Vij (Group Chairman), Mr Ankit Vij (Group President) and Mr Tarun Duneja (Director–Publishing) and all the editorial board and staff members of M/s Jaypee Brothers Medical Publishers, New Delhi, India, for bringing out this book for all the spine lovers.

Contents

CHAPTER

1

Fundamental Anatomic Aspects of the Lumbar Foraminal Zone Applied to the Transforaminal Procedures

Pil Sun Choi

To safely carry out surgical procedures on the lumbar spine, either as open procedures or percutaneously, it is of fundamental importance to have accurate knowledge of the anatomy of the foraminal zone. Specifically, knowledge is required regarding the anatomy of the triangular procedure zone and the triangular safety zone, the relationship between vertebral pedicles and the adjacent neural structures, and the location of the spinal ganglion in the foraminal zone.

Triangular Procedure Zone

The triangular procedure zone, popularly known as triangular safe zone, was first described by Kambin in 1987.[1,2] It consists of a space in the foraminal zone that is delimited anteriorly by the nerve, inferiorly by the upper vertebral plateau of the inferior vertebra, and posteriorly by the upper joint process of the inferior vertebra. The triangular procedure zone is the entry port to the foraminal zone (Fig. 1.1).

Triangular Safety Zone

The triangular safety zone was first described by Mirkovic[5] in 1995 and, subsequently, by Choi[3,4] in 2000. It is a triangular space in the foraminal zone, into which a procedure cannula can be safely introduced without putting the surrounding neural structures at risk, in order to carry out procedures involving transforaminal procedures, such as diskectomy, foraminoplasty, nuclear arthroplasty, static or dynamic anterior lumbar stabilization, etc.

According to Choi, who conducted an anatomical dissection study on fresh human cadavers, the triangular safety zone presents the following characteristics: its lateral limit is the nerve, its lower limit is the upper vertebral plateau of the inferior vertebra, and its medial limit is the spinal dura mater or the nerve root at the lowest lumbar levels, i.e. L4–L5 and L5–S1. The triangular safety zone can admit a procedure cannula of progressively larger external diameter, going from L2–L3 to L5–S1. The smallest mean diameter was 7.55 mm at the L2–L3 level and the largest was 12.59 mm at L5–S1. Thus, these diameters were much

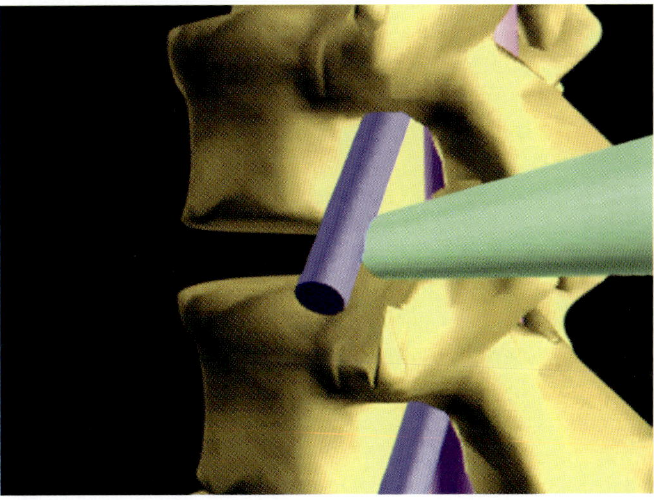

Fig. 1.1 Schematic view of the procedure cannula in the triangular procedure zone. This zone is delimited anteriorly by the nerve, inferiorly by the upper vertebral plateau of the inferior vertebra, and posteriorly by the upper joint process of the inferior vertebra

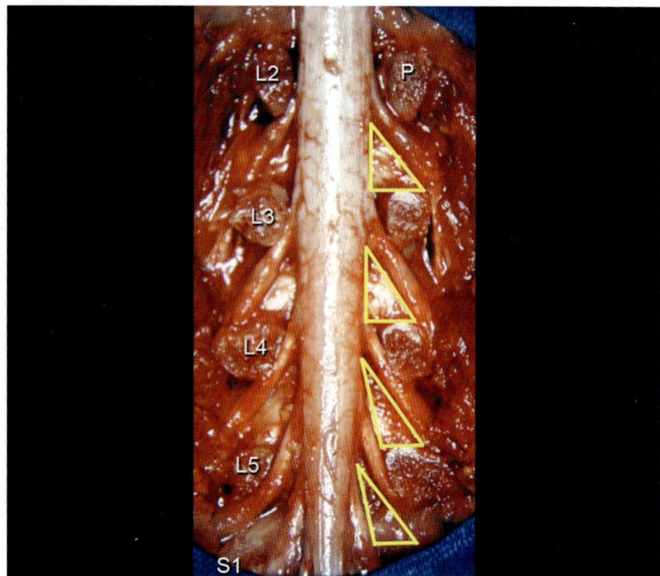

Fig. 1.2 Appearance of anatomical dissection of the fresh lumbar spine after removal of the posterior bone elements at the pedicles of the vertebral arches, showing the triangular safety zone (marked out in yellow): its lateral limit is the nerve; its lower limit is the upper vertebral plateau of the inferior vertebra; and its medial limit is the spinal dura mater or the nerve root at the lowest lumbar levels, i.e. L4–L5 and L5–S1

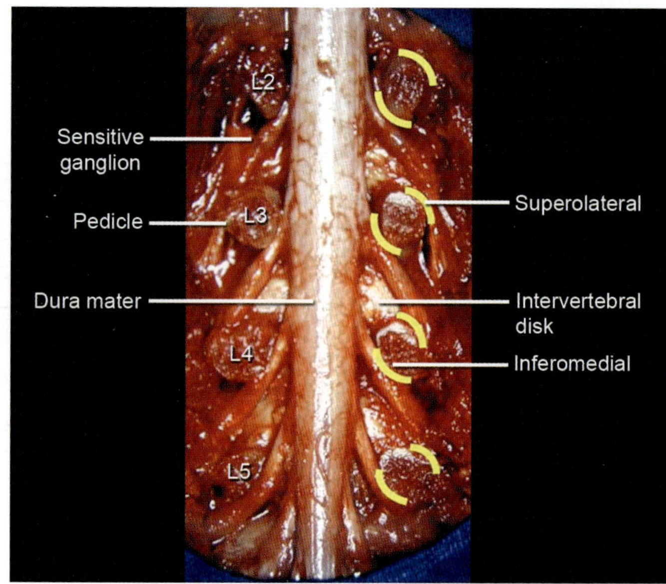

Fig. 1.3 Appearance of anatomical dissection of the lumbar spine after removal of the posterior bone elements at the pedicles of the vertebral arches, showing the relationship between the vertebral pedicles and the adjacent neural structures. The critical areas are the inferomedial and superolateral portions (marked out in yellow)

larger than the diameter of the largest procedure cannula currently used, which is around 6.0–6.5 mm (Fig. 1.2).

Vertebral Pedicle and its Relationship with Adjacent Neural Structures

The vertebral pedicle is considered to be the most important anatomical structure of a vertebra. This became evident over recent years when lumbar spine stabilization started to be performed, with screws introduced through the vertebral pedicles. This greatly increased the stability and diminished the need for supplementary external immobilization following spinal surgery.

Concomitantly, with the increased use of pedicle fixation, the complication rate also started to increase. Among these complications was poor positioning, which invariably would lead to nerve root injury in the foraminal zone and frequently would cause dysesthesia that was difficult to resolve.

According to Matuoka[6] and Choi[3], who conducted an anatomical dissection study on fresh cadavers in 2000 and published in 2002, the lumbar vertebral pedicle increased in size from L2 to L5, both in longitudinal and in transverse diameter, while the transverse diameter of the pedicle is smaller than the longitudinal diameter. The vertebral pedicle is closely related to the nerve root that emerges beneath it: its most distal part is adjacent to the nerve root and its medial edge is adjacent to the dura mater at higher lumbar levels (L2–3 and L3–4) or to the nerve root at lower lumbar levels (L4–5 and L5–S1) (Fig. 1.3).

Location of the Spinal Ganglion

The spinal (sensory) ganglion is considered to be the "brain" of the nerve. It is considered to be the most important and most delicate structure in the foraminal zone. Any damage to this structure may lead to disastrous consequences. For this reason, it is of fundamental importance to know the exact location of this structure in the foraminal zone. In a study conducted by Matuoka[6] and Choi[3], the sensory ganglion occupied the highest portion of the intervertebral foramen (GS 2 and GS 3) in 87% of the cases; the ganglion was surrounded by connective tissue and fat containing foraminal vessels. However, in the upper lumbar region, an intraspinal location is very common, while in the lower lumber region, an extraforaminal location is found, especially at L5–S1 level (Fig. 1.4).

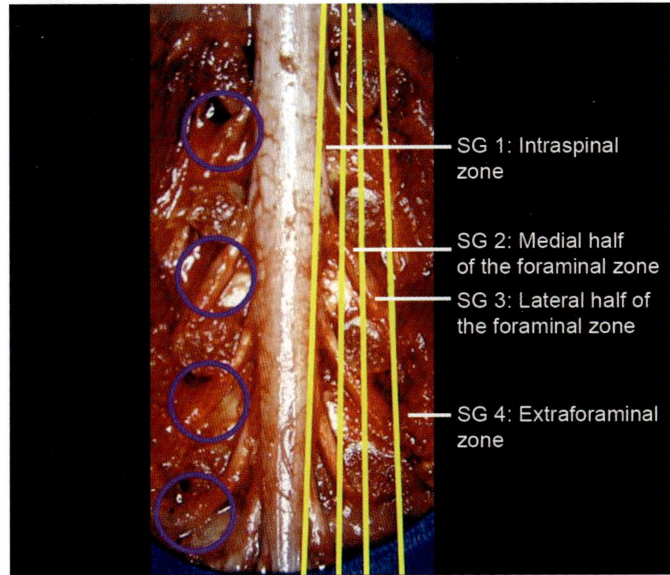

Fig. 1.4 Location of the spinal ganglion in the lumbar region. GS1: intraspinal zone; GS2: foraminal zone (medial half); GS3: foraminal zone (lateral half); GS4: extraforaminal zone. Sensory ganglia (blue circle)

References

1. Kambin P, Brager MD. Percutaneous posterolateral discectomy. Anatomy and mechanism. Clin Orthop. 1987;223:145-54.
2. Kambin P, Zhou L. History and current status of percutaneous arthroscopic disc surgery. Spine. 1996;21:57S-61S.
3. Choi PS. Contribuição ao estudo anatômico da zona triangular de segurança aplicado aos procedimentos percutâneos póstero-laterais lombar. São Paulo, 2000; p. 98. Tese (Mestrado) - Faculdade de Medicina, Universidade de São Paulo.
4. Choi PS, Basile JR. R. Estudo anatômico da zona triangular de segurança aplicada aos procedimentos percutâneos póstero-laterais lombares. Coluna /Columna, 2003;v.2(1):20-6.
5. Mirkovic SR, Schwartz DG, Glazier KD. Anatomic considerations in lumbar posterolateral percutaneous procedures. Spine. 1995;20:1965-71.
6. Matuoka CM. Estudo anatômico do pedículo vertebral lombar e estruturas neurais adjacentes. São Paulo. Tese (Mestrado) - Faculdade de Medicina, Universidade de São Paulo. 2002;65.

CHAPTER

2

Philosophy of Minimally Invasive Spine Surgery

Satishchandra Gore

The surgery for the disk has been in vogue for more than hundred years. Recently, the focus has shifted from late diagnosis to early imaging and early clinical diagnosis and resultant early treatment. Since most of the symptoms follow the degenerative cascade involving the disk and the facet joints and the functional spinal unit in total, it is more predictable now than before. The change of focus has been distinct and noteworthy. It now is mainly on pain. Due to changing social and economic factors, patients also have started asking for solutions to pain, and we have new emerging philosophy of minimalism as applied to treatment of the disk.

The minimalism in disk surgery is not smaller cuts and newer instruments for use through smaller cuts, but it is *doing only what is necessary*.

If we go back in time and look at the patients perception of the surgery on the disk, it is not size of the incision that the patient is bothered about but what a surgeon does inside. The concern is more and real about denervation of muscles, bleeding, scarring, leaving open a defect in nucleus allowing major recurrences and morbidity of the general anesthesia. This concern is amply supported by failed back surgery and its variants. Doing essentially same surgery inside based on philosophy of past is no innovation. Many new variations of same old interlaminar approach have come with mobile tubes, new retractors and longer instruments but are based on same philosophy of operating a unconscious patient and where decision is based on images alone. This thinking also has one major drawback it assumes that in most chronic degenerated disks fusion is needed for pain relief. The alleged relief of pain is due to stability and decompression and replacing disk with bone graft and metal implant . The problems fought with are how to identify what causes pain and it is an unproven idea that stopping movement stops pain. It may work well in cases of gross instability but porting stabilization technology from trauma to degenerative spine is not supported by science.

The emerging and now mostly validated philosophy is visualizing pain generators in lumbar spine *in vivo* and in awake and aware patient after making a primary assessment based on MRI images and supplementing it by using disk probing and imaging with contrast and then acting on it with patients real-time inputs. *In vivo* visualization of the pain generators has made a significant change in our understanding of pain by taking back results of pain generation to clinical assessment and changing our basic perceptions in pain diagnosis.

Clinical assessment and routine imaging studies are not enough for determining the source of chronic back pain and sciatica for surgical planning. As they do not really answer where is pain coming from? Imaging needs to be supplemented by diagnostic and therapeutic injections to elucidate the source of pain. Current imaging creates both false-positive and false-negative clinical conclusions of up to 28%. In transforaminal endoscopic procedures, the ability to visualize and palpate pathoanatomy in the degenerative spine in an awake patient adds greatly to the treatment of painful degenerative conditions. To form theories of pain generation by probing the pathoanatomy in a conscious patient, and treat the pain generator by decompressing, ablating, and irrigating the source of pain, is basic philosophy of minimally invasive physiological transforaminal disk surgery. The ability to visualize pathoanatomy and correlate it with surgical results creates a better understanding of the pain generators in the lumbar spine. The findings also serve to advance and evolve the minimally invasive endoscopic techniques for treatment of the symptomatic degenerative spine (Figs 2.1 and 2.2).

The disk is avascular and cannot heal from injuries. Nutrition is by diffusion through the end plate. The end plate is porous and permeable to nutrients. This permeability and the ability to transport nutrients normally decrease during growth and aging, from diminished blood supply to the intervertebral disk. This occurrence in the second decade appears to initiate tissue breakdow. Permeability also decreases when there is disease due to disk degeneration and end-plate pathology. Nerve fibers normally only penetrate the outer area of the annulus; however, in degenerative disk disease, the nerves progress to the inner annulus and toward the nucleus. Inflammatory and granulation tissues form in and outside the disk, producing pain. The pain can present as (i) leg pain along nerve dermatomes and dynatomes from disk herniation or annular tears, (ii) back pain from disk protrusions, (iii) backache due to facet changes felt along the paraspinal area, (iv) claudication-like leg pain due to unilateral single-level or multilevel lateral canal stenosis, (v) bilateral claudication due to central soft tissue or bony canal stenosis, and (vi) a combination of back pain and sciatica from multiple pain generators (confusing basic standard clinical guidelines). Five of these symptom groups can be distinguished clinically, but because their pathoanatomy usually overlap, it may be necessary to consider new diagnostic and therapeutic methods of evaluation, such as endoscopic probing, and endoscopic evaluation. Symptoms are due to disk and facet changes as components of a functional spinal unit, and both usually cause pain as degeneration progresses. Sacroiliac and piriformis syndromes and related symptoms also contribute to back and leg pain and gaining more attention now.

Minimally invasive diagnostic and surgical techniques that are demonstrated to effectively treat certain painful conditions with minimal morbidity include the following:

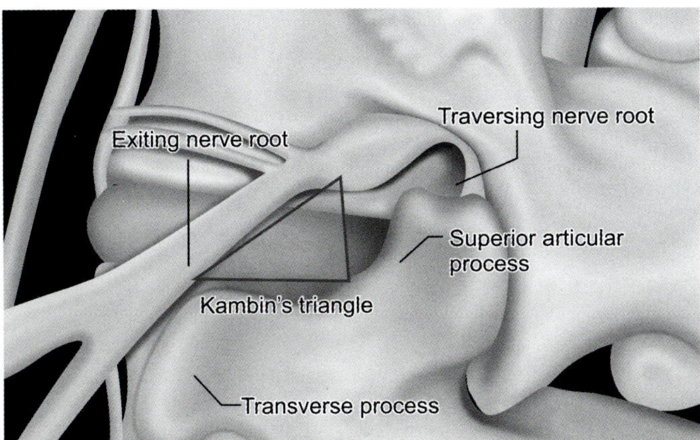

Fig. 2.1 Kambin's triangle

Dorsal Approach

Facet

A

Foraminal approach
Cannula used to shield exiting nerve

Midline

Thecal sac with the traversing nerve root

Laminotomy

Operating cannula passed transforaminally

B

The beveled cannula tip provides a greater operative field

Fig. 2.2 Comparative surgical anatomy

1. Identification of morphological changes for intradiskal therapy: diskography is a critical tool to help correlate pain production with the pathoanatomy visualized. This includes *in vivo* probing,evoking pain from the disc and annulus.
2. Lateral canal volume expansion by endoscopic mechanical and laser-assisted foraminoplasty, also effective in selective cases of listhesis, that is stable or minimally mobile.
3. Facet-related changes treated with denervation of the facet (and possible adjacent musculature responsible for spasm) under endoscopic visualization.
4. Central canal transforaminal or sublaminar decompression by unilateral and contralateral entry with endoscopic visualization.

CHAPTER

3

Sacroiliac Joint Pain Syndrome: Anatomy, Diagnosis, and Treatment—Surgical Laser Thermoneurectomy

John C Chiu

Introduction

- The *chronic low back pain* can be difficult to localize and diagnosed clinically
- Primary function of the *sacroiliac joint (SIJ)* is lending *pelvic* and *lower extremity stability connecting* to *upper body* stability
- SIJ dysfunction can be *caused by* various pathology, including *major lumbar spinal surgery/fusion*

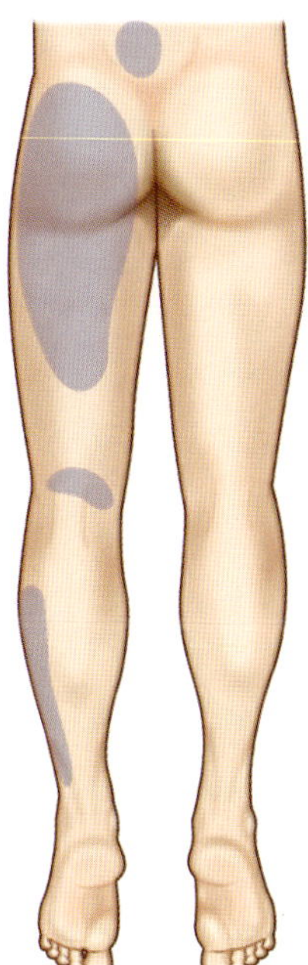

Fig. 3.1 Usual pain pattern seen

- *SIJ pain* contributes up to *25-40% of patients with low back pain* from various causes including minor trauma
- *39%* of patients with *SIJ pain* found to *have low back pain*
- Due to *post-lumbar fusion*-related biomechanical changes which lead to *SIJ* dysfunction/*pain (about 1/3 post fusion patient)*
- SIJ pain can radiate to *the low back, buttocks, abdomen, groin, or legs (Fig. 3.1)*

Anatomy of SI Joint with Nutation

- The *pelvis consists* of the two *ilia* and the *sacrum*
- The *SIJ* is the *largest axial joint* in the body (*17.5 cm^2*)
- The anterior side of the joint is lined with thick hyaline cartilage (Fig. 3.2)

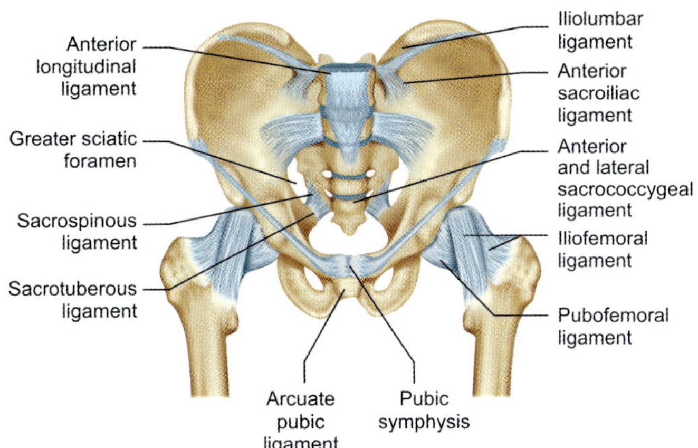

Fig. 3.2 Anterior view of articulations and ligaments of sacroiliac joint and surrounding structures

- The posterior iliac side of the joint is lined with fibrocartilage (Fig. 3.3)
- *Anterior third—true synovial joint*
- The *rest* of the junction is a set of *ligamentous connections.*

Articular Surface of SI Joint

Figures 3.4 and 3.5 illustrate schematically the articular surface of SI joints. Figure 3.5 shows nodding movements of SIJ.

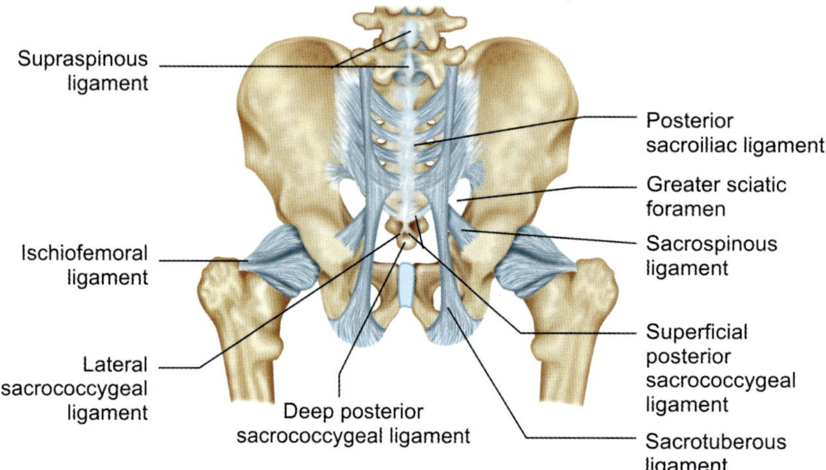

Fig. 3.3 Posterior view of articulations and ligaments of sacroiliac joint and surrounding structures

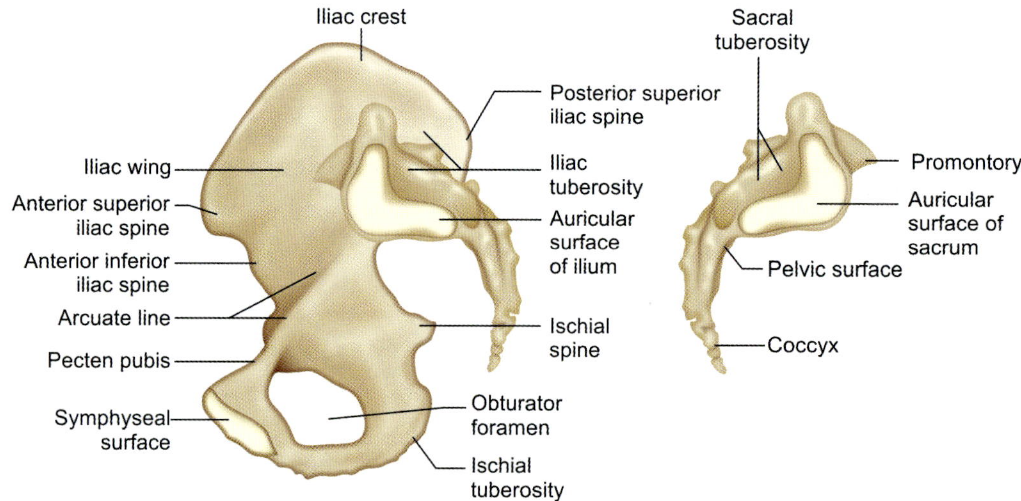

Fig. 3.4 Articular surface of sacroiliac joint

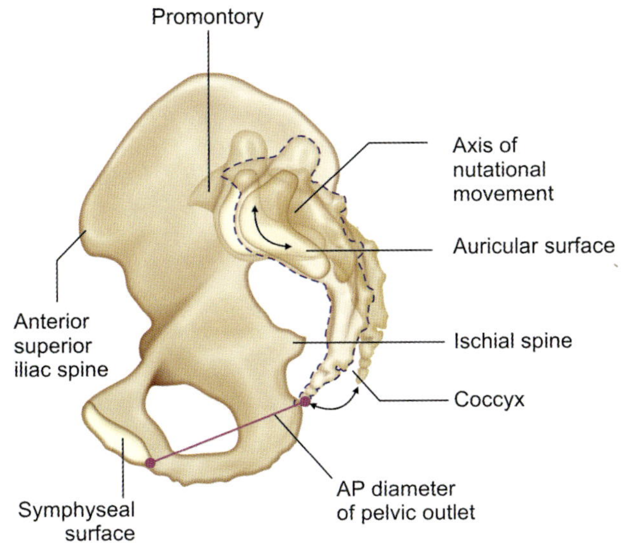

Fig. 3.5 Nutation or rocking, swaying, or nodding motion of SIJ

Pathoanatomy and Pathophysiology

Pathoanatomy

- *Between the sacral and ileum* is a *true SIJ* (Fig. 3.7)
- The biomechanics of SI joint is then a medially directed force six times greater than the lumbar spine but only half the torsion and 1/20th of axial compression load
- The *joint transmits* all the *forces* of the upper body *to the pelvis through the SIJ down to the legs* (Fig. 3.8)
- Currently there is *no standard* SIJ treatment algorithm.

Factors Predisposing SIJ Injury

- Capsular and synovial disruption
- Capsular and ligamentous tension
- Hypomobility or hypermobility

Innervation of SI Joint

- The *innervation of the SIJ* is extremely complex, mostly believed to be as follows (Fig. 3.6):
  - *Posterior innervation* from medial branches of dorsal rami of spinal nerves, L4, L5, S1–3
  - *Anterior innervation*: The L4–S2 ventral rami.

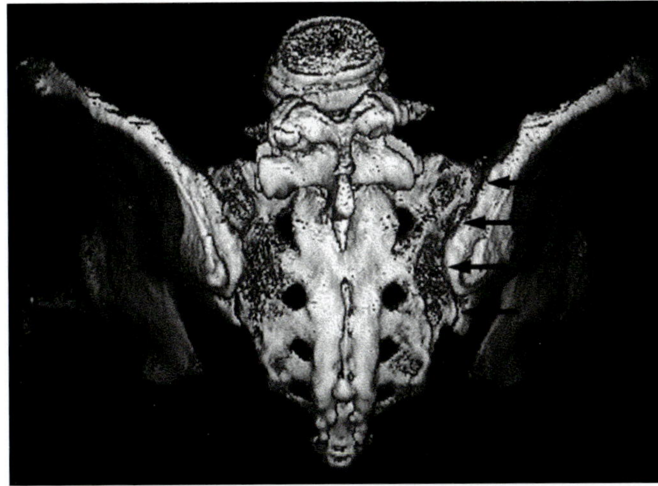

Fig. 3. 7 CT scan of sacroiliac joint from front

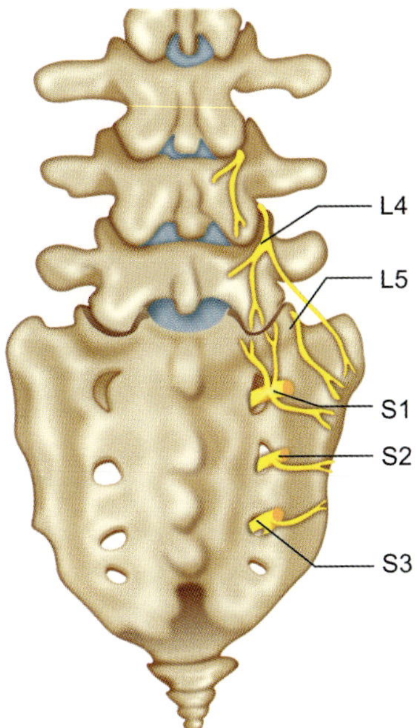

Fig. 3.6 Posterior innervation of sacroiliac joint

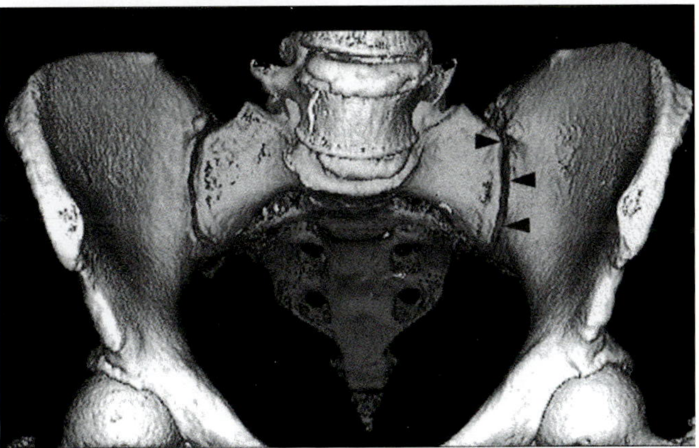

Fig. 3.8 CT scan of sacroiliac joint—posterior view

- Extraneous compression or sharing forces of the joint
- Abnormal joint mechanism
- Microfracture or macrofracture
- Chondromalacia
- Soft tissue injury
- Inflammation
- Joint laxity
- Degenerative joint disease
- History of minor direct trauma with a fall onto the buttocks.

Sacroiliac Joint Dysfunction Syndrome

Causes

- *Often major lumbar spinal surgery and spinal fusion can cause* SIJ dysfunction
- *Various minor traumatic injury to SIJ can initiate SIJ pain* after minor traumatic event, such as *falling onto the buttocks or a slip while pushing* a heavy object
- It is *aggravated* by transitional activities, *such as climbing stairs, getting up from chairs* and getting out of a car (Figs 3.9 and 3.10)
- Aggravated by activities requiring *unequal loading* through the lower extremities or pelvis
- *Pathology of surrounding structures*
- *Capsular* and *ligamentous tension related to* hypomobility or hypermobility, shearing forces, abnormal joint mechanics, fractures, *soft tissue trauma,* inflammation.

How to Diagnose SIJ Dysfunction?

Diagnostic Criteria for SIJ Syndrome

- **Pain in** the region of *SIJ* with possible radiation to the groin, medial buttock and posterior thigh
- *Reproduction of pain* by physical examination technique that stresses the joint—refer to physical signs and *common tests*
- *Elimination of pain with intra-articular injection* of local anesthetics and *nerve blocks*
- An ostentatiously morphological normal joint without demonstration of pathopneumonic radiographic abnormality
- *Point specific tenderness* over the *sacral sulcus* as well as the *posterior superior iliac spine.*

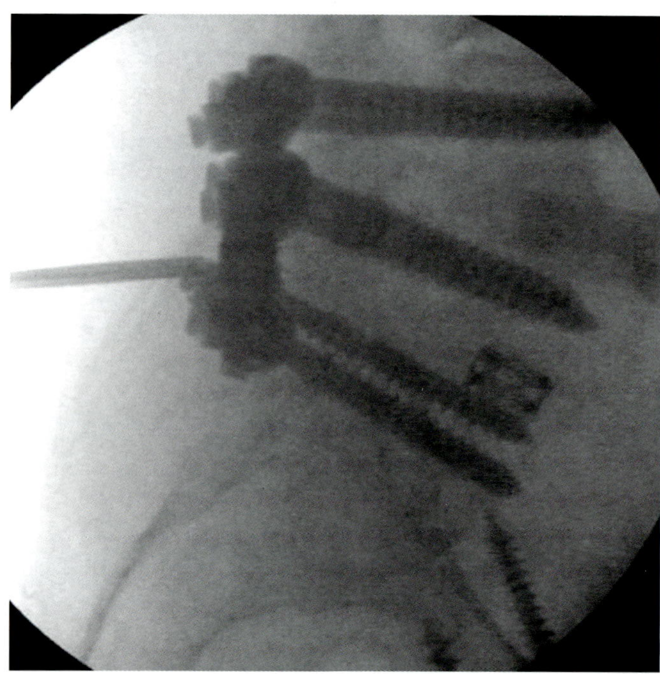

Fig. 3.9 X-rays of lumbar fusion—Lateral view

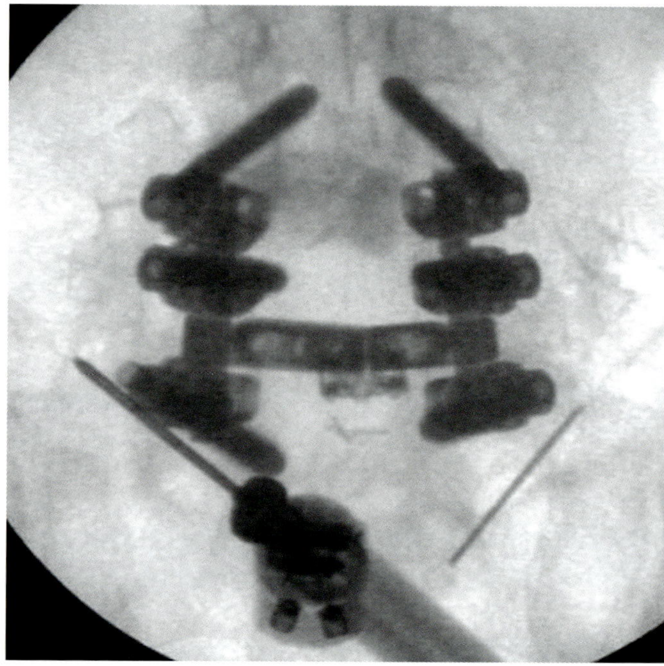

Fig. 3.10 X-rays of lumbar fusion—anteroposterior view

Common Tests

Common Confirmatory Tests and Signs of SIJ Dysfunction

- *Fortin finger test*—patients one finger pointing to the area pain
- Positive result at the site within 1 cm of inferior medial to the *posterior superior iliac spine (PSIS)*
- *Gaenslen test* (Fig. 3.11)
- *Patrick test* (Fig. 3.12)
- *Yeoman test* (Fig. 3.13).

Options for Treatment

Primary Indication for Treatment of SIJ Pain Syndrome

- If *conservative* medications, physical therapy, exercise and acupuncture *fail then,*

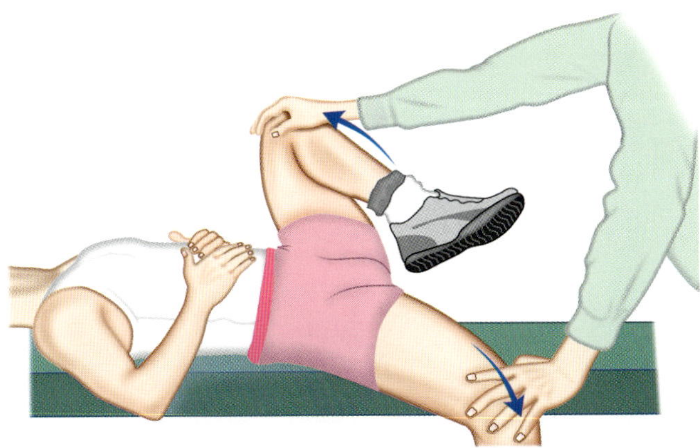

Fig. 3.11 Gaenslen test

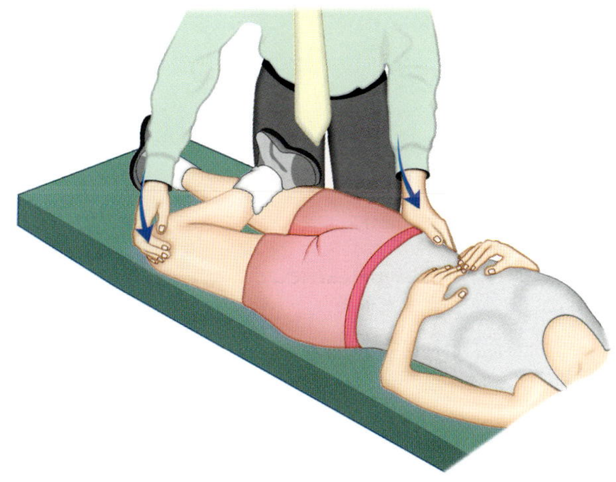

Fig. 3.12 Patrick test

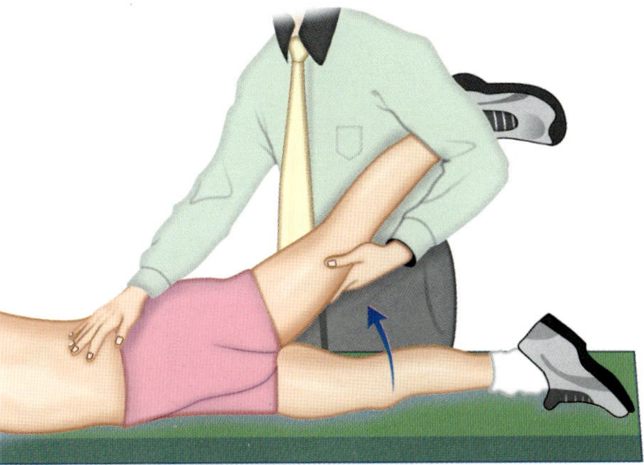

Fig. 3.13 Yeoman test

- *SIJ injections intra-articular and extraarticular*
  - Injection anesthetic medication into the joint confirms whether or not the pain came from the joint
  - The local anesthesia and cortisone can help break a pain cycle or possibly facilitate a rehabilitation exercise program
- If *above fails* and SIJ pain continues to be intractable then,
- *Nerve blocks L4 to S3* are to be performed, if successful then,
- *Laser thermal neurectomy/rhizotomy* for denervation, including endoscopic *microdecompression* and laser neurolysis.

Surgical Procedure/Technique

SIJ Injection and Nerve Blocks

- In the *prone position*
- Under *local anesthesia* with mild IV *sedation*, 22 gauge needle is inserted into the joint under fluoroscopic guidance (Fig. 3.14)
- *Contrast material* (isovue) is injected intra-arctiularly to confirm
- A mixture of *local anesthetics* and *steroids* is injected
- After the injection some *may benefit* by wearing a support belt.

Surgical Laser Thermoneurectomy (LTN) of SIJ

Surgical Technique

- In *prone position*
- The *C-arm fluoroscopic unit* is angled towards the visualized line of the posterior aspect of SIJ

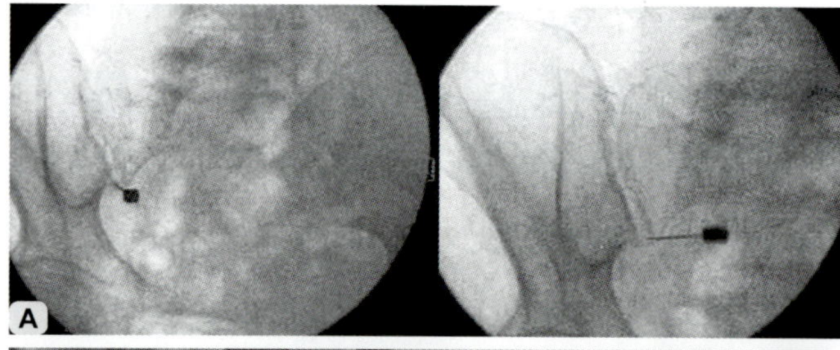

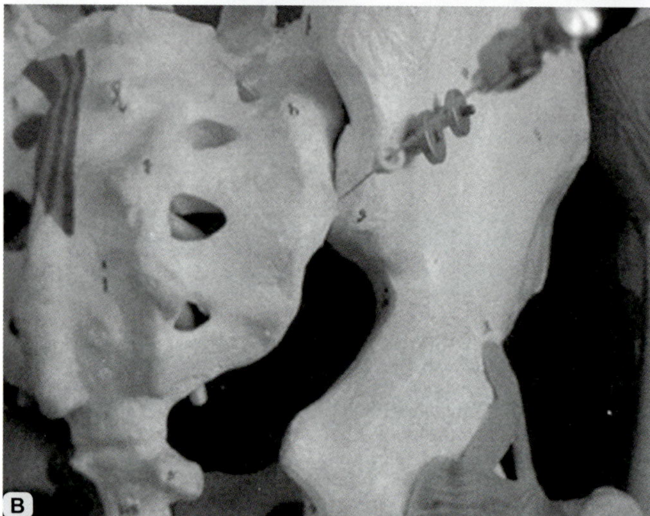

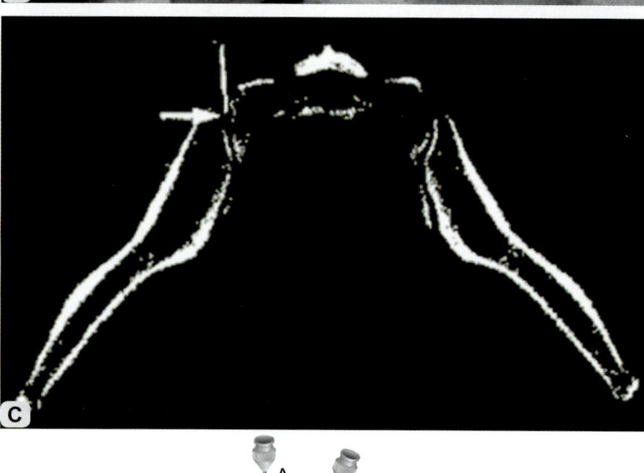

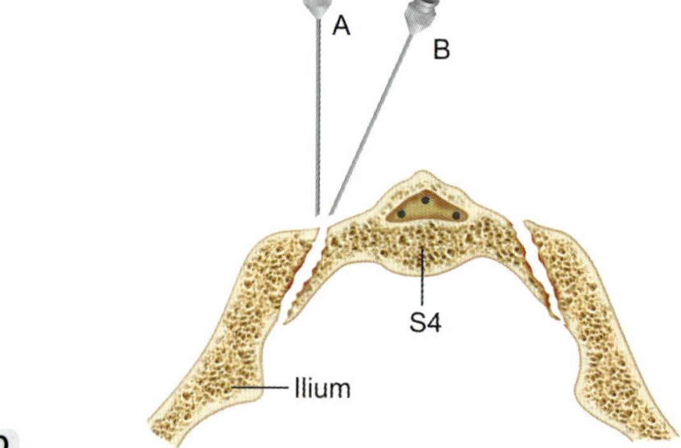

Fig. 3.14 'C'-arm picture, anatomical correlation of sacroiliac block

- The *tube is angled caudally and obliquely* (*15–20 degrees from the opposite side* of the body) from the side opposite to *the SIJ to be denervated* with visualization of posterior SIJ line
- *LTN target* 5 mm to the sacral neural foramen, superiorly and laterally along the foramen for sacral neurectomy of S1, S2, S3 in addition to L4 and L5 medial branch neurectomy for SIJ denervation (Fig. 3.15)
- *Two successful SIJ nerve blocks* are *required before LTN/* rhizotomy.

Surgical Procedure/Technique

Fluoroscopic technique

- The spine is in the *prone position*
- The fluoroscopic beam *aligns the anterior and posterior sacral foramina*
- A photograph of a sacrum from the anterior aspect
- The anterior and posterior foramina align
- *A/P fluoroscopic image* of the sacrum with *alignment of the anterior and the posterior foramina* (Fig. 3.16).

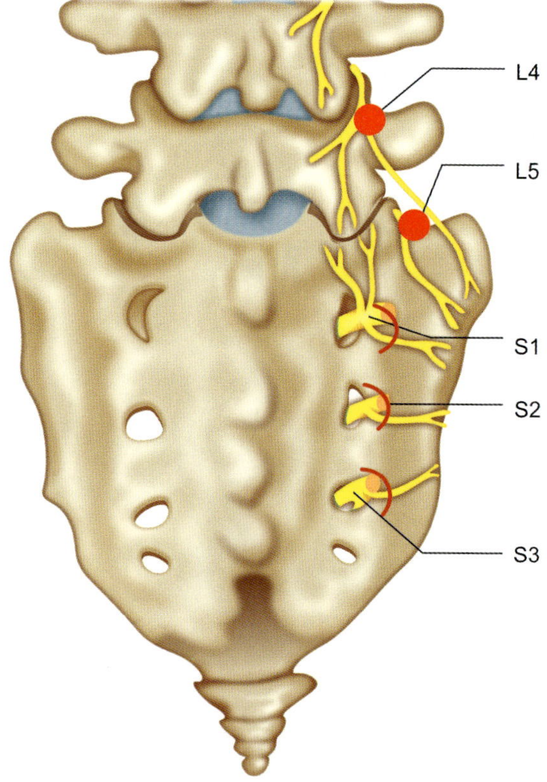

Fig. 3.15 Surgical laser thermoneurectomy targets of S1–S3, lateral branches, and L4–L5 MBR innervating sacroiliac joint

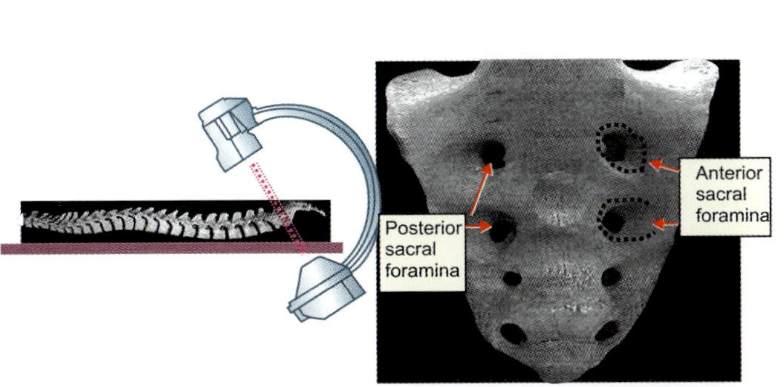

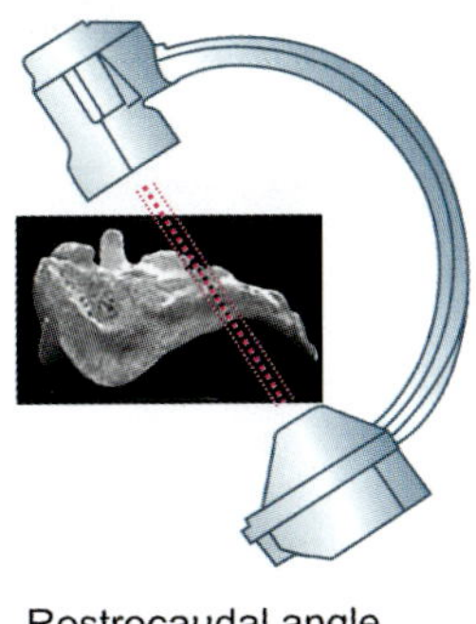

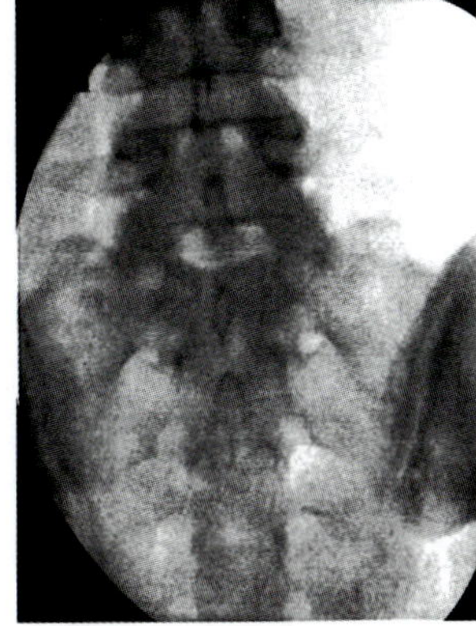

Fig. 3.16 'C'-arm correlation technique

LTN Surgical Technique: Tissue Modulation Technology

Application of *tissue modulation technology* with microdecompression and LTN (laser) and even radiofrequency (Fig. 3.17).

- *Holmium YAG laser* equipment and side firing laser probe are utilized for *LTN* at lower level laser energy for ablation

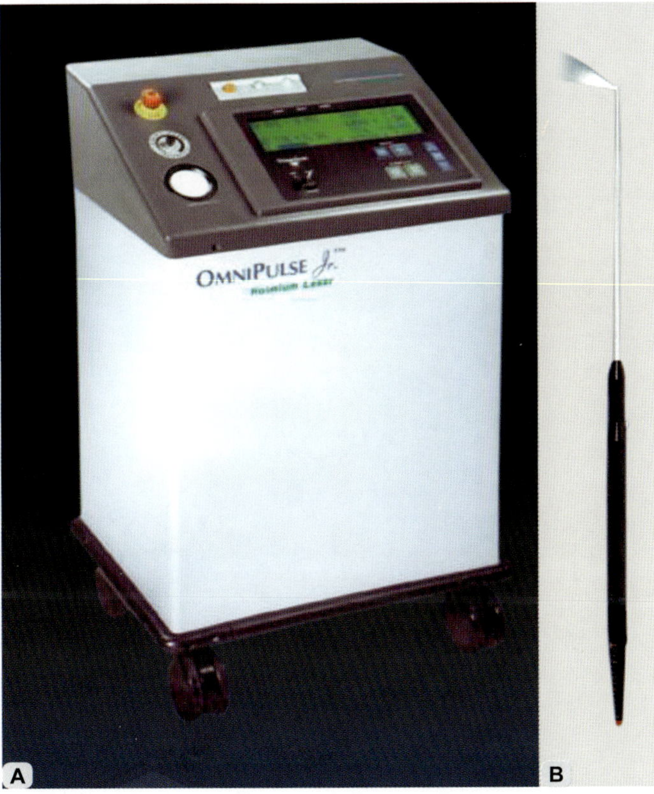

Fig. 3.17 (A) Trimedyne holmium YAG laser generator; (B) Right angle (side firing) laser probe

The Technique

- The red spots and red curved line are the targets (medial branch of posterior roots of L4, L5, S1, S2, S3) for LTN (refer to Fig. 3.15)
- This procedure of laser *denervation* can be successfully performed with *Holmium YAG laser* system at 125 joules (5 watts, 10 hertz) for each site/nerve
- During the *LTN, continuous cold saline irrigation* to *dissipate* the *heat* generated by laser application, caused by the LTN/rhizotomy.

LTN Surgical Equipment

LTN surgical equipments are shown in Figure 3.18.

Surgical Procedure/Technique

- Patient *positioning and localization*
  - In *prone* position on 1–2 pillows
  - Localization – *skin marking* for *portal of entry* and placement of needle under *fluoroscopic guidance* (Figs 3.19 to 3.29).

Postoperative Care

- *Ambulatory* usually in about 30 minutes and discharged subsequently
- May *shower* the following day
- Ice pack is helpful
- *Mild analgesics* and muscle relaxant are needed at times
- *Progressive exercises and able to start PT* the following day (Figs 3.30 and 3.31)
- Rehabilitation complements MISS and motion preservation (Fig. 3.32)
- *Return to work* in 3 days as tolerated (not for heavy work)

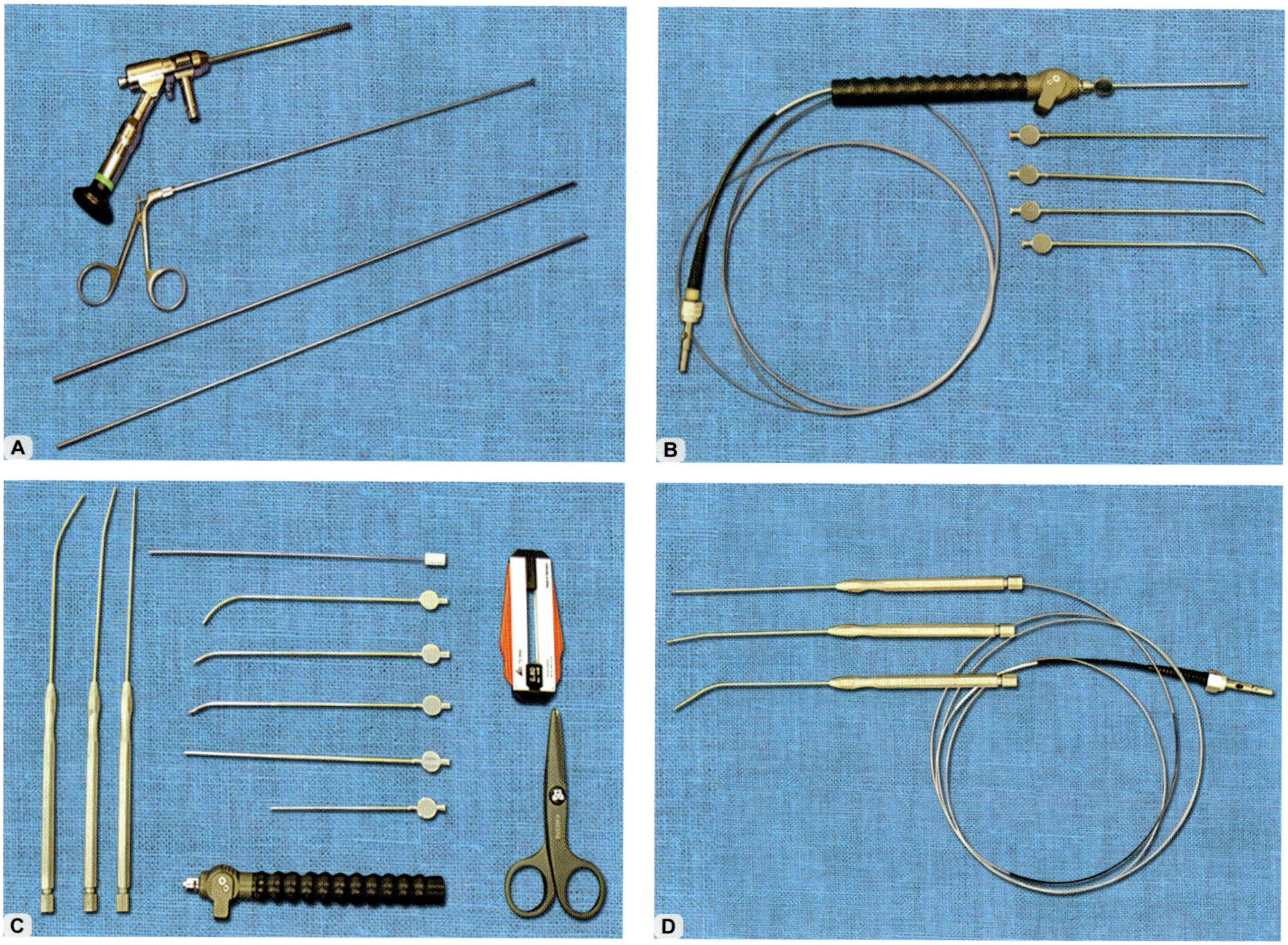

Fig. 3.18 LTN surgical equipment

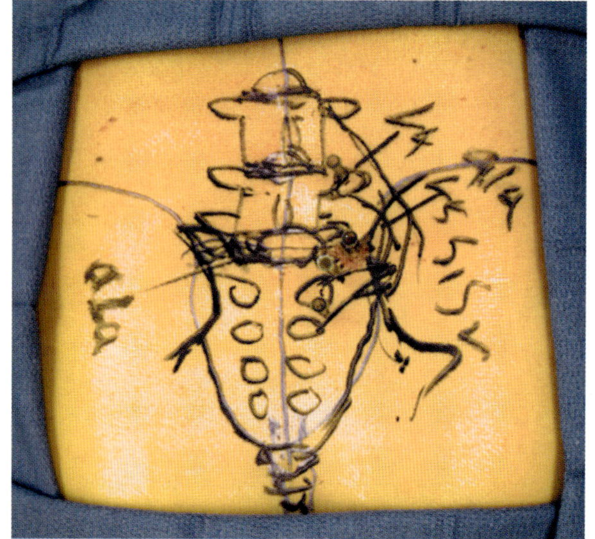

Fig. 3.19 Skin markings for portal entry and needle insertion

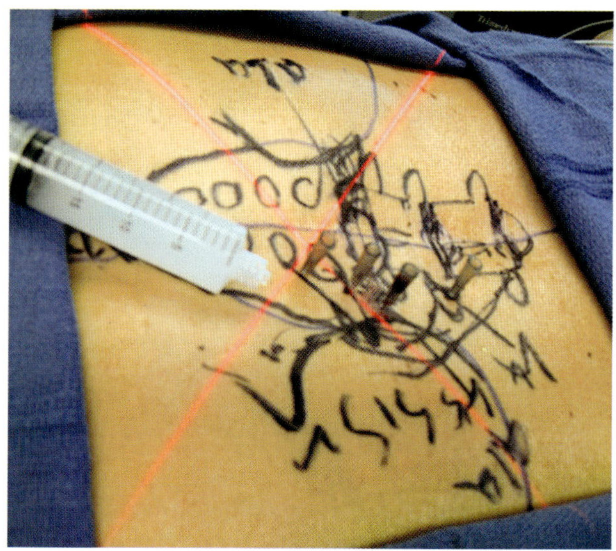

Fig. 3.20 Placement of needle

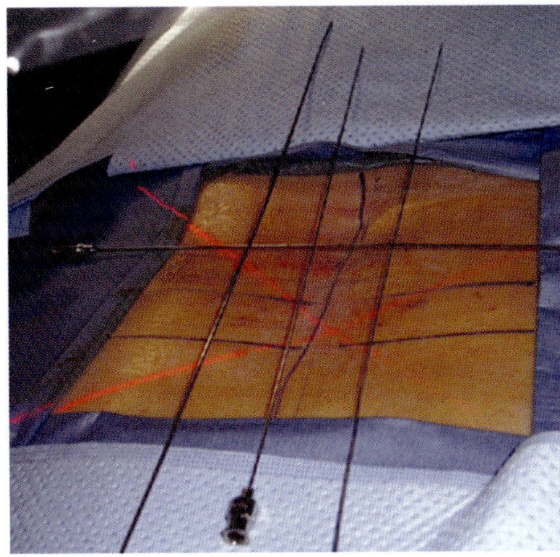

Fig. 3.21 Identifying sacral neural foramen under fluoroscopy

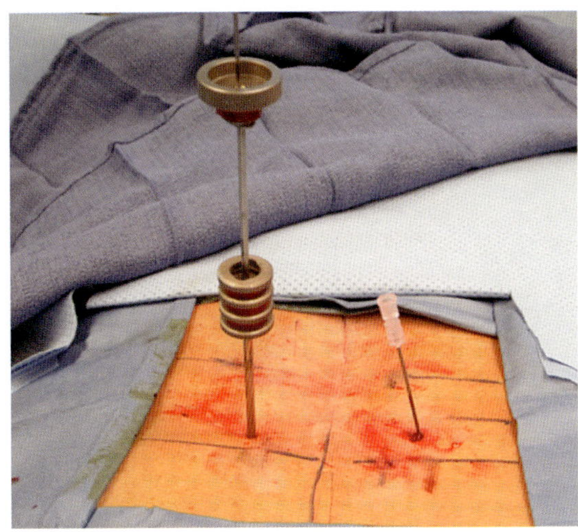

Fig. 3.24 Establishing working channel for microdecompression laser probe insertion

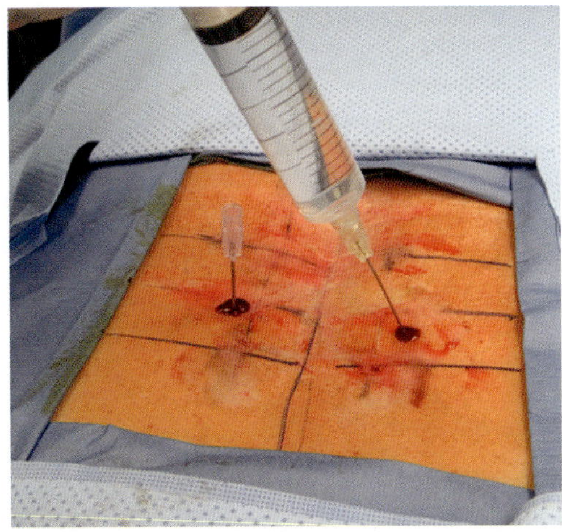

Fig. 3.22 Injection of local anesthetics before denervation

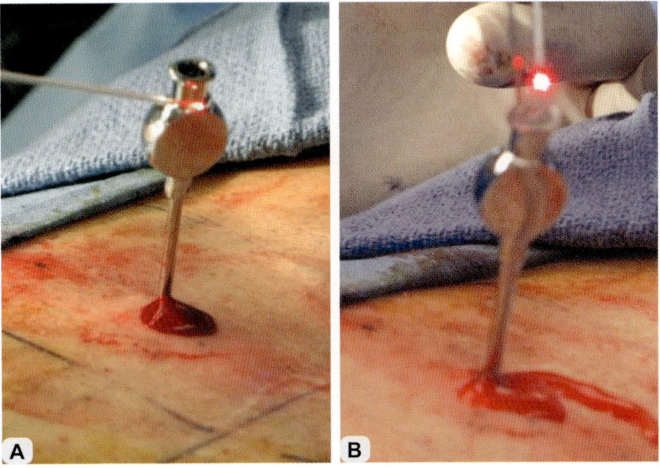

Fig. 3.25 Introduction of working probe channel

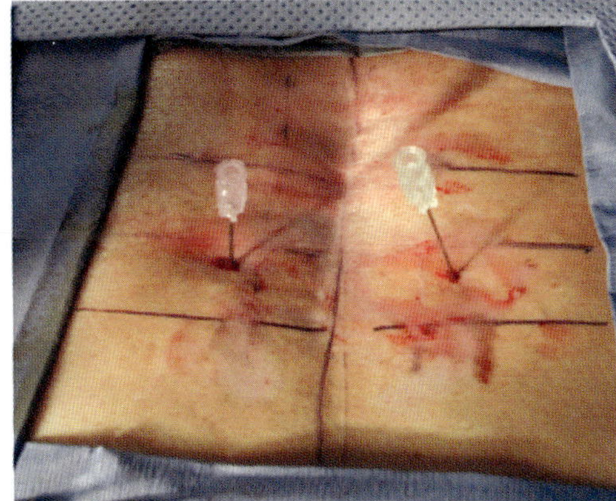

Fig. 3.23 Needle localization for denervation along the neural foramen

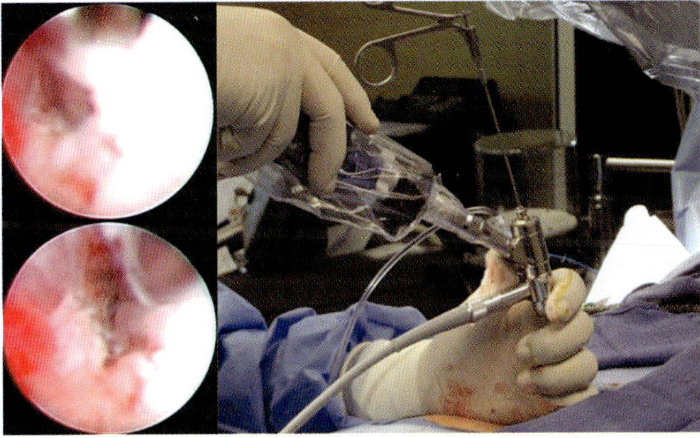

Fig. 3.26 Mechanical endoscopic microdecompression LTN of the L5 medial branch of dorsal root rami

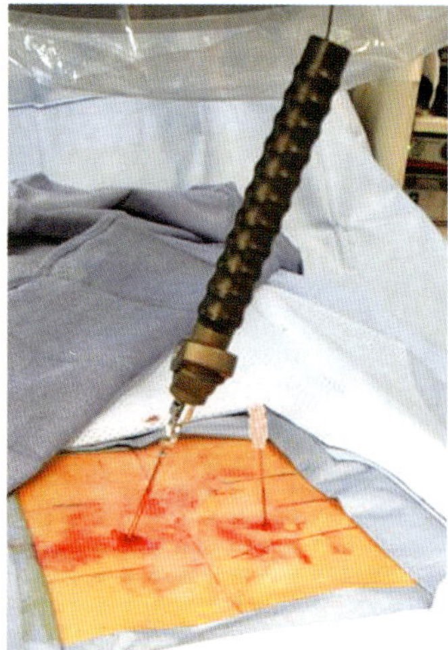

Fig. 3.27 LTN with laser probe in place

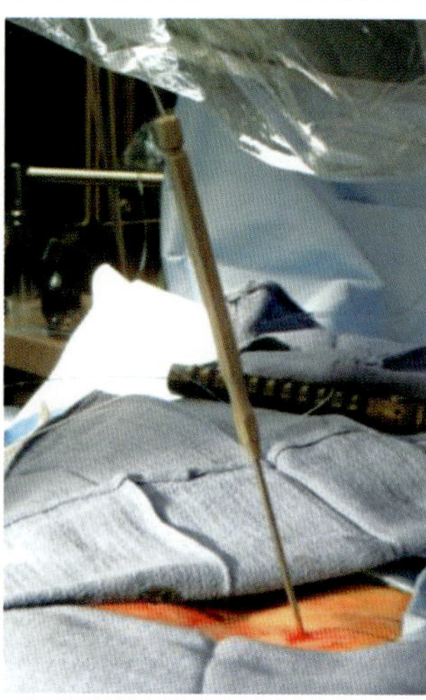

Fig. 3.28 Laser thermoneurectomy

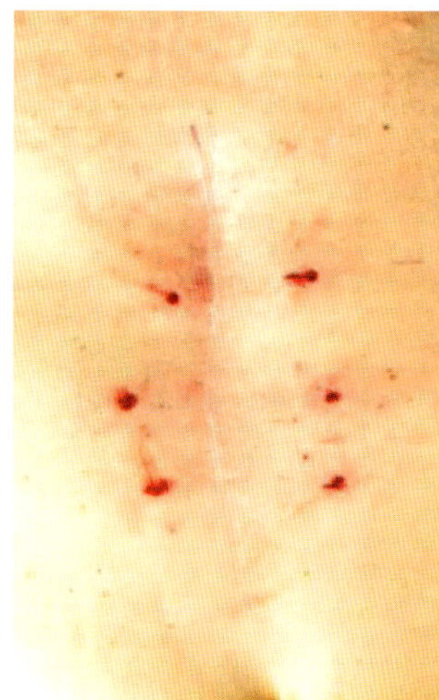

Fig. 3.29 Small surgical wound post LTN

Surgical Outcome for Laser Thermoneurectomy

- In *34 patients*, average follow-up *24 months* (12 months)
- Overall result: 31 (*91.2%*) patients with *good to excellent results*, fair results 3 (8.8%)
- *Response to treatment* evaluated by using: MacNab, modified Mac Nab criteria, ODI, VAS, patient satisfaction scoring, pain diagram and/or patient target achievement score (PTA)
- *Average satisfaction score* – 32 (*94%*) patients
- 3 (8.8%) patients had some mild residual pain
- *Intraoperative and postoperative complication: 0%*
- Preliminary report (Fig. 3.33).

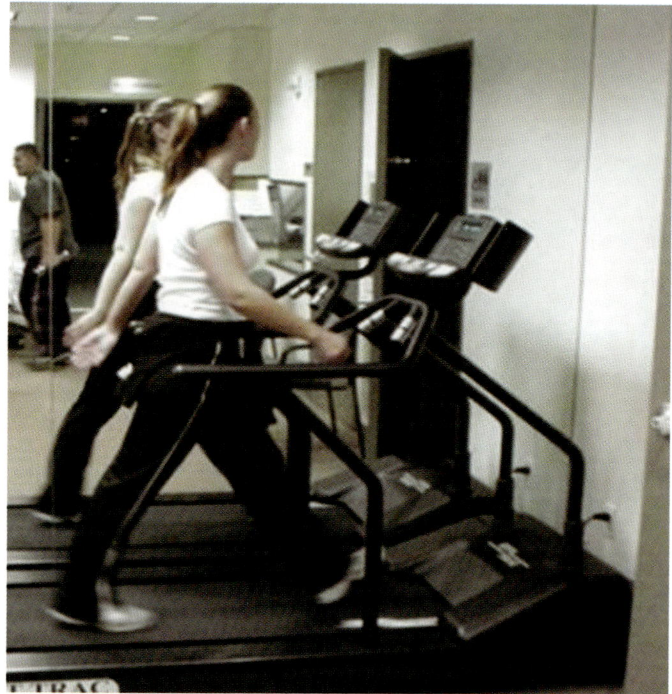

Fig. 3.30

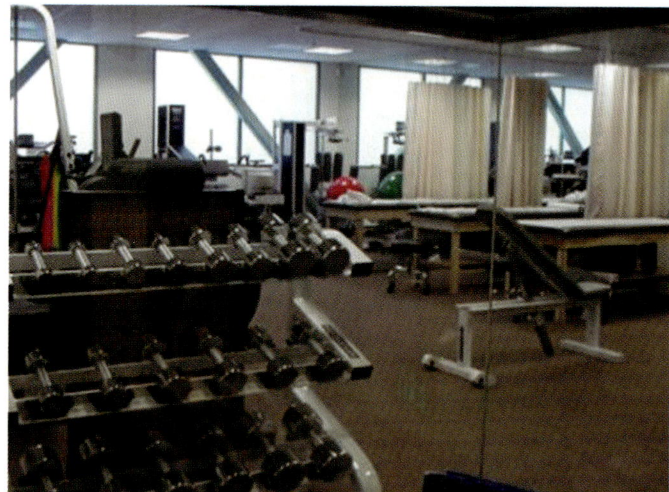

Fig. 3.31

Figs 3.30 and 3.31 Gym for the treatment of the patient

Conclusion

- *Intractable SIJ pain* can be treated *conservatively* with medication, PT, ice, heat, injection and even with *local nerve blocks with some relief*
- *If failure* of conservative treatment and SIJ pain syndrome continues
- It *can be successfully treated with outpatient SIJ nerve blocks and subsequent laser thermoneurectomy (LTN)* with endoscopic rhizotomy/decompression

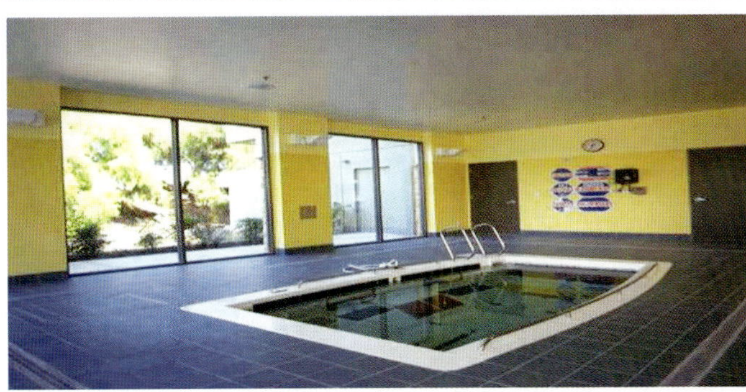

Fig. 3.32 Swimming pool for physiotherapy

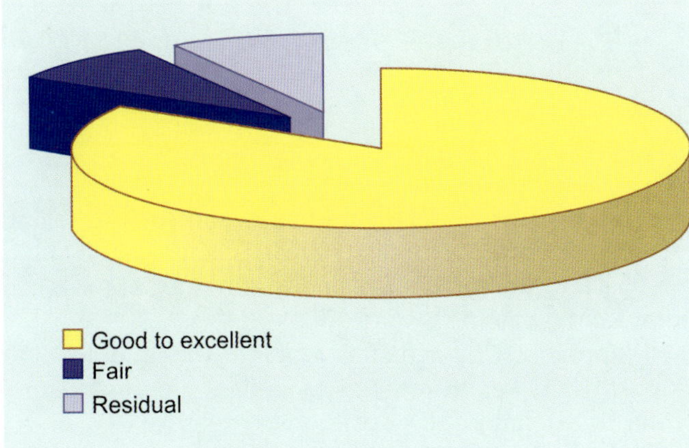

Fig. 3.33 Outcome of surgical LTN

- LTN with microdecompression *of L4–S3 SIJ* appears to be a *safe* and *efficacious outpatient surgical procedure*
- It provides *economical savings and speedy recovery*

Bibliography

1. Chiu J, Clifford T. Microdecompressive percutaneous discectomy: Spinal discectomy with new laser thermodiskoplasty for non extruded herniated nucleus pulposus. Surg Technol Int. 1999;VIII:343-51.
2. Chiu J, Maziad A, Rappard G, et al. Evolving Minimally Invasive Spine Surgery: a Surgeon's Perspective on Technological Convergence and Digital OR Control System. In Szabo Z, Coburg AJ, Savalgi R, Reich H, Yamamotto M (eds): Surgical Technology International XIX, UMP, San Francisco, CA; 2009. pp 211-22.
3. Cohen SR. Sacroiliac joint pain: A comprehensive review of anatomy, diagnosis, and treatment. Aires its Airalg. 2005;101:1440-53.
4. Dreyfuss P, Dreyer SJ, Cole A, Mayo K. Sacroiliac joint pain. J Am Acad Orthop Surg. 2004,12,255-65.
5. Dreyfuss P, Dryer SJ, Griffin J, et al. Positive sacroiliac screening tests in asymptomatic adults. Spine. 1994;19:1138-43.
6. Fenton DS, Czervionke LF (eds). Image-Guided Intervention. Philadelphia: WB Saunders; 2003.
7. Netter FH (ed). Atlas of Human Anatomy. Ciba Geigy Corporation; 1989.
8. Schwarzer AC, Aprill CN, Ilogduk N. The sacroiliac joint in chronic low back pain. Spine. 1995;20:31-7.
9. Waldman SD (ed). Atlas of Interventional Pain Management (2nd ed). Philadelphia: WB Saunders; 2004.
10. Wang LH, Mckenzie-Brown AM, et al. (eds). The Handbook of C-Arm Fluoroscopy-Guided Spinal Injections. Informa Healthcare; 2006.

CHAPTER

4

Treatment for Sacroiliac Joint Pain: A Minimally Invasive Algorithmic Approach

John C Chiu, Ali M Maziad

Introduction

Sacroiliac joint (SIJ) pain contributes up to 25% of patients with low back pain. 25–39% of patients with SIJ pain are found to have low back pain. If the SIJ becomes symptomatic, it may also cause pain in the low back, buttocks, abdomen, groin, or legs. Primary function of the SIJ is lending pelvic and lower extremity stability. It transmits all the forces of the upper body to the pelvis through the SIJ down to the legs.

Chronic low back pain can be difficult to localize and diagnose clinically, as it can be caused by various pathologies. Currently, there is no standard SIJ treatment algorithm for SIJ pain.

We will demonstrate a stepwise treatment approach to SI joint pain.

Anatomy of SI Joint

The pelvis consists of the two ilia and the sacrum connected together through the SIJ which is the largest axial joint in the body (17.5 cm^2). The anterior side of the joint is lined with thick hyaline cartilage while the posterior iliac side of the joint is lined with fibrocartilage. The anterior third of the joint is a true synovial joint but the rest of the junction is a set of ligamentous connections.

The innervation of the SIJ is very complex and mostly believed to be through posterior innervation from medial branches of dorsal rami of spinal nerves, L4, L5, S1–3, and anterior innervations from the L4–S2 ventral rami (Fig. 4.1).

Causes of SIJ Pain

It can be initiated by minor trauma event, such as falling onto the buttocks or a slip. Activities such as climbing stairs, getting up from chairs, and getting out of a car can aggravate the pain.

It is provoked by activities requiring unequal loading through the lower extremities or pelvis, such as skating, gymnastics, golfing, and step aerobics exercise.

Previous back surgery particularly fusion surgery, can alter the mechanics of the lower back region, which may cause abnormal stresses on the joint thus causing or increasing the pain. The pain may refer to the groin, and the entire lower limb, but not the back above the L5 level.

Pathology of surrounding structures: Capsular and ligamentous tension, hypomobility or hypermobility, shearing forces, abnormal joint mechanics, fractures, soft tissue injury, inflammation.

Reproduction of pain by physical examination technique that stresses the joint can help identify SIJ as the cause of pain.

Diagnosis

Point specific tenderness over the sacral sulcus as well as the posterior superior iliac spine. Plain X-rays may detect advanced joint arthritis; however, early degeneration may not be seen on X-rays. Elimination of pain with intra-articular injection of local anesthetics and nerve blocks.

Specific tests for SIJ pain: Patrick test, Fortin, Gaenslen test, Yeoman test.

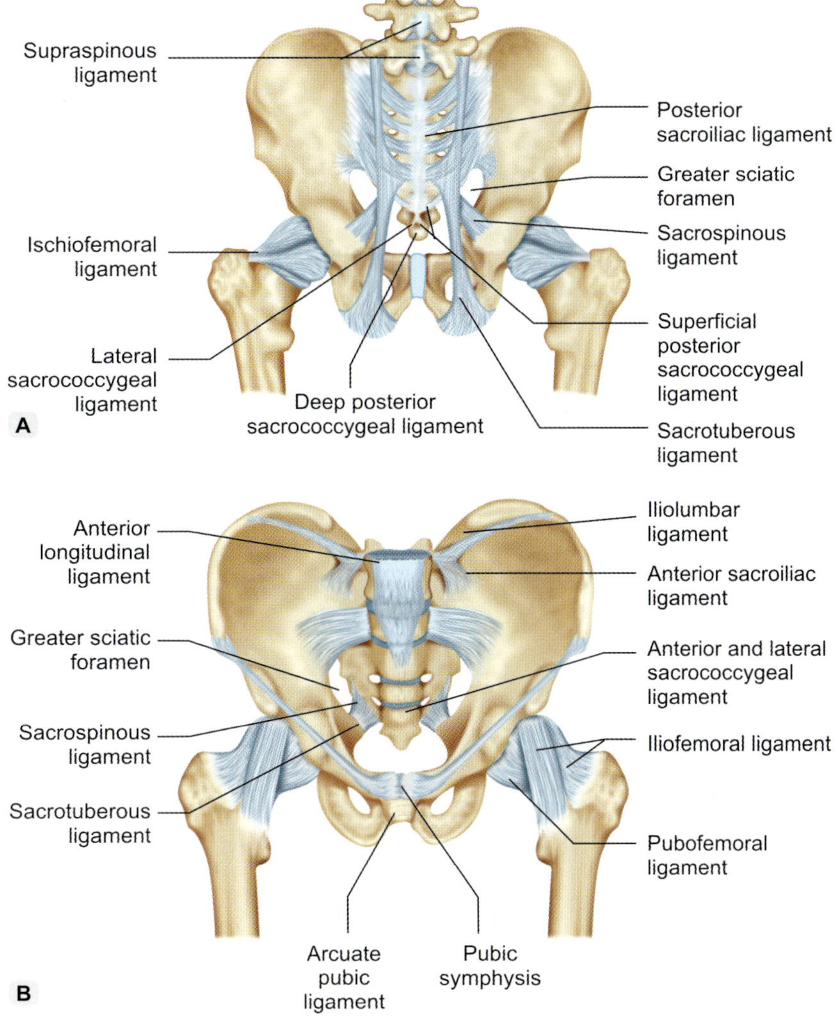

Fig. 4.1 Articulation and ligaments of sacroiliac joint and surrounding structures. (A) Posterior view; (B) Anterior view

Factors Predisposing SIJ Injury or Dysfunction

Capsular and synovial disruption, capsular and ligamentous tension, hypomobility or hypermobility, extraneous compression or sharing forces of the joint, abnormal joint mechanism, microfracture or macrofracture, chondromalacia, soft tissue injury, inflammation, joint laxity, degenerative joint disease, trauma with a fall onto the buttocks, etc.

Treatment of SIJ Pain

- Conservative treatment by medications, physical therapy, and acupuncture should first be attempted. If a good response from those methods is not achieved, further treatment should be attempted which starts by intra-articular joint injections, SI nerve blocks or neurectomies by laser or radiofrequency.
- **SIJ injections intra-articular and extra-articular:** Injection anesthetic medication into the joint confirms whether or not the pain came from the joint

  The local anesthesia and cortisone can help break a pain cycle or possibly facilitate a rehabilitation exercise program.

Technique for SIJ Injection

- Patient is in the *prone position*
- Under *local anesthesia* with mild IV *sedation*, 22 gauge needle is inserted into the joint under fluoroscopic guidance and localization (Fig. 4.2)
- *Contrast material* (isovue) is injected intra-arctiularly to confirm correct needle placement
- A mixture of *local anesthetics* and *steroids* is injected (5–10 cc of 0.25% lidocaine with triamcinalong 30 mg)

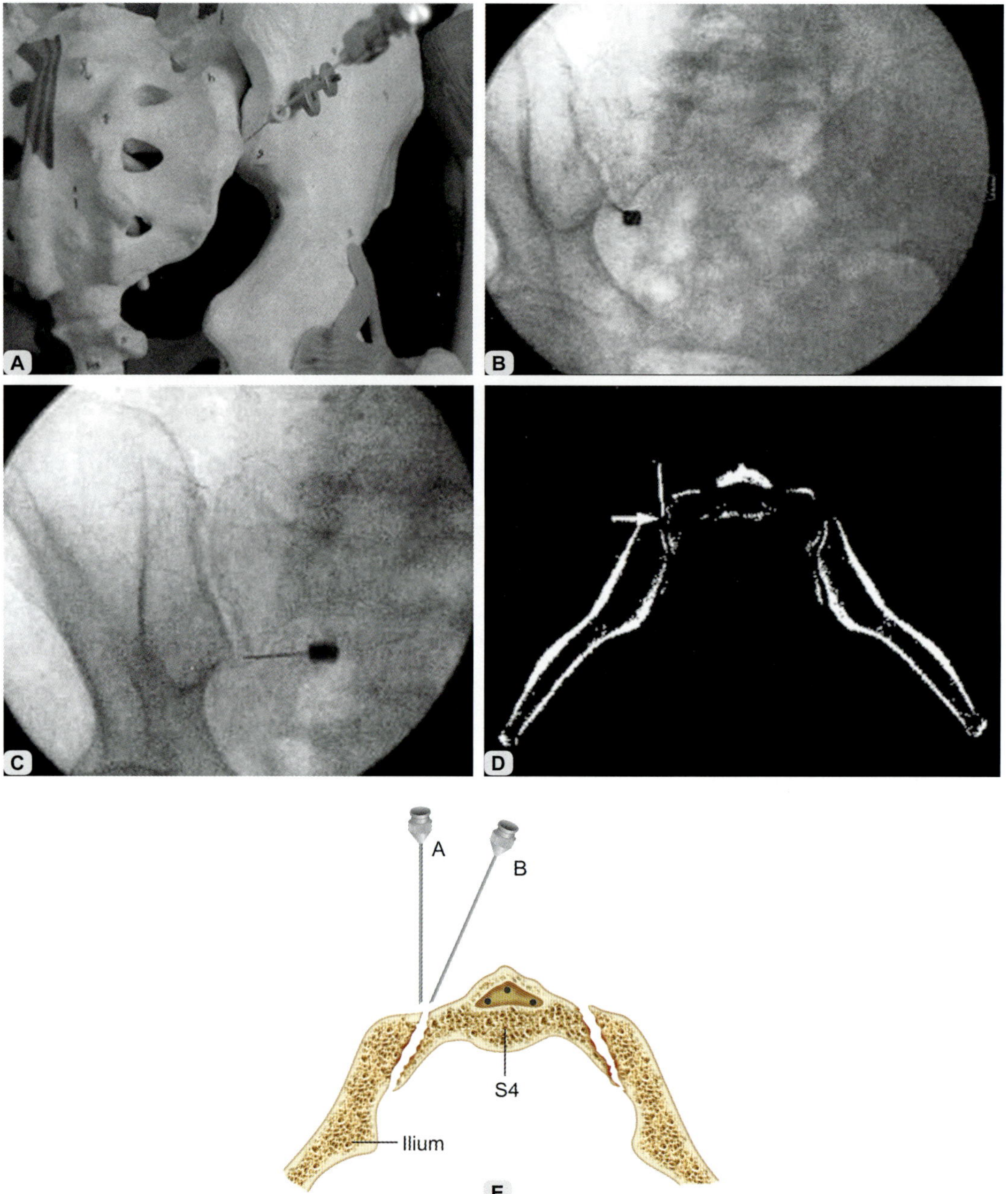

Fig. 4.2 SIJ injection and nerve block

- After the injection some *may benefit* by wearing a SIJ support belt.

Surgical Technique for SIJ Neuroablation

- *Two successful SIJ nerve blocks* are *required before* proceeding with endoscopic microdecompression and *laser thermoneurectomy*/rhizotomy
- Patient in *prone position*
- The *C-arm fluoroscopic unit* is angled towards the visualized line of the posterior aspect of SIJ
- The *tube is angled caudally and obliquely (15–20 degrees from the opposite side* of the body) from the side opposite to the *SIJ to be denervated* with Visualization of posterior SIJ line, 5 mm to the neural foramen, superiorly along the neural foramen laterally (Figs 4.3 and 4.4)

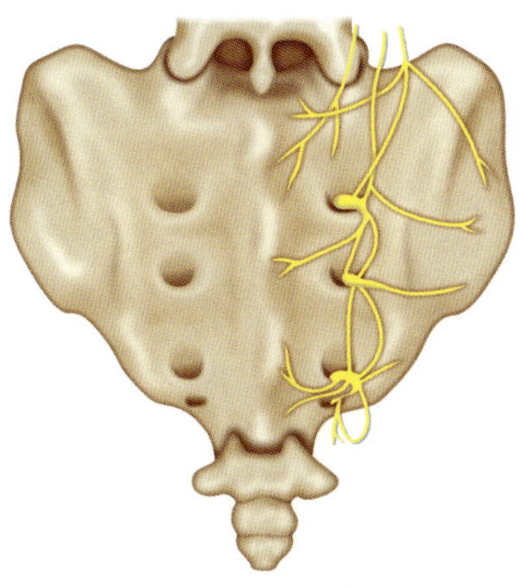

Fig. 4.3 SIJ neuroablation

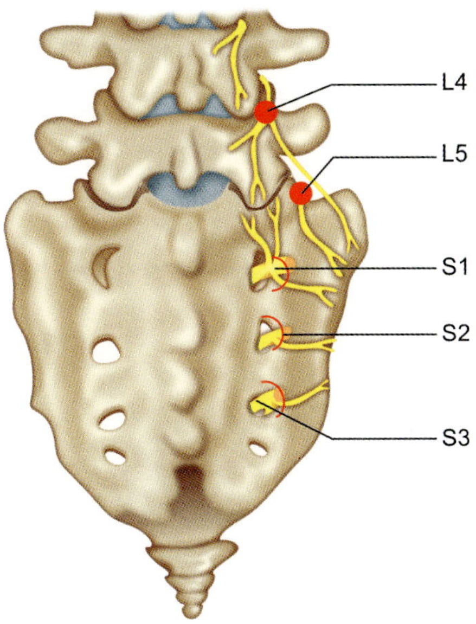

Fig. 4.4 Surgical laser thermoneurectomy targets

Fluoroscopic Technique

- The spine is in the *prone position*
- The fluoroscopic beam *aligns the anterior and posterior sacral foramina*
- A photograph of a sacrum from the anterior aspect
- The anterior and posterior foramina align
- *A/P fluoroscopic image* of the sacrum with *alignment of the anterior and the posterior foramina*
- The *red spots and red curved line* are *the targets for laser thermoneurectomy* (Fig. 4.4)
- This procedure of laser *denervation* can be successfully performed with *Holmium YAG laser* system at 125 joules (5 watts, 10 hertz) for each site/nerve
- Endoscopic guidance can also be used for accurate targeting of the nerves supplying SIJ
- During the *LTN, continuous cold saline irrigation* to *dissipate* the *heat* generated by laser application, caused by the LTN/rhizotomy (Figs 4.5 to 4.8)

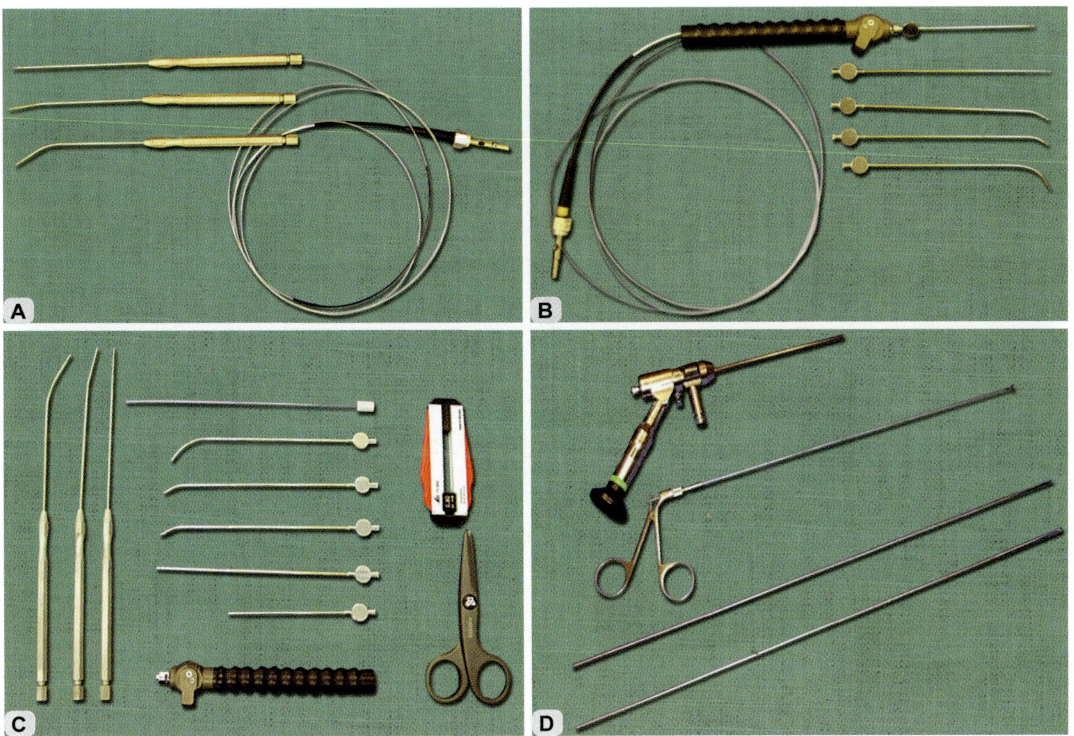

Fig. 4.5 Instruments used for rhizotomy includes laser fibers, different targeting channels, and endoscope

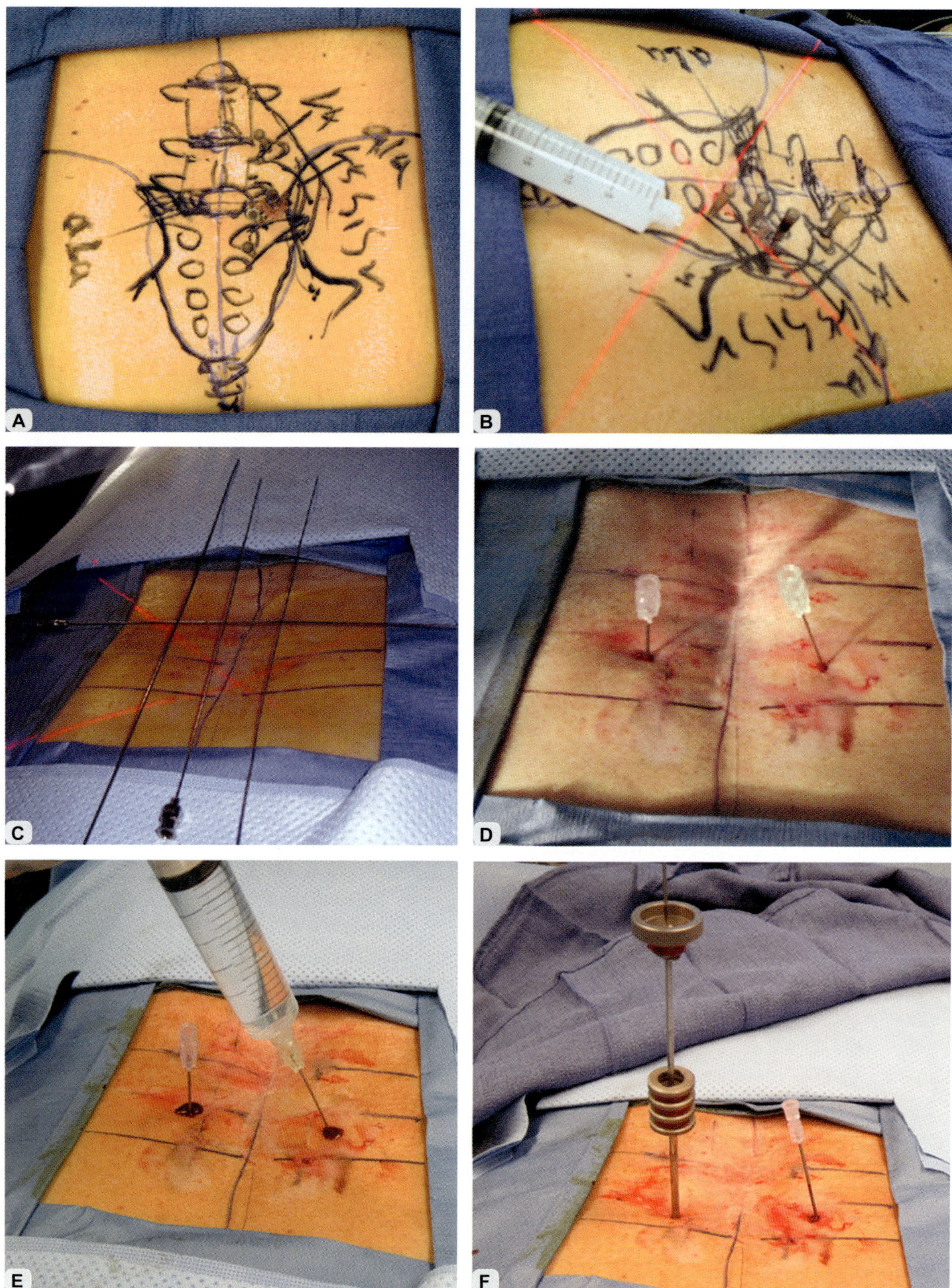

Fig. 4.6 Targeting the nerves supplying SIJ under fluoroscopic guidance

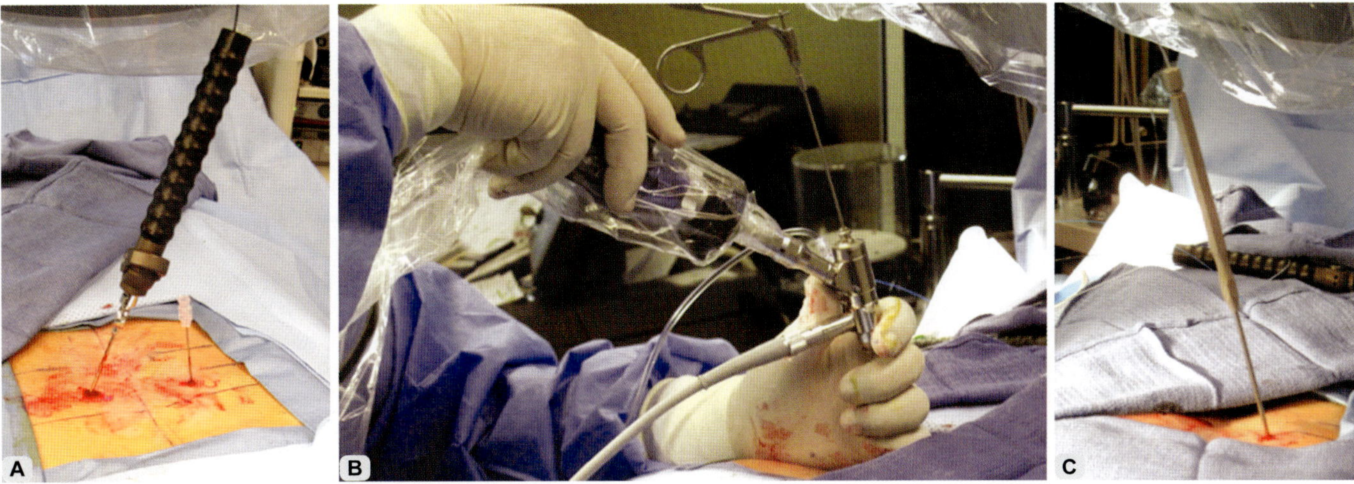

Fig. 4.7 Introduction of working probe channel, endoscopic visualization of nerve

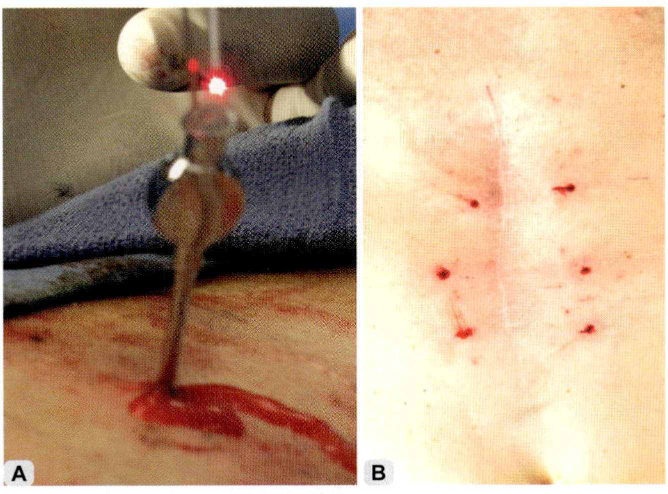

Fig. 4.8 Introduction of laser fiber, picture before closure of puncture wounds

Postoperative Protocol

- *Ambulatory* usually in about 30 minutes and discharged subsequently
- May *shower* the following day
- Icepack is helpful
- *Mild analgesics* and muscle relaxant are needed at times
- *Progressive exercises and able to start PT* the following day
- Rehabilitation complements MISS and motion preservation
- *Return to work* in 3 days as tolerated (not for heavy work).

Surgical Outcome for Laser Thermoneurectomy

- In *34 patients*, average follow-up *24 months* (12 months)
- Overall result: 31 (91.2%) patients with *good to excellent results*, fair results 3 (8.8%)
- Various evaluations of response to treatment: modified Mac Nab criteria, Oswestry disability score/index (ODI), visual analogue pain scale (VAS), patient satisfaction scoring, pain diagram and/or patient target achievement score (PTA) for assessment were utilized
- *Average satisfaction score* – 32 (94%) patients
- 3 (8.8%) patients had mild residual pain and paresthesia, although overall their pain lessened
- *Intraoperative and postoperative complication: 0%.*

Conclusion

SIJ pain can be treated conservatively with medication, PT, ice, heat, injection and local nerve blocks with some relief. If failure of conservative treatment and intractable SIJ pain syndrome continues, it can be successfully treated with outpatient laser thermoneurectomy (LTN) and microdecompression laser thermoneurectomy (LTN) with microdecompression of L3–S3 SI joints. It appears to be a safe and efficacious outpatient surgical procedure for patients who failed conservative treatment. The surgical procedure provides economical savings and speedy recovery.

Bibliography

1. Chiu J, Clifford T. Microdecompressive percutaneous discectomy: Spinal discectomy with new laser thermodiskoplasty for non extruded herniated nucleus pulposus. Surg Technol Int. 1999;VIII:343-51.
2. Chiu J, Maziad A, Rappard G, et al. Evolving Minimally Invasive Spine Surgery: a Surgeon's Perspective on Technological Convergence and Digital OR Control System, In Szabo Z, Coburg AJ, Savalgi R, Reich H, Yamamotto M (eds): Surgical Technology International XIX, UMP, San Francisco, CA; 2009. pp 211-22.
3. Chiu J, Savitz MH. Use of Laser in Minimally Invasive Spinal Surgery and Pain Management. In Kambin P (ed): Arthroscopic and Endoscopic Spinal Surgery – Text and Atlas (Second ed). New Jersey: Humana Press; 2005. Chapter 13, pp 259-69.
4. Cohen SR. Sacroiliac joint pain: A comprehensive review of anatomy, diagnosis, and treatment. Aires its Airalg. 2005;101:1440-53.
5. Dreyfuss P, Dreyer SJ, Cole A, Mayo K. Sacroiliac joint pain. J Am Acad Orthop Surg. 2004;12:255-65.
6. Dreyfuss P, Dryer SJ, Griffin J, et al. Positive sacroiliac screening tests in asymptomatic adults. Spine. 1994;19:1138-43.
7. Fenton DS, Czervionke LF(eds). Image-Guided Intervention. Philadelphia: WB Saunders; 2003.
8. Netter FH (ed). Atlas of Human Anatomy. Ciba Geigy Corporation; 1989.
9. Schwarzer AC, Aprill CN, llogduk N. The sacroiliac joint in chronic low back pain. Spine. 1995;20:31-7.
10. Waldman SD (ed). Atlas of Interventional Pain Management (2nd ed). Philadelphia: WB Saunders; 2004.
11. Wang LH, Mckenzie-Brown AM, et al.(eds). The Handbook of C-Arm Fluoroscopy-Guided Spinal Injections. Informa Healthcare; 2006.

CHAPTER

5

Role of Disc-Fx® for Annulonucleoplasty in the Management of Lumbar Disk Pathology

Naresh Kumar, Sambhav Shah, Siddharth Shah

Introduction

Low back pain (LBP) has a worldwide prevalence of 30 – 40%.[1,2] The total costs due to LBP in the United States exceed $100 billion per year.[3] Approximately 40% of all LBPs have been found to be dikcogenic in origin.[4] Diskogenic back pain may be due to a disk prolapse or degenerative disk disease (DDD). Successful outcomes after diskectomy for a discprolapse have been reported.[5,6] However, it is worth noting that patients with small, contained degenerated disks have been found to be poor candidates for diskectomy as their clinical outcomes are less favorable[7].

Diskogenic pain from DDD has been traditionally managed with either with nonoperative treatment[8] or by major surgical interventions like spinal fusion [9,10] and artificial disk replacement.[11-13] However, major surgical interventions have their own drawbacks. Spinal fusion may be complicated by pseudarthrosis or adjacent segment degeneration.[14-18] High surgical morbidity, risk of implant subsidence, and lack of long-term results are the shortcomings of artificial disk replacement.[19-22] Hence, it is not surprising that several minimally invasive techniques have been developed to treat dikcogenic back pain in recent years.

Disc-Fx® (Elliquence, LLC, Baldwin, NY) is one such minimally invasive system that combines percutaneous manual diskectomy, nucleus ablation, and annular modification procedures at the same time.

Mechanism of Action

Apart from percutaneous manual diskectomy, Disc-Fx® involves application of radiofrequency energy for nucleus ablation and annular modification. This technique utilizes higher frequency of 1.7 MHz provided by the Elliquence Surgi- Max® generator for radiofrequency energy application with two different modulations—bipolar Turbo and bipolar Hemo modes. The Turbo mode allows nuclear ablation, while the Hemo mode allows annular modification with shrinkage.[23,24] The use of higher frequency offers the advantage of reduced heat and minimal tissue alteration.[23,24] The radiofrequency energy is applied using a steerable probe (Trigger- Flex®, Elliquence).

Postmortem studies have shown that an average of 0.8 g of disk material is removed with nuclear ablation with a corresponding reduction in intradiscal pressure.[23] Modulation of the dorsal annulus results in cauterization of inflamed structures, shrinkage of the annulus by 30% and expansion of the epidural space of up to 9%.[23] Moreover, annular modulation may also cause reduction in pain generated by the annular nerve fibers in DDD. Steerable delivery system using Trigger-Flex® permits targeted application in the region of the pathology. Endoscopic visualization in between the steps can help documentation of decompression.

Indications

1. Contained lumbar disk herniations with back and/ or leg pain.
2. Annular tears causing chemical sciatica or back pain.
3. Axial back pain with DDD.

It is recommended that the procedure be undertaken only after failure of conservative treatment for at least three months.

Contraindications

1. Extruded or sequestrated disk
2. Diskopathy with more than 50% loss of height
3. Pfirmann[25] grade <2 or >4
4. Infection
5. Tumors
6. Fracture
7. Pregnancy.

Relative Contraindications

1. High Iliac crest (access to L5 – S1 disk is difficult)
2. Spondylolysis
3. Spondylolisthesis.

Instruments Required

- Surgi-Max® energy source
- Trigger-Flex® bipolar system
- Monitor, camera and light source
- Image intensifier (II)
- Spinal needle 16 G X 8″
- Guide wires (thin and thick)
- Tapered dilator
- Trephine
- Cannula, beveled
- Cannula, straight
- Grasping forceps
- Radiopaque dye (Omnipaque™ 350 (GE Healthcare, Cork, Ireland).

Technique

Disc- Fx® is performed as a daycare procedure under conscious sedation (managed anesthesia care) and local anesthesia. The patient is placed in prone position with bony prominences well padded. The concerned disk level is identified under image intensifier guidance. Using a posterolateral approach, a 16 G/18 G spinal needle is targeted to enter the disc lateral to the superior articular pillar (SAP), yet medial to the exiting nerve root. The trajectory of the needle depends upon the location of the pathology. A 10° – 30° trajectory is commonly used if feasible (at L5 – S1 level such trajectory may not be possible due to the iliac crest). Side of the pathology is the preferred side of needle insertion. For the purpose of description, the procedure is discussed under the following four steps (Figs 5.1 to 5.12):

1. Discography
2. Manual discectomy
3. Nucleus ablation
4. Annulus modulation.

Diskography is performed using a 2 mL mixture of the solution (10 mL solution = 5 mL of Omnipaque dye, 3 mL of saline and 2 mL of indigo carmine) and the results are noted. A guidewire is placed through the needle into the nucleus pulposus, right up to the opposite annulus. A small skin incision of 3 mm is made to accommodate the introduction of the access cannula and soft tissue dilator into the annulus or the disk fragment. An endoscope may be inserted at this point to confirm the correct placement of the cannula.

Manual diskectomy of intra-annular or subligamentary free material is done using small disk forceps or disk rongures.

The Trigger-Flex® probe is inserted and *nucleus ablation* is performed using the bipolar Turbo mode of the Surgi-Max® generator. This produces local heat which shrinks and hardens the nuclear material. Six strokes of ablation are carried out for the nucleus in six different directions. This is followed by extraction of any nuclear material using the grasping forceps. The cavity of the dorsal disk can also be visualized with the use of an endoscope.

Modulation of dorsal annulus is then carried out by placing the steerable Trigger-Flex® probe on the pathological area and using the bipolar Hemo mode. Four strokes of modulation are performed in different directions on the annulus. This ablates any ingrown granulation tissue and nerve endings and shrinks the annular opening.

The epidural space and the nerve root can be visualized through the endoscope and the adequacy of decompression can be confirmed. A 5 cc mixture of steroid with local anesthetic (triamcinolone acetonide + marcaine) is infiltrated into the annulus at the end of the procedure. All the aforementioned steps are carried out under image intensifier. The approximate procedure time is 30 – 40 minutes. Post-procedure, the patient is observed for development of any neurological deficit or procedure-related problems and is allowed to be discharged the same day.

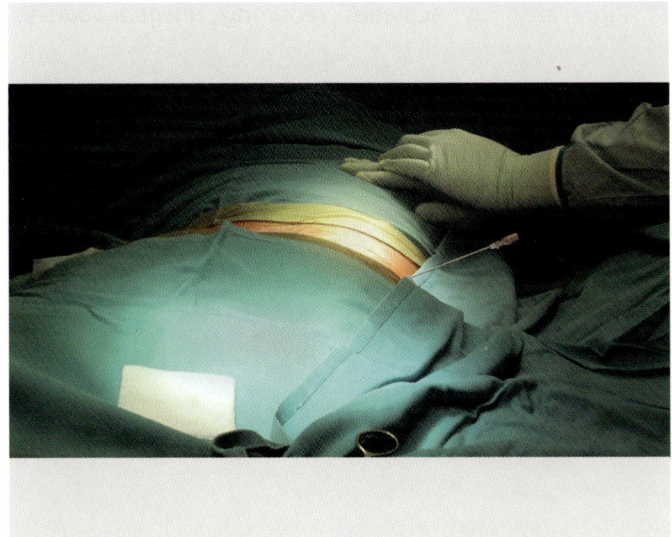

Fig. 5.1 Insertion of the needle for diskography

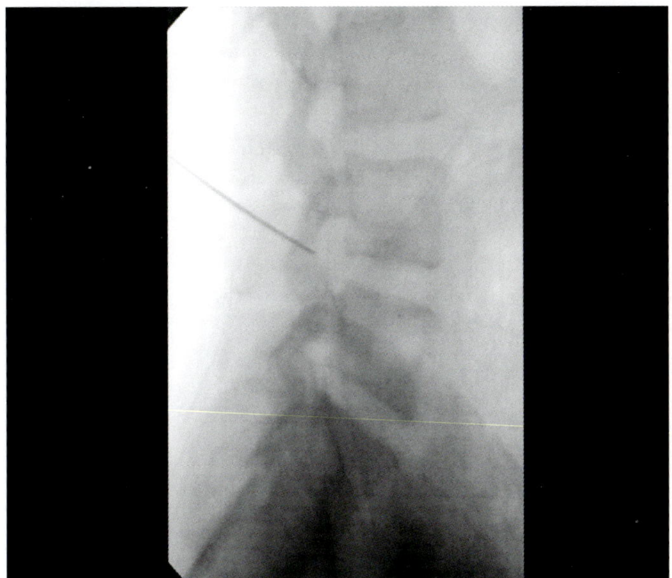

Fig. 5.2 Needle is being directed to the disk space under image intensifier guidance

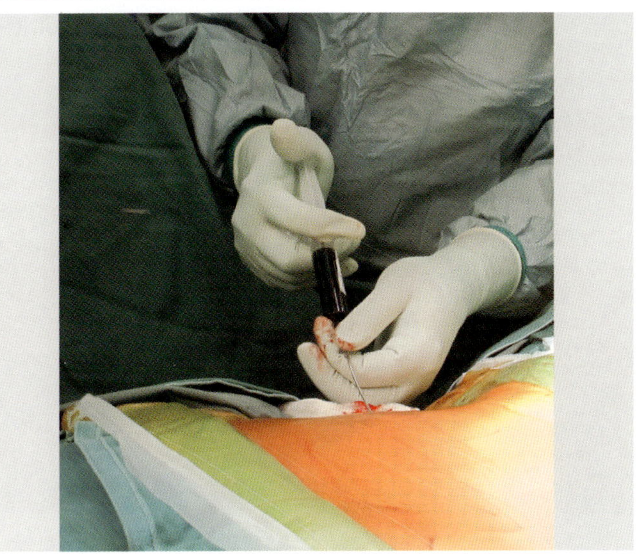

Fig. 5.3 Injection of contrast agent for diskography

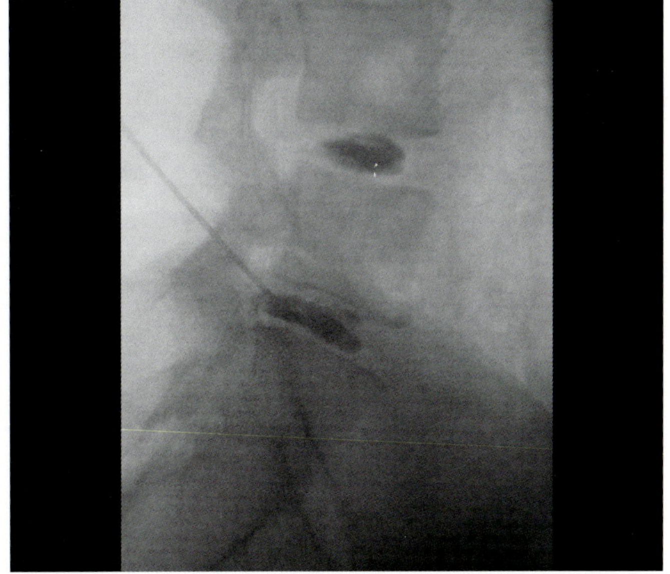

Fig. 5.4 Diskogram showing 'cottonball' appearance at the control disk-L4/5 and 'fissured' appearance at the L5 – S1 disk—symptomatic disk

Advantages

1. Minimally invasive technique
2. Tissue-sparing approach
3. Can be done under conscious sedation
4. Visualized endoscopic discectomy (if endoscope is used).
5. Targeted application of manual diskectomy and thermal energy.
6. Small diameter of the working cannula (3 mm) prevents irritation of the dorsal root ganglion (DRG) in the foramen.
7. Low risk of infection
8. Avoidance of postoperative scarring and fibrosis
9. Faster recovery and early return to work.

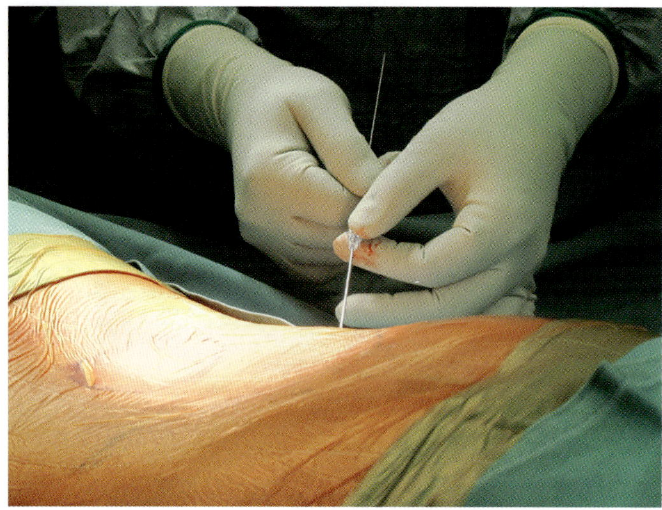

Fig. 5.5 Insertion of the guidewire for Disc- Fx® through the needle

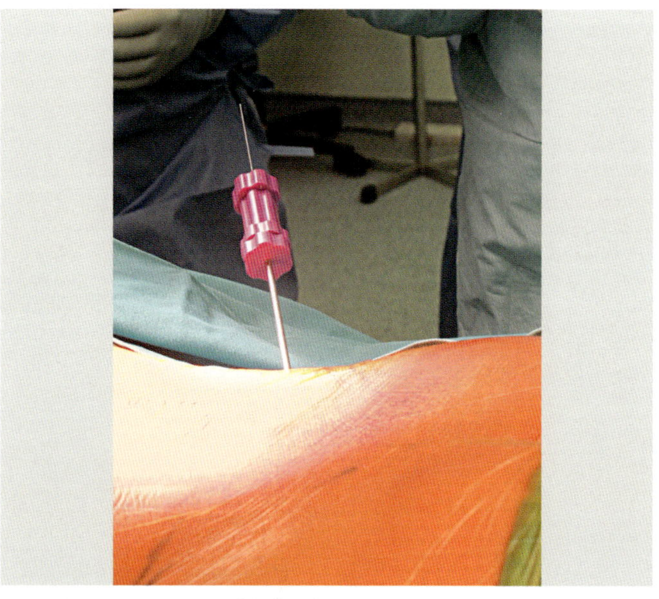

Fig. 5.6 Insertion of the working cannula over the guidewire

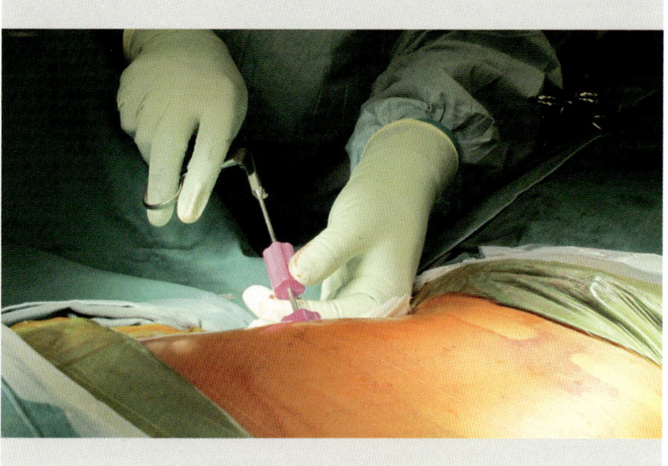

Fig. 5.7 Percutaneous manual diskectomy through the working cannula

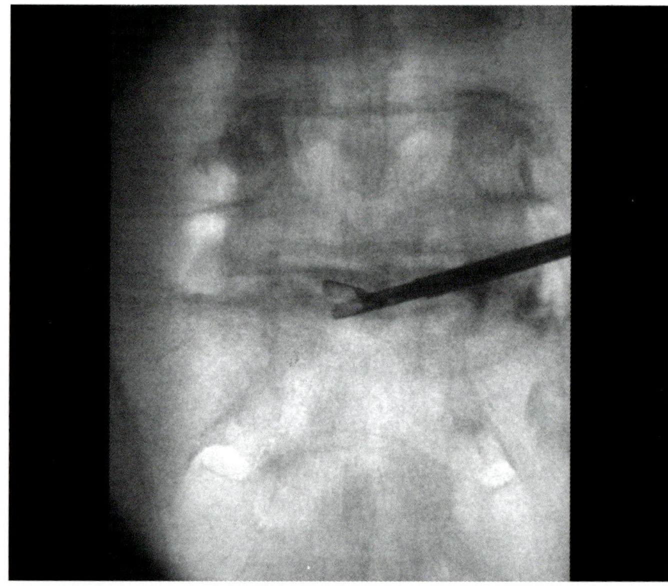

Fig. 5.8 Percutaneous manual diskectomy under image intensifier

Disadvantages

1. Limited scientific data
2. Limited access to L5 – S1 disk in patients with high iliac crest.
3. Minimal annulotomy is required. Hence, there is a theoretical risk of reherniation.
4. Inability to visualize the pathology, if endoscope is not used.
5. Special disposable instrument set is required adding to the cost of the procedure.
6. Learning curve for surgeons unfamiliar with percutaneous procedures.

Evidence

In a comparative study of Disc-Fx® (25 patients) against fenestration and decompression (25 patients) for contained

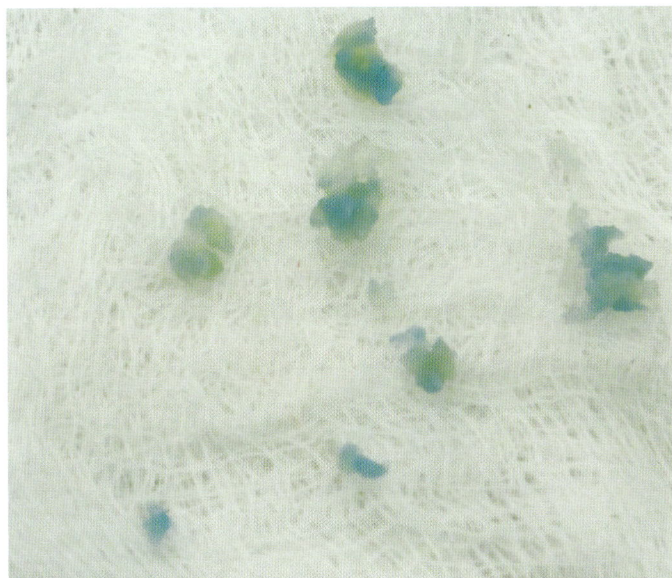

Fig. 5.9 Disk material removed after discectomy.

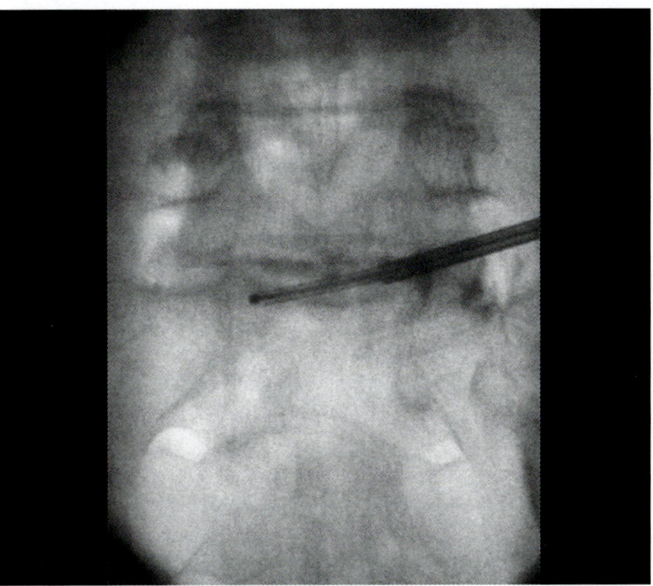

Fig. 5.11 The steerable Trigger- Flex® probe as seen under image intensifier.

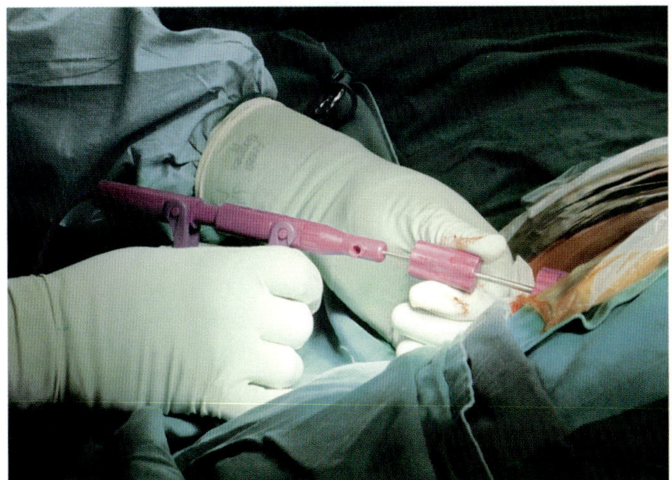

Fig. 5.10 Insertion of the Trigger- Flex® probe through the working cannula

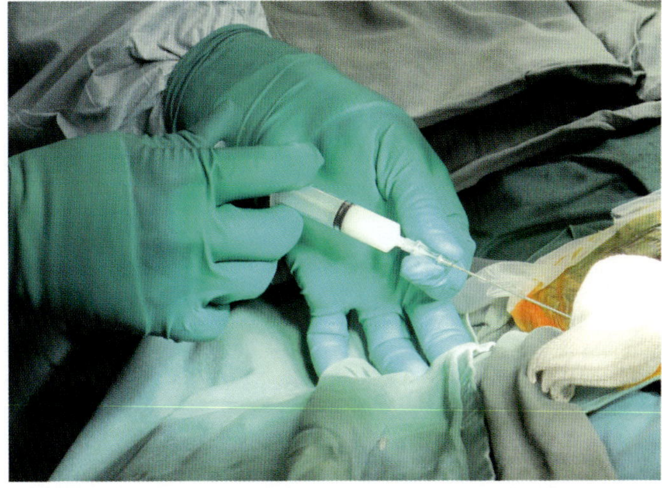

Fig. 5.12 Injection of steroid+ local anesthetic mixrure into the disk annulus after completion of the annulonucleoplasty

lumbar disk herniation with unilateral radicular pain, Liao et al.[26] found that the operation time, blood loss and length of hospital stay in the Disc- Fx® group was significantly lesser than the latter (p = 0.01). The Oswestry disability index (ODI) and visual analog scale (VAS) scores were significantly better than the respective preoperative scores in both the groups at 12 months after surgery (p = 0.01) and there was no significant difference between the two groups (p = 0.05).

In a retrospective evaluation of 130 patients treated with Disc- Fx® at 198 levels, Ramirez et al.[27] reported a complication rate of 4.5% which included dural puncture, radiculitus, and diskitis. The re-intervention rate was 3.8%. The mean return to work after surgery was eight days and the mean pre-operative VAS of 7.6 reduced to 1.6 at three years.

In a prospective controlled study of 72 patients undergoing Disc- Fx®, Stefan Hellinger[23] reported that the VAS-back and leg pain showed significant improvement from 8.5 pre-operatively to 3.3 at six months. The original MacNab index showed excellent and good results in more than 70% patients at six months. All patients were ready to undergo a similar procedure again, if necessary and would recommend the procedure to others.

Summary

To summarize, Disc-Fx® is a newer minimally invasive procedure with potential applications in the management of selective group of patients with contained lumbar disk herniation or degenerative disk disease that fail to respond to conservative treatment. While early results of the procedure are promising, high quality evidence with a longer follow-up is lacking.

References

1. Papageorgiou AC, Croft PR, Ferry S, et al. Estimating the prevalence of low back pain in the general population. Evidence from the South Manchester Back Pain Survey. Spine (Phila Pa 1976). 1995;20:1889-94.
2. Skovron ML, Szpalski M, Nordin M, et al. Sociocultural factors and back pain. A population-based study in Belgian adults. Spine (Phila Pa 1976). 1994;19:129-37.
3. Katz JN. Lumbar disc disorders and low-back pain: socioeconomic factors and consequences. J Bone Joint Surg Am. 2006;88 (Suppl 2):21-4.
4. Kallewaard JW, Terheggen MA, Groen GJ, et al. Discogenic Low Back Pain. Pain Pract. 2010;10:560-79.
5. Mirza SK, Deyo RA. Systematic review of randomized trials comparing lumbar fusion surgery to nonoperative care for treatment of chronic back pain. Spine (Phila Pa 1976). 2007;32:816-23.
6. Weinstein JN, Lurie JD, Tosteson TD, et al. Surgical versus nonoperative treatment for lumbar disc herniation: four-year results for the Spine Patient Outcomes Research Trial (SPORT). Spine (Phila Pa 1976). 2008;33:2789-800.
7. Dora C, Schmid MR, Elfering A, et al. Lumbar disk herniation: do MR imaging findings predict recurrence after surgical diskectomy? Radiology 2005;235:562-7.
8. Singh V, Derby R. Percutaneous lumbar disc decompression. Pain Physician. 2006;9:139-46.
9. Gerges FJ, Lipsitz SR, Nedeljkovic SS. A systematic review on the effectiveness of the Nucleoplasty procedure for discogenic pain. Pain Physician. 2010;13:117-32.
10. Manchikanti L, Derby R, Benyamin RM, et al. A systematic review of mechanical lumbar disc decompression with nucleoplasty. Pain Physician. 2009;12:561-72.
11. Pfirrmann CW, Metzdorf A, Zanetti M, et al. Magnetic resonance classification of lumbar intervertebral disc degeneration. Spine (Phila Pa 1976). 2001;26:1873-8.
12. Lee JS, Hobden E, Stiell IG, et al. Clinically important change in the visual analog scale after adequate pain control. Acad Emerg Med. 2003;10:1128-30.
13. Copay AG, Glassman SD, Subach BR, et al. Minimum clinically important difference in lumbar spine surgery patients: a choice of methods using the Oswestry Disability Index, Medical Outcomes Study questionnaire Short Form 36, and pain scales. Spine J. 2008;8:968-74.
14. Chen YC, Lee SH, Chen D. Intradiscal pressure study of percutaneous disc decompression with nucleoplasty in human cadavers. Spine (Phila Pa 1976). 2003;28:661-5.
15. Chen YC, Lee SH, Saenz Y, et al. Histologic findings of disc, end plate and neural elements after coblation of nucleus pulposus: an experimental nucleoplasty study. Spine J. 2003;3:466-70.
16. Lee MS, Cooper G, Lutz GE, et al. Histologic characterization of coblation nucleoplasty performed on sheep intervertebral discs. Pain Physician. 2003;6:439-42.
17. O'Neill CW, Liu JJ, Leibenberg E, et al. Percutaneous plasma decompression alters cytokine expression in injured porcine intervertebral discs. Spine J. 2004;4:88-98.
18. Bokov A, Skorodumov A, Isrelov A, et al. Differential treatment of nerve root compression pain caused by lumbar disc herniation applying nucleoplasty. Pain Physician. 2010;13:469-80.
19. Mirzai H, Tekin I, Yaman O, et al. The results of nucleoplasty in patients with lumbar herniated disc: a prospective clinical study of 52 consecutive patients. Spine J. 2007;7:88-92; discussion -3.
20. Gerszten PC, Welch WC, King JT, Jr. Quality of life assessment in patients undergoing nucleoplasty-based percutaneous discectomy. J Neurosurg Spine. 2006;4:36-42.
21. Cohen SP, Williams S, Kurihara C, et al. Nucleoplasty with or without intradiscal electrothermal therapy (IDET) as a treatment for lumbar herniated disc. J Spinal Disord Tech. 2005;18 Suppl:S119-24.
22. Singh V, Piryani C, Liao K, et al. Percutaneous disc decompression using coblation (nucleoplasty) in the treatment of chronic discogenic pain. Pain Physician. 2002;5:250-9.
23. Hellinger S. Disc-FX – A Treatment for Discal Pain Syndromes Combining a Manual and Radiofrequency-assisted Posterolateral Microtubular Decompressive Nucleotomy. European Musculoskeletal Review. 2011;6(2):100-4.
24. Hellinger S, Liao X, Mermelstein L, Kumar N, Nucci R, Ramirez J. Radiofrequency assisted lumbar semi- endoscopic manual discectomy using the Disc- Fx system- Preliminary results of various ongoing clinical outcome studies worldwide. European Musculoskeletal Review. 2011;6(4):265-71.
25. Pfirrmann CW, Metzdorf A, Zanetti M, et al. Magnetic resonance classification of lumbar intervertebral disc degeneration. Spine (Phila Pa 1976). 2001;26:1873-8.
26. Liao X, Jiang J, Xiong DL at al. the comparison of clinical outcomes of percutaneous lumbar discectomy with Disc- fx system with fenestration and decompression for contained lumbar disc herniation (LDH) with radicular pain. Chinese J Pain Med. 2011;17(1):25-29.
27. Ramirez JF, Sierra JM. Rugeles JG et al. Thermodiscoplasty with RF: An alternative to the management of discogenic pain. Presented at: 4th Congress of the Inter American Society for Minimally Invasive Spine Surgery, Cartagena, 12th May 2011.

CHAPTER

6

Pearls and Tricks of Endoscopic Minimally Invasive Spinal Surgery

John C Chiu, Ali M Maziad

Introduction

Disk degeneration is a common problem affecting many middle-aged individuals that increases in severity with age. Lack of exercise, bad postural habits, obesity, and repetitive trauma may accelerate the process and can lead to early onset of symptoms. Depending on the number of spinal segments involved and the degree of degeneration, symptoms can range from mild muscular aches to severe neural compression that can compromise movement and sensation severely up to a point of disability.

Treatment usually follows a hierarchy of steps or algorithm ranging from rest and medical treatment to extensive major surgery. Due to the nature of conventional spine surgery, large incisions and extensive deep tissue dissection are mandatory to gain access to the site of pathology.

Following open procedures, delayed recovery, which maybe incomplete, is expected. Extensive muscle dissection becomes a source of pain for those patients and recovery can take months before the patient adapts to the pain due to surgery and until the patient's spine achieves fusion.

Quite often, posterior fusion alone is not sufficient to achieve a sound biomechanical fusion. Anterior inter-body fusion may be needed which in turn poses more surgical trauma and risks if done transabdominally.

Patients are often reluctant to proceed with conventional extensive surgery due to its risks. Thanks to recent advances in imaging, endoscopic and laser systems, minimally invasive spinal surgery[1-3] can be safely and effectively performed with far lesser risks.

The goal of minimally invasive spinal surgery is to decompress nerve roots and disk bulges as well as provide more room for the thecal sac (in cases of spinal canal stenosis) through small access portals without destabilizing or interfering with the structure of the spine. In cases with gross instability of the spine, patients may still require spinal fixation. However, if the patient is high risk or refuses open surgery, minimally invasive spinal surgery with grid positioning system (GPS) should be the alternative surgical treatment.

We have applied the new concept of GPS[1] to precisely localize the lesion or target preoperatively and to aid in the localization of the foramen during surgery as well.

In this chapter we will demonstrate how GPS aids and facilitates[1] minimally invasive spinal surgery[4-12] in effectively alleviating the symptoms[13-22] associated with degenerative disk disease and neurological compression with lesser risks and speedier recovery.[23-33]

We will also point out the pearls and tricks that we have gathered over the years, which can help the surgeons avoid many pitfalls and perform an effective procedure with less risks to the patient.

Surgical Indications[7-12]

- Intractable low back pain with radiation down the leg (radicular pain)
- Symptoms of spinal neurogenic claudication
- Compressive and symptomatic radiculopathy with sensory and motor impairment

- Disk extrusion or sequestration with predominantly back or leg pain
- Nonradicular low back pain persistence despite facet joint injection
- Lateral recess stenosis with dynamic compressive or noncompressive radiculopathy
- Prior failed conventional surgery with perineural scarring and failed back syndrome and junctional disk degeneration and disk herniation following fusion
- No improvement of symptoms after a minimum of 12 weeks of conservative therapy
- Grade 1 spondylolisthesis
- Diffused multilevel disk degeneration that would otherwise require very extensive open surgery.

Pearls

- Quite often, patients may present with multiple degenerated disks on imaging studies particularly MRIs which have high false-positive results. Thus, it is very crucial to obtain a detailed history from the patient and perform a full physical examination "before" attempting to read MRIs and other studies, which are readily available in today's practice. This approach will ensure that the surgeon builds a hypothesis regarding the actual pathology that is causing the patient symptoms
- A trial of conservative treatment, such as exercise, medications, physiotherapy, injections of trigger points or facet joints are very useful in excluding muscular and facet joint pathology as the primary cause of symptoms. Usually a mixture of short-acting anesthetic (lidocaine), longer acting anesthetic (marcaine) and steroids (dexamethasone) can help relief some of the patients symptoms
- Provocative diskograms may be useful in cases where disk pathologies are suspected. Reproduction of symptoms when patients are under mild sedation confirms the source of back pain or radiculopathy and provides a more solid indication for performing surgery. Epidural steroid injections can be performed in the same setting provide some relief until the definitive surgery is performed
- As in any type of surgery, preoperative planning is key to a successful surgery. Confirming the site of "symptomatic" pathology with the patient and the side of pain will avoid simple yet big mistakes, such as operating on the wrong side or level
- Many of the patients complaining of spine problems, particularly the elder population may have concomitant osteoporosis which aggravates to the symptoms of back pain. As a routine, we perform bone density studies on patients above 60 years and start antiresorptive treatment if T-score is below –2.5 SD
- It is also important to notice any vertebral anomalies, such as extra-ribs, sacralization of lumbar vertebra, lumbarization of sacral vertebra, absent vertebra, etc. If such anomalies are encountered, we advice obtaining a full x-ray study of the spine to accurately count the vertebrae and ribs in order to avoid operating on the wrong level, (Fig. 6.1).

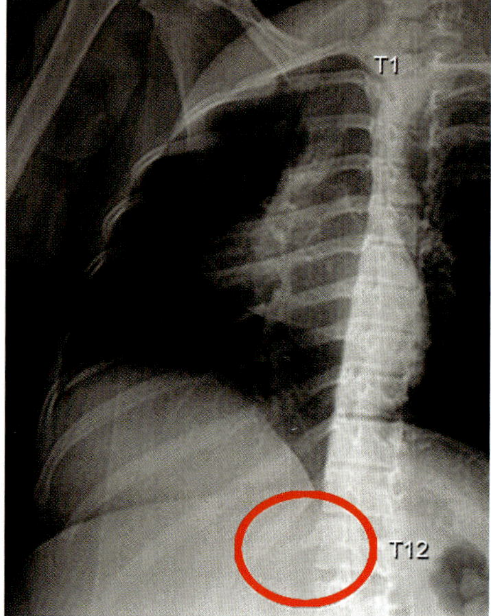

Fig. 6.1 A patient with single rib at T12—obtain full X-ray of thoracic spine to ensure proper count.

Contraindications

- Cauda rquina syndrome
- Tumors
- Gross instability of the degenerative spine (spondylolisthesis grades 2 and 3)
- Post traumatic unstable spinal fractures

Pearls

In those cases, minimally invasive spinal surgery (MISS) may not be the complete answer to the problem due to the biomechanical concerns or aggressive nature of the pathology; however, it may be the only alternative to an extensive open procedure if the patient's general condition does not allow an open procedure.

Anesthesia and Positioning[7-12]

Unlike conventional surgery, minimally invasive spine surgery can be effectively done under local anesthesia and IV conscious sedation, which helps avoid complications of general anesthesia.

We have modified our technique so that the patient is positioned in the lateral decubitus with the painful leg up. Compared to prone position, the lateral position reduces intra-abdominal pressure, venous pressure, pelvic congestion and risk of DVT as well as pulmonary complications as it maintains a better lung reserve. It also provided better airway control. If a bilateral surgery is to be performed, the patient is positioned on one side first and then the flipped to the other side.

Pearls

- Positioning of both hips and knees in 90 degrees of flexion reduces the traction on the nerve roots and provides a safer procedure
- Anti-DVT stockings should be used with all patients even the young population to avoid vascular stagnation
- Proper padding of boney prominences helps to avoid pressure sores.
- When placing patient in the prone position (for thoracid diskectomy) use a well padded frame that positions the patient in flexion to open the disk spaces posteriorly
- EMG needles should be placed to monitor any muscular activities due to nerve irritation
- Taping the patient to the table firmly in the operative position will avoid movement during surgery. The slightest movement or change in position may make the procedure much more difficult and would require repositioning
- It is important to have a paramedical team who understands the procedure well, this will ensure that no radio-opaque structures are placed in the field of surgery and will save operative time
- This procedure is highly reliant on fluoroscopy. Thus having a well trained C-arm technologist can save a lot of valuable time for the surgeon and the patient and avoid unnecessary radiation exposure.
- Placing preoperative imaging studies in a visible location in the OR preferably on wide digital screens can be very helpful in identifying the exact site of pathology during surgery particularly in multi-level procedures (i.e. central, paracentral, far lateral disks, boney spurs, ligamentum flavum hypertrophy, etc.)
- Utilizing the advanced technology of intraoperative surgical informatics systems, such as Surgmatix ® which is specifically designed for minimally invasive spinal surgery can make the procedure more patient-centric and help the surgeon as well as the OR staff to continuously monitor all aspects of surgery (Patient vitals, BIS, EMG, C-arm, endoscope, laser machine log, etc.) and thus provide a safer procedure for the patient. (Fig. 6.2).

Continuous Intraoperative Monitoring[9-12]

Sterile needle electrodes are placed for continuous intraoperative neurophysiological electromyographic (EMG) monitoring. EMG monitoring is absolutely needed to avoid the risk of nerve root injury during MISS procedures. In addition EEG surface monitoring is utilized to optimize anesthesia and reduce anesthetic requirements.

Full monitoring of the patient's vitals is also recommended even if procedure is done under local anesthesia.

Localization of Pathology by Using Grid Positioning System[1]

Grid Positioning System is an anatomical grid system utilized to accurately determine the exact position of the protruded or extruded disk fragment in a 24 zone grid. Understanding of the map of 24 zones of grid position in the lumbar vertebrae in relation to other anatomical landmarks such as the pedicle, lamina sand thecal sac is critical and important to guide the surgical approach and to perform precise endoscopic MISS.

Depending on the position of the protruded disk, different transforaminal trajectories (either ipsilateral or contralateral to the lesion) can be used to create a portal of entry and gain access to the pathology. Central lesions can also be accessed through interlaminar approach. Accurate preoperative localization of the lesion is important in order to precisely reach the lesion and avoid undue trauma to the nerves, vessels, dorsal root ganglia, dura and even the spinal cord.

The location of the lesion or target can be precisely localized within the grid of the GPS system (Fig. 3). Twenty four different zones (A, B, C, D and 1, 2, 3) of the lumbar spine are located in the grid at these zones.

The four vertical zones of the lumbar vertebrae are:

A. Extraforaminal
B. Foraminal

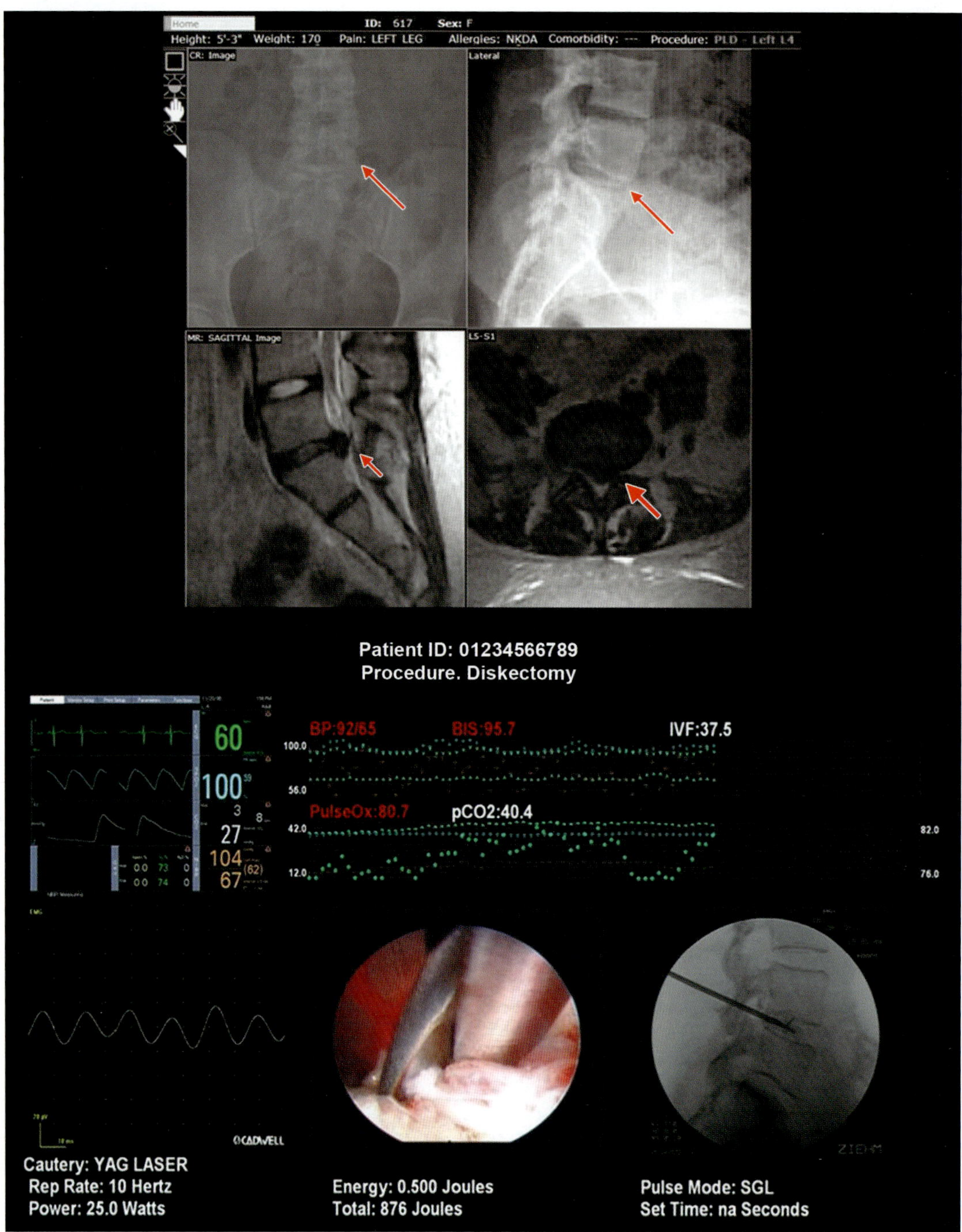

Fig. 6.2 Surgmatix preoperative and intraoperative digital monitoring screens

C. Subarticular
D. Paracentral (Right and left)

The three horizontal levels of the lumbar vertebrae are:

1. At the level of the disk
2. Between the disk and the pedicle, at the level of the neuroforamen.
3. At the level of the pedicle.

Surgical Equipment, Instruments (Fig. 6.4), and Preparation[7-11]

The following surgical instruments are necessary to perform endoscopic laser, and/or lumbar foraminoplasty, or both:

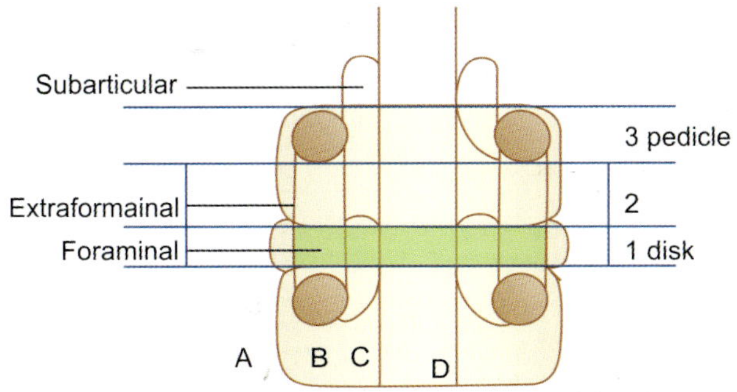

Fig. 6.3 Grid positional system (GPS) with various zones

- Digital fluoroscopic equipment (C-arm) and monitor
- Radiolucent C-arm/fluoroscopic carbon-fiber surgical table
- Endoscopic tower equipped with digital videomonitor
- Wide-angle percutaneous posterolateral foraminoscope 6-degree, operating sheath 6 mm OD, 3 mm working channel
- Set of serial/progressive dilators, and cannula in graduated sizes (3.5 – 5.8 mm); a set of progressive cannula with duck bill extensions (with various lengths 5 – 10 mm on one side), to retract and to protect neural structures from neural trauma intraoperatively
- Aggressive toothed trephine set in graduated sizes
- 9.9 mm tubular retractor system with a gradual dilator set
- Wide angle endoscopes, 0 degree and 30 degrees, 4 mm OD (Karl Storz)
- Trephine, curette, grasper and spoon forceps, 2 mm rotating bone punch (rongeurs), rasp, and burr
- Lumbar dikcectomy sets (2.5, 3.5, 4.7 mm)
- Endoscopic grasping and cutting forceps, probe, knife, scissors, diskectomy rongeurs, and curette (Fig. 6.4)
- Suction irrigation instruments (Diskectomes) either manual or mechanical
- Holmium: yttrium aluminum garnet (YAG) laser or radiophrequency generators
- Holmium 550 µm laser bare fiber with flat tip and right angle (side-firing) probes with and without irrigating system of various sizes, and 2 mm sidefiring irrigating laser probe.

Pearls

We cannot stress enough on the importance of having a well equipped theatre as well as instrumentation that is specifically designed for this type of procedure. A very simple matter such as an incompletely radiolucent surgical table, can make the procedure much more difficult to perform. Likewise, using instruments that are not designed for endoscopic procedures, will make it much more tedious to perform and may pose more risks to the patient.

Surgical Procedure

Intraoperative Determination of Portal of Entry by Grid Positioning System[1]

C-arm fluoroscopy is used to identify the lumbar levels requiring surgery. The midline of the spine (by connecting the lumbar spinal processes under fluoroscopy) and foraminal line of the spine (by connecting the neuro-foramen under fluoroscopy) are first identified by using a flexible stylette under fluoroscopy.

A transverse disk space-line (representing the horizontal disk plane), is drawn under fluoroscopy, starting at the foramen line by using a flexible stylette and intersecting with the midline of the spine.

The portal of entry for lumbar spinal surgery is marked on the transverse disk space-line with a marking pen. The distance of the point of the portal of entry from the midline varies with the height and weight of the patient. In an average-sized patient it is approximately 12 cm at the affected disk level. The more obese the patient, the greater the distance of the portal of entry point is from the midline in order to accommodate for excess subcutaneous fat.

Operative Technique[9, 11]

- Following GPS localization, local anesthetic is injected along the surgical trajectory the Kambin safety triangle to treat disk herniations (Figs 6.5 to 6.11). A long stylette is introduced through the identified entry point (as explained above) (Fig. 6.12). The stylette is directed towards the disc through the Kambin triangle (Safety zone) (Fig. 6.5). The Kambin triangle is the site of surgical access for posterolateral endoscopic lumbar diskectomy. It is defined as a right angled triangle over the dorsolateral disk. The hypotenuse is the exiting nerve, the base (width) is the superior border of the caudal vertebra, and the height is the traversing nerve root and dura
- Serial dilators are introduced guided by the stylette to reach the disk space (Fig. 6.13A).
- Provocative dikcogram is done to confirm disc pathology (Fig. 6.13B).
- Different types of graspers, trephines and curettes are utilized to mechanically decompress the disk material guided by fluoroscopy and endoscopy (Figs 6.13C to G, 6.14, and 6.17C)

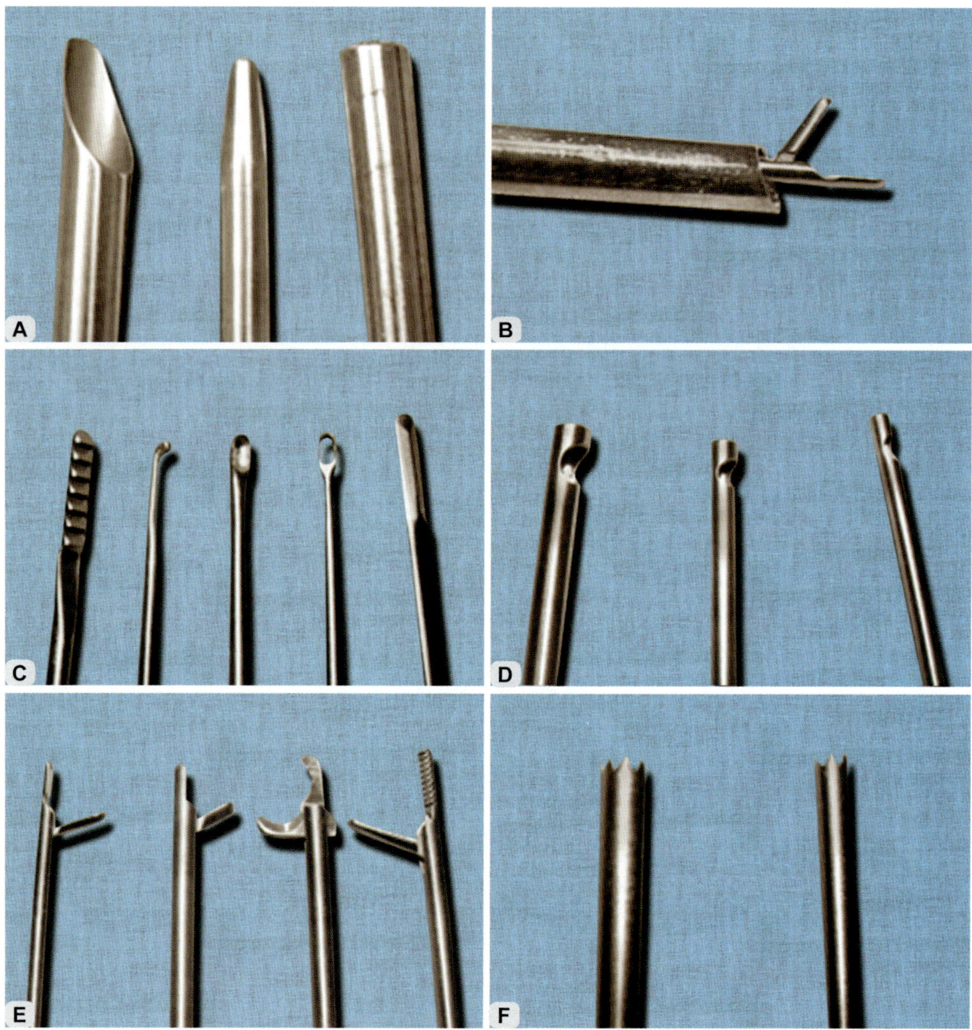

Fig. 6.4 Different microdiskectomy instruments: duck bill tubular retractor with dilator, endoscopic grasper, rasps, curettes, diskectomes, cutter, and grasper forceps and trephine

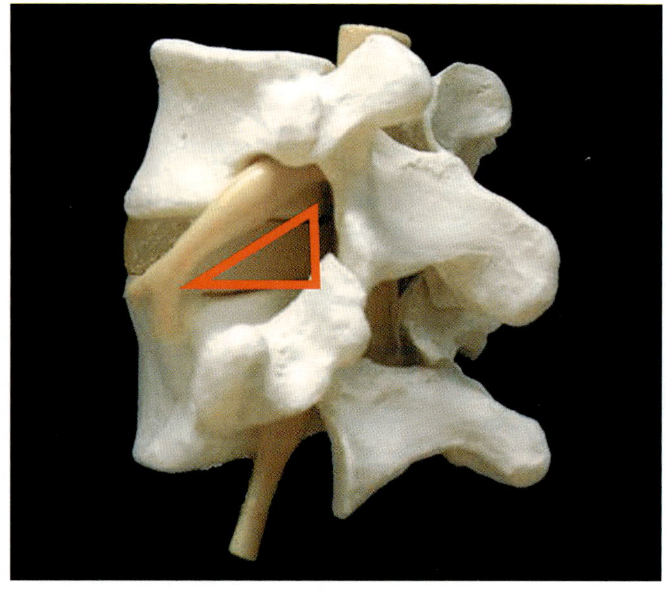

Fig. 6.5 Kambin safety triangle

- Bony spurs can also be trimmed using rongeurs, curettes or high power laser (Fig 6.15).
- Following mechanical decompression, holmium YAG laser is used for thermodiskoplasty of the disk which helps to shrink the disk bulge, denervation of the pain fibers, seal the opening in the annulus fibrosis and coagulate bleeding vessels in vertebral endplates. Applying laser in an inverted cone shape maneuver helps cover a wider area inside the disk through a small skin incision (Fig. 6.15).
- After laser application, diskectome is used for suction irrigation of disk debris (Fig. 6.16).
- Steroid and anesthetic injection intradiskally and along the surgical tract is done as a final step to reduce postoperative pain and inflammation (Fig. 6.17A).
- A single stitch is used to close the skin puncture (Fig. 6.17C).

At times, two levels can be accessed through a single skin puncture by changing the trajectory of the entry (Fig. 6.10).

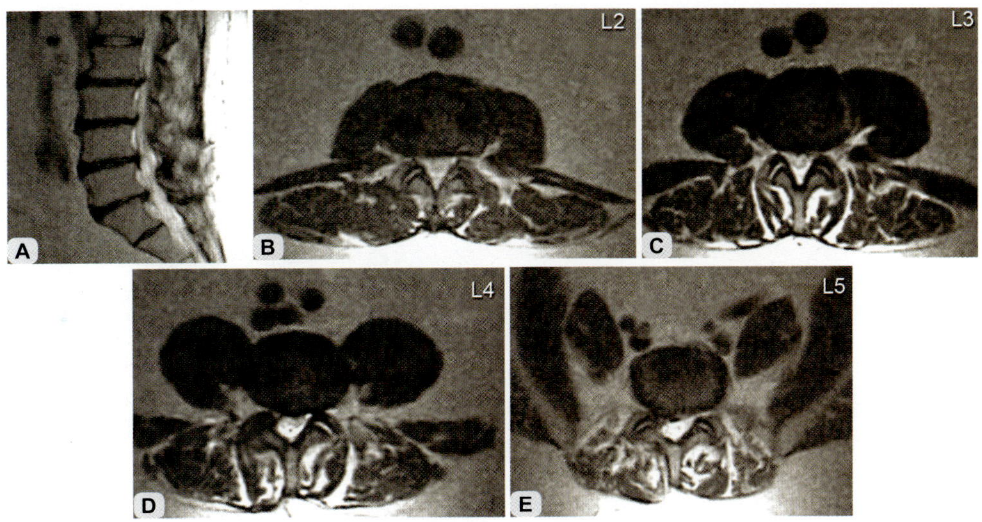

Fig. 6.6 Sagital T2 view MRI showing (A) multi-level disk protrusions and canal stenosis (B to E) with bilateral nerve roots compression

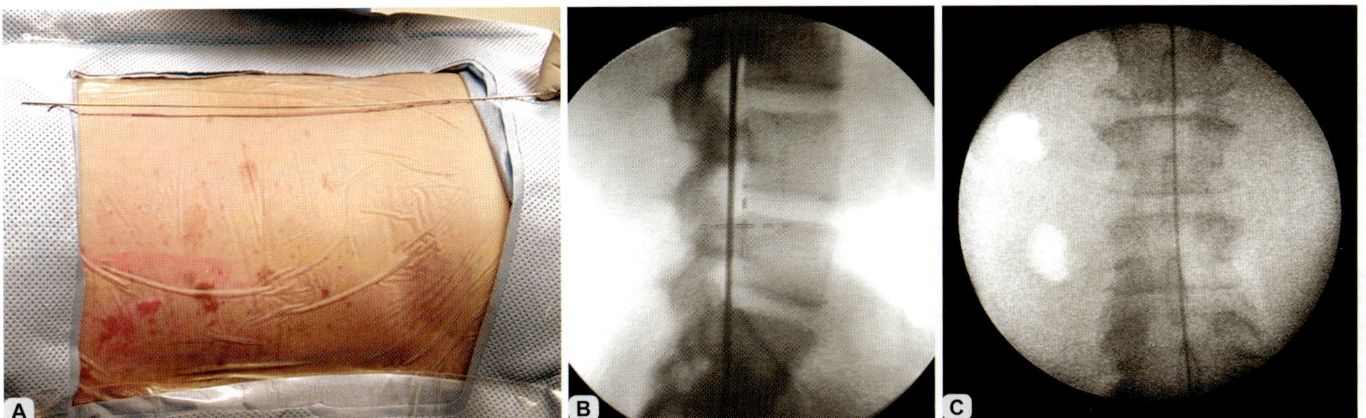

Fig. 6.7 (A) Identifying the foraminal line on patient; (B) Fluoroscopic lateral view; (C) Fluoroscopic midline or lateral foraminal line (on AP view)

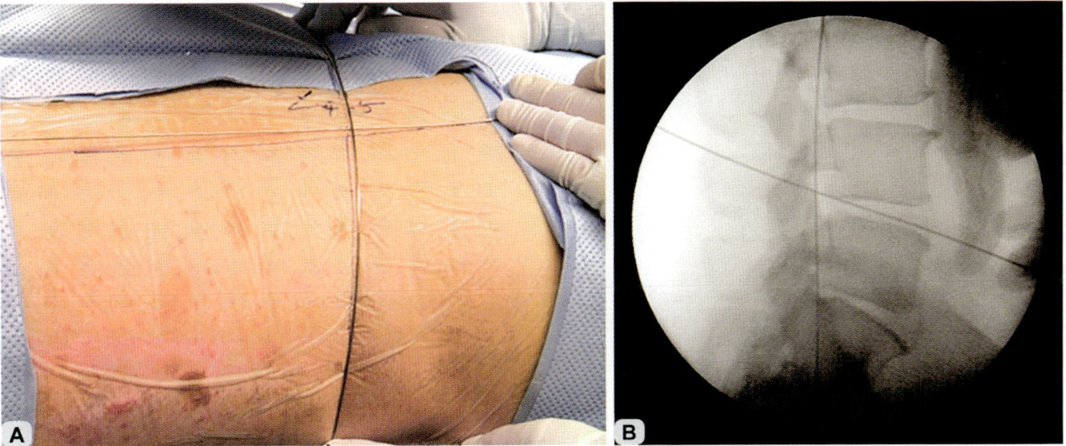

Fig. 6.8 Flexible stylette is used to identify the intersection of the L4/5 disk space line with the foraminal line, on patient and under fluoroscopy

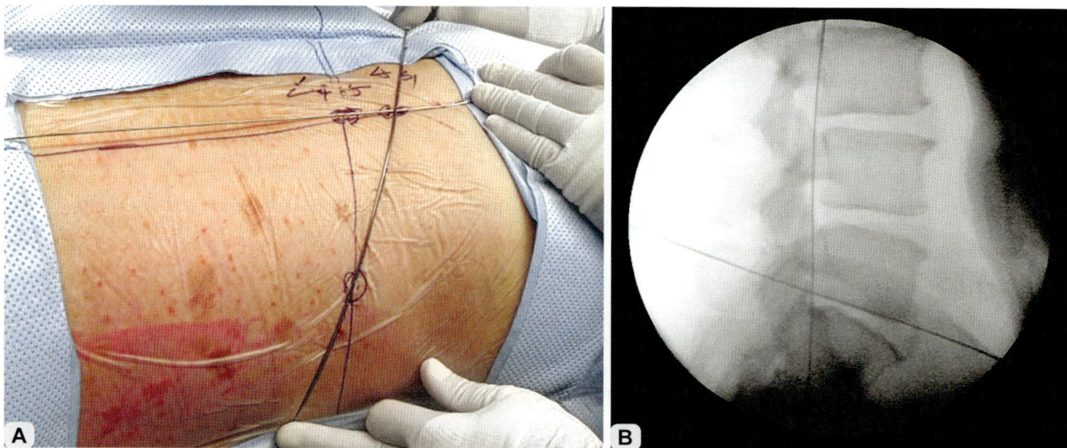

Fig. 6.9 L5/S1 disk can be accessed through the same skin puncture entry through a steeper angle, on patient and under fluoroscopy

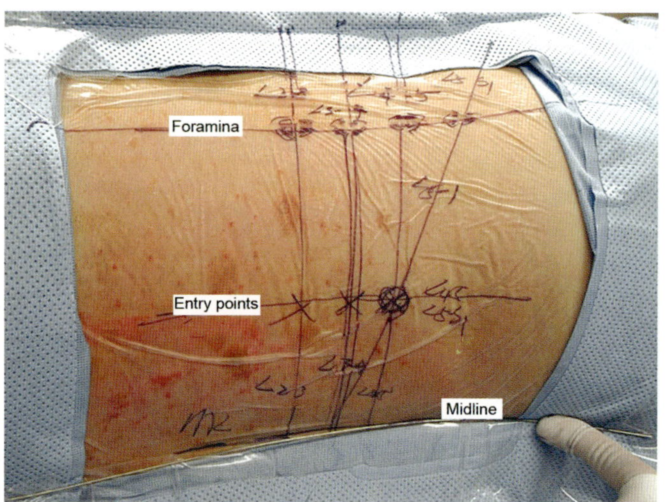

Fig. 6.10 Completed grid positional system

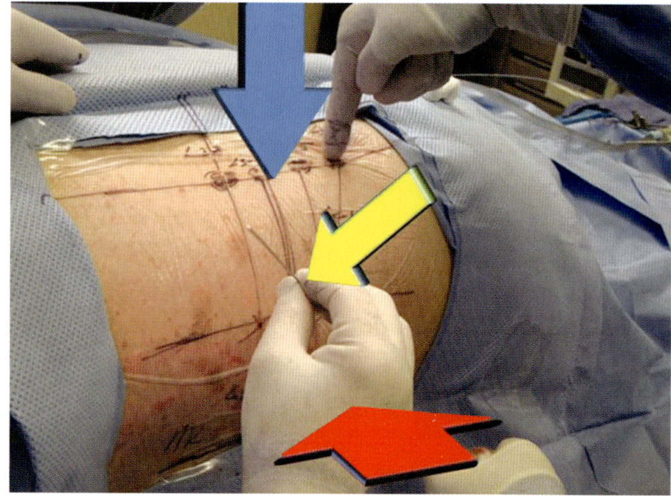

Fig. 6.12 Stylette is introduced at an angle of approximately 45 degrees accurately toward the foramen in the GPS grid, under fluoroscopy.

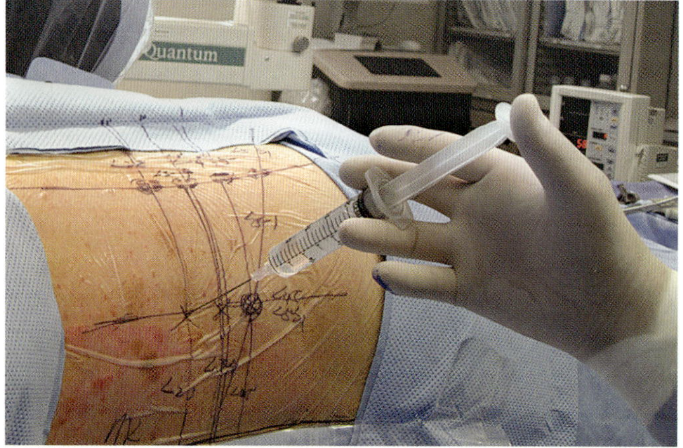

Fig. 6.11 Local anesthetics is injected for each portal entry point

For the thoracic region, the patient is placed in the prone position and the portal can be achieved as follows:

The portal of entry is to be marked at 4–5 cm away from the midline at the mid-thoracic area (T5 – T8 inclusive) at the respective thoracic disk level, 6 – 7 cm from the midline at the lower thoracic area (T9 – T12 inclusive), and at the upper thoracic area (T1 – T4 inclusive).

The needle is incrementally advanced under C-arm fluoroscopic guidance at a 35 – 45 degree angle from the sagittal plane, targeting toward the center of the disk, into the "safety zone," between the interpedicular line medially and the rib head at the costovertebral articulation laterally and medial to costotransverse junction. During the needle insertion, one must keep the needle tip immediately along the medial aspect of the rib head to avoid entering the spinal canal medially, and medial to the costovertebral junction to avoid pleural puncture (Fig. 6.18).

Once a working channel has been established, diskectomy is done in a similar fashion as outlined for the lumbar region.

For the cervical region, the technique is a little different, since we approach the disk from the front .

The portal of entry (operating portal) is at the medial border of the right sternocleidomastoid muscle, where firm pressure is applied digitally in the space between that muscle and the trachea, pointing toward the vertebral surface. The larynx and trachea are displaced medially while the carotid artery laterally. The anterior surface of the cervical spine is palpated with the fingertips (Fig. 6.19).

A standard 18 gauge spinal needle is passed transdermally into the disk space and its position confirmed fluoroscopically. A diskogram is done at this point using a radiopaque contrast material to confirm the level. A 3 – 4 mm skin incision is made and a narrow guidewire 12-inch stylette is passed through the spinal needle, which is then removed. A 2.5 mm or 3.5 mm internal diameter cannula/dilator is introduced over the stylette and into the disk interspace. Once a working channel has been established, diskectomy is done in a similar fashion as outlined above for the lumbar region.

Pearls

- C-arm guidance for every step of the procedure is extremely crucial even when endoscope is used. AP and lateral C-arm images provide a 3D orientation for instruments in relation to vital structures and organs. A single fluoroscopy shot that is thought to be unnecessary and thus not taken may result in a catastrophe if a sharp instrument is advanced in the bowel or great vessels. We tend to call it "Eye of wisdom" since it is wiser to take an extra shot when in doubt that to take the risk of injuring a vital structure

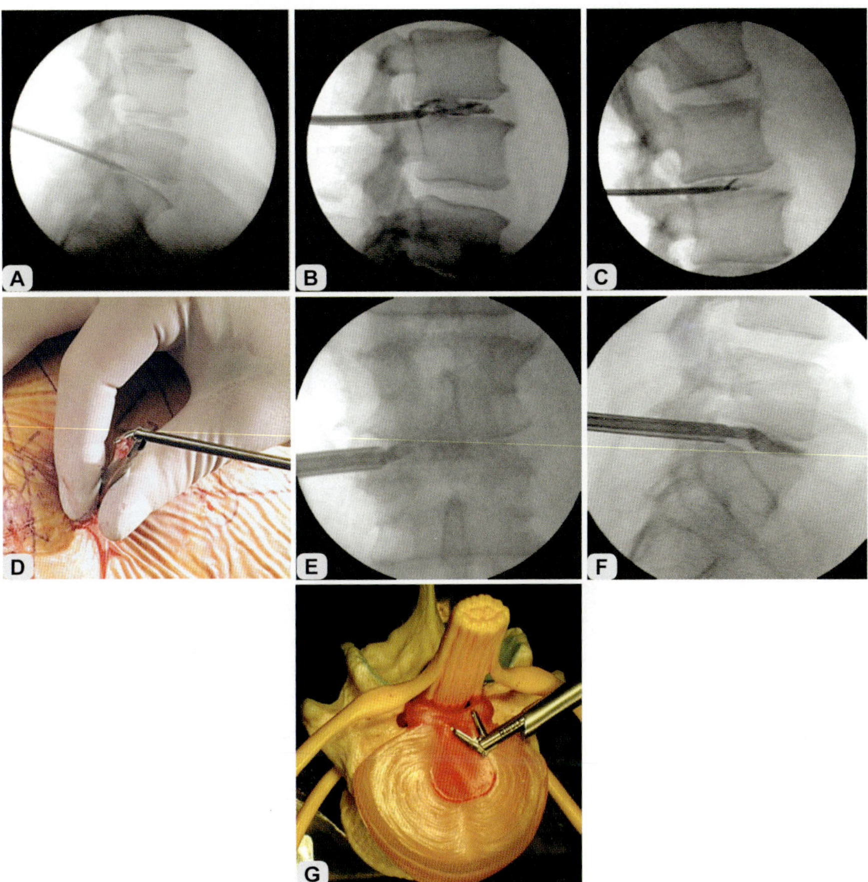

Fig. 6.13 Microdecompressive lumbar diskectomy fluoroscopic views of (A) stylette and dilator; (B) Discogram confirming disk degeneration; (C) grasping forceps; (D to G) Using a special flexible articulating angle grasper to reach posterior protruded herniated disk not reached by a conventional grasper

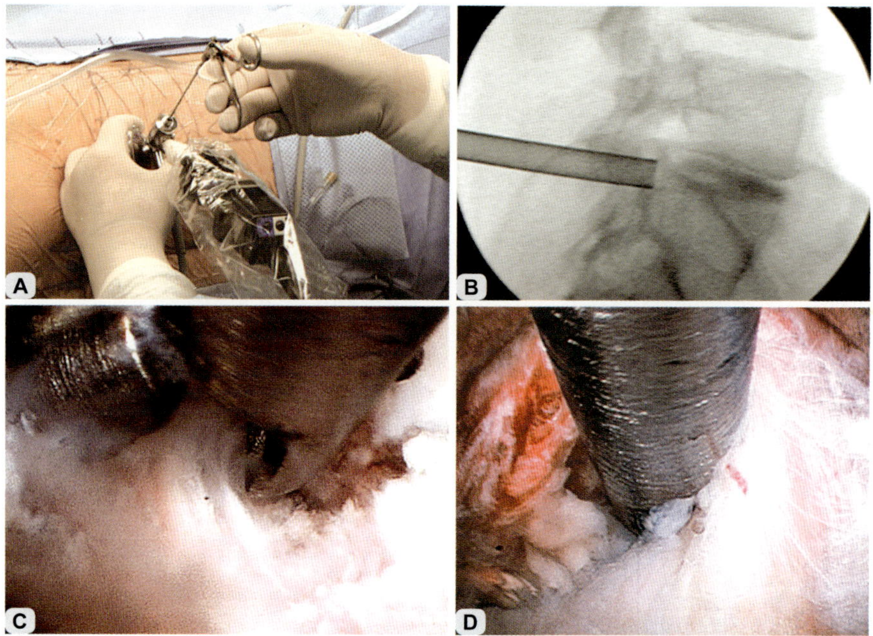

Fig. 6.14 Performing endoscopic disk microdecompression

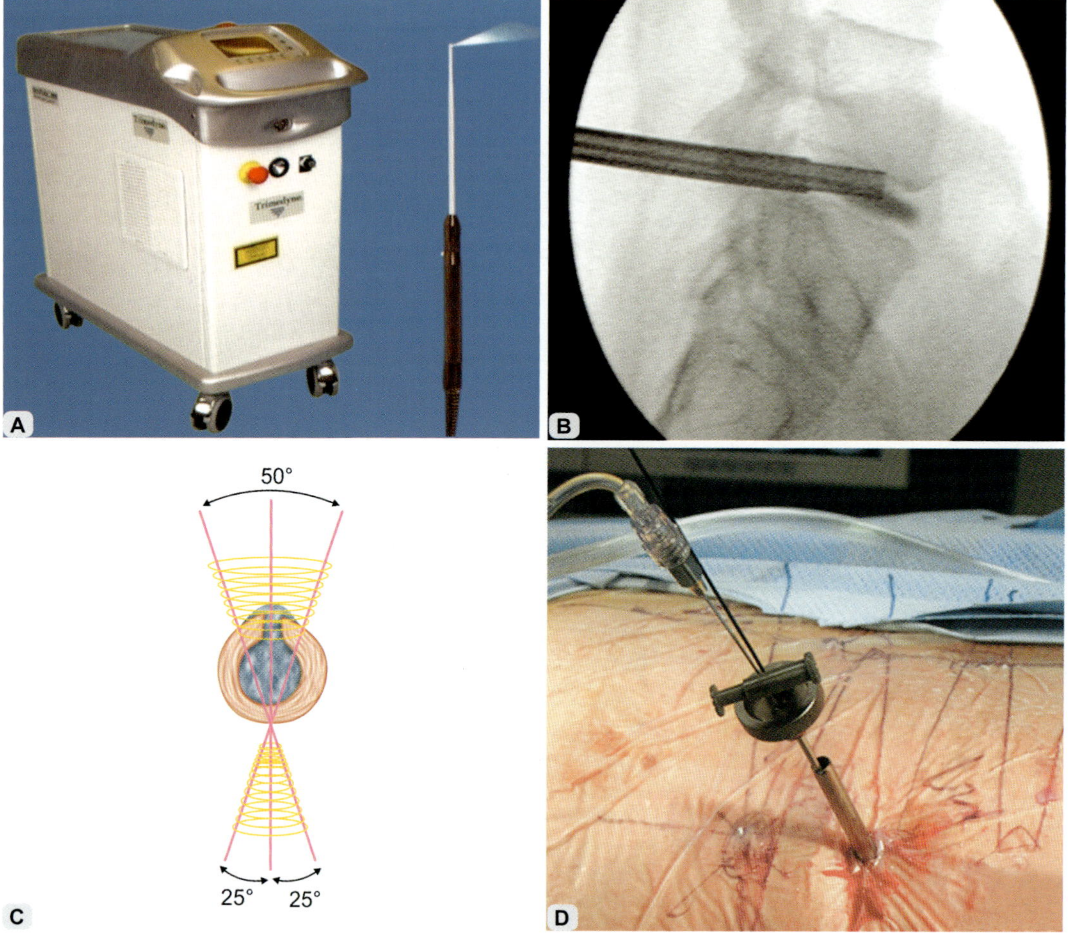

Fig. 6.15 (A) Holmium YAG laser generator; (B) Probe on fluoroscopic view; (C) Inverted cone shape maneuver; (D) Laser thermodiskoplasty procedure

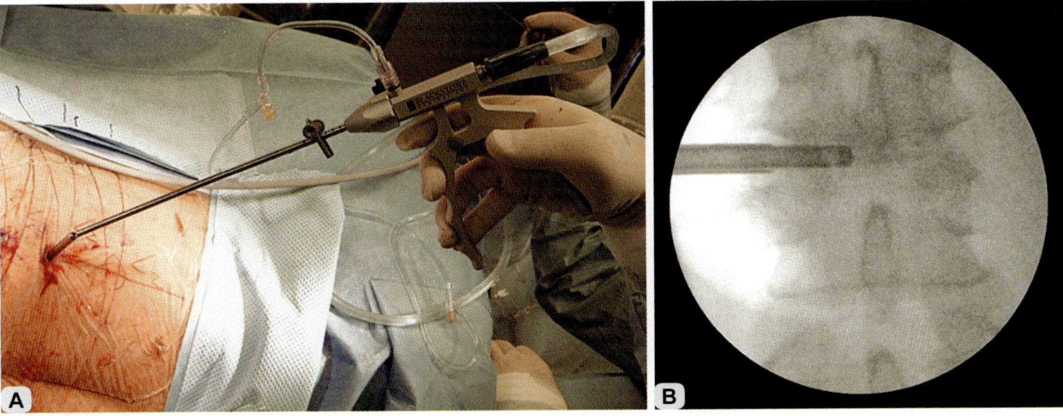

Fig. 6.16 (A) Diskectome for irrigation and suction of debris after laser application; (B) Fluoroscopic view

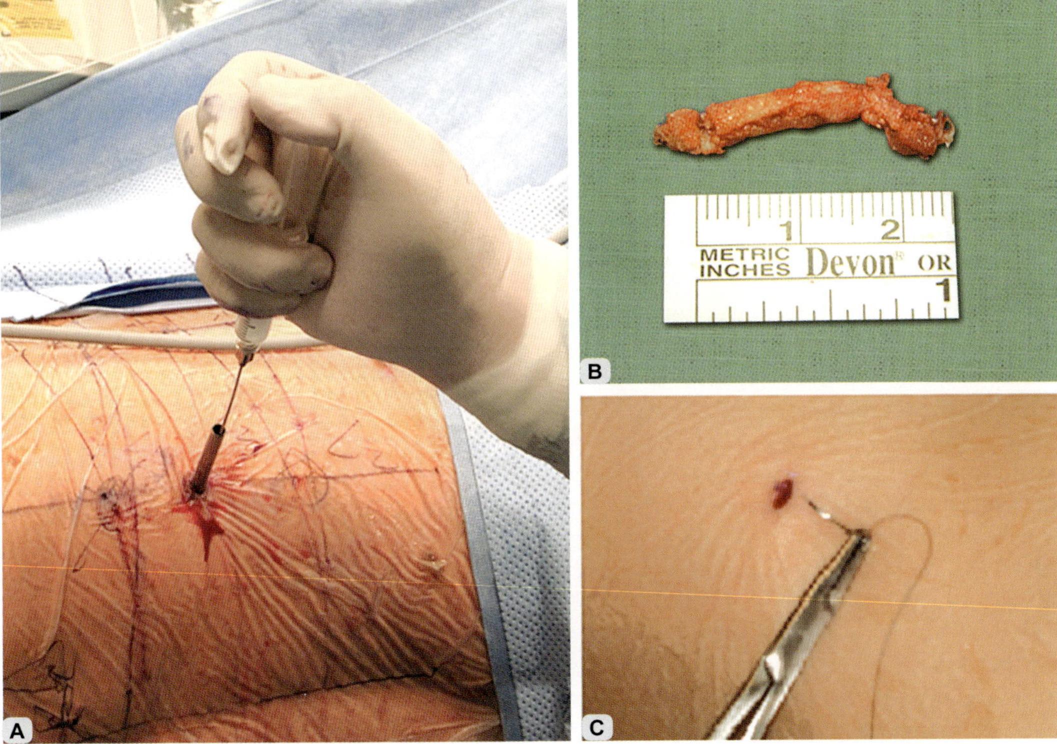

Fig. 6.17 (A) Steroid and anesthetic injection into the disk as final step to reduce postoperative pain and inflammation; (B) Excised disk material and calcified osteophytes of the affected level; (C) Single stitch to close the skin puncture wound

- It may be necessary to adjust the alignment of the C-arm in order to obtain a true AP and lateral views particularly in patients with degenerative scoliosis or kyphosis. Such adjustments should be done until parallel endplates are obtained to ensure a safe trajectory to the disk
- When performing cervical procedures, we prefer to have a systolic blood pressure of 130 mm Hg (5 – 10 mg of ephedrine can achieve this) during initial insertion of the needle. This helps palpate the carotid vessels more easily. Also, placing a nasogastric tube, helps palpate the esophagus
- Placing a pillow under the patient beneath the scapulae can help extend the neck and open up the disk space. Applying traction on both shoulders using adhesive tapes can also provide better visualization of the cervical spine particularly in the lower cervical region and at the cervicothoracic junction by moving the shoulders more inferiorly.

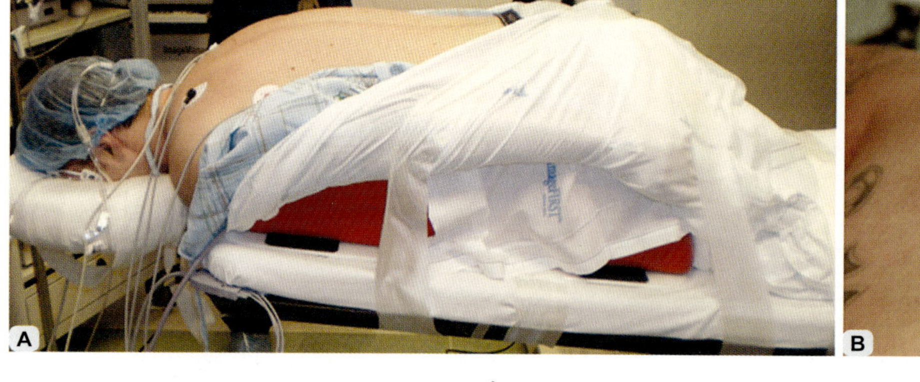

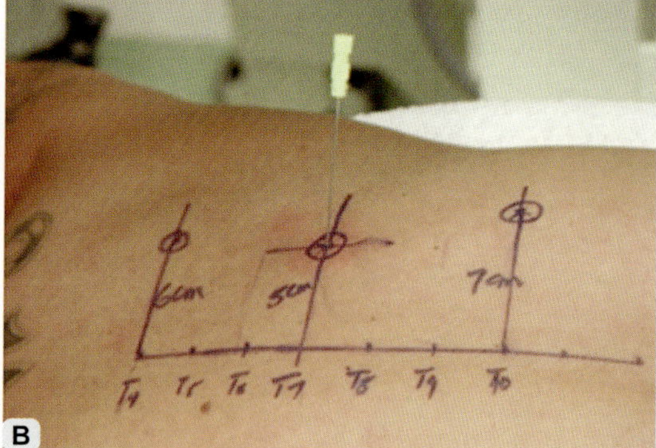

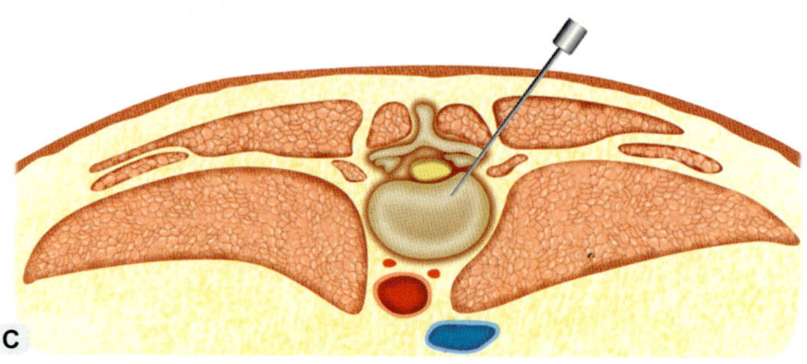

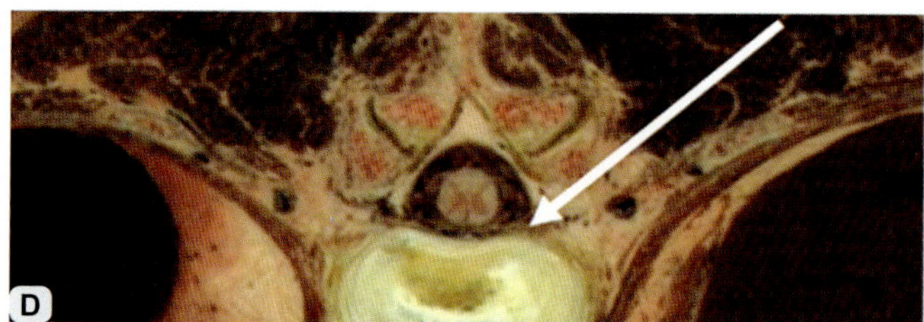

Fig. 6.18 (A) Position; (B) Marking; (C and D) Trajectory of needle introduction

- When performing thoracic surgery, it is always important to count and confirm the surgical level counting from both the cervicothroacic as well as thoracolumbar junction. It is also important to obtain postoperative chest X-rays to detect early pneumothorax even if patient is asymptomatic
- Dilating structures using tube systems is always better than cutting. It can help reduce intraoperative bleeding as well as postoperative scarring. Thus gives an overall less painful and quicker recovery with a better functional outcome.
- Laser application should correlate with the size and location of the disk. We usually use 900 – 1200 Joules for lumbar disks, 500 – 700 Joules for thoracic disks, and 200 – 400 Joules for cervical disks. Special care should be taken to avoid injury of nerve roots when applying laser especially in the foramen.

Postoperative Care[8-11]

Ambulation begins immediately after recovery, and the patient is usually discharged one hour after surgery. They may shower the following day. Applying an ice pack is helpful. Nonsteroidal anti-inflammatory drugs (NSAIDs) are prescribed, and mild analgesics and muscle relaxants as needed. Patients return progressively to usual activities in ten days to three weeks, provided heavy labor and prolonged sitting are not involved.

Case Illustrations

Case 1: Lumbar Spine

A 63-year-old patient with morbid obesity and insulin-dependent diabetes mellitus suffered from spinal canal stenosis and multiple level disk protrusions at L2/3, L3/4, L4/5, and L5/S1. The largest disk was at L5/S1, >6 mm as illustrated below. His weight is 280 lbs and height 5′ 8″ (Figs 6.6 to 6.17 and 6.20).

The patient complained of back pain and radicular symptoms including the anterior and surface of both thighs and legs, and back of the foot with more severe pain on the right side associated with some neurogenic claudication.

Previously the patient refused open surgery with fusion, because of increased risk in morbid obese and diabetic patients and requiring a multilevel extensive open spinal fusion.

After reviewing his MRI scans (Fig. 6.6) minimally invasive endoscopic microdecompression surgery was recommended to the patient as a solution for his spinal condition. He agreed to proceed with MISS surgery.

It can be very time consuming to reach the foramen in obese patients since the fat distribution gives a false orientation of the actual location of the spine in relation to the skin surface. By using the GPS system to triangulate the 3D orientation of the foramen under fluoroscopy, the height, width and depth of the soft tissue in relation to the foramen

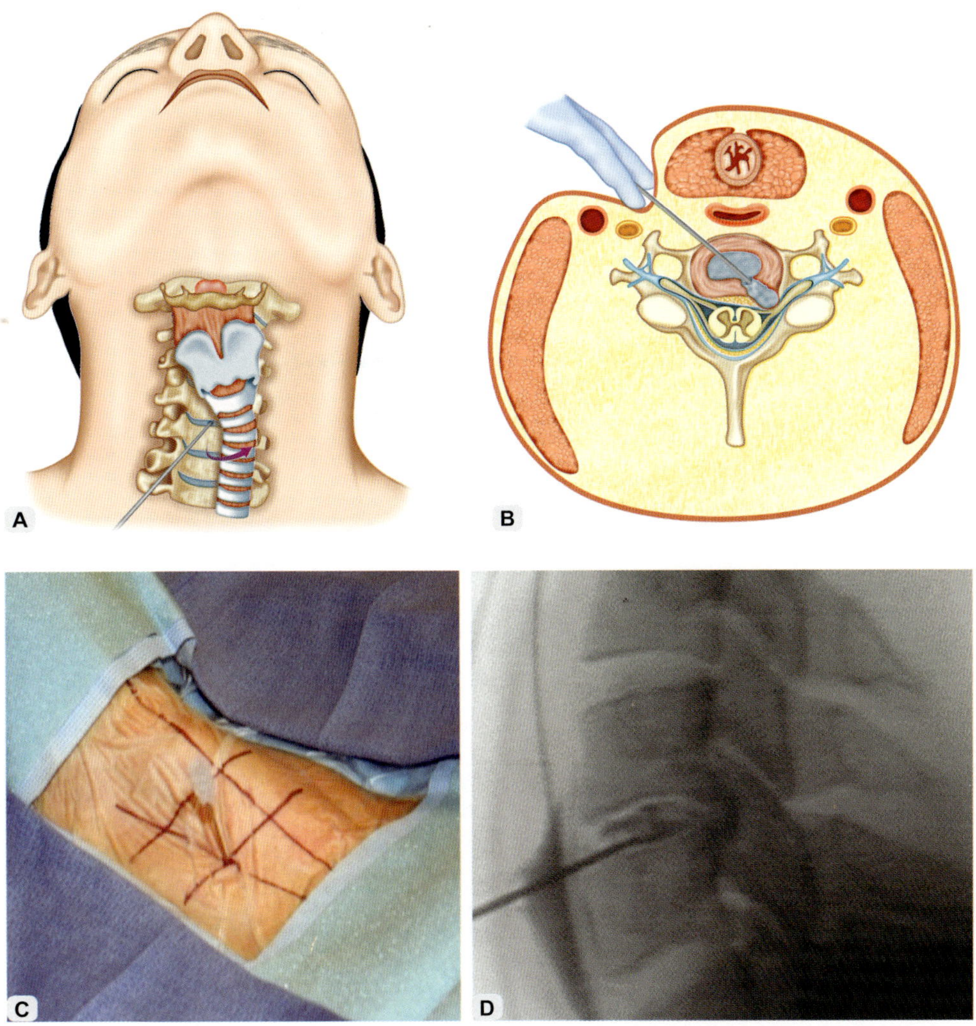

Fig. 6.19 Demonstrate the technique for creating a portal of entry

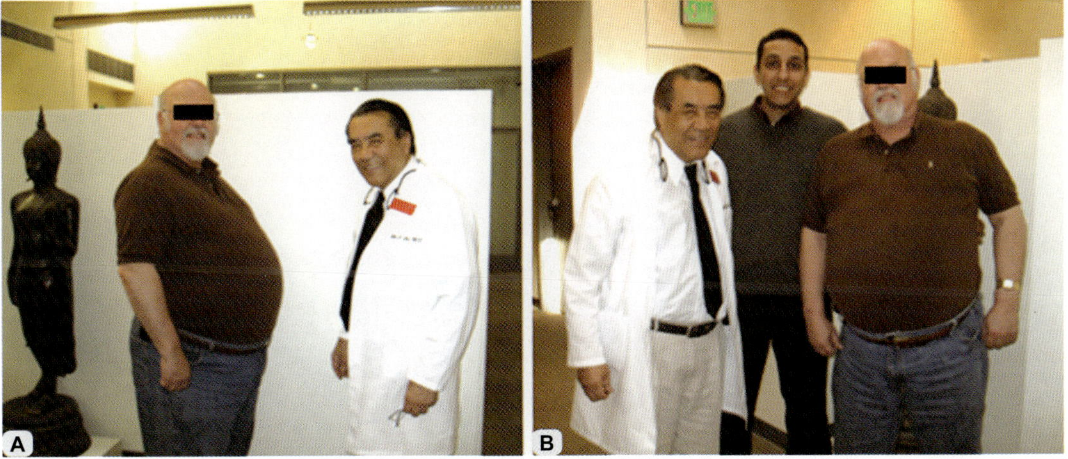

Fig. 6.20 Morbidly obese patient immediately following successful multilevel GPS microdecompressive lumbar diskectomy

was determined the microdecompression was successfully performed. Bilateral L2 – L5 endoscopic microdecompressive discectomy (Figs 6.7 to 6.17 and 6.20) was performed in the lateral decubitus position on two sittings of less than 1 hour for each side to avoid a prolonged single procedure.

The patient reported marked relief of his back symptoms and lower limb numbness on the next postoperative day with a better range of motion and ambulation.

Note: L4/5 disk portal of entry point can be used to access both L4/5 and L5/S1 disks by applying different angles to the trajectory of the stylette, perpendicular (for L4/5 disk) vs. steeper angle (for L5/S1 disk).

Case 2: Cervical Spine (Figs 6.21 to 6.23)

A 22-year-old male martial arts player is suffering from persistent neck and left upper extremity pain, with increasing numbness of fingers in left hand. MRI reveiled herniated cervical disk at C5/6. The patient previously refused to do an open procedure. Therefore, AECM surgical treatment of

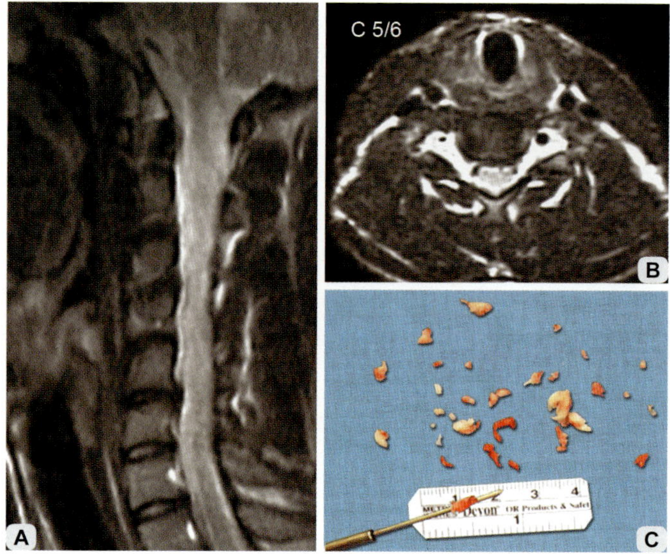

Fig. 6.21 (A and B) MRI showing disk bulges at C5 – 6 (C) Removed disk material

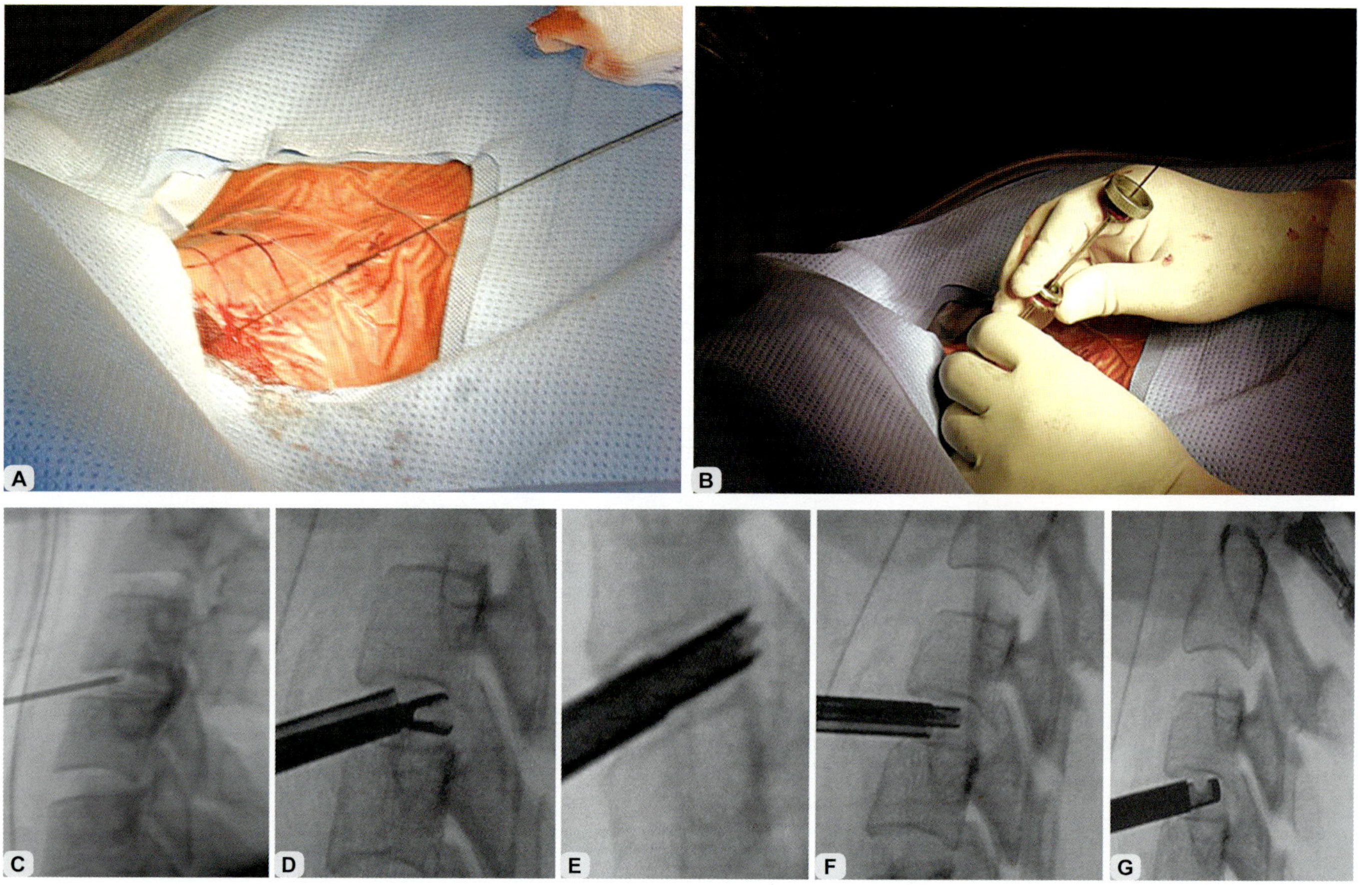

Fig. 6.22 (A and B) Stylette insertion; (C) working channel; (D to G) Grasper, trephine, laser fiber and diskectome

the C5 – C6 herniated disk and foraminal decompressive diskectomy was recommended. The outpatient surgery was performed successfully.

Case 3: Thoracic Spine

A 20-year-old male athletic suffering from persistent mid thoracic pain and increasing numbness along the left 9th rib and T9 dermatome following a motorcycle accident. MRI reviled herniated thoracic disk at T8/9. Physical therapy, analgesics, and epidural steroid injections did not alleviate his discomfort. The patient previously refused to do an open procedure due to the invasive nature of the procedure, so endoscopic discectomy was suggested for treatment (Figs 6.24 to 6.27).

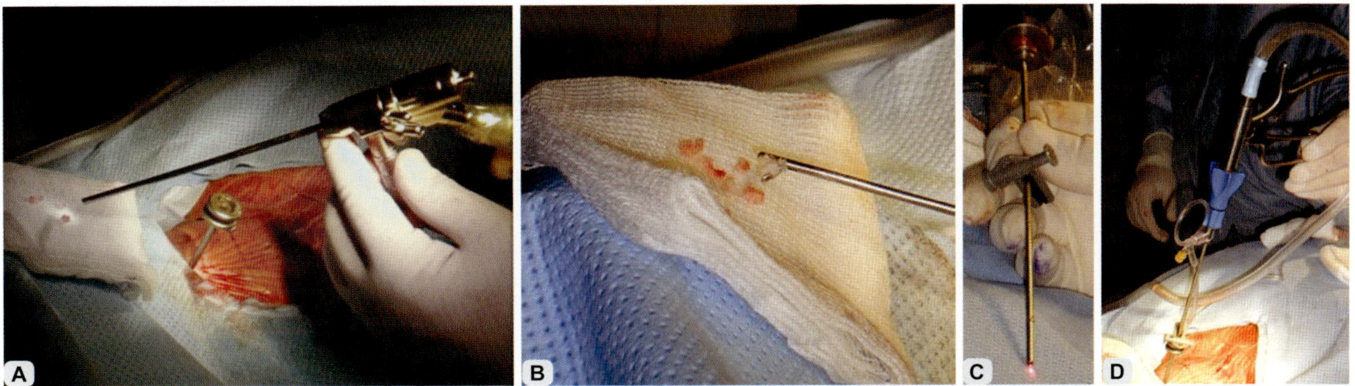

Fig. 6.23 Endoscopic disketomy and laser diskoplasty and suction irrigation

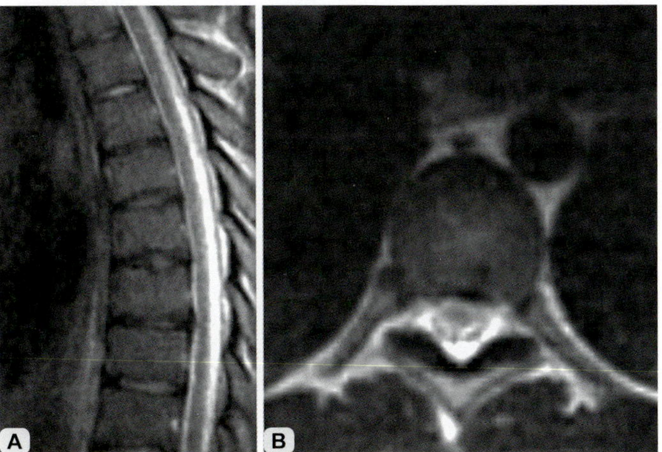

Fig. 6.24 MRI showing a disk herniation at T8/9

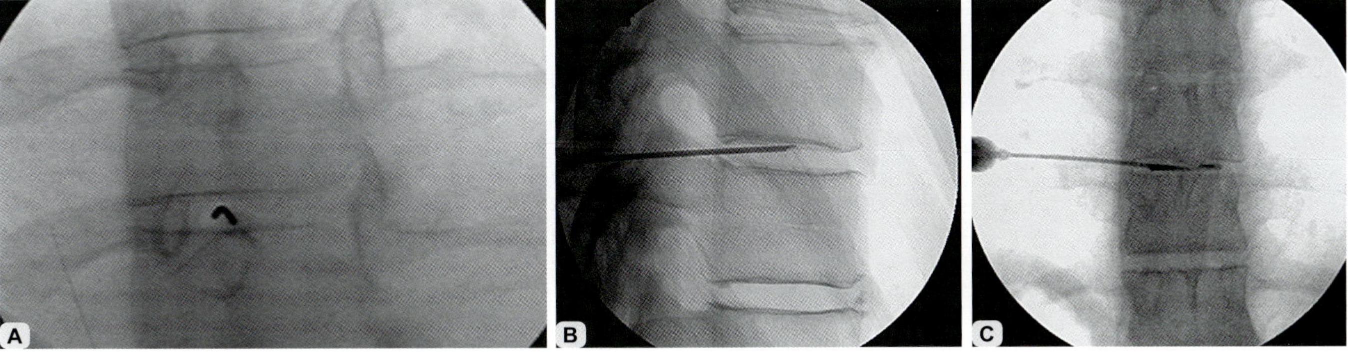

Fig. 6.25 Needle placement into "safety zone" at the neuro foramen between interpedicular line and the rib head followed by diskography

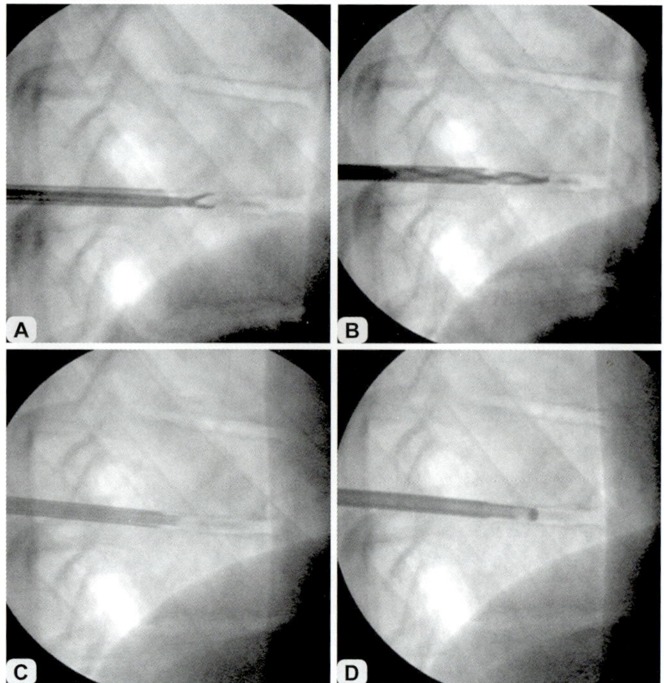

Fig. 6.26 Grasper, drill, laser, and diskectome

Discussion

We have developed a step-by-step localization system (Grid Positioning System or GPS) to facilitate the precise surgical approach toward the lesion or target for MISS procedure. Utilizing GPS dramatically improves accuracy, reduces the operative time and adds an extra-advantage on an improved surgical outcome particularly in high risk medical patients. Minimally invasive endoscopic microdecompression for herniated lumbar disks and spinal stenosis can effectively treat disk pathologies and spinal stenosis and alleviate patient symptoms. However, accurately localizing the spinal foramen and lesion can be a challenging task for the inexperienced surgeon particularly in cases with abnormal anatomy following previous open surgery or spinal deformities, such as degenerative scoliosis. More commonly localizing the spinal foramen can be difficult in morbidly obese patients where the topographic anatomy related to the spine is quite different from the norm. Again, GPS facilitates the MISS process.

MISS with GPS guidance combines different modalities for addressing spinal pathology; aggressive mechanical decompression, laser application, disk suctioning and pharmacological treatment of the disk by steroids and anesthetics to reduce inflammation. It can effectively treat spinal pathology at multiple levels without having to worry about the potential complications of extensive exposures, prolonged surgery, infection, implant failure, potential junctional disk herniation often associated with conventional spinal surgeries. It also provides significant economic savings as no hardware implants are required, recovery is much faster, easier, and fewer medications are needed.

Furthermore, this is the only logical solution for many elderly patients (even octogenarians and beyond) who suffer symptoms caused by spinal stenosis and disk problems in order to avoid major surgery. The results of this operation can be an extremely gratifying experience for both the patient and the surgeon.

Although MISS with GPS guidance is not the answer to all spinal problems, we believe it can address many of the problems related to spine degeneration without destabilizing the spine or compromising the flexibility of the motion segment if clinically appropriate, we recommend treatment with MISS followed by several months of recovery and re-evaluation before a patient undergoes an irreversible fusion surgery.

The MISS procedure requires a knowledgeable and competent surgeon with a thorough understanding of the surgical anatomy of the spine. Therefore, we believe

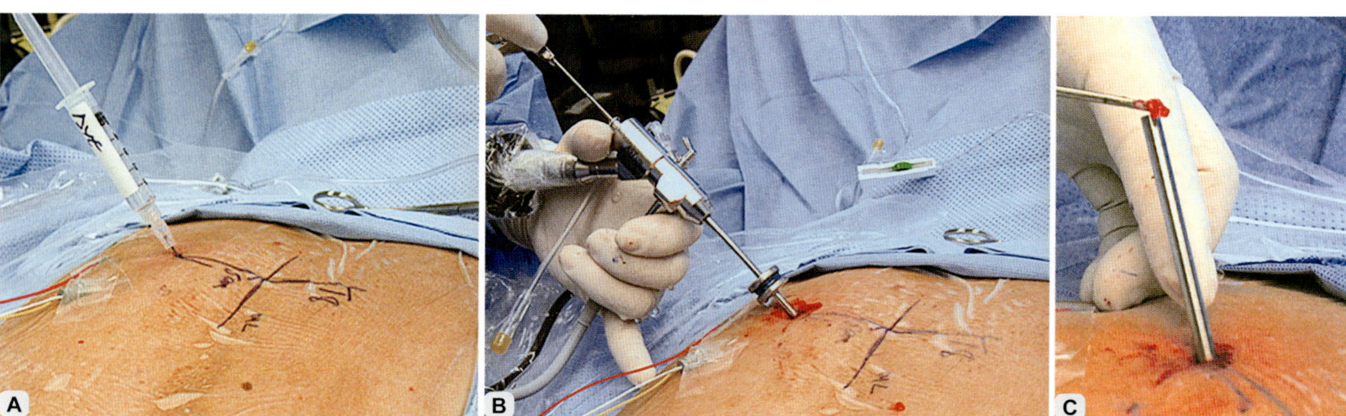

Fig. 6.27 Endoscopic disketomy thoracic spine

that previous surgical experience with conventional open procedures can actually help the surgeon better understand this type of surgery compared to surgeons without such experience. A minimally invasive spine surgeon must have surgical training with hands-on experience with an expert in the field in order to go through the steep surgical learning curve.

Minimally invasive spinal can be performed on different regions of the spine with slight variation in the technique. With the current fast-paced advancement in surgical technology, more applications for MISS will emerge in the near future.[1]

Conclusion

Following the techniques and tips outlined in this article can aid surgeons in performing minimally invasive spinal surgery procedures in a safe and effective way, and it can help the surgeon facilitate the MISS process by quickly identifying the surgical portal of entry to the disk or target without compromising vital anatomical or neural structures and accomplish needed spinal microdecompression. GPS is of particular value especially in medically high risk patients, including the morbidly obese and even those with prior surgeries. MISS procedures can be very effective in surgical treatment of degenerative spine in different spinal regions especially, if proper patient selection and sound MISS techniques are utilized.

References

1. Chiu J, Maziad A. Rappard, G et al. Evolving Minimally Invasive Spine Surgery: a Surgeon's Perspective on Technological Convergence and Digital OR Control System. In Szabo Z, Coburg AJ, Savalgi R, Reich H, Yamamotto M (eds) Surgical Technology International XIX, UMP, San Francisco, CA. 2009. p.211-22.
2. Chiu J. Surgeon's Perspective and Consideration: OR Digital Technology Convergence and Control System for Minimally Invasive Spine Surgery, Presented at Special Session, Minimally Invasive Spine Surgery, CARS 2008, Computer Assisted Radiology and Surgery 22nd International Congress and Exhibition, Barcelona, Spain, Proceedings. 2008;23-8.
3. Chiu JC. A surgeon's perspective on digital technological convergence and control system for minimally invasive spine surgery, abstract published in Computer Assisted Radiology and Surgery, Proceedings of the 24th International Congress and Exhibition, Geneva, Switzerland, Volume 5, Supplement 1: S5-S10, DOI 10.1007/211548-0101-0431-x - Springer Verlag, Heidlberg, Germany; 2010.
4. Chiu J. Digital Technology Convergence and Control System: Minimally Invasive Spine Surgeon's (MISS) Perspective and Technological Consideration, "Interdisciplinary PACS" The Second Iranian Imaging Informatics Conference Syllabus, Tehran, Iran; 2008; p.30-1.
5. Chiu J. Therapeutic Application of Surgical ePR Control System Beyond Radiology PACS, presented at the SPIE Medical Imaging Advanced PACS Based Imaging Informatics and Therapeutic Applications, Orlando, Fl, February 8-12, 2009.
6. Chiu J, Savitz, MH. Use of Laser in Minimally Invasive Spinal Surgery and Pain Management. In Kambin P (ed): Arthroscopic and Endoscopic Spinal Surgery – Text and Atlas. Second Edition. New Jersey: Humana Press; 2005. Chapter 13. p. 259-69.
7. Chiu J. Anterior Endoscopic Cervical Microdiscectomy. In Kim D, Fessler R, Regan J (eds): Endoscopic Spine Surgery and Instrumentation. New York: Thieme Medical Publisher; 2004. Chapter 5 p. 48-58.
8. Chiu J. Posterolateral Endoscopic Thoracic Discectomy. In Kim D, Fessler R, Regan J, (eds) Endoscopic Spine Surgery and Instrumentation. New York: Thieme Medical Publisher; 2004. Chapter 11 p.125-36.
9. Chiu J, Clifford T, Princenthal R. Junctional Disc Herniation in Post Spinal Fusion Treated with Endoscopic Spine Surgery: In, Szabo Z, Coburg AJ, Savalgi R, Reich H, Yamamotto M, (eds): Surgical Technology International XIV, UMP, San Francisco, CA. 2005. p. 305-15.
10. Chiu J. Endoscopic Assisted Microdecompression of Cervical Disc and Foramen. In Szabo Z, Coburg AJ, Savalgi R, Reich H, Yamamotto M, (eds): Surgical Technology International XVII, UMP, San Francisco, CA; 2008, p. 269-79.
11. Chiu J. Endoscopic Assisted Lumbar Microdecompressive Spinal Surgery with a New Smart Endoscopic System. In Szabo Z, Coburg AJ, Savalgi R, Reich H, Yamamotto M, (eds): Surgical Technology International XV, UMP, San Francisco, CA; 2006, p. 265-75.
12. Chiu, J. Cervical Endoscopic Microdecompressive Discectomy and Foraminal Decompression, Presented at the annual meeting of the Rome Spine Society, Rome, Italy. 2009;6:265-75.
13. Savitz MH, Chiu JC, Yeung AT. History of Minimalism in spinal medicine and surgery. In: Savitz MH, Chiu JC, Yeung AD (eds). The practice of minimally invasive spinal technique. Richmond, VA: AAMISMS Education, LLC. 2000;pp.1-12.
14. Chiu JC The Decade of Evolving Minimally Invasive Spinal Surgery (MISS) and Technological Considerations. The Internet Journal of Minimally Invasive Spinal Technology. 2008; 2(3).
15. Liu BJ, Law YY, Documet J, Gertych A, Image-Assisted Knowledge Discovery and Decision Support in Radiation Therapy Planning, Computerized Medical Imaging and Graphics. 2007;31:4-5:pp 311-21.
16. Hijikata S. Percutaneous nucleotomy: A new concept technique and 12 years' experience. Clin Orthop. 1989;238:9-23.
17. Ascher PW, Choy D. Application of the laser in neurosurgery. Laser Surg Med. 1986;2:91-7.

18. Kambin P, Saliffer PL. Percutaneous lumbar discectomy: reviewing 100 patients and current practice. Clin Orthop. 1989;238:24-34.
19. Schreiber A, Suezawa Y, Leu HJ. Does percutaneous nucleotomy with discoscopy replaces conventional discectomy? Eight years of experience and results in treatment of herniated lumbar disc. Clin Orthop. 1989;238:35-42.
20. Chiu J, Endoscopic Assisted Lumbar Microdecompressive Spinal Surgery with a New Smart Endoscopic System. In, Szabo Z, Coburg AJ, Savalgi R, Reich H, Yamamotto M (eds): Surgical Technology International XV, UMP, San Francisco, CA. 2006; p.265-75.
21. Destandau J. Endoscopically assisted microdiscectomy. In: Savitz MH, Chiu JC, Yeung AD (eds): The practice of minimally invasive spinal technique. Richmond, VA: AAMISMS Education, LLC. 2000; pp.187-92.
22. Chiu J. Evolving Transforaminal Endoscopic Microdecompression for Herniated Lumbar Discs and Spinal Stenosis: In Szabo Z, Coburg AJ, Savalgi R, Reich H, (eds): Surgical Technology International XIII, UMP, San Francisco, CA. 2004;pp.276-86.
23. Chiu J. Endoscopic Lumbar Foraminoplasty In: Kim D, Fessler R, Regan J (eds): Endoscopic Spine Surgery and Instrumentation. New York: Thieme Medical Publisher. 2004;Chapter 19: pp.212-29.
24. Chiu J, Clifford T, Princenthal R. The new frontier of minimally invasive spine surgery through computer assisted technology. In Lemke HU, Vannier MN, Invamura RD (eds), Computer assisted radiology and surgery, CARS 2002. Berlin: Springer-Verlag. 2002;p.233-7.
25. Chiu J, Clifford T. Microdecompressive percutaneous discectomy: Spinal discectomy with new laser thermodiskoplasty for non extruded herniated nucleus pulposus. Surg Technol Int. 1999;VIII:343-51.
26. Chiu J, Stechison M, Percutaneous Vertebral Augmentation and Reconstruction with an Intervertebral Mesh and Morecelized Bone Graft: In Szabo Z, Coburg AJ, Savalgi R, Reich H, Yamamotto M (eds) Surgical Technology International XIV, UMP, San Francisco, CA. 2005;p.287-96.
27. Chiu JC, Hansraj K, Akiyama C, et al. Percutaneous (endoscopic) decompressive discectomy for non-extruded cervical herniated nucleus pulposus. Surg Technol Int. 1997;VI:405-11.
28. Kambin P, Casey K, O'Brien E, et al. Transforaminal arthroscopic decompression of lateral recess stenosis. J Neurosurg. 1996;84:462-7.
29. Chiu JC, Clifford T. Multiple herniated discs at single and multiple spinal segments treated with endoscopic microdecompressive surgery. J Minim Invasive Spinal Tech. 2001;1:15-9.
30. Knight M, Goswami A. Endoscopic laser foraminoplasty. In: Savitz MH, Chiu JC, Yeung AD (eds): The practice of minimally invasive spinal technique. Richmond, VA: AAMISMS Education, LLC. 2000;pp.337-40.
31. Clifford T, Chiu JC, Rogers G. Neurophysiological monitoring of peripheral nerve function during endoscopic laser discectomy: J Minim Invasive Spinal Tech. 2001;1:54-7.
32. Chiu J. SMART Endolumbar System for Microdecompression of Degenerative Disc Disease, presented at the Practical Course on Minimally Invasive Technique in Spinal Surgery, Russian Spinal Cord Society, Moscow Russia. 2007;April 26-29.
33. Chiu J, Complications and Avoidance in Endoscopic Spine Surgery, presented at the North American Spine Society Minimally Invasive Spine Technique: Hands-on Course, Barrow Neurological Institute (BNI), Phoenix, AZ.

CHAPTER

7

Transformaminal Diskectomy on Difficult L4 – L5 and L5 – S1 Hernias

Daniel Gastambide

DIFFICULT L4 – L5 HERNIAS

Preliminary Points

- The patients position and complications are the same as for the L5 – S1 approach
- You have to evaluate the width of the foramen and the best angle to extract the hernia without wounding the dura mater. Indeed, if the foramen is large, you can penetrate the dura inadvertently (Figs 7.1 and 7.2).

Techniques

An L4 – L5 hernia is not usually difficult to operate. Sometimes, it can prove difficult in the case of pusillanimous patients. In this case, you must take more time to obtain a more efficient effect with the sedation.

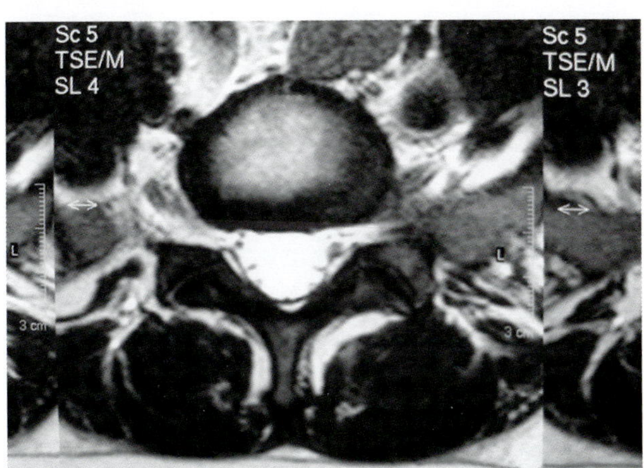

Fig. 7.1 Large dura

The hernia can be almost excluded in the medullar channel (Figs 7.3 to 7.5) and then you have to penetrate the foramen at 70 degrees from the sagittal plane, as in the case of an L5 – S1.

The triangular working zone can be small, and you have to be very careful when passing along the exiting root so you do not wound it.

Sometimes, you can insert a trephine to abrase the anterior side of the facet (posterior side of the foramen) and then take out the hernia.

Sometimes, you get a big fragment of two colors blue for the side inside the disk and white or red for the side in the epidural space.

More often you do not immediately find this big fragment and you have to look for it in the epidural space by using the endoscope.

An enormous articular facet can be difficult to abrase or pass around. You have to persevere in reaching the hernia.

Tricks Concerning the Instruments

You should check the quality of the forceps. Some manufacturers make forceps with one of the jaws which opens at 70 degrees (Fig. 7.6).

This makes it easier to clasp a hernia and to pull on it in the epidural space.

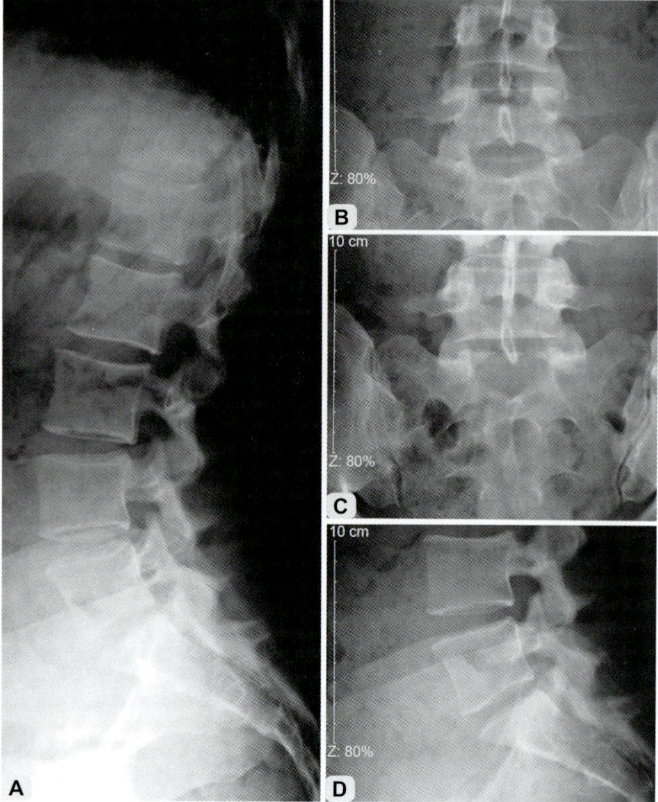

Fig. 7.2 Large foramen

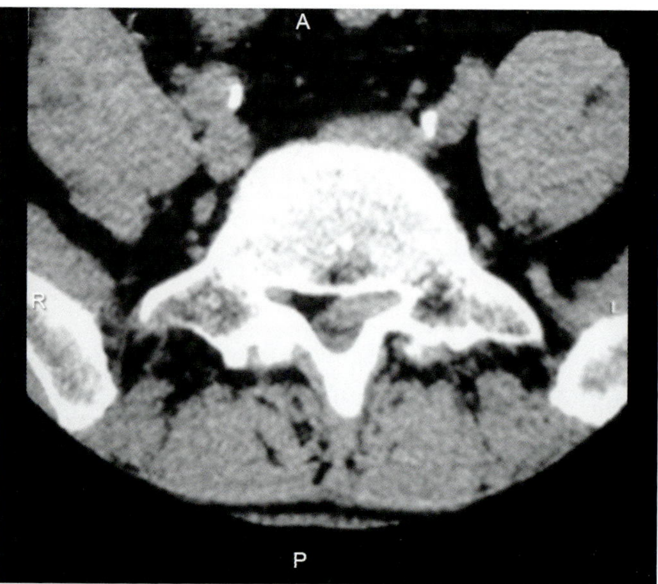

Fig. 7.4 Same patient, larger view

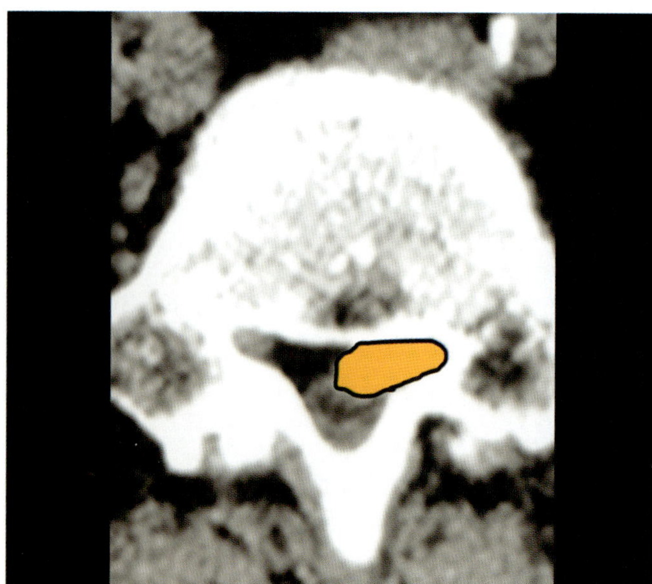

Fig. 7.3 Hernia descending in the recess until the middle of the medular channel

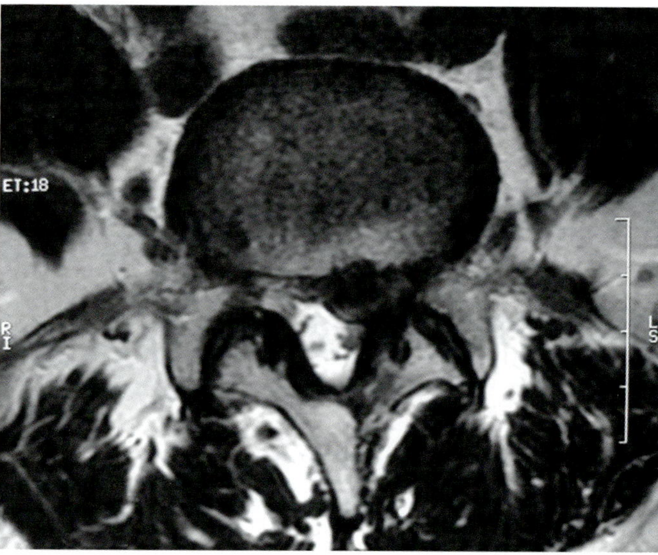

Fig. 7.5 MRI of the same patient. This shows the advantage of having both a CT scan and an MRI to decide of the best approach to use

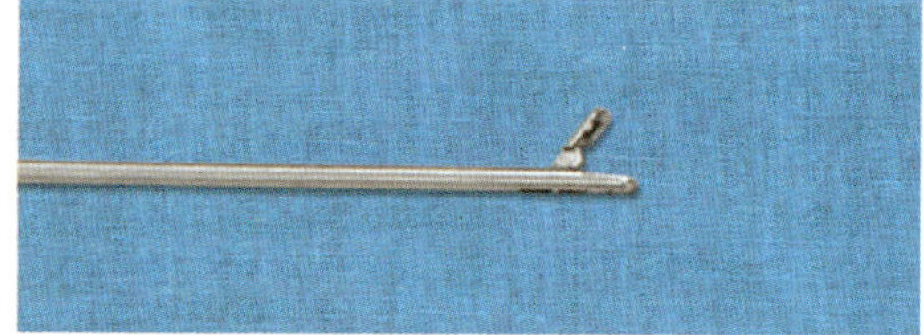

Fig. 7.6 Forceps with jaws opened at 70 degrees

DIFFICULT L5 – S1 HERNIAS

Tips and Tricks about Transforaminal Diskectomy on L5–S1 with a High Iliac Crest

Preliminary Points

- Explain the aim of the sedation to the anesthesiologist (Fig. 7.7), because sometimes, the drugs can have a paradoxical effect on the patient and make him agitated
- If possible, prescribe premedication yourself to the patient, thus, adapting the type of medication to his sensibility and to his degree of anxiety
- Prescribe antibiotics 24 hours prior to the operation, because the disk is white without direct vascularization, and antibiotics penetrate it very slowly
- You must have a good monitor (Fig. 7.8)
- A good endoscope (Fig. 7.9)
- Good tubes (Fig. 7.10) (adapting each one to the next, with a degressive length),
- Good forceps (Fig. 7.11) and a good C-arm (Fig. 7.12) with orthogonal views, a printer for the C-arm, an arthro-pump with an injectible serum (Fig. 7.13)
- Gentalline (40 mg/L) with adrenaline (half a mg/L).

Introduction

The first reflex you have when you see a high iliac crest on an L5 – S1 hernia is to think you will operate it using a posterior approach. However, I personnally prefer to use a percutaneous approach on a high iliac crest for two reasons:

- There is less risk of radicular lesion than in the case of an endoscopic interlaminar approach
- The endoscopic transforaminal technique is the most used for lumbar hernias for "endoscopist" surgeons.

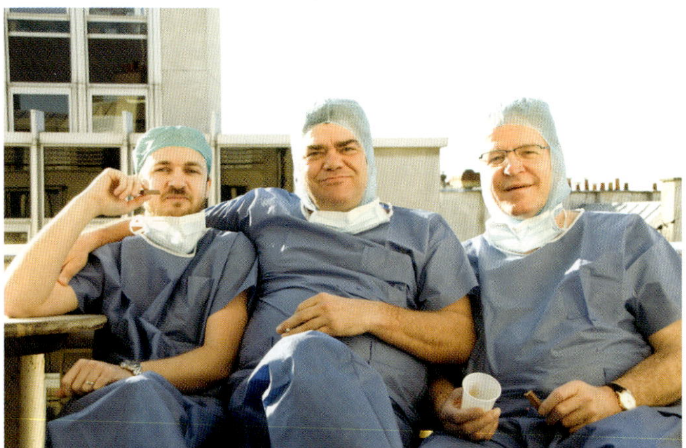

Fig. 7.7 A united surgical team, anesthesiologist on the left, surgical assistant in the middle, and the author on the right

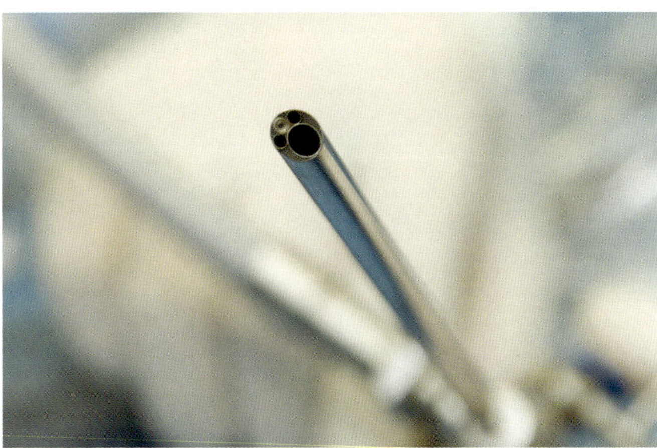

Fig. 7.9 The tip of the endoscope with four channels, one for the forceps, one for the light and for the camera, and two for the water flow

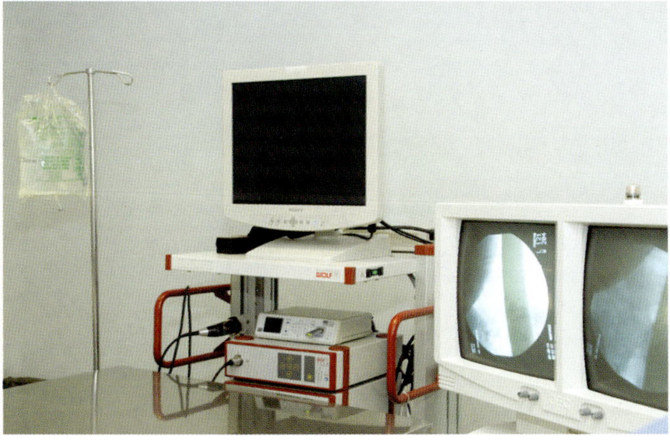

Fig. 7.8 A good monitor

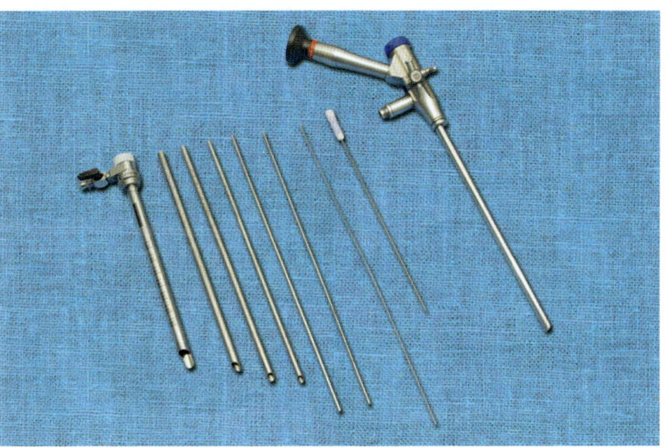

Fig. 7.10 Good dilating and working tubes

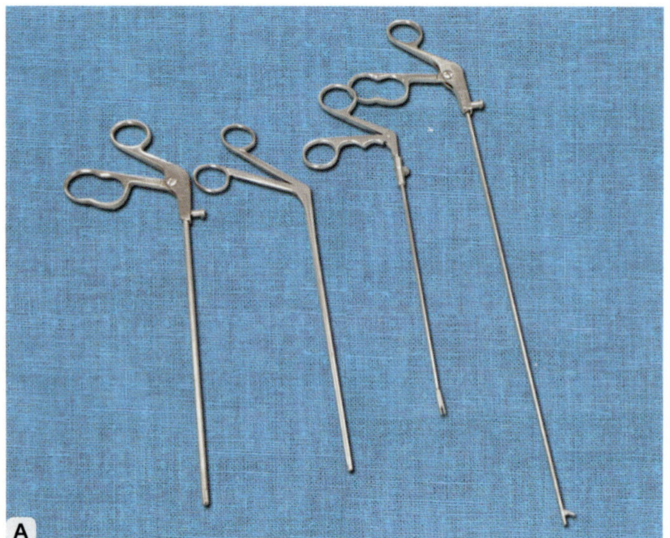
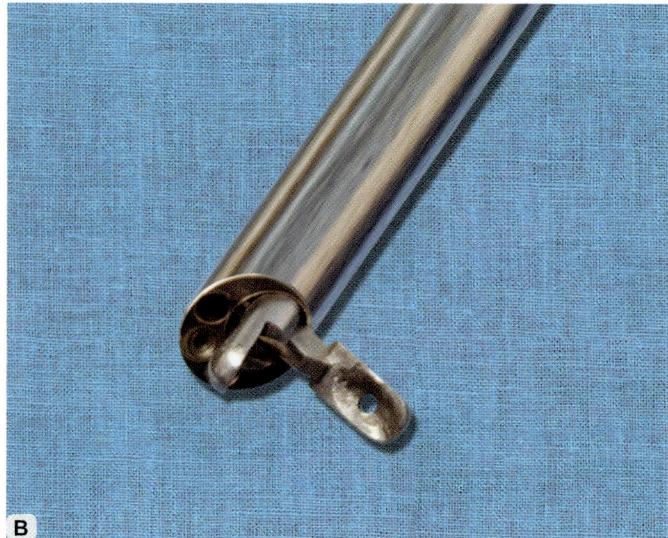

Fig. 7.11 A good forceps

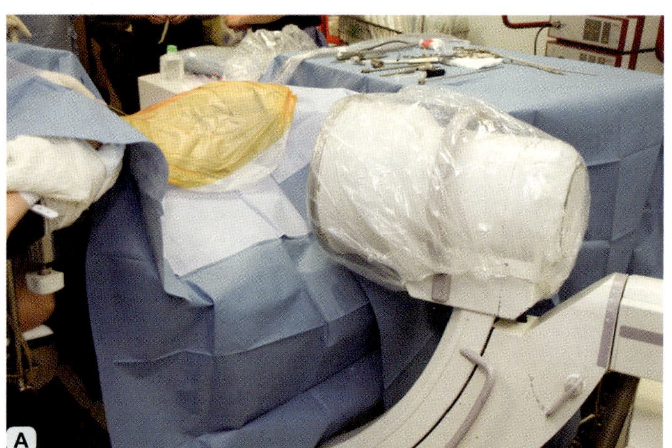
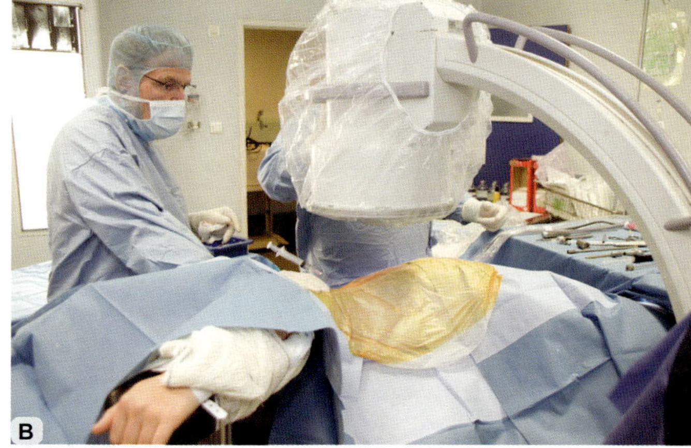

Fig. 7.12 A good C-arm. (A) Lateral view; (B) AP view

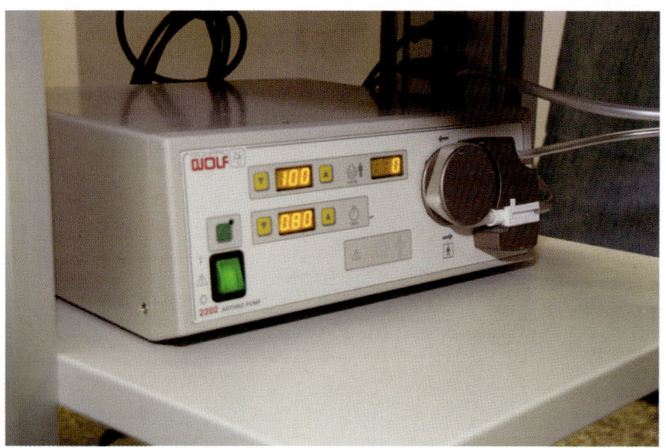

Fig. 7.13 A good arthro-pump

Operation

You have to install the patient in a lateral position for several reasons:

- First of all, it is easier for the anesthesiologist to survey the patient
- This position is more comfortable for the patient
- You can try to open the intervertebral space by placing the contralateral external buttock in one of the operating table's curves; a buttock under the flank is not usually tolerated
- Sometimes, it is difficult to stabilize the knees with a cushion more so if the patient moves during the operation (Fig. 7.14)

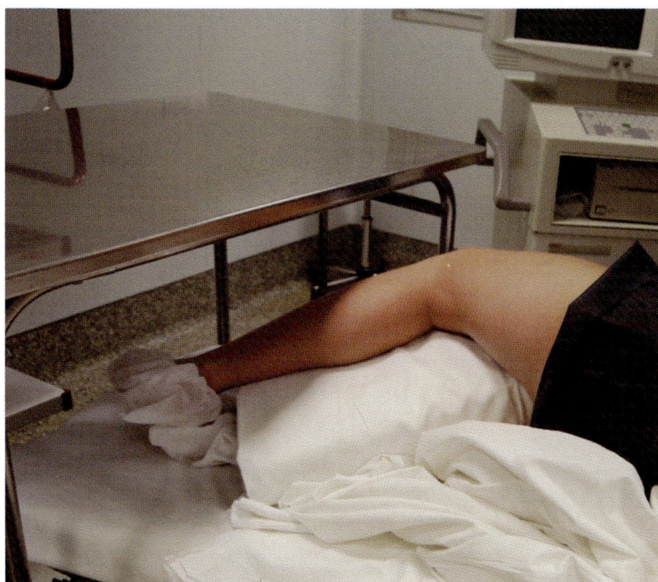

Fig. 7.14 A cushion placed between the knees

- To avoid the patient moving during the operation, you can put a special band around him; however, by doing so, it could prove difficult to reposition the patient after an unexpected displacement
- You may be tempted to ask the anesthesiologist to put the patient to sleep so he or she does not react to the nociceptive stimuli. However, by doing so, you would put the security of the operation at risk and can easily paralyse the feet elevators

You have to evaluate the L5 – S1 slope (Figs 7.15 and 7.16) on the lateral X-ray and CT scan. It's often higher than 30 degrees and is high enough to insert the first needle (Fig. 7.17).

The skin landmarks have to be very precise (Fig. 7.18). You have to penetrate the disk at an angle of 70 degrees to the sagittal plane. This means that you make two orthogonal marks with a metallic instrument using anteroposterior and lateral X-rays (Fig. 7.19), projecting the tip of the instrument on the foramen.

Of course, you must first inject the skin with lidocaine through a very thin needle.

Then you insert the 18 G needle very slowly to spread the lidocaine on its way (Fig. 7.20). After this you have to feel the anterior border of the facet's capsule with the tip of this needle and then you slide along it, across the foramen until you feel you have reached the disk.

If you want to make a local anesthesia in the epidural space, only use 0.5% lidocaine. This will create a hypoesthesia without any motor deficits, and it is a secure method because the patient will react to the nociceptive stimuli.

Seeing that you are inserting a 22 G curved needle in the disk through an 18 G needle which remains behind the disk, you must check that your needle is properly in the disk by carrying out a diskography (Fig. 7.21), which evaluates the degree of degeneration and colors the disk in blue with indigo carmine mixed with an opaque X-ray solution.

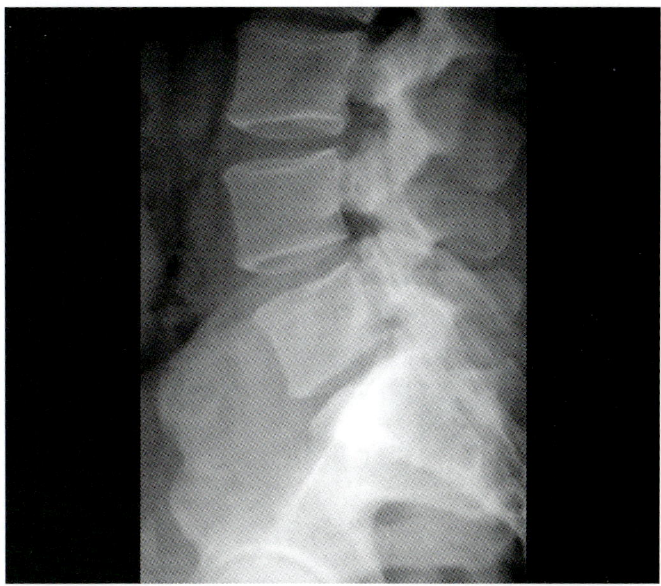

Fig. 7.15 An important slope

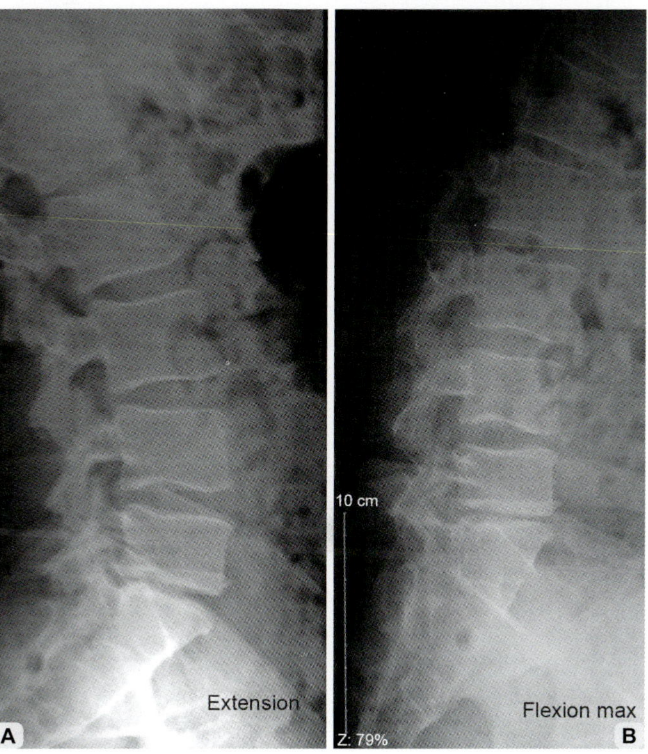

Fig. 7.16 A less important slope

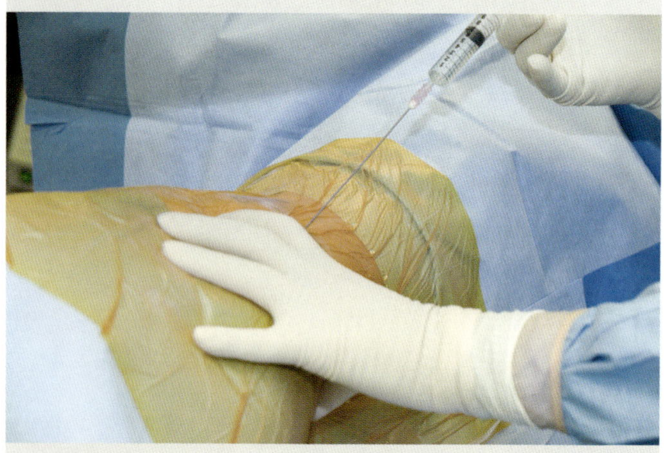

Fig. 7.17 First needle is inserted at 30 degrees to the horizontal plane of the disk

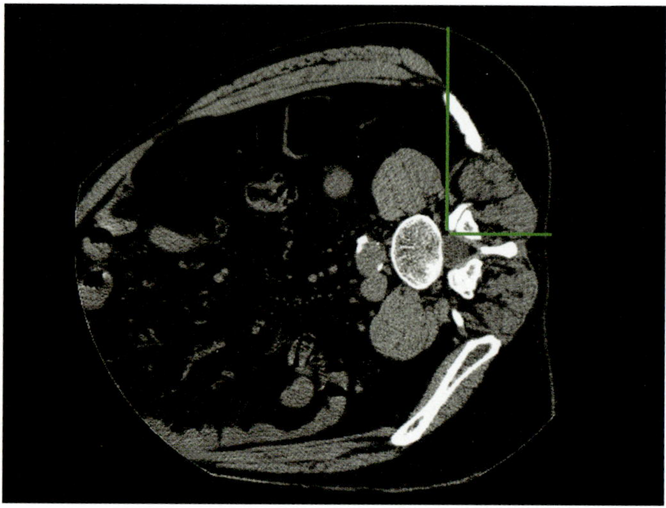

Fig. 7.19 CT scan of the patient on the right side with virtual landmarks in green

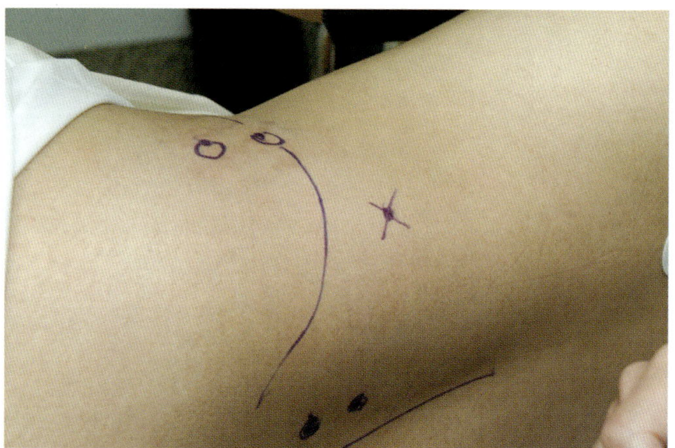

Fig. 7.18 Skin landmarks where you will penetrate the disk at 70 degrees to the sagittal plane

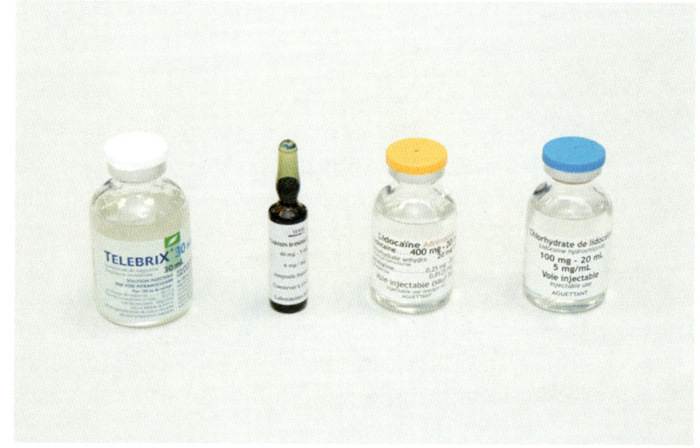

Fig. 7.20 Telebrix and Indigo carmine (dilution 1/10) will be injected in the disk. Before this, you inject adrenalined lidocaine 5% along the way (bottle with orange cap) and you can use 0.5% lidocaine around the root (bottle with blue cap)

This often shows where the hernia is. Having penetrated the disk with the 22 G needle, you will then be able to push the 18 G needle in a more precise and slightly curved trajectory around the 22 G in the disk.

The bevelled tip of the 18 G needle often has to be axially rotated in order to obtain a smooth penetration in the disk without scraping the superior vertebral plateau.

Then you pull out the 22 G needle and insert a thin Kirshner-wire with a rounded tip inside the 18 G needle.

You pull out the 18 G needle, controlling on the X-ray monitor that you do not pull out the K-wire at the same time.

Then, you push in the dilators (Fig. 7.22).

You can insert them into the disk at an angle of about 25 degrees. After having done this, you control that you have penetrated the disk and not the S1 bone. If the patient feels too much pain, you have to insert the endoscope to see the L5 exiting root which is often on the anterosuperior side. Because of this, when you insert the bevelled dilator, you have to open the bevel in an anterosuperior direction to leave some space for the exiting root. You always have to check the exiting root through the scope (Fig. 7.23).

Then, you can use the last working tube with a rotating axial movement to smoothly push the exiting root away.

Variations of the Birth of Rami Communicantes

Sometimes this rotating movement can prove painful for the patient because of the thickness or adhesions of the ganglion (the anatomy of the anastomotic branches of the

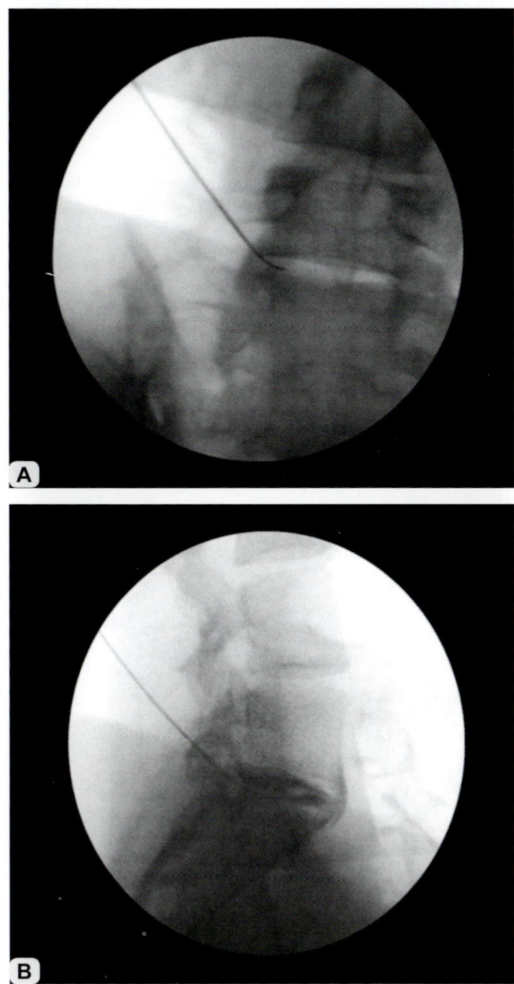

Fig. 7.21 On the AP view you can see the needle that will reach the middle of the disk which you inject with opaque solution. Here, there is a leak behind the sacrum. In a previous trial, the same needle went towards the rim of the disk and did not opacify it properly. Therefore, the opacification of the anterior rim of the disk happened incidently

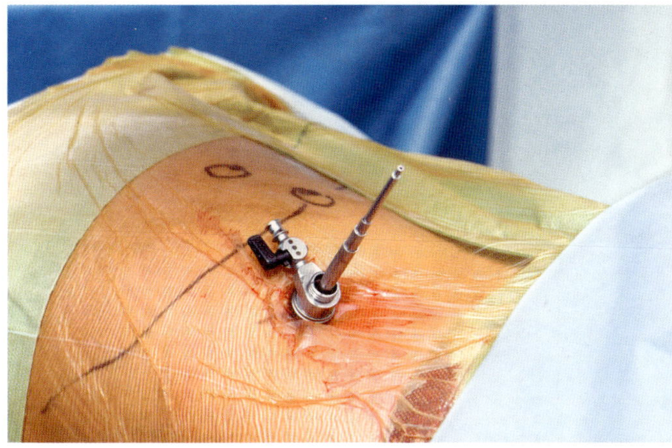

Fig. 7.22 Dilators and working tubes fitted into each other

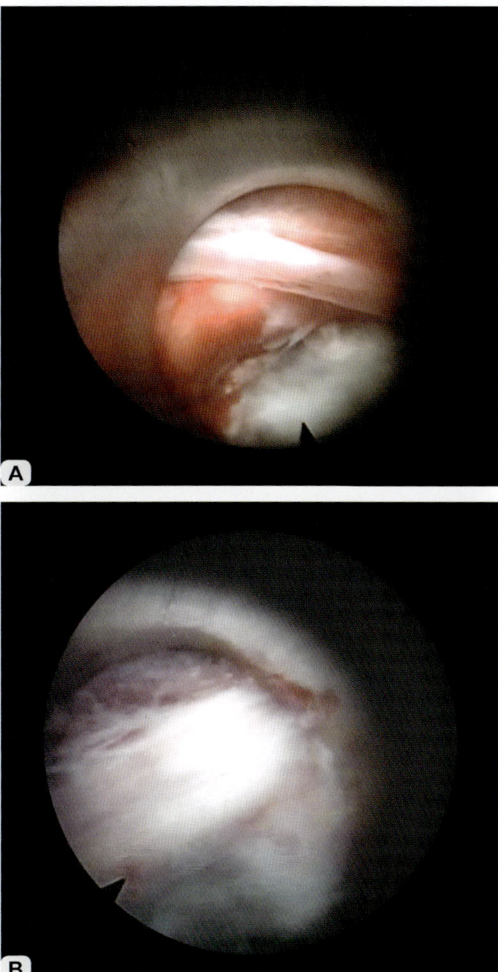

Fig. 7.23 Exiting root as seen through endoscope

ganglion is essentially variable) (Fig. 7.24). Then you have to check the anterosuperior half of your view and smoothly slide your instruments along the posteroinferior rim of this exiting root.

If you can push the working tube into the disk without creating any pain, you can use 4 – 5 mm forceps without scope to extract thicker fragments faster (Figs 7.25 and 7.26).

Often at the end of the procedure and sometimes at the beginning, you can see the epidural fat (Fig. 7.27) or directly the dura mater, which pulses at the same rhythm as the arthro-pump. Then you can verify whether the descending root is free or not.

If you fear that fragments have remained above, below, or behind the L5 or S1 wall (Fig. 7.28), you can place one of your forceps jaws along the posterior wall to check that there are not any other fragments behind the vertebra. X-ray control is always necessary.

At the end of the procedure, you check that the hernia has been properly extracted by inserting the endoscope.

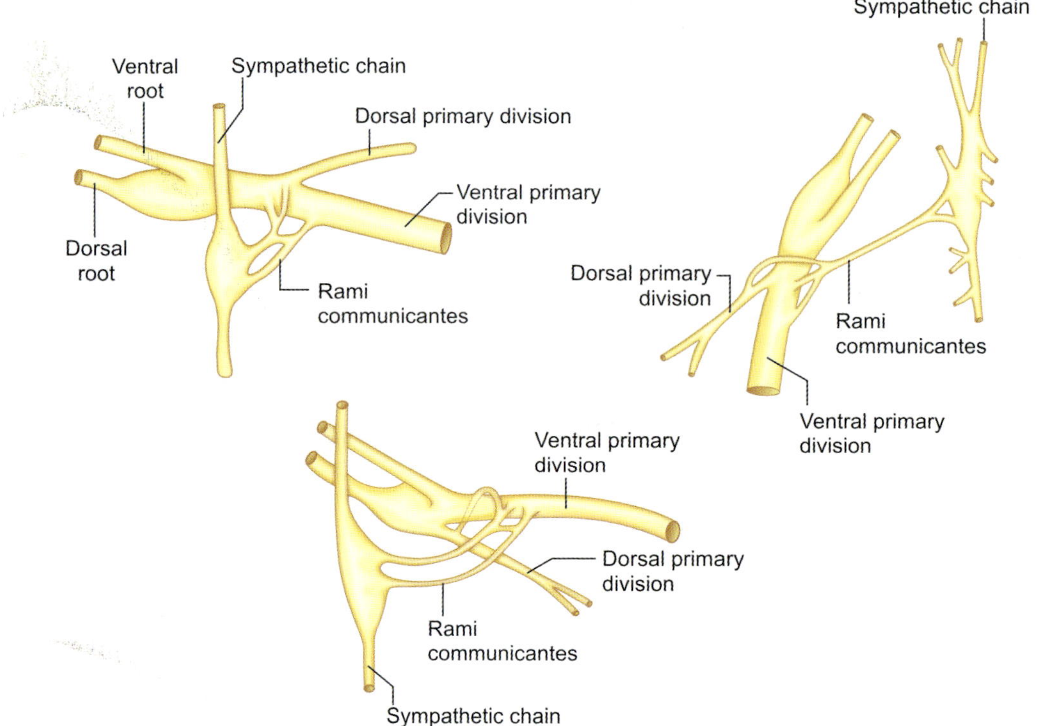

Fig. 7.24 Variability of the birth of sympathetic nerves (white and gray rami communicantes) (*Courtesy*: Ramji DASS. Sympathetic components of the dorsal primary divisions of human spinal nerves, 493-501 Department of Anatomy, New York University College of Medicine)

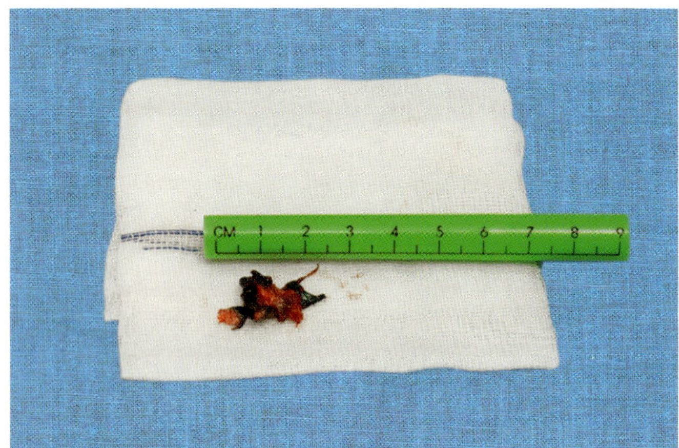

Fig. 7.25 Red and blue fragment

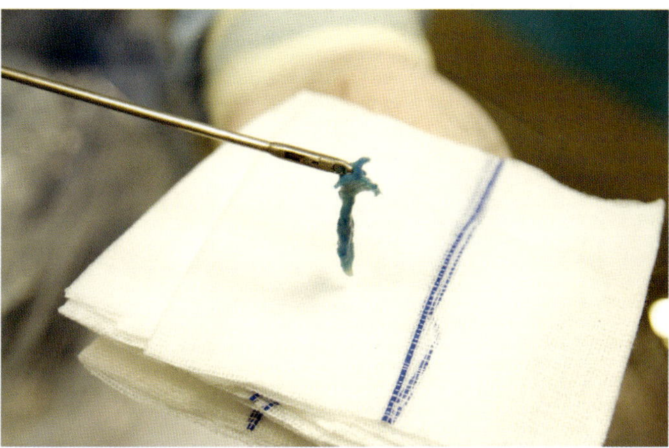

Fig. 7.26 Blue fragment

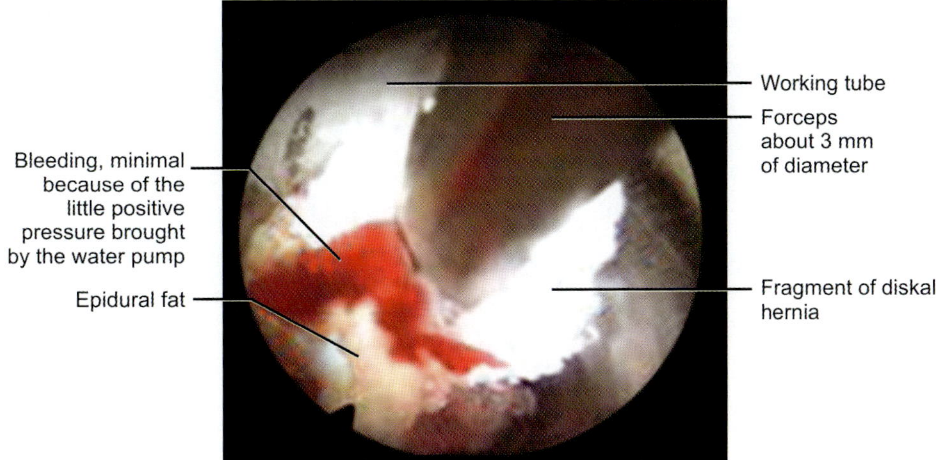

Fig. 7.27 Epidural fat around the dura

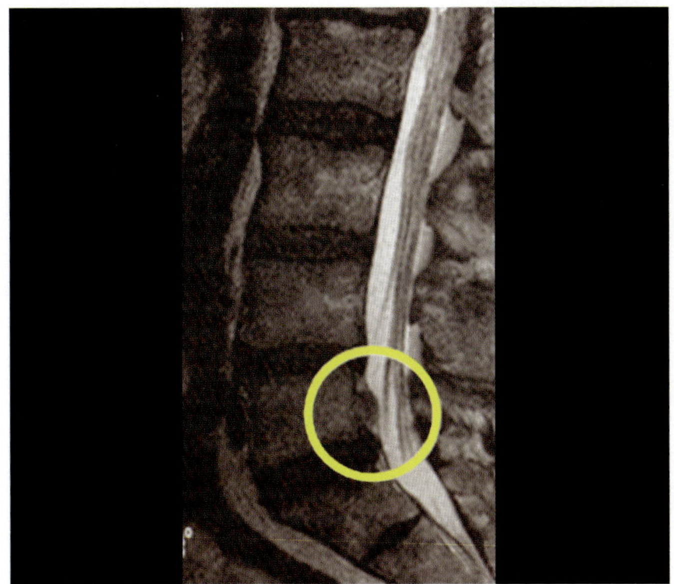

Fig. 7.28 Fragments remaining behind the L5 vertebra

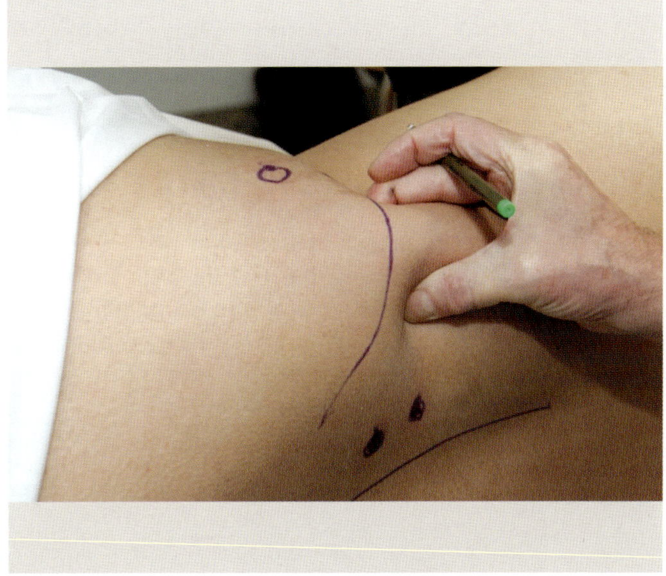

Fig. 7.29 Love handles

More specifically, it can be difficult to operate on obese patients who have a thickness of 5 cm of fat around the iliac crest (love handles) (Fig. 7.29).

This requires that you penetrate the skin much higher so you can cross the crest without remaining in the external face of the iliac wing.

Essential Points

- It will be easier to penetrate the disk if it is more inclined
- The orthogonal points must be properly marked laterally and frontally
- Never direct the needle towards the front without controlling the lateral view
- Never cross the middle of the vertebra
- Never put the patient to sleep.

Operation Complications

In rare cases, if you do not know the quality of the material, you can break one of the forceps jaws in the disk, and it can be difficult to extract it from the disk using the same transforaminal approach. In about five cases during my first years of practice, I was always able to take it out by using another forceps.

The irradiation time for the patient is not important because he or she is only operated once and the dose is no more than a long-distance flight where passengers are exposed to gamma and X-rays from the sun's activity. The nurses and anesthesiologist have to wear a lead gown. As for yourself, if you wish to wear a lead gown, you can only operate for about half an hour because of your body heat. A partial gown exists for your pelvis.

The "*hormesis*" effect, or beneficial effect of low dose of radiation, is an ongoing issue. Many factors are at play : age, tissue and cell sensitivity for example.

Bleeding can be prevented by increasing the flow of the arthro-pump but do keep in mind that this can create excessive pressure in the epidural space with bad consequences on the skull, with head and neck aches.

Coagulation by radiofrequency can be useful but is not compulsory unlike the arthro-pump which is absolutely necessary if you want to be able to see something.

WHEN TO MAKE A FUSION ON A FAR LATERAL HERNIA?

About 7% (3 – 11%) of most hernias are far lateral hernias. If you are lucky, you immediately find this type of hernia under the exiting root with your endoscope (Figs 7.30 and 7.31). You must not be misled by the simplicity of the operation because the disks degree of degeneration is more important than in other types of hernias: reoperations for relapse or indications for fusion are at least three times more frequent in this case than for paramedian hernias (Fig. 7.32).

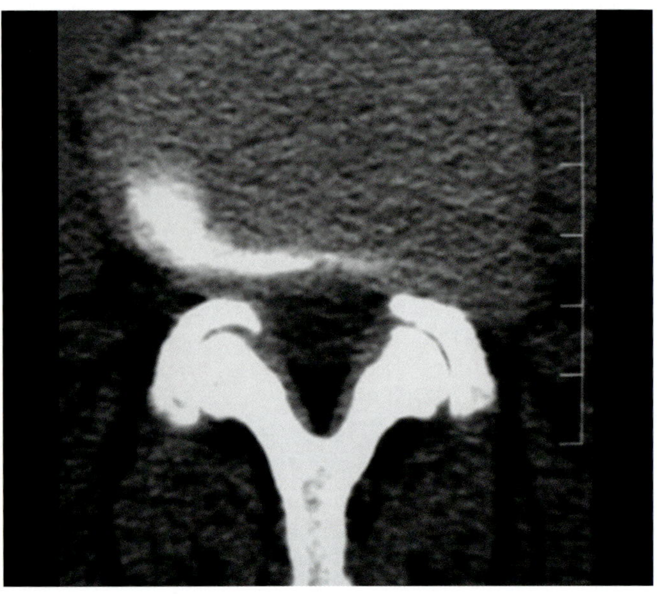

Fig. 7.30 Lateral hernia, extraforaminal

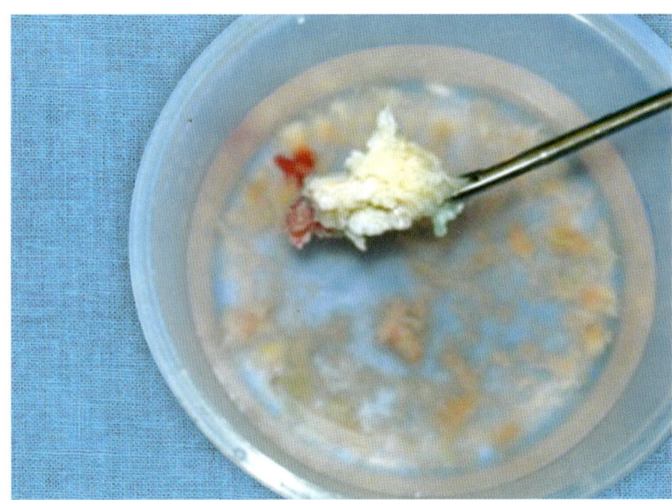

Fig. 7.31 Big fragment 3 cm long. The blue part on the left was colored with indigo carmine during the diskography. At the bottom of the recipient, you can see the other small fragments extracted from the disk

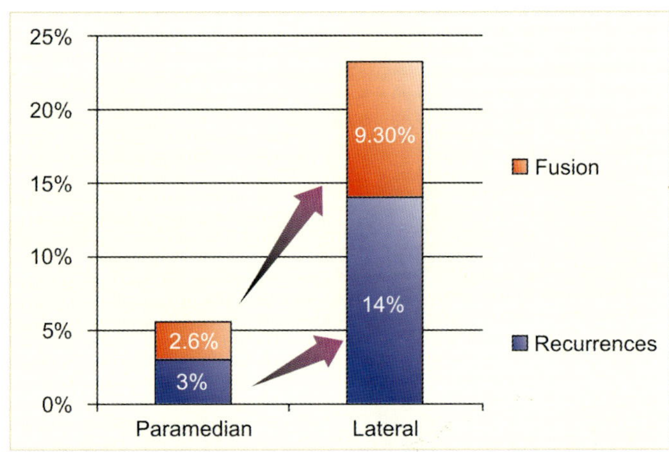

Fig. 7.32 Reoperations according to the type of hernia

You have to be able to indicate an arthrodesis more easily in this type of hernia when you hesitate to do a fusion. If the disk is less than half the normal height, if there is a Scheuermann disease and if the patient is more than 70 years of age, you can carry out a fusion without reservation.

PERCUTANEOUS LUMBAR CAGES IN THE CASE OF CRITICAL SPINE SURGERY

In rare cases, you have to operate on very old patients with a contraindication of general anesthesia due to heart failure or vascular brain strokes. In this case, you must think about using a percutaneous procedure with cages and screws.

You must evaluate if the patient can remain prone for more than one hour without tracheal intubation.

The first phase of the operation is to install the cages on each side of the intervertebral space. You obliquely penetrate the external part of the foramen and one half of the disk on each side under C-arm control.

You have to trace a vertical skin landmark along the middle of the back, horizontal landmarks on the level of the disks and vertical landmarks at 5, 6 and 7 cm from the first vertical midline (Fig. 7.33). Then you choose the best way to reach the anterior part of the disk near the midline. You carry out a local anesthesia on one side, insert the needle and feel the capsule of the zygapophyseal joint in which you inject lidocaine 2%, half a cc. After this, you cross the foramen in the triangular working zone and inject lidocain 0.5% in the disk if it is painful.

Having inserted the guidewire, you insert the dilators (Fig. 7.34). You prepare the disk with a trephine (Fig. 7.35) and curette.

Figure 7.36, after having dilated and pushed the exiting root to the side (see the marker around the root), you can insert the cage.

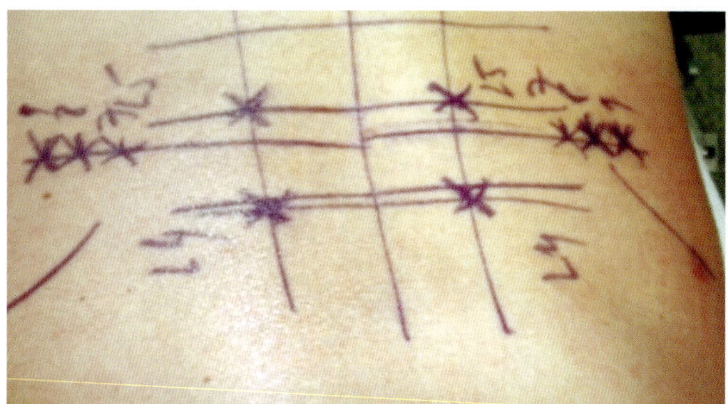

Fig. 7.33 Skin landmarks made under 'C' arm control

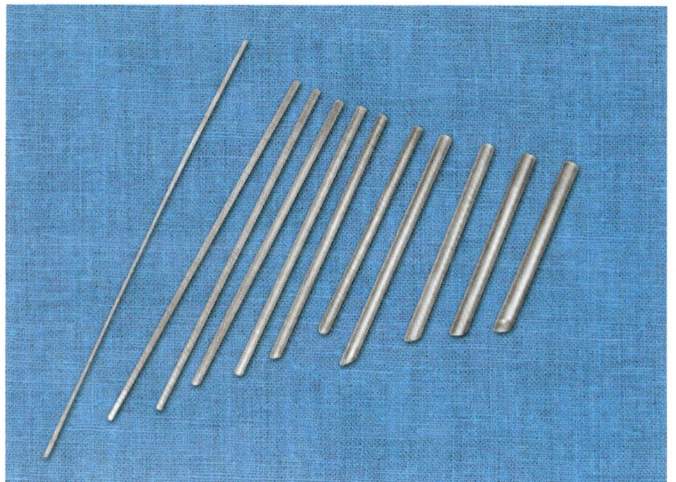

Fig. 7.34 A set of dilators

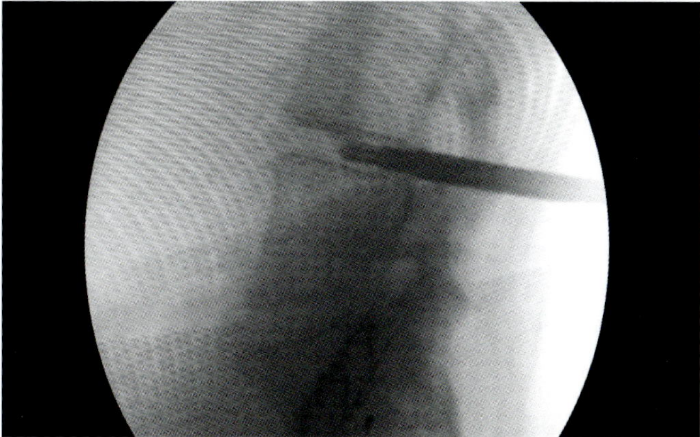

Fig. 7.35 Trephine preparing the disk

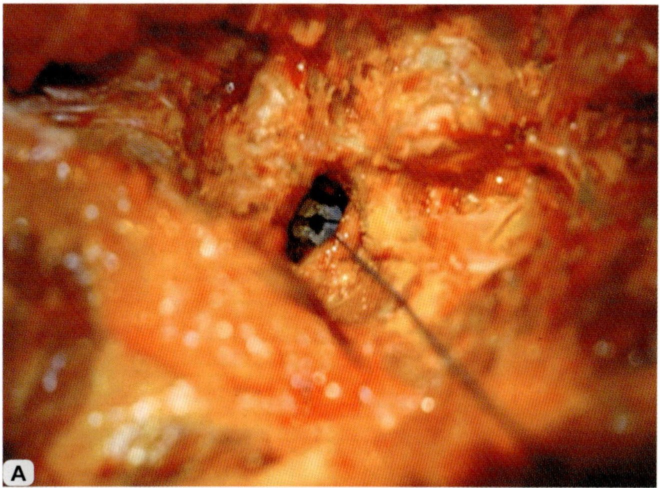

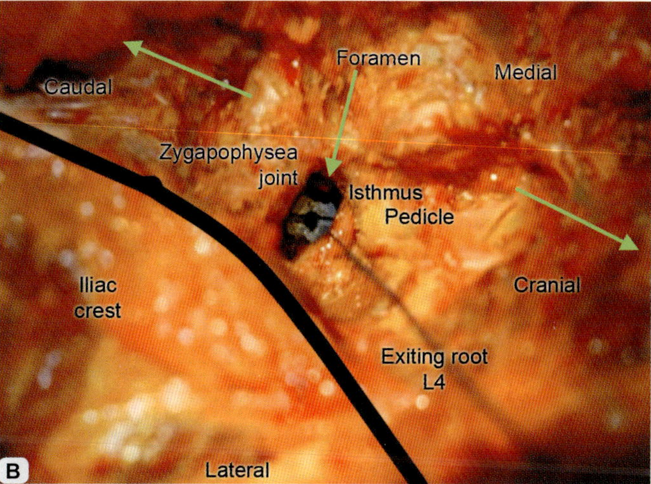

Fig. 7.36 (A) The triangular zone between the zygapophyseal joint and the exiting root and at the bottom, you can see the back of the cage (dissection); (B) Same dissection

After six to seven millimeters of dilation, you have to push the exiting root to the side until you can reach a gap, which is big enough to insert the last dilator you have chosen (Fig. 7.36). For example, if you want to install a cage of 10 mm of width and height, your last dilator has to be 14 mm of diameter.

If the disk height is of 5 mm, you choose a cage of 6 mm in height and a dilator of 8 mm in diameter (Fig. 7.37).

Sometimes, it is difficult to insert the last dilator, and it may be preferable to push the cage in directly after having prepared the disk plateaux (Fig. 7.38). Obviously, the cages are full of bone substitute. If you have chosen to use a bone remodeling protein (BMP), you fill the cage with it.

Then you percutaneously insert the plates (Fig. 7.39). You have to check the hardness of the bone, particularly when you push a perforator into the posterior side of the superior zygapophysal joint so the instrument penetrates it in the middle of the vertebral body, creating a space to insert a pedicular screw through a percutaneous plate.

Tips and Tricks

The plate's bed between the capsules and the muscles has been made by a special instrument introduced obliquely until it reaches the underlying zygapophyseal joint (Fig. 7.40).

Sometimes, the operation can take too much time and the patient starts to move. Therefore, your landmarks are constantly changing and makes the operation quite difficult.

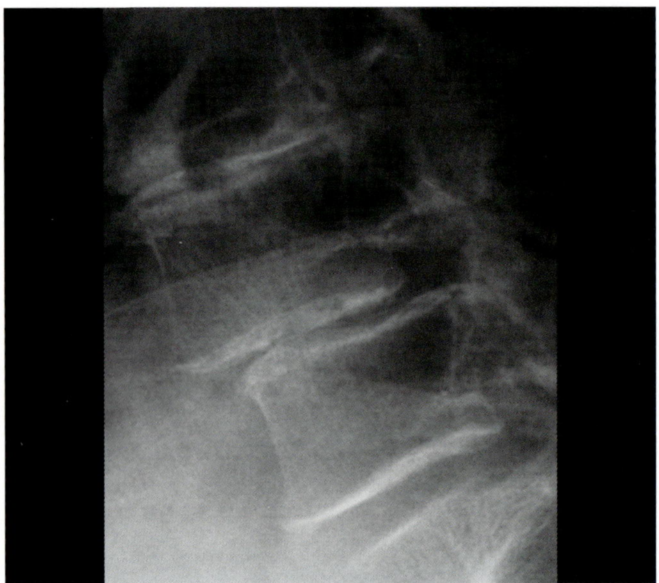

Fig. 7.37 Spondylolisthesis with diminishing of the intervertebral height, 91 year-old female

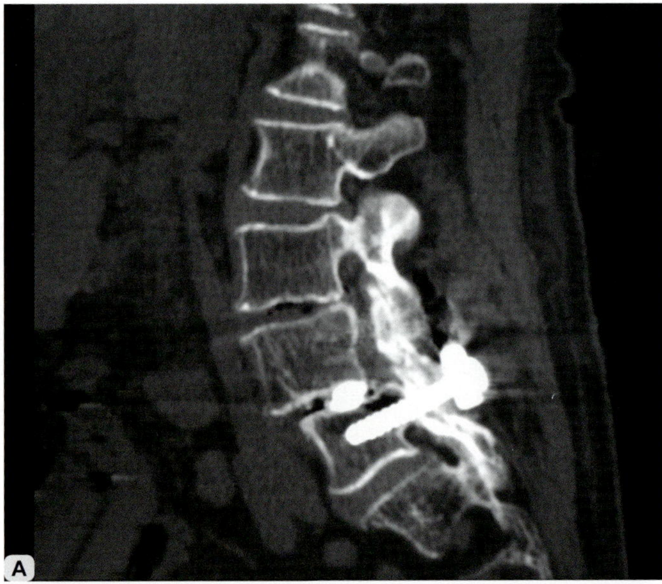

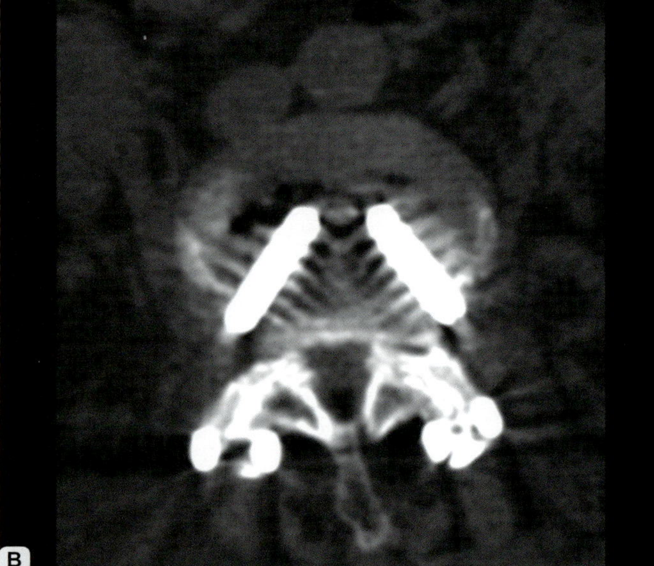

Fig. 7.38 (A) CT scan sagittal reconstruction, same patient; (B) CT scan axial reconstruction, two cages and two plates with the head of one screw on the left, same patient

Complications

If you wish to carry out a percutaneous procedure, you have to keep in mind that the patient has to be awake if you don't want to make an open procedure.

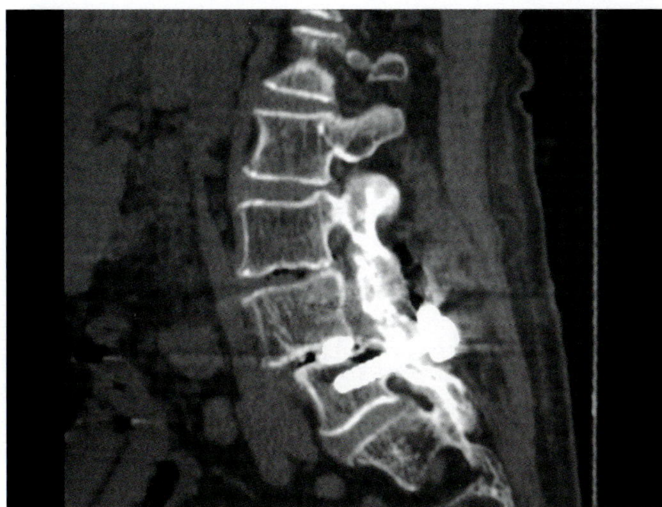

Fig. 7.39 CT scan , sagittal reconstruction of the L4 – L5 space with a partial reduction of the spondylolisthesis with plates, same patient

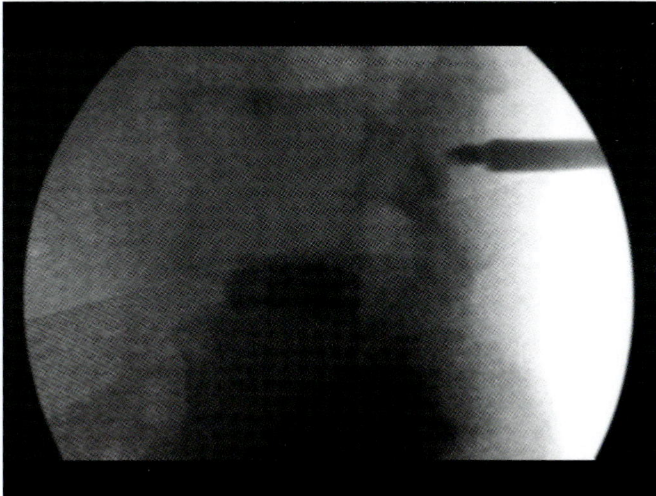

Fig. 7.40 Special instrument reaching the underlying zygapophyseal joint

Bibliography

1. Cameron J. Radiation increased the longevity of British radiologists, British Journal of Radiology. 2002;75:637-40.
2. Fred A. Mettler, Jr, Arthur C. Upton, Medical Effects of Ionizing Radiation, Third Edition Chapter 12, Saunders Elsevier; 2008. p.474-6.
3. Personal presentation, IITS-AMCICO International Congress, Cancun 2011.
4. Personal presentation, ISMISS Congress, Zurich 2011.
5. Roux A, Bronsard N, Blanchet N, de Peretti F. Can fluoroscopy radiation exposure be measured in minimally invasive traima surgery? Revue de chirurgie orthopédique er traumatologique. 2011;97:p644-51.

CHAPTER

8

Prevention of Development of Postoperative Dysesthesia in Transforaminal Percutaneous Endoscopic Lumbar Diskectomy for Intracanalicular Lumbar Disk Herniations (Floating Retraction Technique)

Jiyoung Cho, Ho-Yeon Lee, Sang-Ho Lee

Introduction

Percutaneous endoscopic lumbar diskectomy has been evolving from a state-of-the-art procedure into a more standard technique for treatment of extruded and/or migrated lumbar disk herniations, even stenosis. However, reliable methods of preventing possible complications, such as incomplete decompression, infection, and postoperative dysesthesia (exiting DRG injury) are not yet established. Postoperative dysesthesia (POD) is a complication peculiar to PELD and does not occur during microscopic diskectomy for intracanalicular herniated lumbar disk. Once POD occurs, even if only temporarily, the negative effect on the patient's daily life obscures the benefits of PELD as a minimally invasive procedure. Thus, prevention of POD is the key to successful and widespread use of PELD.

Indications

This technique could be applied in any circumstance in which transforaminal percutaneous endoscopic lumbar diskectomy (PELD) is used, especially for intracanalicular disk herniations.

Goal of Surgery

The goal of this procedure is to avoid development of post-operative dysesthesia (exiting dorsal root ganglion (DRG) injury) in PELD for intracanalicular herniated lumbar disk.

Treatment Options and Critical Decision Points

Plan 1: Floating retraction technique (FRT)
Plan 2: Foraminoplastic technique (FPT)
Plan 3: Diskography technique (parallel to disk space) (DT).

About 10 years ago, DT was the standard technique. When performing paraspinal approach, a guidewire was inserted into the disk and cut under the skin to obtain an anatomic orientation around the foramen, which was not familiar at that time (Figs 8.1 and 8.2). The DRG was usually

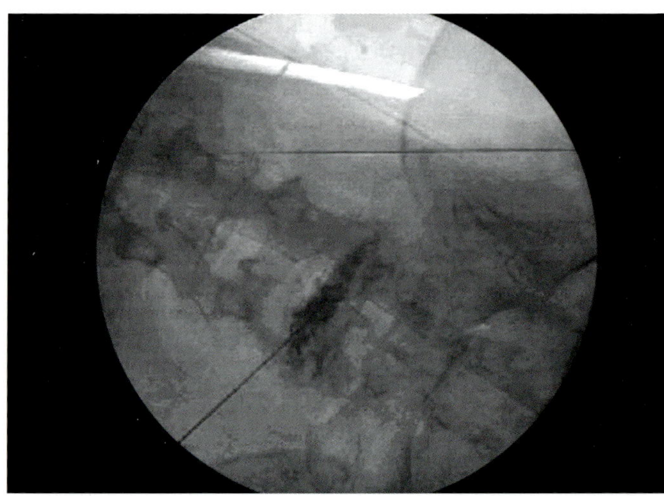

Fig. 8.1 Preoperative diskography was done with standard technique (Needle was parallel to disk space)

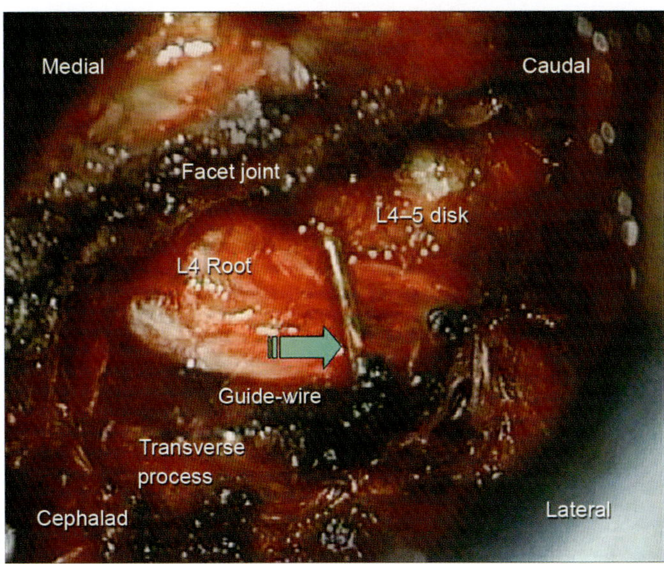

Fig. 8.2 A guidewire (arrow) was compressing dorsal root ganglion

compressed or even pierced by guidewires. (Fig. 8.2 arrow). Similarly, during PELD, an obturator or cannula being passed along the guidewire can touch or compress the DRG, supposing that there was no extraforaminal disk herniation, and DRG position was normal. This could explain the high incidence of POD in patients with a laterally extended degenerated facet joint. Thus, FPT (Plan 2) or FRT (Plan 1) should be selected to accomplish gentle insertion of the cannula without touching the DRG.

Removal of a portion of the superior facet is the main component of FPT and is accomplished with special twisted drills, a round cutter, or an endoscopic drill. This technique is quite useful at the L5 – S1 level and in cases of disk herniation with foraminal stenosis. However, it is time consuming and requires special equipment.

In contrast, FRT (Plan 1) is a simple modification of DT. It does not require extratime or special tools. There are three differences between FRT and DT: final guidewire location, trajectory in the foramen, and location of the skin entry point. In DT, the tip of the guidewire should be located at the center or in the posterior 1/3 of the disk (intradiskal location). In FRT, the ideal location of the guidewire is medial, at the superior border of the lower pedicle on the anteroposterior (AP) view, and at the superior pedicular notch on the lateral view (epidural location). Because the guidewire is not fixed by an annulus, pressure to the DRG caused by the cannula subsequent to the obturator may be lower than that in cases in which a fixed guidewire is used.

Floating Retraction Technique

Preparation

The patient is placed in a prone position on a radiolucent frame. The C-arm is positioned so that it is true lateral and AP without any change of the bed or C-arm angle. The patient's entire back is then prepped and draped in a sterile fashion with the C-arm.

Approaches

Skin Entry Point

The skin entry point is located at the intersection of the lines extrapolated from point A to point B on the AP and lateral views (Figs 8.3 and 8.4). Point A is at the superomedial border of the lower pedicle on the AP view and at the base of the superior vertebral notch of the lower vertebra on the lateral view. Point B is at the lateral margin of the superior facet of the lower vertebra on the AP view and at the cranial 1/3 of the superior facet on the lateral view. The usual skin entry point is located at the level of the upper pedicle on the lateral view and at a point calculated by adding the digits of the vertebra number + 2 cm lateral from the mid-line on the AP view. Hence, the usual skin entry point of L4 – 5 is the L4 pedicle on the AP view and 11 cm (4 + 5 + 2) from the midline. The usual skin entry point of L2 – 3 is the L2 pedicle and 7 cm (2 + 3 + 2) from the midline. This placement reflects the fact that the facet is located more medially at this level, and the thecal sac expands to eventually fill the entire spinal canal, moving upward. Thus, the laterality is

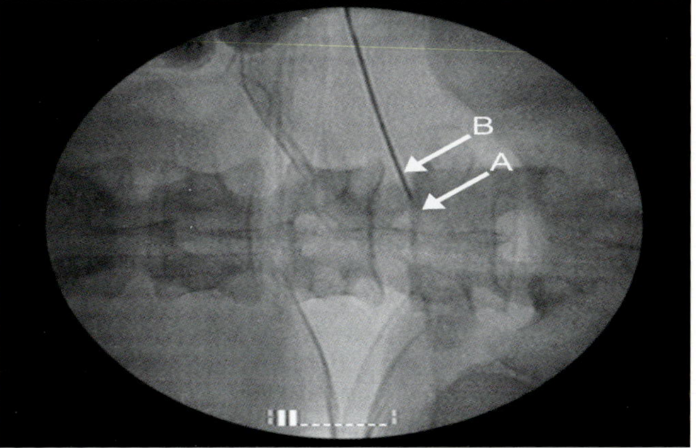

Fig. 8.3 C-arm AP view; point A: superomedial border of the lower pedicle, point B: the lateral margin of the superior facet of the lower vertebra

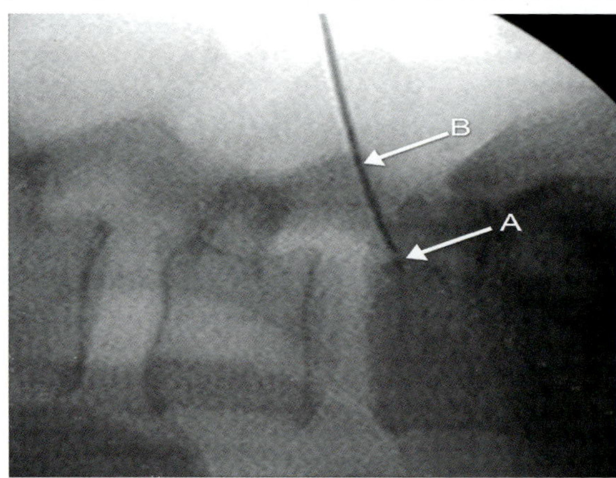

Fig. 8.4 C-arm lateral view; point (A) the base of the superior vertebral notch of the lower vertebra, point; (B) the cranial 1/3rd of the superior facet of lower vertebra

not the absolute value; it can be changed according to the patient's body shape or the location of the lesion.

In contrast, the facet is located more laterally at the L5 – S1 level, and the lateral portion of the spinal canal is generally not filled with thecal sac. Special attention should be paid to the L5 – S1 level. At this level, point B is at the inferior portion of the pars interarticularis on the AP view and at the tip of the superior facet of S1 on the lateral view. The usual skin entry point for L5 – S1 is the L5 pedicle on the AP view and 9 – 10 cm from the mid-line, to avoid fencing from the iliac crest.

Once the skin entry point has been determined, local anesthetic is infiltrated throughout a 2 cm by 2 cm area centered on the predetermined skin entry point.

Finding the Exact Pathway from the Skin Entry Point to Point B

A 23 G spinal needle is useful for this purpose. Because it is not strong to be steered easily in the muscle, it should be withdrawn to skin depth to locate the correct pathway. The exact angle and direction to point B can be found by repeated needling with lidocaine infiltration. This needling must be performed on the lateral view. Dural puncture may be the most serious complication of needle insertion under the lateral C-arm view. If the surgeon makes sure to pull out the spinal needle before injecting lidocaine, dural puncture by the 23 G needle is not a problem. However, needling under the AP view results in contamination from pierced intestine, especially in thin, less muscular female patients. A facet block on the superior-lateral synovial recess is helpful in diminishing operative pain. The 23 G spinal needle can be left *in situ* as a vanguard during 18 G needle insertion.

From Point B to Point A

A 6-inch-long 18 G spinal needle is inserted to touch point B under the lateral view, and placement is then checked in the AP view. The needle is passed from point B to point A, guided by the surgeon's hand feeling the bone (between the lateral facet capsule and the lateral aspect of the superior facet), under the lateral view and checked in the AP view at point A. (Fig. 8.5). Once placement is confirmed, 1 – 1.5 cc of 1% lidocaine is injected into the foraminal epidural space, and a guidewire is inserted through the needle. At point A, the guidewire should touch the bone and not pierce the annulus.

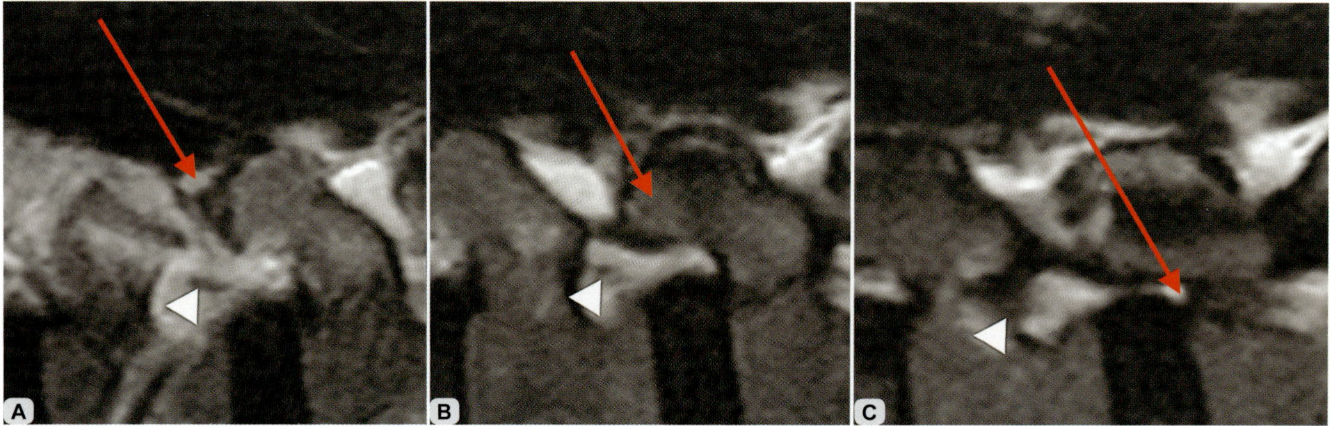

Fig. 8.5 T2 weighted sagittal views of foramen. (A) Lateral pedicular line; (B) mid-pedicular line; (C) medial pedicular line. Head of arrow in Figure A is the point B in Figures 8.3 and 8.4, and that in Figure C is the point A in Figures 8.3 and 8.4. Arrow head is the exiting root

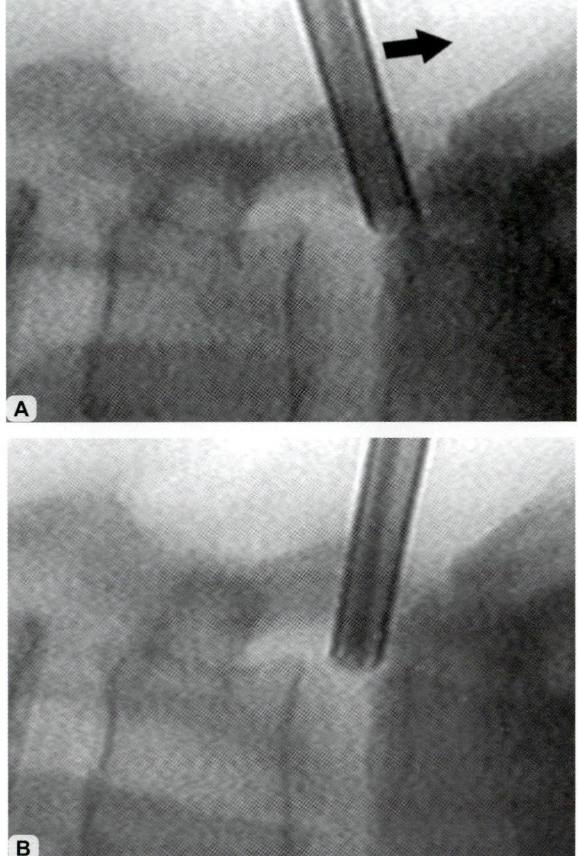

Fig. 8.6 (A) Cannula opening is facing lower pedicle; (B) Cannula opening is in working position after changing angle

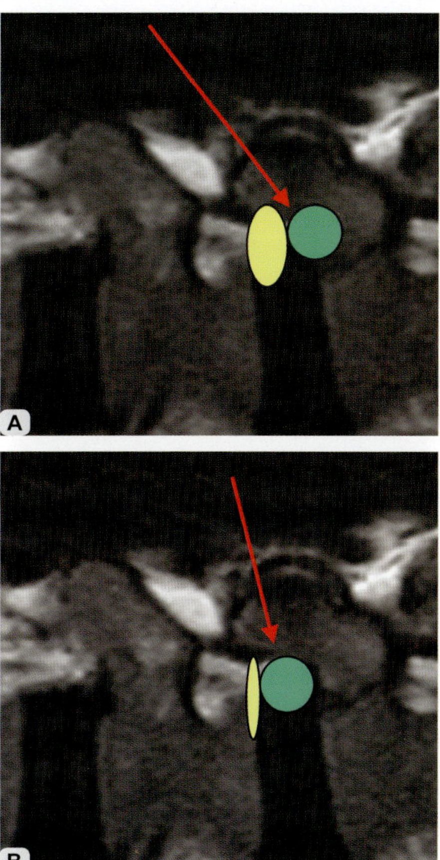

Fig. 8.7 Arrow is the direction of cannula. (A) The round circle is the opening of cannula facing pedicle; (B) The elliptical circle represents perineural fat after changing the direction of cannula (arrow), perineural fat (elliptical circle) is compressed

The dilator is introduced into the foramen along the guide-wire, followed by the cannula, both under the AP view. When the dilator and cannula pass point B, the surgeon warns the patient of sharp back pain. The warning may reassure the patient that the pain is expected and does not indicate that something is wrong. At this time, the cannula opening is still facing the upper medial portion of the lower pedicle. Just changing the angle of the cannula by gently pushing in can place the cannula in a more medial position with gentle retraction of the perineural tissue in the foramen (Figs 8.6 and 8.7).

Discussion and Practical Points

An interesting technical difference is present between microdiskectomy (MD) and PELD, relating to the blind phase of the two procedures. Partial hemilaminectomy to the traversing root is not performed blindly in MD, but the surgeon has no direct vision while probing under the nerve root. In contrast, full endoscopic direct vision is possible during diskectomy, but there is no direct visual control during cannula insertion, which is equivalent to the laminectomy phase of MD. If minor neural injury occurs during the blind phase of MD, it happens on the traversing root, which is already compromised by the herniated disk, and is usually well tolerated. In PELD, the injury happens on the fresh exiting DRG, not the root, and the patient complains of a new symptom (POD), even if the traversing root has been successfully decompressed. This POD has been reported by less than 5% of patients in published case series and is not a life-threatening complication like vessel injury or infection.[1–3] However, it is a complication related to the percutaneous approach itself, and it could be not only the first but also the last learning barrier[4] because it breaks the patient's expectation of a simple endoscopic discectomy in a clinical setting. Despite this peculiar complication, percutaneous endoscopic diskectomy is becoming more common because the postoperative course is shorter than that for microscopic diskectomy.[5] In addition, the most advanced microdiskectomy with the use of a tubular rectractor has not yet achieved a lower incidence of paraspinal muscle injury than is associated with conventional diskectomy (Love's method).[6]

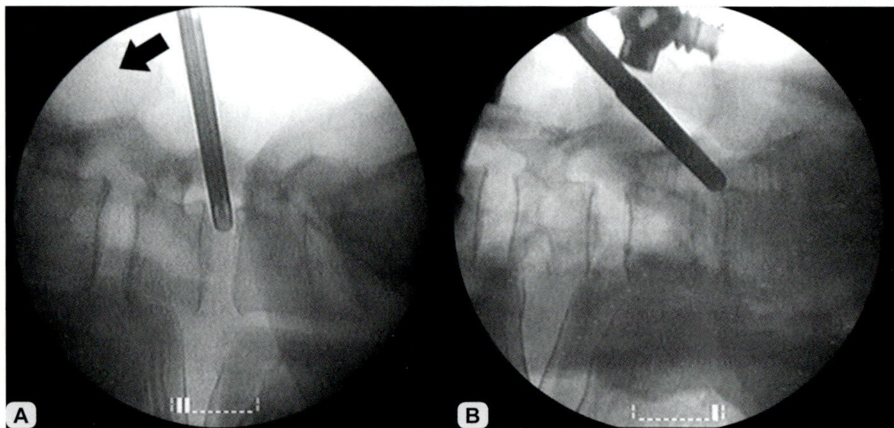

Fig. 8.8 (A) Cannula is placed intradiskal position; (B) Cannula is placed in the epidural space after levering

The occurrence of POD in the patients of even the most experienced surgeons could be explained by the findings of a cadaveric study of DT (parallel to disk space).[7] In that study, the exiting nerve was found to be 2 – 3 mm (mean, 2.3 mm) from the annulotomy hole made by a 2.7 mm diameter diskoscope. Supposing a 7 mm cannula is used at the same center, the exiting nerve is 0.15 mm compressed or 0.75 mm away from the cannula. If some tissue connected to the exiting nerve (e.g. vessel, furcal nerve) is pulled into the gap between the obturator and cannula, traction injury to the exiting nerve can develop after it passes the annulus level. In addition to the possible occurrence of POD, manipulation of the cannula angle is also restricted due to the proximity of the exiting nerve. This restriction results in limitation of indications for the procedure (huge herniations, migrated fragments).[8,9] Thus, DT is easy but is a mere legacy of the intradiskal era.

To overcome the disadvantages of DT, endoscopic surgeons have been trying foraminal enlargement (FPT) or use of two trajectories in one foramen with small cannulae.[8,10,11] These two techniques require extra-equipment or effort, whereas FRT involves only a simple change of the DT procedure, suitable for epidural work.

A noteworthy study has been published by a surgeon who performed PELD with FRT for 126 patients with intracanalicular herniation in a single year.[12] There were no instances of POD or of conversion to microdiskectomy. A dramatic improvement of Oswestry disability index (from 73% to 9%) was also observed.[13] In this series, the extent of canal compromise or migration of the herniated disk is comparable to that in two other series in which DT was used, but no failure was observed in high-grade canal compromise or high-grade migration.[8,9] Especially in cases of low-grade downward migration very close to the pedicle in the lateral recess, disk removal and decompression of the lateral recess area were easily accomplished with a ventral decompression technique.[12,14,15]

In fact, the path of FRT in the foramen is midway of two trajectories in one foramen, as described by Ditsworth (Fig. 8.8).[2] Through this ambiguous path, a large cannula can provide sufficient angles of view in the spinal canal, equivalent to those available with a tube retractor in microdiskectomy, without exiting DRG injury.

References

1. Ruetten S, Komp M, Merk H, Godolias G. Use of newly developed instruments and endoscopes: full-endoscopic resection of lumbar disc herniations via the interlaminar and lateral transforaminal approach. J Neurosurg Spine. 2007;6:521-30.
2. Tsou PM, Yeung AT. Transforaminal endoscopic decompression for radiculopathy secondary to intracanal noncontained lumbar disc herniations: outcome and technique. Spine J. 2002;2:41-8.
3. Yeung AT, Tsou PM. Posterolateral endoscopic excision for lumbar disc herniation: Surgical technique, outcome, and complications in 307 consecutive cases. Spine. 2002;27:722-31.
4. Yeung AT, Yeung CA. Minimally invasive techniques for the management of lumbar disc herniation. Orthop Clin North Am. 2007;38:363-72. abstract vi.
5. Mayer HM, Brock M. Percutaneous endoscopic discectomy: surgical technique and preliminary results compared to microsurgical discectomy. J Neurosurg. 1993;78:216-25.
6. Muramatsu K, Hachiya Y, Morita C. Postoperative magnetic resonance imaging of lumbar disc herniation: comparison of microendoscopic discectomy and Love's method. Spine. 2001;26:1599-605.

7. Osman SG, Marsolais EB. Posterolateral arthroscopic discectomies of the thoracic and lumbar spine. Clin Orthop Relat Res. 1994;304:122-9.
8. Lee S, Kim SK, Lee SH, Kim WJ, Choi WC, Choi G, Shin SW. Percutaneous endoscopic lumbar discectomy for migrated disc herniation: classification of disc migration and surgical approaches. Eur Spine J. 2007;16:431-7.
9. Lee SH, Kang BU, Ahn Y, Choi G, Choi YG, Ahn KU, Shin SW, Kang HY. Operative failure of percutaneous endoscopic lumbar discectomy: a radiologic analysis of 55 cases. Spine. 2006;31:E285-90.
10. Ahn Y, Lee SH, Park WM, Lee HY, Shin SW, Kang HY. Percutaneous endoscopic lumbar discectomy for recurrent disc herniation: surgical technique, outcome, and prognostic factors of 43 consecutive cases. Spine. 2004;15:E326-32.
11. Ditsworth DA. Endoscopic transforaminal lumbar discectomy and reconfiguration: a postero-lateral approach into the spinal canal. Surg Neurol. 1998;49:588-97.
12. Lee HY, Ahn Y, Lee S, Lee SH. Percutaneous endoscopic lumbar discectomy. J Korean Assoc for the Study of Spinal Pain. 2004;5:71-7.
13. Kim DY, Lee SH, Lee HY, Lee HJ, Chang SB, Chung SK, Kim HJ. Validation of the Korean version of the Oswestry disability index. Spine. 2005;30:E123-7.
14. Lee HY, Ahn Y, Kim DY, Shin SW, Lee SH. Percutaneous ventral decompression for L4-L5 degenerative spondylolisthesis in medically compromised elderly patients: technical case report. Neurosurgery. 2004;55:E455-9.
15. Lee HY, Lee SH, Shin SW. Percutaneous ventral decompression for degenerative lumbar spondylolisthesis in medically compromised geriatric patients. JDRS. 2005;16:133-6.

CHAPTER

9

Percutaneous Endoscopic Lumbar Diskectomy for Migrated Herniations

Fujio Ito, Yasushi Miura, Motohide Shibayama, Shu Nakamura, Shoji Ikeda, Minoru Yamada, Tomohiko Yamada

Introduction

Percutaneous endoscopic lumbar diskectomy (PELD) is a spine surgery involving a 7 mm incision under local anesthesia that requires a one-night stay. There are three basic variations of PELD: the transforaminal (TF) approach, which is a method of operating through the intervertebral foramen, the interlaminar (IL) approach, utilizing the interlaminar space, and the extraforaminal (EF) approach for lateral lumbar disk herniation.[1] In conventional surgical procedures for migrated herniation, surgeons in the early stage of the learning curve are more likely to cause complications, such as insufficient hernia removal, epidural space hemorrhage, dura mater injury, and adhesive radiculitis. We have developed novel techniques to avoid these. The migration of lumber disk hernia (LDH) was classified into four grades: disk-level LDH, slight-migrated LDH, moderate-migrated LDH, and severe-migrated LDH. The "half-and-half technique" of the TF approach was used for disk-level and slight-migrated LDH, in which the tip of a beveled cannula was positioned to equally face both the inside of the intervertebral disk and the epidural space. The inside-out technique was employed to initially remove the nucleus pulposus from the intervertebral disk to depressurize it and then remove the hernia from the epidural space. Although the half-and-half technique was initially performed on moderate-migrated LDH above the L4/5 disk, preparatory foraminoplasty was additionally performed, if required, to remove several millimeters of the superior articular process so as to incorporate the epiduroscopic technique, which permits introduction of an endoscope into the epidural space.[2] Moderate-migrated LDH from the L5/S level were treated with the IL approach to remove the upper edge of the lamina, followed by partial laminoplasty in which the interlaminar space was enlarged to freely direct the endoscope downward. Severe downward-migrated LDH from the L4/5 to L5/S levels were treated with a method combining the TF approach to resect the upper third of the hernia from the L4/5 level and the IL approach to remove the lower two thirds from the L5/S level.[3]

For severe upward-migrated LDH at the L3/4 and L4/5 levels, we have developed a novel translaminar approach to bore a 9 mm hole in the lamina. The following discusses these applied PELD techniques.

Materials

Background of Patients

We performed percutaneous endoscopic lumbar diskectomy (PELD) on 1,181 cases of lumbar disk herniation between April 2007 and October 2010. The patients were 320 women and 748 men with an average age of 48.3 ± 16.1. The patients who received PELD were those not exhibiting much improvement after receiving at least six weeks of conservative treatment, such as block injections, NSAID, and rehabilitation, those having difficulty in moving their bodies due to severe pain, or those clearly exhibiting progressive neurological symptoms who received a definitive diagnosis based on MRI, CT, or functional X-ray. Those with central stenosis, a lateral recess of 3 mm or less, and an intervertebral foramen of 7 mm or less, and those who indicated instability under functional X-ray were excluded from the above.[1]

In this study, we selected from the above patient pool 320 subjects who had at least two grams of hernia removed for analysis. Those were large central hernia at the disk level and migrated LDH with an average extracted amount of 2.72 ± 0.75 g (the largest was 6.3 g). The breakdown of the subjects was 252 men and 68 women with the youngest aged 14 years old and the oldest aged 93 years old. The TF approach was used for 200 cases, the IL approach for 68 cases, the EF approach for 26 cases, and the novel dual approach for 26 cases. The duration of surgery was 78.09 ± 30.45 minutes. The breakdown of the cases in terms of intervertebral disk level was 107 cases at the L5/S level, 174 cases at the L4/5 level, 26 cases at the L3/4 level, 12 cases at the L2/3 level, and one case at the L1/2 level. We were able to follow up 305 of the above cases with observations and evaluations at one month, three months, and six months from surgery. We examined the results of the surgery and the newly developed techniques.

The results were assessed according to a modified Macnab's method by having the patients check applicable boxes in a questionnaire. "Excellent" indicates the patient is free of pain and able to work and practice sports unhindered. "Good" indicates that the patient can work without any limitation despite experiencing occasional pain and numbness but not to the extent that requires a painkiller. "Fair" indicates that the patient exhibits some degree of improvement but requires occasional medication and block injections and has some limitations on functioning in daily life. Conditions in this grade may require a reoperation. "Failure" indicates the condition of the patient has not improved or exhibits such deterioration that it significantly hinders the patient's daily life and requires a reoperation. Lower limb pain, which is the main symptom, was assessed according to the visual analog scale (a VAS of "0" indicates absence of pain and "10" indicates unbearable pain).

Classification of Hernia Migration (Fig. 9.1)

The direction of migration was classified into two groups, downward or upward, with each graded according to severity into slight, moderate, or severe migration.[4]

Zone 0 (the disk level) corresponds to no vertical migration, accounting for 153 of the 305 cases. Those were cases of unilateral large hernia, central large hernia, and off-center hernia with double root damage. A majority of the hernias were at this zone.

Zone 1 (slight-downward) corresponds to the location within the upper 5 mm of the lower vertebral body – 65 cases fell into this category.

Zone 2 (moderate-downward) indicates the area from 5 mm below the upper edge of the lower vertebral body to the lower edge of the pedicle – 35 cases fell into this category.

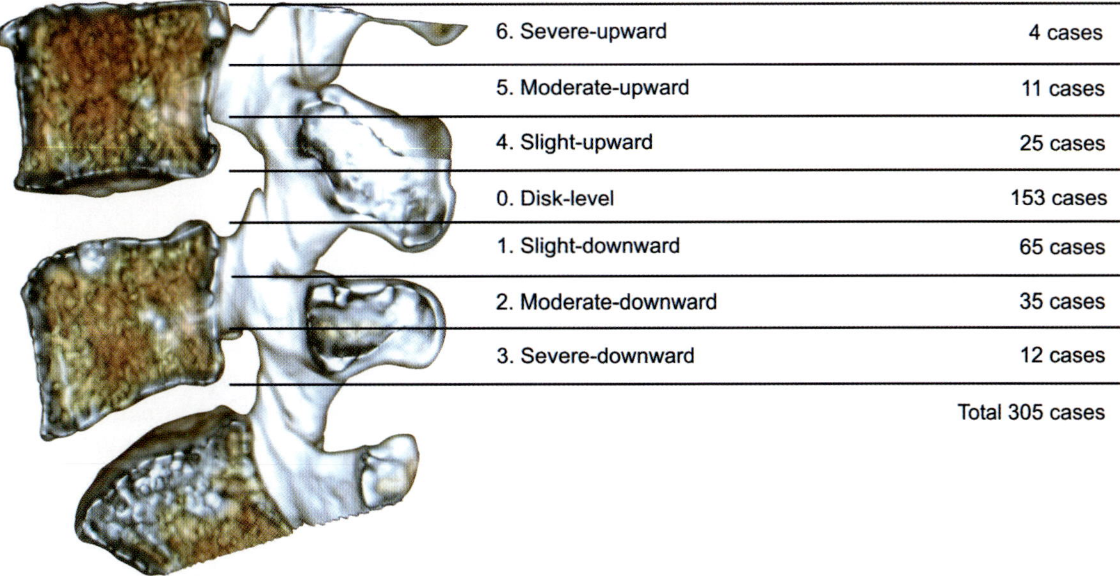

Fig. 9.1 Grades of migrated herniation. Zone 0. disk-level: no vertical migration. Zone 1: Slight – downward: within upper 5 mm of the lower vertebral body. Zone 2: Moderate-downward – from 5 mm below upper edge of the lower vertebral body to the lower edge of the pedicle. Zone 3: Severe-downward – below lower edge of the lower pedicle. Zone 4: Slight-upward – within lower 5 mm of the upper vertebral body. Zone 5: Moderate-upward – from 5 mm above the lower edge of the upper vertebral body to the center of the pedicle. Zone 6: Severe-upward – above the center of the upper pedicle

Zone 3 (severe-downward) indicates that the hernia hangs down to or below the lower edge of the lower pedicle. We identified 12 ca ses of these hernias extending from the L4/5 level to the L5/S level.

As for upward migratory zones:

Zone 4 (slight-upward) indicates the location within the lower 5 mm of the upper vertebral body – 25 cases fell into this category.

Zone 5 (moderate-upward) corresponds to the area from 5 mm above the lower edge of the upper vertebral body to the center of the pedicle – 11 cases fell into this category.

Zone 6 (severe-upward) corresponds to the area above the center of the upper pedicle – 4 cases.

Surgical Techniques Developed

Half-and-half Technique for Disk-level (Zone 0) and Slight-migrated LDH (Zones 1 and 4)

This technique is applied to cases with no migrations at the disk level and those within upper 5 mm of the lower vertebral body. The location of needle insertion and the needle trajectory are measured preoperatively based on MRI or CT cross-sectional images. A far lateral approach is adopted in which insertion is made at the most lateral point possible of the trunk. At the same time, it is essential that the trajectory is such that it may not damage the retroperitoneum or the viscera[5]. An 18 G needle is pointed to the intervertebral foramen and brought into contact with the superior articular process. The needle is then introduced into the epidural space. The axillary regions of the exiting and traversing roots are safe areas and inexperienced surgeons are required to confirm that the location is safe by epidurography. Preferably, the needle point should penetrate the intervertebral disk parallel to the posterior edge of the vertebral body as seen in a lateral image of the fluoroscopy, and it should preferably be at the central region of the intervertebral disk as seen from the anteroposterior view. Half of the beveled cannula is positioned inside the intervertebral disk while the other half is positioned to peer into the epidural space. When performing the inside-out technique, the dorsal portion of the intervertebral disk and part of the fibrous annulus are resected to create space. Next, the tip of the cannula is pointed to the epidural space and the hernia mass is extracted using forceps with 5 mm long blades. The fibrous annulus often pinches the protruding hernia mass. When the dura mater or the traversing root begins to float in response to the fluctuation of the perfusate pressure, then that signals the end point (Fig. 9.2).[2]

An Epiduroscopic Technique for Moderate-downward Migrated LDH at L4/5 or above (Zone 2)

Unless sequestrated, it is possible to extract a moderate-migrated LDH at the L4/5 disk or above by pulling it out by its end, with forceps. However, these LDH tend to break off during the attempt. We have developed an epiduroscopic technique that allows for tool manipulation within the epidural space. Going straight to the epidural space is risky. Accordingly, the standard procedure involves initially creating space within the intervertebral disk and then performing the inside-out technique. In most cases, foraminoplasty is required to reach the epidural space.[6] After withdrawing the cannula to the entrance of the intervertebral foramen, the intervertebral foraminal ligament is vaporized with a holmium laser under the endoscope, and the intervertebral foramen side of the superior articular process is resected with an appropriate tool, such as a high-speed drill or a trephine. If a moderate-downward migrated hernia mass exits inside the pedicle, additional removal of part of the upper portion of the pedicle or the posterior edge of the lower vertebral body will facilitate manipulation of the cannula. All of these operations are conducted under endoscope (Fig. 9.3).

Interlaminar Approach Involving Partial Laminoplasty for Moderate-downward Migrated L5/S LDH (Zone 2)

The anatomical characteristics of the L5/S1 include a high iliac crest, and large L5 transverse processes, with a narrow space between the transverse processes of L4 and L5. Additionally, the diameter of the intervertebral foramen inversely corresponds proportionately to the lumbosacral angle by becoming smaller. The above situation makes it difficult to employ the TF approach for the L5/S LDH. Fortunately, the IL approach is a viable option due to the large intervertebral space.[7] When using the IL approach, the needle is advanced from the skin located on the center of the L5/S along the medial wall of the lamina until the yellow ligament is penetrated, after-which an epidurography is performed. Then, after the needle is confirmed to be in the shoulder portion of the S1 root, the yellow ligament is split and dilated with a sequential dilator and the S1 root is inwardly retracted with a tubular retractor. There are cases, however, in which the cannula cannot be freely manipulated downward like a joystick. If this occurs, the upper edge of the S1 lamina is trimmed with a high-speed drill, a 2 mm wide chisel or a trephine. Partial laminoplasty is then performed to enlarge the interlaminar space, which

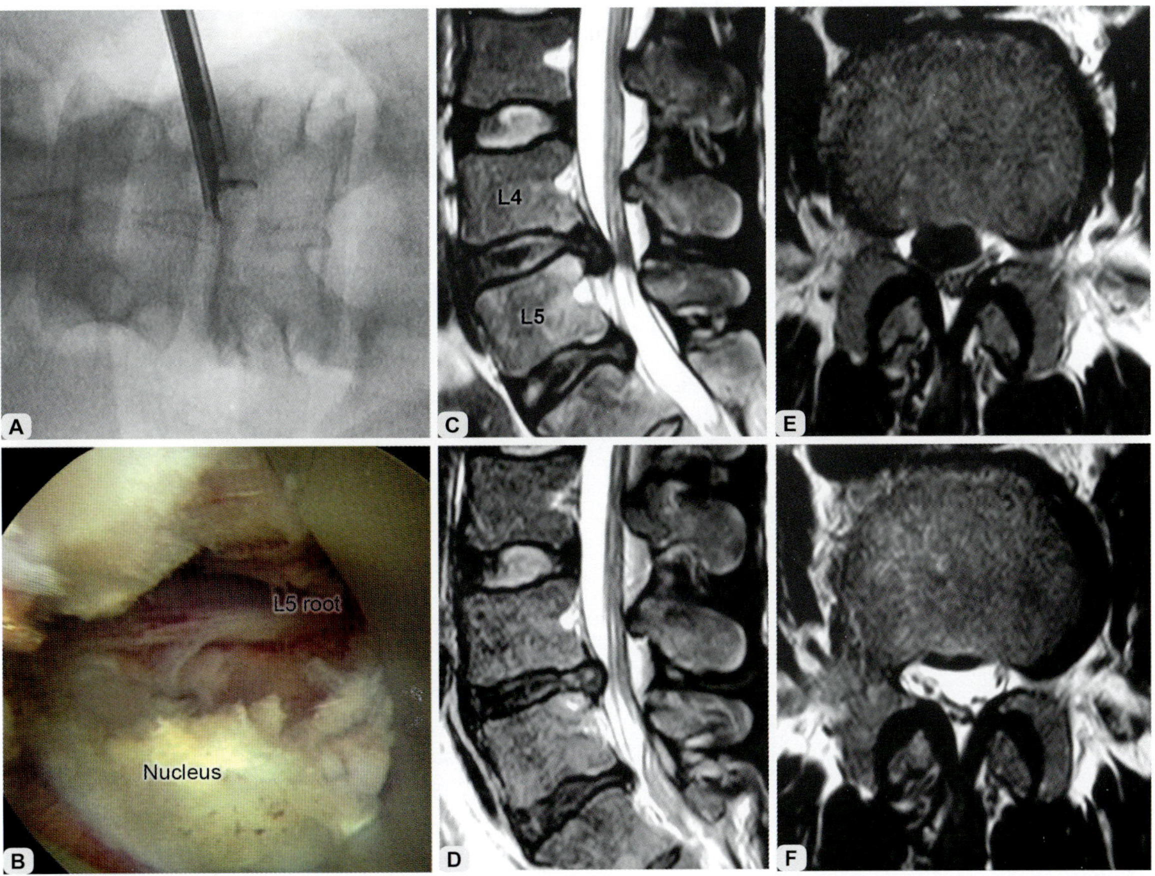

Fig. 9.2 Slight-downward migrated L4/5 hernia. (A) Extracting a hanging hernia mass using forceps with 5 mm long blades; (B) Decompressing ventral side of traversing root with the half-and-half technique; (C and D) Sagittal images of preoperative and postoperative MRI; (E and F) Axial images of preoperative and postoperative MRI

allows forceps to advance sufficiently downward so that the moderate-downward migrated LDH may be removed (Fig. 9.4).

Combination of TF (L4/5) and IL (L5/S) Approaches for Severe-downward Migrated L4/5 Hernia (Zone 3)

In standard posterior surgeries (MED and MD) on severe-downward migrated L4/5 LDH, performing a hemilaminectomy in order to reach the L5/S level is generally unavoidable. In PELD, the half-and-half technique of TF is employed to initially extract the upper third of the hernia starting from the L4/5 level going downwards. The IL approach as applied to the L5/S level is then employed for the extraction of the lower two thirds of the hernia.[8] A cannula is inserted from below and pointed upwards to the remaining portion of the hernia at the shoulder of the S1 root. The endoscope is advanced to the ventral side of the axillary region of the L5 root while gradually going upwards, extracting the remainder of the hernia (Fig. 9.5).[3]

Epiduroscopic Technique for Moderate-upward Migrated LDH at L4/5 or above (Zone 5)

For moderate-upward migrated LDH at the L4/5 or above, the epiduroscopic technique is employed to advance the cannula up toward the axillary region of the traversing root and the exiting root to remove the hernia mass. Since the upper lumbar vertebrae have a larger intervertebral foramen, foraminoplasty is not always required. In the lower lumbar vertebrae, however, foraminoplasty needs to be performed to reach the epidural space. Foraminoplasty for moderate-upward migrated LDH involves removing the ventral side of the upper portion of the superior articular process. If osteophytes are present on the lower posterior edge of the upper lumbar vertebrae as they often are, it is

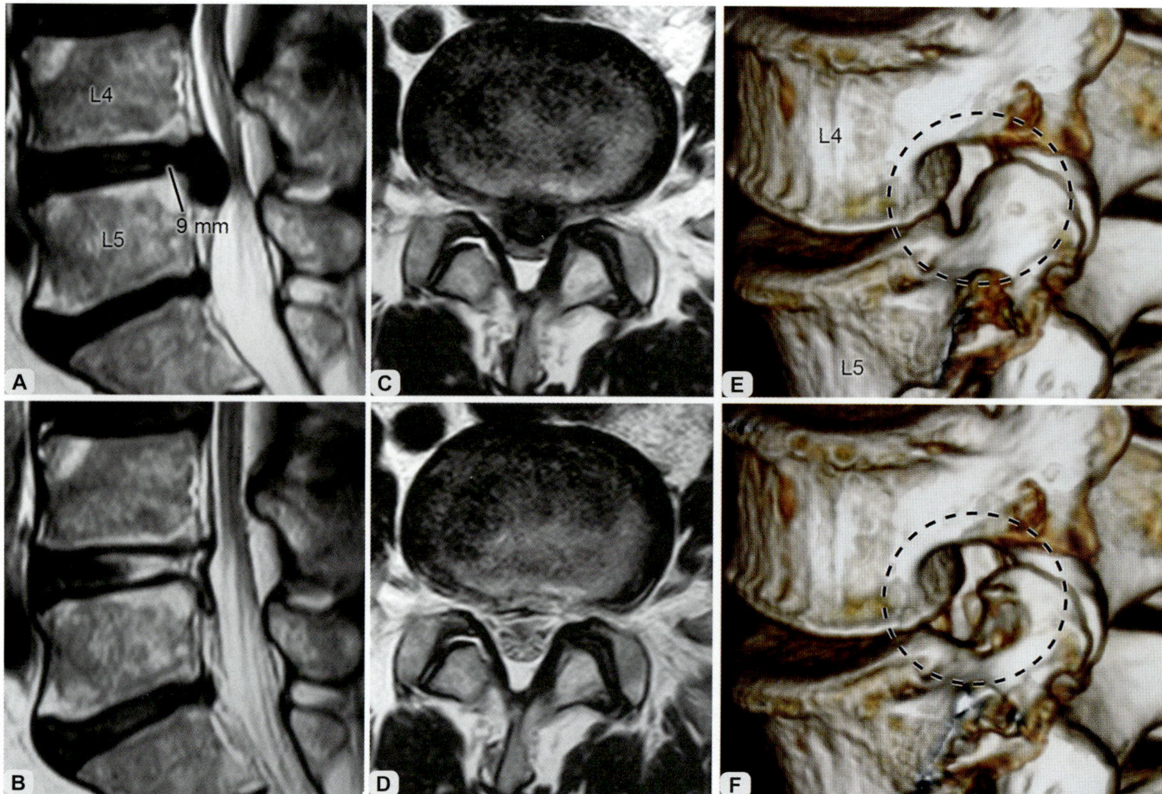

Fig. 9.3 Foraminoplasty for moderate-downward migrated L4/5 hernia. (A and B) Sagittal images of preoperative and postoperative MRI; (C and D) Axial images of preoperative and Postoperative MRI; (E) A small foraminal space prevents entry of the cannula; (F) The foraminal space is enlarged by resecting the superior articular facet, upper portion of vertebral pedicle and posterior edge of L4 vertebral body

additionally required to resect the osteophytes with a 3 mm wide trephine or a 2 mm wide chisel in order to facilitate insertion of the cannula into the epidural space (Fig. 9.6).

Epiduroscopic Technique for Severe-upward Migrated LDH (Zone 6) with Spondylolisthesis

Even in cases of severe-upward migrated LDH with spondylolisthesis, the anteroposterior width of the intervertebral foramen tends to be sufficiently large enough to permit easy insertion of the cannula tip into the epidural space. However, the absence of both instability and cauda equina disorders due to slippage are prerequisites for this procedure. At the L4/5 level, because the intervertebral foramen space is larger on the dorsal side of the L4 root, the tips of the forceps can reach the upper edge of the L4 vertebral body immediately under the endoscope (Fig. 9.7).

Translaminar Approach for Severe-upward Migrated LDH (Zone 6)

When performing the TF approach, it is not possible to reach the upper location of the severe-upward migrated LDH without spondylolisthesis. Instead, a 9 mm hole is made in the lamina through which to insert a cannula to enter the epidural space on the shoulder of the traversing root. With hernias at the L4/5 level, the patient's skin is marked slightly above the center of the affected side of the lamina under fluoroscopy and the needle is positioned onto the lamina. Several millimeters of muscle are scraped off the lamina with the tip of a flat-ended cannula to expose the cortical layer of the lamina bone. A trephine with a 5 mm diameter is used to penetrate the inner bone cortex of the lamina with a loss of resistance with reference to a lateral view under the fluoroscopy. Subsequently, the hole is enlarged with a drill with a maximum 9 mm diameter to easily insert a 7 mm beveled cannula to the shoulder side of the L5 root.

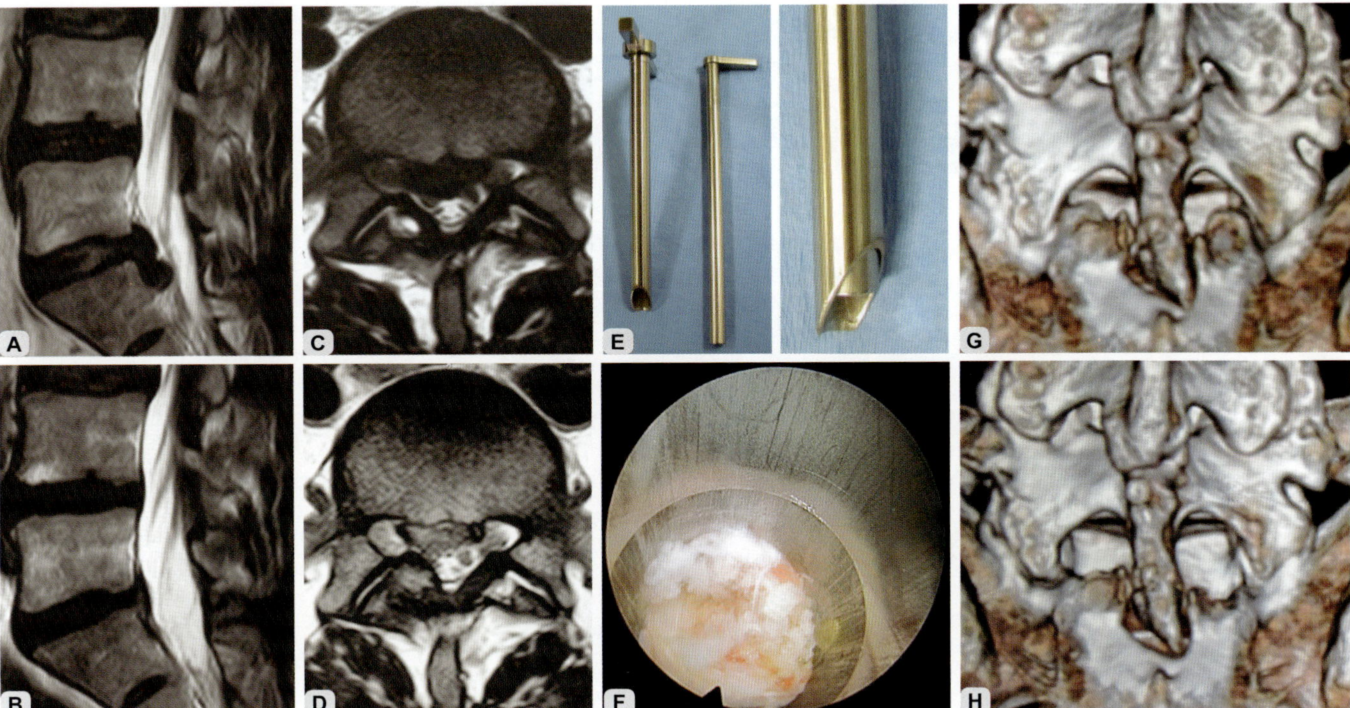

Fig. 9.4 Partial laminoplasty for moderate-downward migrated L5/S hernia. (A and B) Sagittal images of preoperative and postoperative MRI; (C and D) Axial images of preoperative and postoperative MRI; (E) A cylindrical semicircular chisel designed by Dr.Nakamura (9 mm φ) (Left : cylindrical semicircular chisel, Center : 8 mm φcannula, Right : the chisel encasing the cannula); (F) Partial laminoplasty using the cylindrical semicircular chisel under percutaneous endoscopy; (G and H) Preoperative and postoperative 3D-CT images showing partial laminoplasty to widen lateral-inferior portions of both L5/S1 level interlaminar spaces

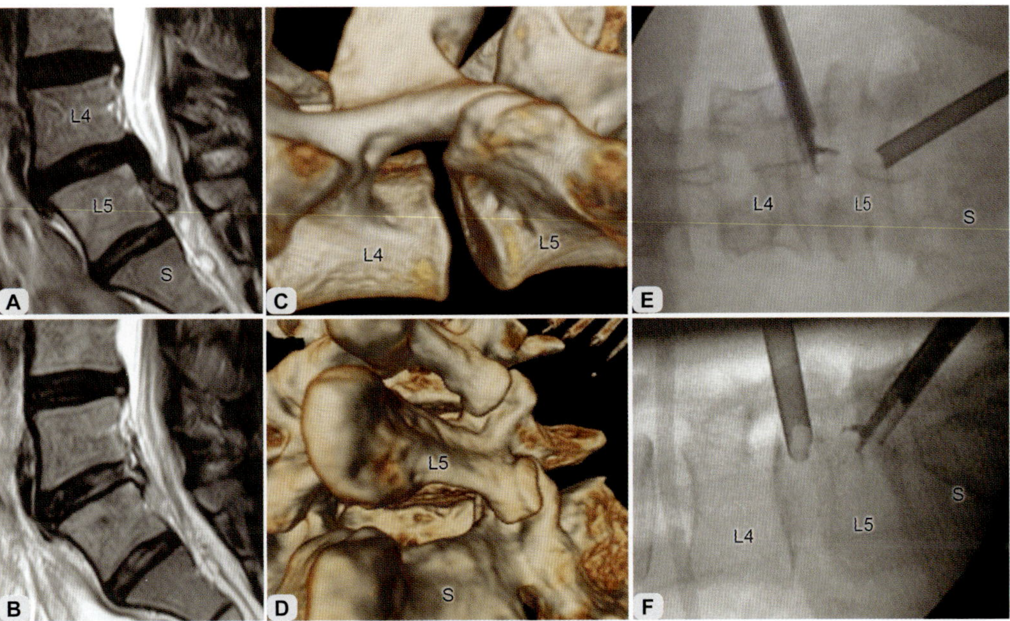

Fig. 9.5 Combination of transforaminal (L4/5) and interlaminar (L5/S) approaches for severe-downward migrated L4/5 hernia. (A and B) Sagittal images of preoperative and postoperative MRI; (C and D) Endoscopic trajectory of transforaminal (TF) and sInterlaminar (IL) approaches; (E and F) Anterior-posterior and lateral views of dual approach. Using transforminal approach to remove upper 1/3 rd of the nucleus at L4/5. Using interlaminar approach to remove lower 2/3 rd of the nucleus at L5/S

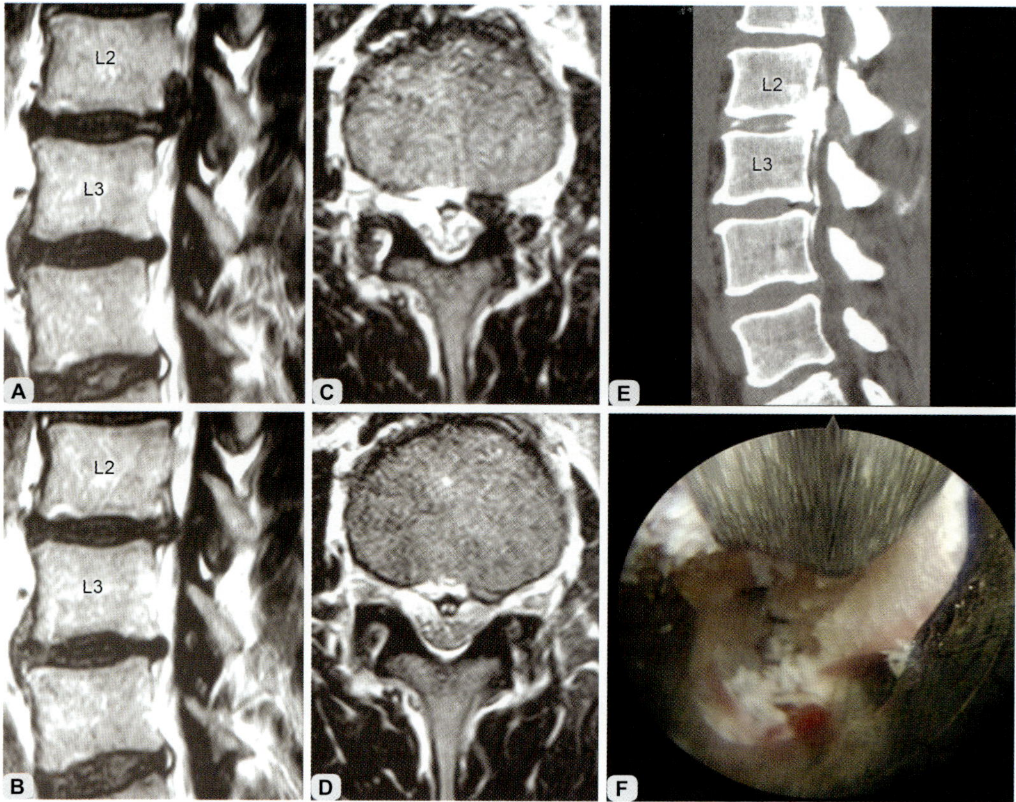

Fig. 9.6 Epiduroscopic technique for moderate-upward migrated L2/3 hernia. (A and B) Sagittal images of preoperative and postoperative MRI; (C and D) Axial images of preoperative and postoperative MRI; (E) Disko-CT sagittal image; (F) Foraminoplasty to remove superior articular facet with trephine

This procedure can be completed in about 15 minutes. No yellow ligament exists at this site; instead, epidural fat and dura mater are present. At this site, the beveled cannula (which also serves as a tubular retractor) is introduced into the epidural space. As the dura mater and the L5 root are retracted inwardly with the cannula, the hernia is extracted by applying a vertical joystick-like manipulation. It is possible to extract the top of the hernia to the branch point of the L4 root and the L5 root. As for the tail, the portion up to the lower edge of the L5 vertebral body can be extracted (Fig. 9.8). While the translaminar approach can be used to extract severe-upward migrated LDH at the L3/4 and L4/5 levels, this approach is difficult for the upper lumbar vertebrae L1/2/3, since there is not sufficient space at the shoulder to permit retraction of the dura mater. As for severe migration in an upper lumbar vertebra, it may be possible to employ the TF approach to retract the herniation with curved blade forceps. However, it may break off during the procedure. If there is a possibility of leaving remnants, the procedure is immediately switched to MED under general anesthesia to perform hemilaminectomy.

Results

The satisfaction ratings ("excellent" and "good" combined) of initial surgeries according to a modified Macnab's method decreased as the degree of migration increased, with the level of satisfaction registering the relatively high figure of 90% (138/153) for zone 0 (disk level), 88% (57/65) for zone 1 (slight-downward), and 71% (25/35) for zone 2 (moderate-downward). A similar tendency of a gradually decreasing level of satisfaction was observed among upward migrated herniations; the satisfaction rating for zone 4 (slight-upward) was 84% (21/25) and 73% (8/11) for zone 5 (moderate-upward). Since a special combination technique was employed for zone 3 (severe-downward), the level of satisfaction was highest at 100% (12/12). As for zone 6 (severe-upward), although the figure was 75% (3/4), the number of cases was too small for meaningful statistical examination. Generally, the more severe the migration was the more often remnants and oversights resulted to increase the percentage of reoperations. This occurred

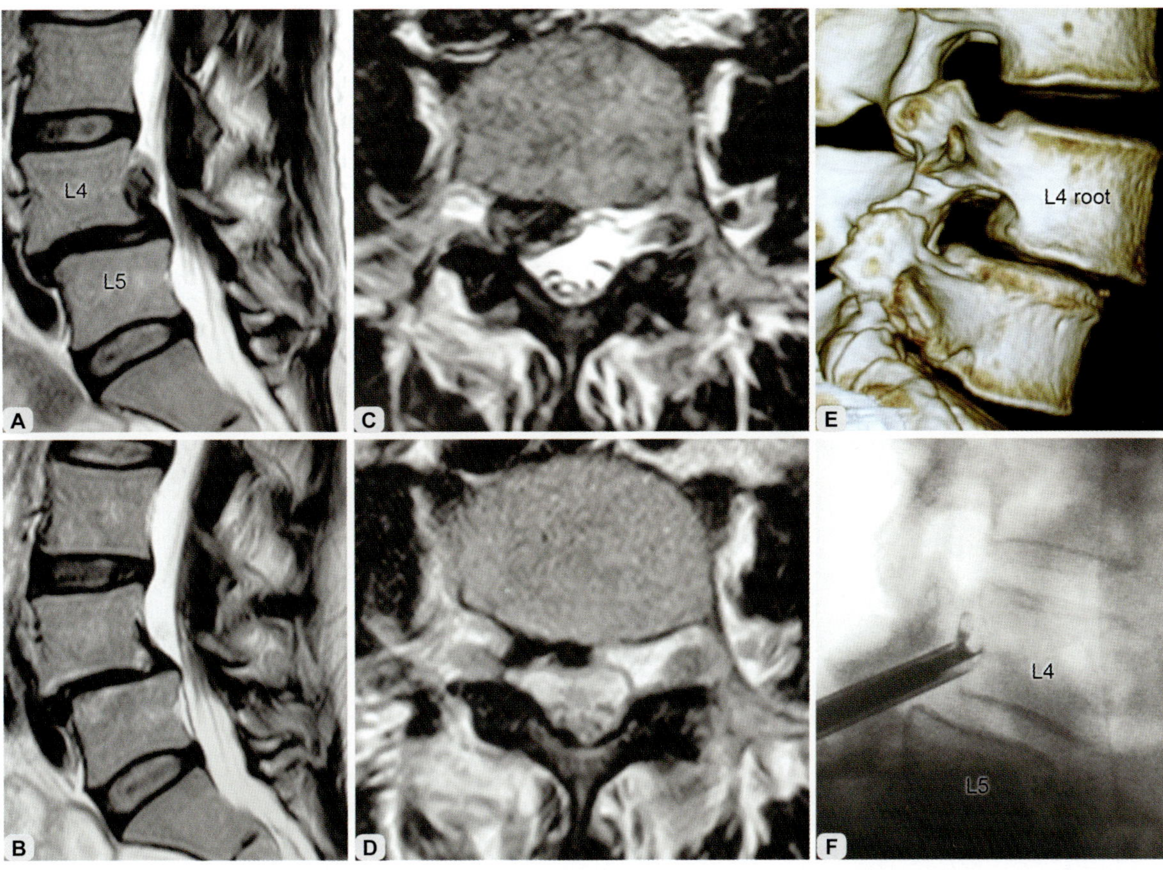

Fig. 9.7 Severe-upward migrated herniation with spondylolisthesis. (A and B) Sagittal images of preoperative and postoperative MRI; (C and D) Axial images of preoperative and postoperative MRI; (E) Foramen is enlarged between the anterior–posterior space due to spondylolysthesis; (F) Forceps can be easily used in the posterior space of the exiting root

more with beginner surgeons with steeper learning curves, with the advanced surgeons compensating for beginners' unsatisfactory results by performing PELD or MED in reoperations. The satisfaction ratings for reoperations were inversely proportional to the degree of migration and averaged 66%. The final satisfaction rating, combining those of the initial operations and the revision operations, was 94% (Table 9.1). The VAS for sciatica, which is the main symptom of herniation, was preoperatively 7.11 ± 2.64, which decreased to 2.59 ± 2.61 (paired t-test, $p < 0.005$) one month after the operation, 2.1 ± 2.43 ($p < 0.05$) after three months, and 1.6 ± 2.07($p < 0.01$) after six months.

Discussion

Migration is inseparable from herniation, and it is necessary to determine which technique should be used for the hernia's extraction and how much of it can be extracted. We have pictorially classified hernias and developed techniques suitable for different types of herniations. These new techniques, originally developed because of unsatisfactory results, such as hernia remnants, are more sophisticated than conventional ones and involve risks for novice surgeons. To avoid risks, the half-and-half technique used in the TF approach and the epiduroscopic technique for moderate migration is based on the inside-out technique.[9] These offer high levels of safety as the initial manipulation takes place immediately below the hernia mass (located between the dura mater and the fibrous annulus), rather than immediately below the dura and nerve roots. According to the half-and-half technique, the cannula can be safely manipulated with a lever after the fibrous annulus is cut off, allowing extraction of the hernia mass in the epidural space immediately under the endoscope. In the epiduroscopic technique, foraminoplasty is essential to partially resect the superior articular process due to the possibilities of epidural space hemorrhage, nerve damage, and perioperative pain. The operation is started within the intervertebral disk and the intervertebral foramen is enlarged by foraminoplasty, which allows the cannula to pass to the outer layer of the fibrous annulus. This in turn enables extraction of the

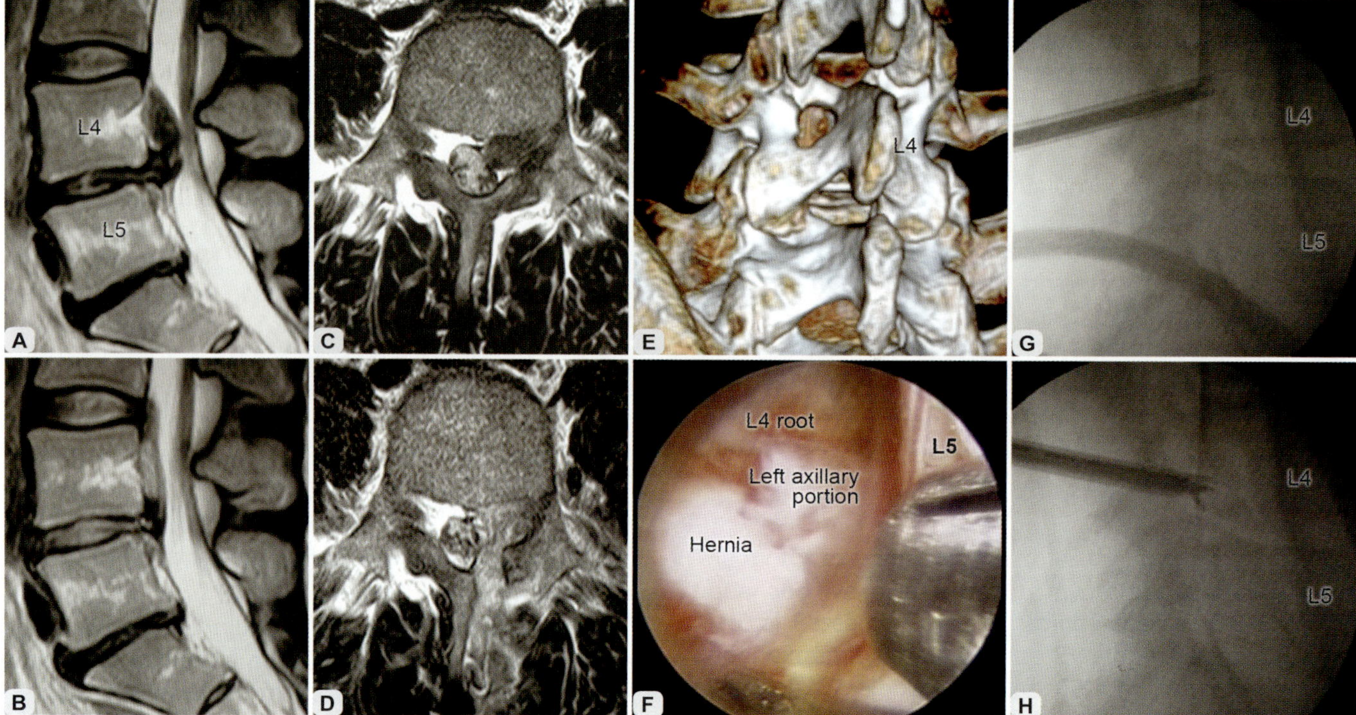

Fig. 9.8 Translaminar approach for severe-upward migrated herniation; (A and B) Sagittal images of preoperative and postoperative MRI; (C and D) Axial images of preoperative and postoperative MRI; (E) Must bore a 9 mm hole in the vertebral lamina; (F) A herniotomy is performed in the axillary region around the L5 and L4 roots; (G and H) Forceps can be manipulated up and down along the posterior wall of the L4 vertebral body

migrated LDH. The cannula is oriented downward if the herniation is migrated caudally, and oriented upward if it is migrated cephalically. In MED and MD, removal of the lamina or substantial osteotomy of the inferior articular process has been unavoidable. However, the introduction of our special techniques of PELD has eliminated the need for excessive osteotomy. The TF and IL combination approach for severe-downward migrated LDH from the L4/5 level does not require resection of the lamina. Rather, under endoscopy, this approach can extract a hernia mass extended from the L4 vertebral body's upper edge toward its lower edge. The results of the twelve cases were all satisfactory. According to the translaminar approach for severe-upward migrated LDH, the cannula is inserted directly to the outer side of the epidural space through a 9 mm diameter hole. Then, the hernia can be extracted under endoscopy by joystick manipulation of forceps along nearly the entire height of the vertebral body whilst retracting the traversing root with the cannula itself. However, since there is little space that the cannula can enter on the outer side of the dura mater of the upper lumbar vertebrae (L1/2/3), the translaminar approach cannot be employed for herniation at these sites. Accordingly, curved blade forceps are used instead. If there still is a fear of leaving remnants, it can be preferable to use MED.[10,11]

We followed up the cases with evaluations of the procedures and their effectiveness for up to six months. The cases of moderate migration exhibited poorer results than those of slight migration, with similar tendencies repeated in the postoperative MRI evaluations. This is attributable to the fact that beginners left behind remnants and broke apart hernia mass. Accordingly, we believe that as a surgical option for highly migrated hernias, MED is more suitable for beginners than PELD since extensive osteotomy is possible in MED. After becoming an "old hand" with 100 or more cases of disk-level operations under his/her belt, a surgeon may begin to employ high-level techniques, such as foraminoplasty, partial laminoplasty, the TF and IL combination, and the translaminar approach, to produce improved results while offering less invasive surgical options to the patients.

Note that in all the cases, we have obtained informed consent from the patients for this clinical publication as well as for the use of data in papers and academic meetings.

Summary

The degree of migration of lumbar disk herniations (LDH) was graded into disk-level, slight, moderate, and severe. The first

Table 9.1 Satisfaction rating. Initial operation and revision operation

Grade of migration	*Exellent*	*Good*	*Satisfied group*	*Fair*	*Failure*	*Unsatisfied group*	*Reoperation*	*Satisfactory of reoperation (%)*	*Total*
6. Severe-upward	3 (75%)	0 (0%)	3 (75%)	1 (25%)	0 (0%)	1 (25%)	0 (0%)		4 (1%)
5. Moderate-upward	4 (36%)	4 (36%)	8 (73%)	1 (9%)	2 (18%)	3 (27%)	3 (27%)	1 (9%) (33%)	11 (4%)
4. Slight-upward	10 (40%)	11 (44%)	21 (84%)	2 (8%)	2 (8%)	4 (16%)	3 (12%)	2 (8%) (67%)	25 (8%)
0. Disk-level	85 (56%)	53 (35%)	138 (90%)	6 (4%)	9 (6%)	15 (10%)	12 (8%)	9 (6%) (75%)	153 (50%)
1. Slight-downward	30 (46%)	27 (42%)	57 (88%)	3 (5%)	5 (8%)	8 (12%)	8 (12%)	6 (9%) (75%)	65 (21%)
2. Moderate-downward	10 (29%)	15 (43%)	25 (71%)	3 (9%)	7 (20%)	10 (29%)	9 (26%)	5 (14%) (56%)	35 (11%)
3. Severe-downward	8 (67%)	4 (33%)	12 (100%)	0 (0%)	0 (0%)	0 (0%)	0 (0%)		12 (4%)
Total	150 (49%)	114 (37%)	264 (87%)	16 (5%)	25 (8%)	41 (13%)	35 (11%)	23 (8%) (66%)	305 (100%)

Assessment according to a modified Macnab's method
Excellent: the patient is free of pain and able to work and practice sports unhindered.
Good: the patient can work without any limitation despite experiencing occasional pain and numbness but not to the extent that requires a painkiller.
Fair: the patient exhibits some degree of improvement but requires occasional medication and block injections and has some limitations on functioning in daily life. Conditions in this grade may require a reoperation
Failure: the condition of the patient has not improved but exhibits such deterioration that it significantly hinders the patient's daily life and requires a reoperation

two grades were treated with the half-and-half technique of a transforaminal approach in which the subannular nucleus and the epidural prolapsed nucleus were extracted in the inside-out manner whilst maintaining the intradisk and the epidural space in the same field of vision. Foraminoplasty was performed on moderate migrations at the L4/5 level or above and an epiduroscopic technique was used to enable tool manipulation within the epidural space. Partial laminoplasty was performed on moderate-migrated LDH at L5/S to enlarge the interlaminar space, enabling tubular joystick manipulation. A combination technique of the transforaminal and interlaminar approaches was employed on severe-downward migrated LDH from the L4/5 to L5/S levels. For severe-upward migrated LDH at the L3/4 and L4/5 levels, a translaminar technique was employed to bore a 9 mm hole in the lamina. The aforementioned techniques are suitable for advanced surgeons and beginners are strongly advised to perform any of the above under the guidance of supervisory surgeons.

References

1. Fujio Ito, et al. Percutaneous Endoscopic Lumbar Disc Herniation Extraction—Clinical Examination of 197 Cases—, The Journal of Japanese Society of Lumbar Spine Disorders. 2009; 15(1): 180-9.
2. Fujio Ito, Miura Y, Nakamura S, et al. Percutaneous endoscopic lumbar discectomy (PELD) —Transforaminal approach and indications— Asian Journal of Neurosurgery. 2008; 11: 41-6.
3. Choi G, Prada N, Modi HN, et al. Percutaneous endoscopic lumbar hernietomy for high-grade down-migrated L4-L5 disk through an L5-S1 interlaminar approach: a technical note. Minim Invas Neurosurg. 2010; 53:147-52.
4. Lee S, Kim SK, Lee SH, et al. Percutaneous endoscopic lumbar discectomy for migrated disc herniation: classification of disc migration and surgical approaches. Eur Spine J. 2007; 16(3): 431-7.
5. Ruetten S, Komp M, Godolias G, et al. An extreme lateral access for the surgery of lumbar disc herniation inside the spinal canal using the full-endoscopic uniportal transforaminal approach- technique and prospective results of 463 patients. Spine. 2005; 30(22): 2570-8.
6. Choi G, Lee SH, Lokhande P, et al. Percutaneous endoscopic approach for highly migrated intracanal disc herniations by foraminoplastic technique using rigid working channel endoscope. Spine (Phila Pa 1976). 2008; 1; 33(15): E508-15.
7. Ruetten S, Komp M, Merk H, et al. Full-endoscopic interlaminar and transforaminal lumbar discectomy versus conventional microsurgical techunique. Spine. 2008; 33(9): 931-9.
8. Fujio Ito, et al. Minimally Invasive Percutaneous Endoscopic Spine Surgery, J Spine Res. 2010; 1: 1674-81.
9. Fujio Ito. Percutaneous Endoscopic Lumbar Discectomy (PELD)-Transforaminal and Interlaminar approaches-Essential Practice of Neurosurgery, Access Publishing Co,. Ltd. 2010; 939-46.
10. Fujio Ito. Percutaneous Endoscopic Lumbar Disc Herniation Extraction — Three Techniques and Adaptations— The Central Japan Journal of Orthopaedic Surgery & Traumatology. 2008; 51:1053-61.
11. Fujio Ito. Percutaneous Endoscopic Lumbar Discectomy for central large herniation. The Central Japan Journal of Orthopaedic Surgery & Traumatology. 2011; 54: 637-46.

CHAPTER

10

Percutaneous Posterolateral Endoscopic Treatment for Spinal Infection

Manabu Ito

Introduction

There is a tendency that the numbers of patients with spinal infections are increasing in developed countries.[1,2] The reasons for the increase of spinal infections are : (i) aged population is rapidly growing, (ii) immunocompromized hosts are increasing due to the development of medical management, (iii) patients with diabetes mellitus are increasing, and (iv) there are increasing numbers of spinal surgeries in recent years. Spinal infection sometimes leads patients to serious general conditions, which have significant impacts not only on the patients but also on their relatives and societies.[3] Since conventional spinal surgeries for spinal infection are too invasive to those with multiple comorbid medical problems, there have been significant needs for both patients and medical care providers to develop less invasive surgical procedures for spinal infection. In this chapter, a minimally invasive treatment using percutaneous posterolateral spinal endoscopic procedures will be introduced and discussed.

Treatment Options for Spinal Infection

The principle of treatments for spinal infection is administration of antibiotics which are effective to the causative organisms. By taking culture samples from blood or tissues from the infected sites, the causative organisms and optimal antibiotics are to be determined before starting treatments. For most common forms of pyogenic spinal infection, the first generation of Cephalosporins should be administered intravenously with a relatively high dose by an interval of 6 hours. A recent animal study showed that even Linezolid, the most effective drug with a small molecule size for MRSA infection, does not penetrate into the intervertebral disk due to its avascular nature.[4] Any interventions, therefore, will be needed to enhance the blood flow to the intervertebral disk to obtain better penetration of antibiotics for effective treatment of spondylodiskitis.

Conventional major surgical treatments consisting of debridement of infected tissues followed by bone grafting and spinal instrumentation have been indicated for patients who have severe destructive changes at the anterior column with progression of local kyphosis and epidural abscess causing neurological deteriorations.[5] Since the anterior column of the spine is the primary focus in most cases of spinal infection,[6] anterior debridement and anterior fusion with iliac bone or fibula have been considered as the best surgical option for treatment of spinal infection. Though the use of spinal instrumentation has been advocated especially for patients with tuberculous spinal infection, there are increasing numbers of articles showing that the metal implants can be used even for patients with pyogenic infections if complete debridement of infected tissues can be conducted.[7-9] However, complication rates related to these spinal reconstruction surgeries in patients with pyogenic spinal infection and multiple comorbidities were reported very high exceeding 40%.[10]

There has been a minimally invasive treatment for spinal infection to drain the abscess by placing and leaving a tube at the area of infection.[11] This procedure is effective to reduce the pressure inside the abscess and bring rapid pain reduction to the patients. Another benefit of this procedure is able to take tissue samples directly from the infection sites for culture examinations. A limitation of this procedure, however, is a difficulty in curetting the bony endplates of the surrounding vertebral bodies and increasing the penetration of antibiotics in the intervertebral disk by enhancing blood flow. Therefore, there has been a significant need for any kinds of minimally invasive procedures, which can enhance the blood flow at the sites of infection.

Application of Percutaneous Endoscopic Lumbar Diskectomy (PELD) for Debridement of Infected Tissues

Percutaneous endoscopic diskectomy originated from Hijikata's percutaneous lumbar diskectomy.[12] His technique was adopted by Kambin and Yeung in the United States of America and revised to the posterolateral spinal endoscopic system named by "YESS" which stands for "Yeung's Endoscopic Spinal System".[13,14] This system allows surgeons to use holmium YAG laser, radiofrequency, automated shavers as well as many types of rongeurs. This technique has been widely spread in many Asian countries except Japan for treatment of lumbar disk herniation.

The benefits of this procedure for treatment of spinal infection are, (i) debridement of infected tissues can be done with a 1 cm skin incision, (ii) curettage of bony endplates and vertebral bodies around the infection site is possible so that blood flow can be enhanced in the intervertebral disk, which enables better infiltration of antibiotics at the site of infection, (iii) a bipotal technique can allow surgeons to perform irrigation and drainage at the same time, (iv) drain tubes can be placed at the end of the procedure so that postoperative drainage at the site of infection can be maintained, (v) this procedure is minimally invasive so that it can be applied even for patients with multiple comorbid medical problems, and (vi) direct sampling of the infected tissues can increase the possibility to identify the causative organisms.

The indications of PELD for spinal infection include any types of spinal infections such as pyogenic, tuberculous or non-tuberculous mycobacterial, fungal or others.[15-17] The best indication is an early phase of spinal infection with minimal destructive changes of the spinal column. If non-surgical treatments using antibiotics and orthosis were not successful in one or two weeks, this technique can be an excellent option to identify the causative organisms and make effective debridement possible at the infected sites in a minimally invasive way.

Surgical Procedures of PELD for Spinal Infection[15]

Selection of Patients

Patients with spinal infection at the thoracic and lumbar spine without either severe destructive changes or severe local kyphosis are best candidates for this surgery. This surgery is not indicated for patients with cervical spinal infection, because the safety of this procedure for the cervical spine is not validated yet. And those with severe destructive changes and presence of severe local kyphosis at the thoracolumbar spine are not the candidates for this surgery due to a high possibility of progression of local kyphosis after this procedure at the thoracolumbar junction with severe destructive changes. For these patients, it is more reliable to perform conventional spinal reconstruction surgery using iliac bone or fibula to reconstruct the collapsed anterior spinal column. For those with spondylodiskitis with severe destructive changes at the lower lumbar spine, however, PELD can be a good treatment option because postoperative collapse would not be of clinical problem in the lower lumbar spine, which may be due to the significant load-sharing on the posterior elements of the spine, not on the anterior column in this area.

Surgical Approach to the Sites of Infection

For treatment of the lumbar spine, forty-five degree oblique angle is the best direction to place the surgical tools at the sites of infection. The reason for this is that forty-five degree can allow surgeons to access and debride the largest area of the infected intervertebral disks. To obtain this insertion angle, the insertion points of the surgical tools should be marked on the skin surface in the lumbar spine 8 – 10 cm away from the midline. If its trajectory is too steep, the surgical tools would reach only the lateral parts of the spine and the disks could not be resected efficiently. If the trajectory is too shallow, there is an increasing risk to damage the neural structures. The basic principle is that the surgical tools should be placed at the triangular working zone, which is formed by the exiting nerve root, traversing nerve root and transverse process. If the disk space is severely collapsed on radiographs, however, the safest way to the exiting nerve roots is to place a working sleeve from the base of the caudal transverse process and then retract the exiting nerve root to the cephalad direction. For infections at L5/S1, large facet joints and wide transverse process sometimes hinder the placement of the surgical tools. Under these circumstances, bony surface of the ala should be resected with trephines to make a room for surgical tools. Though removal of the L5 transverse process is another choice, the surgeons should keep in mind that the L5 nerve root is located just underneath the transverse process. For patients with infection at the thoracic spine, the insertion point of the surgical tools should be more medial than that for the lumbar spine. The points of 4 – 5 cm away from the midline are recommended after checking preoperative CT images of the thoracic spine. The location of the aorta and relation between the path of the surgical tools and the lung should be checked by preoperative CT images. A single portal approach, not from the side of the aorta but from the contralateral side of it, is safe to those with spinal infection at the middle thoracic spine.

Anesthesia

For treatment for the lumbar spine, intravenous anesthesia using diazepam and fentanyl is used in combination with local anesthesia. The reason for keeping a patient awake is to make sure of the safety to the lumbar nerve roots. As soon as the surgical instruments touch the nerve roots, the patient can quickly respond to the irritation to the nerves. The outermost annulus at the infected intervertebral disk is inflamed and so sensitive that it produces significant pain when touched by the surgical instruments. The surgeon should ask the anesthesiologist to deepen anesthesia with adding intravenous anesthetics while touching the outermost annulus during procedures. Once the cannula passed the outermost annulus and the working sleeve is firmly placed on the annulus away from the neural structures, patients can be put to sleep with a higher dose of anesthetics.

Settings of Operation Room

A patient is placed prone on a U-shaped frame on a Jackson table. A C-arm is used for AP and lateral image controls. If the surgeon stands on the left side of the patient, the displays of C-arm and endoscopy should be located on the opposite side (Fig. 10.1). A biportal approach is recommended for better debridement of infected tissues and to make outflow of the irrigation water on one side and inflow on the other side. For the thoracic spine, it is safe not to place the portal on the side of the aorta.

Surgical Procedures (Figs 10.1 and 10.2)

A disk needle, a guide wire, a dilator and a working sleeve is securely placed successively. Once a working sleeve is correctly placed at the posterolateral corner of the disk, an endoscopy is inserted into the working sleeve to make sure that a nerve root is not seen in the endoscopic view. A thinner trephine is inserted to penetrate the annulus, which is followed by a thicker trephine to make a bigger hole for insertion of rongures and other surgical devices. The tips of the instruments should be monitored frequently by lateral view of C-arm. Debridement of infected disk materials and removal endplates should be done as much as possible and then shavers are used to remove more bone from the adjacent vertebral bodies. For the lumbar spine, the trajectory of the working sleeve should be 45 degrees oblique in order to allow surgeons to achieve maximum debridement of infected sites. For the thoracic spine, the insertion point of the surgical tool is more medical than that for the lumbar spine, which can be determined by the preoperative planning based on CT images. After removal of infected tissues as much as possible thorough the two portals, pressurized irrigation with more than two litters of saline should be carried out. Complete connection between the both portals at a disk level is important for irrigation at the infected sites. One portal is used for inflow and the other is for outflow of the water. After irrigation, a drain tube with 5 mm in thickness is inserted through a portal. Then another drain tube is placed on the other side if needed. Though continuous irrigation can be done postoperatively, the needs for postoperative continuous irrigation may not be so high after this minimally invasive procedure. In our series, postoperative continuous irrigation was done for only 2 patients out of 100 patients, who had a significant wide range of infection involving multiple vertebral bodies and surrounding tissues.

Postoperative Management

A patient can ambulate with a soft lumbar orthosis or a hard TLSO at postoperative one day according to the general conditions. The type of orthosis is dependent on the degree of preoperative destructive changes of the spine. Drain tubes are placed for 1 or 2 weeks according the amount of pus and exudate. In most patients with pyogenic spondylodiskitis, the tubes can be removed within 2 weeks because the amount of pus will decrease day by day after surgery. On the other hand, for tuberculous infection, the duration of drain tube placement may become much longer than that for pyogenic infection. Since drain tubes are placed just below the exiting nerve roots and progression of local kyphosis at the level of infection may occur, the most frequent complication after PELD procedure is irritation to the nerve roots by drain tubes. If the irritation to the nerves became evident, drain tubes should be removed immediately not to lead to neurological deficits.

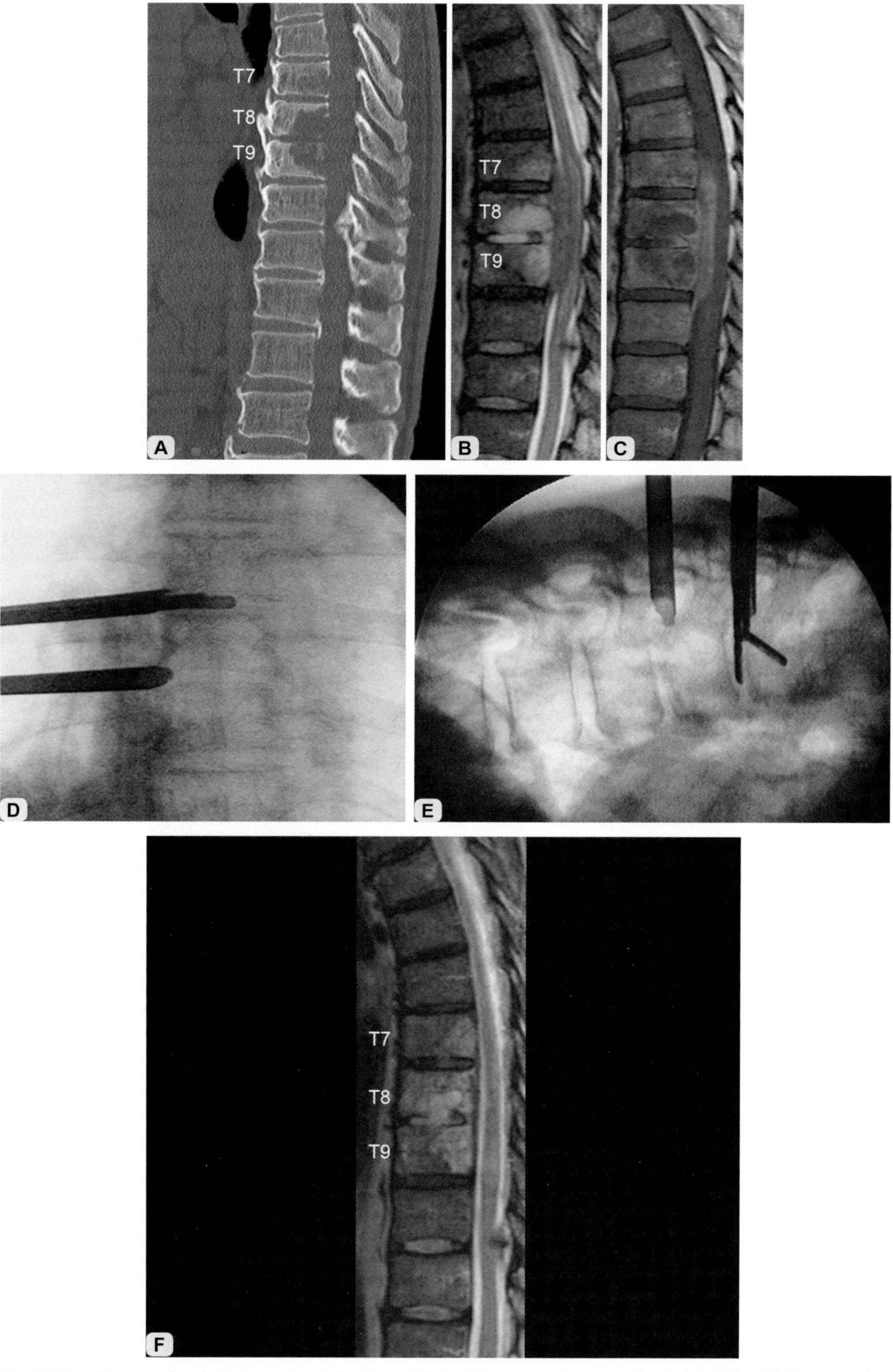

Fig. 10.1 61 years of male. Tuberculous infection at T7-9 with progressive neurological deficits. (A) Preoperative CT image showed bony lesions at T7 to T10 without local kyphosis; (B) Preoperative T1 weighted MR image showed epidural abscess compressing the thoracic spinal cord; (C) Preoperative Gd enhancement image showed typical rim-enhancement; (D) AP view of intraoperative C-arm to make sure of the location of the tip of instrument; (E) Lateral view of intraoperative C-arm; (F) T2 weighted MR sagittal image at postoperative 1 month showed complete disappearance of epidural abscess and there was no sign of further progression of kyphotic deformity

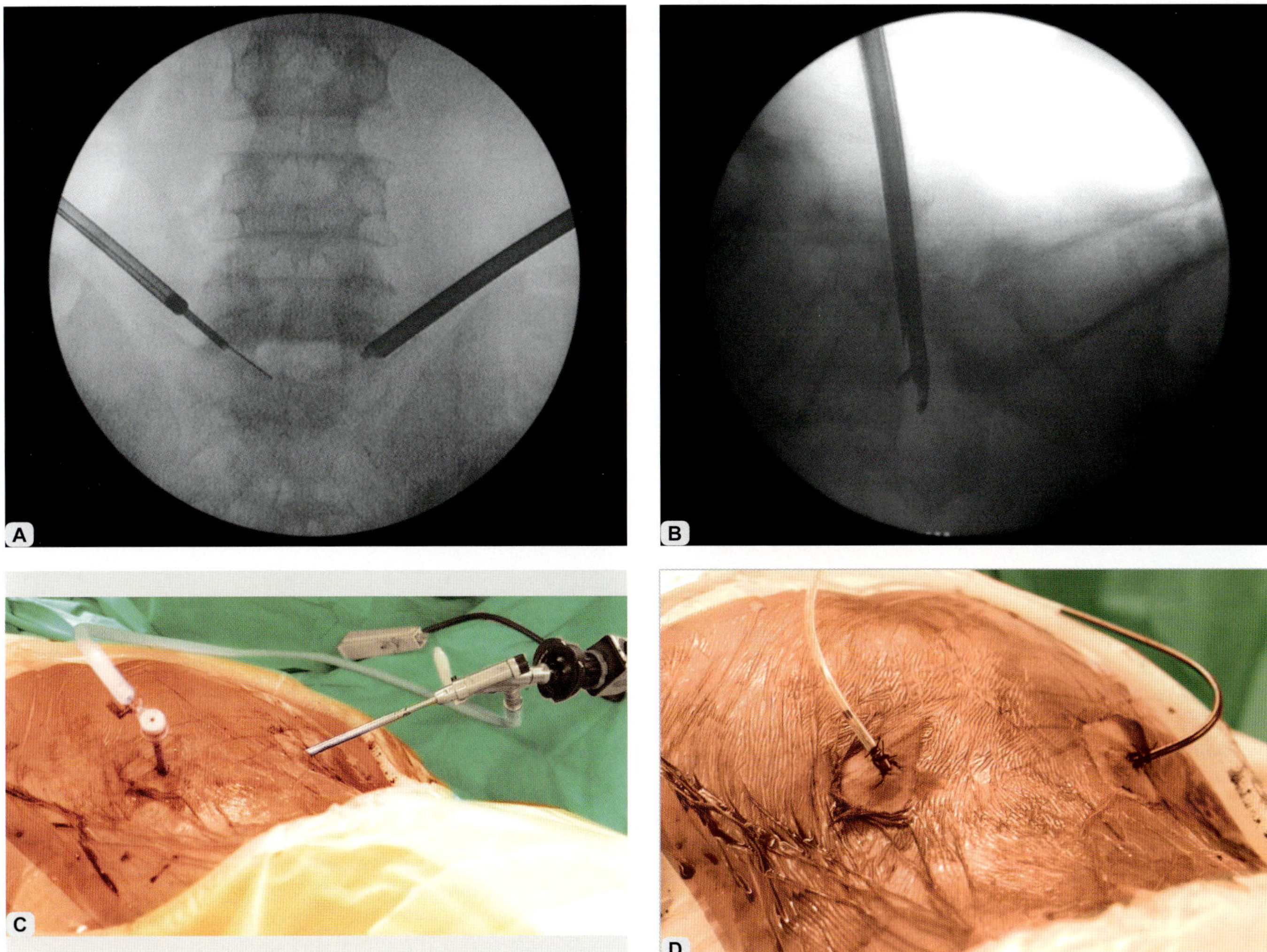

Fig. 10.2 Percutaneous posterolateral endoscopic spinal surgery. (A) Placement of surgical tools for L5/S1. The tools should be placed below the L5 nerve roots; (B) Debridement of infected disk materials and curettage of endplates should be done to make sure of bleeding from the surrounding intact bone; (C) Irrigation should be performed by two portals, one of which is for in-flow of water and the other for out-flow; (D) Drain tubes are placed at the end of the procedures

Clinical Results

Seventy patients with spinal infections had been treated in our institute from the beginning of 2001 to the end of 2008. The areas of infection were the thoracic spine in 5 patients, the thoracolumbar spine in 10, the lumbar spine in 43 and the lumbosacral spine in 12. There were 44 patients who had comorbid medical problems, such as malignant tumor, collagen disease treated with long-term steroids, diabetes mellitus, and others. CRP rated 4.65 mg/dL in average before surgery, 1.59 mg/dL at postoperative 1 week and 0.73 mg/dL at postoperative 2 weeks. Low back pain dramatically dropped down from 86/100 before surgery to 26/100 at postoperative 1 week. Causative organisms were successfully detected by this procedure in 49 patients out of 10 (detection rate: 70%). Seventeen patients (35%) were MRSA infection. During follow-up, relapse of spinal infection was observed in 7 patients (10%) who had serious comorbid medical problems, such as malignancy and collagen diseases. In terms of surgery-related complications, five patients showed nerve root irritation due to the placement of drain tubes, which recovered completely after removing them. Four patients needed additional spinal reconstruction surgery due to the progression of local kyphosis at the surgical sites, most of which were severe destructive changes at the thoracolumbar junction before surgery.

Discussion

Minimally invasive spinal surgery can be a treatment option for patients with poor general conditions due to their serious medical problems. Conventional spinal reconstruction surgery using bone graft and instrumentation for spinal infections had high complication rates exceeding 40%.[10] Our minimally invasive technique could lower the complication rates down to 13% and there were no serious complications at postoperative periods. Since there are difficulties to maintain the general conditions of these ill patients after conventional major surgery, this minimally invasive approach to spinal infection is of benefit not only for patients but also for medical care providers who are taking care of the patients after surgery.

There have been clinical reports of percutaneous drainage for pyogenic spinal infections.[12] Most of these reports showed favorable clinical outcomes and less complication rates compared to conventional major surgical treatments. The limitation of this procedure is that it cannot enhance blood flow at the infection sites due to its inability to curette the endplates and vertebral bodies. The intervertebral disk is avascular, and it is difficult to distribute antibiotics to the entire intervertebral dicks only with intravenous administration.[4] Even brand new antibiotics, such as Linezolid, could not be delivered to the nucleus pulposus and annuls fibrosis.[4] Avascular nature of the intervertebral disk hinders the effects of antibiotics and makes it difficult to cure spinal infection. By curetting the endplates and vertebral bodies around the infection site to induce bleeding, the concentration of antibiotics could increase over the MIC (minimally inhibitory concentration) which may have a higher possibility to subside spinal infection.

This new endoscopic procedure is best indicated for the early phase of spinal infection regardless of organisms. Our clinical results showed that not only pyogenic but also tuberculous and even fungal infections can be treated successfully by this minimally invasive endoscopic procedure. In spite of the benefit of this procedure, spinal infection with severe destructive changes is out of indication. These conditions should be treated with conventional bone grafting and spinal instrumentation to restore spinal alignment and provide the collapsed spine with better stability.

The basic principle for treatment of spinal infection is to use of the most sensitive antibiotics to the target organism from the early beginning of treatment.[18] Without using effective antibiotics, spinal infection cannot be eradicated. This minimally invasive endoscopic procedure helps antibiotics penetrate into the entire disk spaces more efficiently than without. This procedure is applicable not only to primary spinal infections but also to postsurgical spinal infections.[19]

Conclusion

This chapter introduces a minimally invasive percutaneous posterolateral endoscopic debridement and irrigation procedure for various kinds of spinal infections. This procedure is best indicated for patients with an early phase of spinal infection. To identify the causative organisms and debride the infected tissues, this procedure can be applied for patients when conventional conservative treatments become ineffective in 1 or 2 weeks. This procedure can be applied for patients with multiple comorbid medical problems, because this procedure does not put any harm to those with poor general conditions.

References

1. Grammatico L, et al. Epidemiology of vertebral osteomyelitis (VO) in France: analysis of hospital-discharge data 2002-2003. Epidemiol Infec. 2007;136:653-60.
2. Pigrau C, et al. Spontaneous pyogenic vertebral osteomyelitis and endocarditis: incidence, risk factors, and outcome. Am J Med. 2005;118:1287,e17.
3. Hadjipavlou, A.G., et al. Hematogenous pyogenic spinal infections and their surgical management. Spine. 2000;25:1668-79.
4. Komatsu M, et al. Penetration of linezolid into rabbit intervertebral discs and surrounding tissues. Eur Spine J. 2010;19(12):2149-55.
5. Myloma E, et al. Vertebral osteomyelitis: a systematic review of clinical characteristics. Semin Arthritis Rheum. 2009;39(1):10-7.
6. Emery SE, et al. Treatment of hematogenous pyogenic vertebral osteomyelitis with anterior debridement and primary bone grafting. Spine. 1989;14(3):284-91.
7. Fukuta,S. et al. Two-stage(posterior and anterior) surgical treatment using posterior spinal instrumentation for pyogenic and tuberculotic spondylitis. Spine. 2003;28:E302-8.
8. Oga M, et al. Evaluation of the risk of instrumentation as a foreign body in spinal tuberculosis. Clinical and biologic study. Spine. 1993;18(13):1890-4.
9. Carragee EJ, Iezza A. Does acute placement of instrumentation in the treatment of vertebral osteomyelitis predispose to recurrent infection: long-term follow-up in immune-suppressed patients. Spine. 2008;33(19):2089-93.
10. Carragee EJ. Instrumentation of the infected and unstable spine. A review of 17 cases from the thoracic and lumbar spine with pyogenic infections. J Spinal Disord. 1997;10:317-24.

11. Yu WY, et al. Percutaneous suction aspiration for osteomyelitis. Report of two cases. Spine. 1991;16(2):198-202.
12. Hijikata S. Percutaneous nucleotomy. A new concept technique and 12 years' experience. Clin Orthop Relat Res. 1989;238:9-23.
13. Kambin P, et al. Transforaminal arthroscopic decompression of lateral recess stenosis. J Neurosurg. 1996;84(3):462-7.
14. Yeung AT. Minimally invasive disc surgery with the Yeung endoscopic spine system. Orthopaedic Surgery. Surg Tech Inter 8. 1999;P1-11.
15. Ito M, et al. Clinical outcome of posterolateral endoscopic surgery for pyogenic spondylodiscitis. Results of 15 patients with serious comorbid conditions. Spine. 2007;32(2):200-6.
16. Ito M, et al. Minimally invasive surgical treatment for tuberculous spondylodiscitis. Minim Invasive Neurosurg. 2009;52(5-6):250-3.
17. Iwata A, et al. Fungal Spinal Infection Treated with Percutaneous Posterolateral Endoscopic Surgery -A report of four cases-. Minim Invasive Neurosurg. In press 2012.
18. Brodke DS, et al. Infections of the spine. Chapter38. Orthopedic Knowledge Update Spine 3 (ed by Spivak JM et al), AAOS. 2006;367-75.
19. Jimenez-Mejias ME, et al. Postoperarive spondilodiskitis: etiology, clinical findings, prognosis, and comparison with nonoperative spondylodiskitis. Clin Infect Dis. 1999;29:339-45.

CHAPTER

11

Microendoscopic Decompression Using Tubular Retractor System for Lumbar Canal Stenosis

Arvind G Kulkarni, Sambhav Shah

Introduction

Lumbar canal stenosis is the leading cause of leg pain in elderly patients. Lumbar canal decompression is the commonest spinal operation in this age group. Microendoscopic decompression provides minimal access posterior lumbar decompression through a 2 cm incision with minimal bone removal and soft tissue trauma. Decompression of the central canal as well as ipsilateral and contralateral lateral recesses and foramina can be adequately carried out through the same portal.[1-6]

Indications and Contraindications

Lumbar canal stenosis is secondary to ligamentum flavum hypertrophy, facet arthropathy with hypertrophy and osteophyte formation. Central canal, subarticular and lateral recess stenosis can be decompressed using this technique with minimal bone removal, thus, maintaining stability of the motion segment. Large synovial cysts can also be safely addressed. It is contraindicated in cases of stenosis associated with instability. However, selected cases of grade I degenerative spondylolisthesis with no demonstrable instability is not a contraindication. Inexperience with the procedure can lead to inadequate decompression and complications.

Advantages

Being a minimally invasive procedure there is less soft tissue trauma as compared to conventional decompression. This is evident by low levels of Interleukin 6 and C-RP levels (markers of inflammation) in patients operated using the tubular system[1,2] in comparison to open surgery or microlumbar surgery. Decompression is achieved without stripping any soft tissue and injury to the posterior ligamentous complex, thus aiding stability (Fig. 11.1). Decompression of the central canal and bilateral lateral recesses and foramina can be achieved through one keyhole. The contralateral anatomy is thus preserved. The side of port of entry is chosen based on patient symptoms, facet inclination on the axial MRI and spinal alignment.

Minimal morbidity and pain as well as excellent cosmesis are hallmarks of this procedure. There is minimal blood loss, almost zero-infection rate, reduced hospital stay and cost. Patients can be mobilized in a few hours (2 – 3 hours) following the surgery. It is cosmetically more appealing whilst accomplishing the same goal.[3,4] The greatest beneficiaries of this procedure are patients with high BMI, who would otherwise need long incisions even

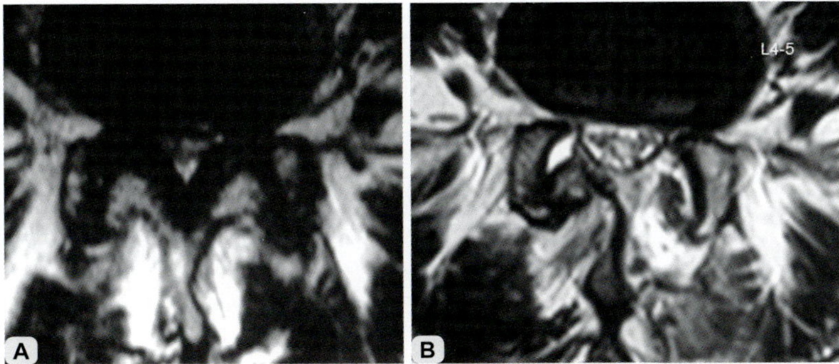

Fig. 11.1 (A) Preoperative axial MRI showing severe central canal and lateral recess stenosis bilaterally; (B) Postoperative MRI showing adequate decompression bilaterally while maintaining soft tissue and posterior ligamentous and bony integrity

for a single level surgery. It also avoids a wrong level surgery as the entry of the tubular retractor is done under image intensifier guidance.

Disadvantages and Complications

There is a steep learning curve to this procedure. Initially the surgical time and complications may be higher. However, with experience decompression can be safely and quickly performed. Small dural tears can be managed with masterly inactivity, but large tears may need the usage of fibrin glue to seal the tear (Fig. 11.2). A laterally placed portal can lead to violation of the medial facet while executing ipsilateral decompression requiring fusion. Surgery can also be time consuming if multilevel decompression is required with more exposure to radiation. Spinous process fracture may occur while drilling the base. Special instrument sets are required to carry out this procedure.

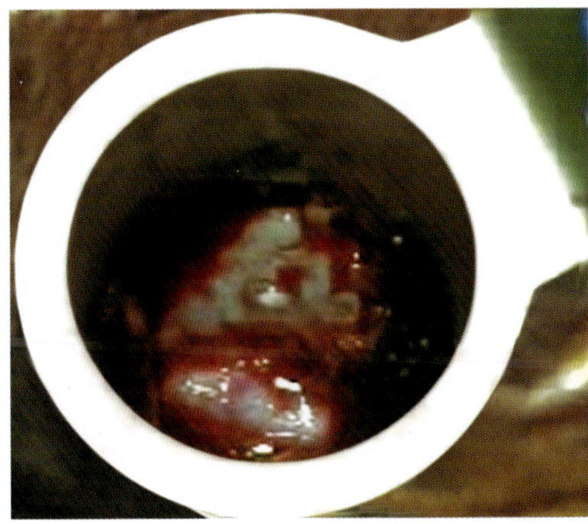

Fig. 11.2 Intraoperative image showing dural tear and glistening CSF

Preoperative Workup

MRI is mandatory before operating upon the patient to identify the location of stenosis. Presence of dynamic instability on preoperative radiographs and MRI is a contraindication to this procedure. The surgeon should be precise about the location of the pathology as the exposure is limited. A thorough clinical examination should be done and should correlate with the radiographic findings.

Anesthesia

General anesthesia.

Position

Patient is positioned on a radiolucent table in prone position with bolsters below the chest and iliac crest keeping the abdomen free to reduce intravenous pressure in the epidural plexus. A head high of 10 – 15 degrees should be given to avoid venous engorgement in the eyes (Fig. 11.3). The foot end of the table should be flexed as the patient may slip off, as the head end of the table is raised. Pressure points should be well padded. Patient should be firmly strapped to the table to avoid slippage while turning the table. Breaking the table at the level of the surgery helps in opening up the interlaminar area. The surgeon should stand on the side that he chooses to decompress depending on the MRI findings and the leg symptoms. Lateral recess decompression is

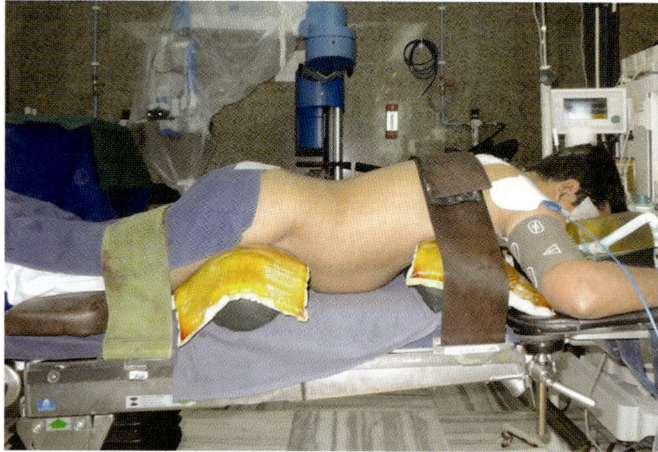

Fig. 11.3 Patient positioning—10 – 15 degree head prevents venous engorgement in the eyes and keeps the working portal perpendicular, especially at L4 – 5 and L5 – S1 owing to the lordosis

easier achieved by approaching from the opposite side as it provides a better trajectory. The table mount and flexible arm of the tubular system should be tightly secured before the incision.

Technique

Using lateral fluoroscopy imaging a 20 G spinal needle is inserted at the level of the involved disk space bisecting it. The needle is inserted about 1.2 cm lateral to the midline and position confirmed with image intensifier. About 5 cc of 0.5% bupivacaine diluted in 15 cc of saline is infiltrated for preemptive analgesia. A 2 cm incision is then centered over the needle and deepened till the fascia. Although the diameter of the tube (working portal) is 18 mm, it is better to take a slightly longer (2 cm) incision to get a better looking scar. A guidewire with a blunt end is then inserted under fluoroscopy guidance. The target site is the inferior lamina of the superior vertebrae. Initial dilator is then inserted over the guidewire and the wire is removed. The initial dilator is used to sweep off the paraspinal muscle mass and palpate the bony landmarks (Fig. 11.4). The spinous process medially and the facet joint complex laterally are felt as two mountains with the lamina as the valley in-between. Sequential dilators are then inserted while confirming the target site under fluoroscopy. The dilators have graduations marked on them to determine the depth of the tube. The marking on the final dilator at the level of skin provides the depth of the tubular retractor. If the marking is between 4 and 5 then a no 5 tubular retractor should be used. Tubular retractor, which is 18 mm in diameter, is then docked with the flexible arm as the final working channel. The working channel should be kept as perpendicular to the floor to

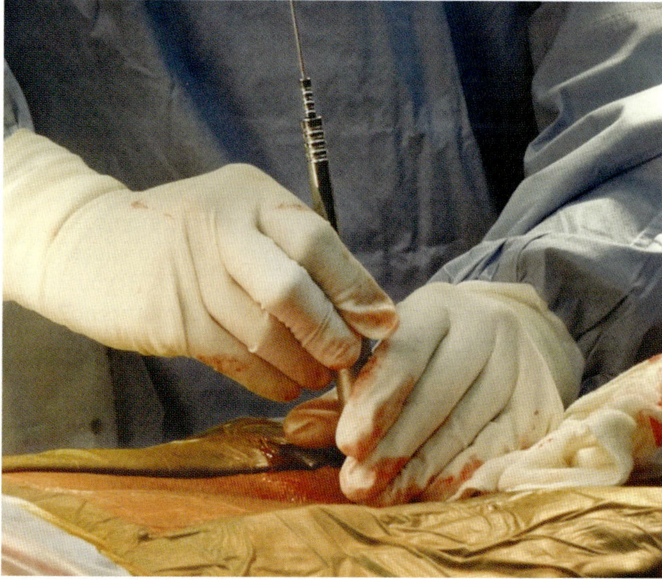

Fig. 11.4 Insertion of serial dilators over guidewire

maintain an easy working position for the surgeon. This can be achieved by raising the head end of the table. This is essential for decompressing the L4 – 5 and L5 – S1 levels owing to the lumbar lordosis. Microscope is then brought into the field (Fig. 11.5). As an alternative an endoscopic camera can also be attached to the tubular retractor.

Soft tissue is separated using a long cautery tip till the lamina can be visualized. An excellent exposure is one, wherein a part of the inferior lamina and flavum is visualized (Fig. 11.6). Lamina is then burred using a 4 mm cutting burr, till the junction of the inner cortex and ligamentum flavum is encountered (Fig. 11.7A). Flavum is separated from the lamina by using a bayonet-handle angled curette. Ipsilateral laminotomy is completed using a no 2 Kerrison ronguer, leaving the flavum intact. Intact flavum protects the dural sac from injury whilst drilling the opposite side. In order to decompress the opposite side the line of vision must extend underneath the spinous process and interspinous ligament across the midline. This is achieved by, aiming the tubular retractor medially and tilting the table away from the operating surgeon, towards the opposite side (Wanding). This helps in providing a better visualization of the lateral recess of the contralateral side. The inner cortex of the contra-lateral lamina till the hypertrophied medial margins of the opposite facet joint are drilled with a high-speed burr, beginning at the base of the spinous processes and proceeding laterally within the canal (Fig. 11.7B). This de-roofs the canal and exposes the flavum entirely. The insertion of the flavum is then detached using a no 4 Penfield. The intervening ligamentum flavum is removed piece meal thus decompressing the dural sac and the

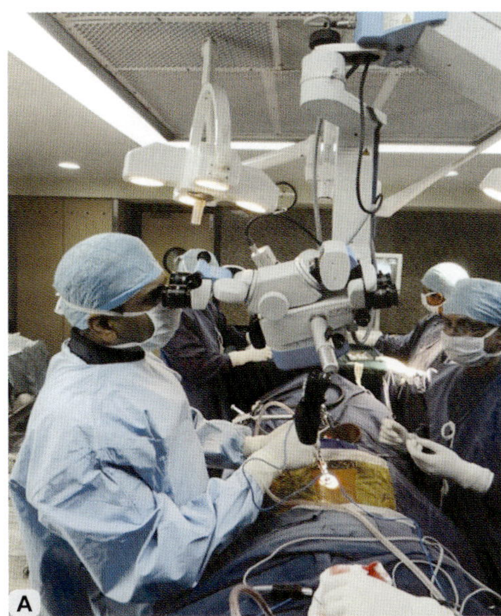

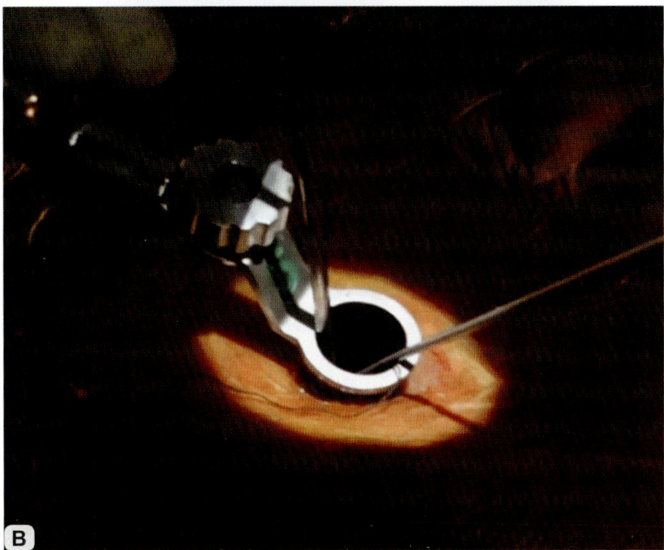

Fig. 11.5 (A) Intraoperative picture showing microscope set up and positioning of surgeon and staff; (B) Working portal -18 mm diameter tube

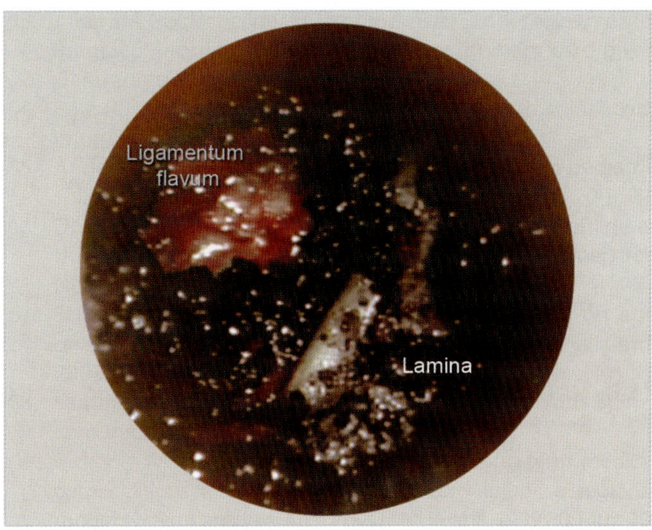

Fig. 11.6 Target site while inserting the dilators – inferior portion of the superior lamina

opposite side nerve toot. This successive resection is carried laterally until the contralateral caudal pedicle is visualized. Using a curved Kerrison the lateral recess is decompressed effectively. A dural retractor or a nerve hook can be used to confirm if adequate decompression has been achieved. The nerve root is traced form its exit from the dura till it exits out of the foramen (Fig. 11.8). Changing the direction of the tube superiorly and inferiorly and tilting the operating table aids in achieving this (Fig. 11.9). This technique preserves the contralateral anatomy. The tube is then turned back medially and table turned towards the surgeon and the ipsilateral side is decompressed similarly. The nerve root on this side is similarly traced.

Bleeding is controlled using a combination of bipolar cautery, bone wax and gel-foam. Fascia and subcutaneous tissue are closed using 2 – 0 vicryl. Skin is closed using 3 – 0 monocryl. Steristrips are applied hold the skin edges together. Waterproof dressing is applied. If another level is

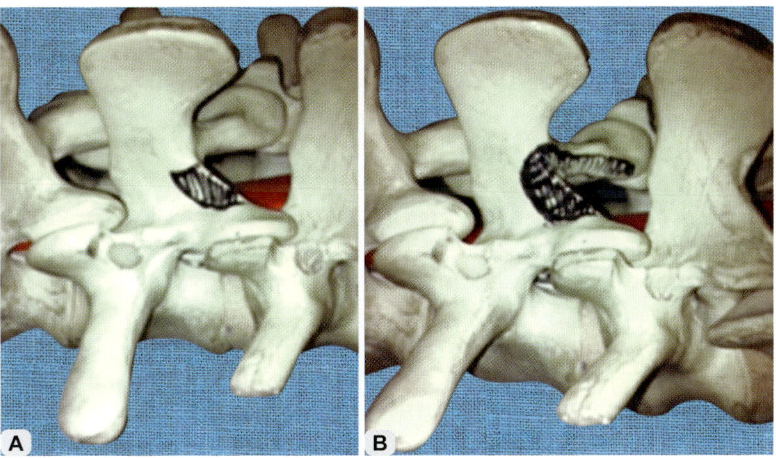

Fig. 11.7 Extent of bone to be removed for (A) Ipsilateral and (B) Contralateral decompression

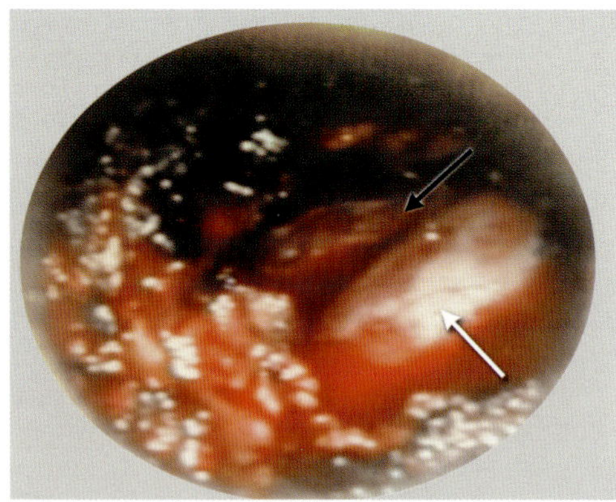

Fig. 11.8 Intraoperative picture after the tube was tilted medially and table tilted away from the surgeon (wanding). The base of spinous process and lamina are burred and flavum removed. Picture shows the dura (white arrow) with the contralateral nerve root (black arrow) decompressed and free

to be decompressed the same procedure is repeated again. It is sometimes possible to decompress L4 – 5 and L5 – S1 levels through the same incision owing to the lordosis.

Postoperative Schedule

Patient is mobilized the same evening and is discharged the next day. Only one dose of intravenous antibiotic is given the same night. Injectable analgesics are given on the day of surgery and oral antibiotics the next day onwards. Patient is weaned off oral analgesics by the 5th day postoperatively. Bathing is allowed immediately. Patient is allowed to go back to light duty work and is not allowed to lift heavy weights after 10 days. A gradual back strengthening program is started after 6 weeks. The scar usually shrinks to a size of 1.0 – 1.5 cm after healing (about 3 months) (Fig. 11.10).

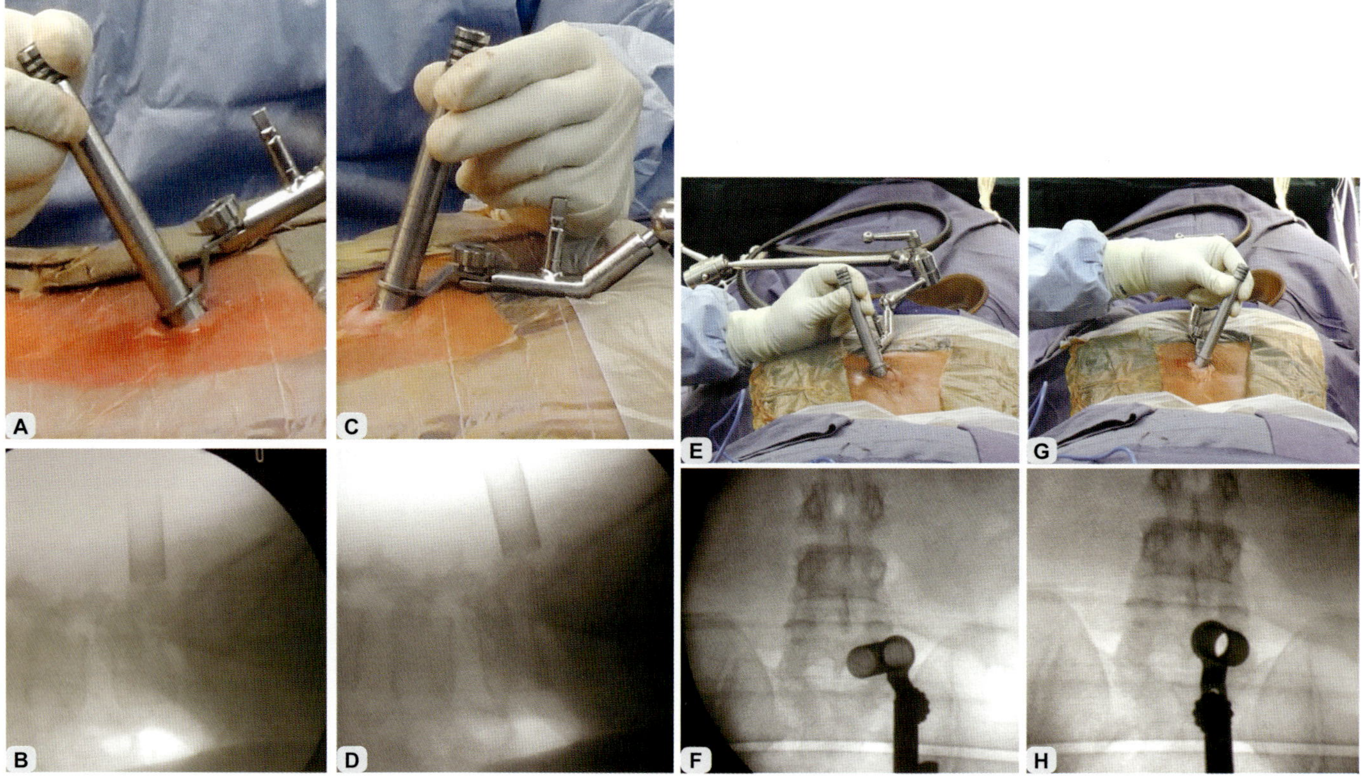

Fig. 11.9 The position of working portal can be shifted superiorly, inferiorly, medially and laterally, depending on the work area. Images showing different directions of the working channel, with intraoperative C-arm images

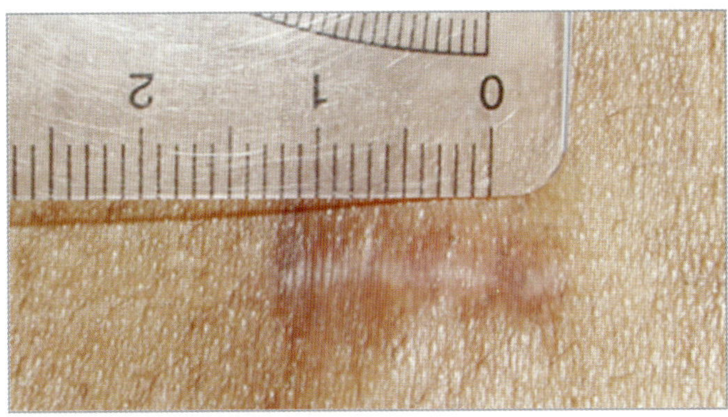

Fig. 11.10 Postoperatively final scar shrinks to 1 cm

Key Points

- Adequate contralateral decompression can be achieved through the same incision
- L4 – 5 and L5 – S1 levels may be approached through the same incision.
- Guidewire should be inserted with the blunt side as to avoid penetration in the canal.
- The tubular retractor should be deeply seated on the lamina and can be angulated in any direction.
- Patient should be tightly secured to the table to safely tilt the table.
- Small dural tears can be managed with masterly inactivity or by using fibrin glue. Large tears may require open surgical repair.
- Curved Kerrison rongeur aids in lateral recess decompression.
- Long and bayonet instruments are required for a better visual field through the microscope.

Must Have Instruments

1. Tubular dilators and retractors
2. Long bayonet instruments
3. Operating table that can tilt in all directions.
4. Curved Kerrison
5. Long cautery tip
6. High speed cutting burr
7. Nerve root retractor
8. Nerve hook
9. Gelfoam and long tip bipolar cautery
10. Fibrin glue.

References

1. Houten JK, Tandon A. Comparison of postoperative values for C-reactive protein in minimally invasive and open lumbar spinal fusion surgery. Surg Neurol Int. 2011;2:94.
2. Schick U et al. Microendoscopic Lumbar Discectomy versus open surgery: an introp EMG study. European Spine J. 2002;11(1):20-6.
3. Khoo LT, Fessler RG. Microendoscopic decompressive laminotomy for the treatment of lumbar stenosis. Neurosurgery. 2002;51:S146-54.
4. Katayama Y, Matsuyama Y, Yoshihara H, Sakai Y, Nakamura H, Nakashima S, et al. Comparison of surgical outcomes between macro discectomy and micro discectomy for lumbar disc herniation: A prospective randomized study with surgery performed by the same spine surgeon. J Spinal Disord Tech. 2006;19:344-7.
5. Larry Khoo, Fessler Richard. Microendoscopic Decompressive Laminotomy for the Treatment of Stenosis. Neurosurgery. 2002;Suppl 51:146-54.
6. David Rosen, John O, et al. Minimally invasive Lumbar Spinal Decompression in the Elderly. Outcomes of 50 patients aged 75 years and older. Neurosurgery. 2007;Suppl 60:503-10.

CHAPTER

12

How Much Cement is Enough for Vertebroplasty to Reduce Adjacent Vertebral Fractures in Osteoporotic Vertebral Fractures?

Arvind Bhave

Materials and Methods

Included patients were those suffering from subacute osteoporotic vertebral compression fractures (OVCF) of duration more than 4 weeks. Most of them were offered vertebroplasty, after having gained no relief from conservative treatment comprising of rest in bed, NSAIDs and braces. These patients had progressive increase in pain and disabilities.

Clinical Examination

1. Local bony tenderness over spinous process, indicating that the pain is attributable to the fractured vertebral level. VAS scores 7 or above for back pain affecting activities of daily living (ADL).
2. Detailed neurological examination to look for sensory and motor changes and radiculopathies to confirm that there is no neurologic deficit due to compression of spinal cord or nerves.

Investigations

1. *Laboratory tests:* Blood investigations for complete blood count, diabetes control and coagulation indices. Appropriate additional tests were done for the primary disease, if any, causing the OVCF.
2. *X-rays:* of the spine in AP and lateral views; preferably standing lateral view in flexion and extension.
3. *CT scan:* The CT scanning with 3D, sagittal and coronal reconstructions was done in a few cases as they were helpful in assessing the complex vertebral fractures. Thin reconstructed sections could show the fracture and the integrity of the posterior vertebral wall.
4. *MRI:* This is one of the most important investigations in the evaluation of the OVCF. Bone marrow edema or end plate edema seen on the MRI are important positive prognostic markers in the disease. The magnetic resonance tomogram is helpful to assess all the involved fracture levels, to define the inter-vertebral clefts, and to aid in giving information about pathological fractures. High density signals on T-2 weighted or short-tau inversion recovery (STIR) sequences signify intra osseous edema. (Fig. 12.1) Involvement of the pedicle or soft tissue or in epidural space may indicate malignancy or infection. Signal changes in the vertebral body are predictive of high positive outcome with vertebroplasty. STIR sequence is the most sensitive in identifying acute

fractures.

Imaging modality of choice is MRI of spine as it is:

- Highly sensitive
- Increased signals in T2 sequence indicate an acute fracture, because the edema causes an increased signal T1 STIR T2.[1-3] High intensity signal on STIR MRI has been shown to have a 100% association with the OVCF correction predictor for the vertebral body fracture correction.[4]

Results

Total 137 vertebroplasties in 104 patients were studied. 34 patients were males and 71 were females in the age group of 50 – 90 years. Levels operated were from D5 to L4 (Table 12.1).

The 137 levels operated were as depicted in Table 12.2.

All the vertebroplasties were done using continuous 'C' arm image guidance. Local anesthesia and sedation was used for all the patients. Devised used was 'AB needle for vertebroplasty'. Patients were advised 2 hours bed rest post-operatively. Most of them could use toilet facilities on the same day and were discharged on the next day. Average PMMA filled was 2.2 – 4.0 mL in thoracic vertebrae and about 3.5 – 5.0 cc in lumbar vertebrae, equivalent to about less than 30% but more than 16% volume of the vertebral bodies.

It can be seen (Table 12.3 and Fig. 12.1) that as compared to pre-procedural VAS pain score, there was significant ($p < 0.000$) reduction in VAS pain score among the patients immediately after 1 hour of the procedure, and it sustained even after 1 hour of the procedure. In other words, we can say that there was significant improvement in the pain of the patients after the procedure.

All the patients were followed up regularly every month for the next 3 months and then at 6 monthly intervals. They were examined clinically for local tenderness, reduction of pain [VAS scores] and follow up radiographs to confirm that there was no adjacent vertebral fracture. Minimum follow up was for 2 years and maximum follow up was for up to 8 years.

Discussion

Pain relief is main goal of Vertebroplasty. Incidence of new vertebral fractures in study by Lindsay and Silvermann stated 20% risk of new vertebral fractures in the first year.[5]

Table 12.1 Distribution of gender in the study population

Patients	*Males*	*Females*	*Total*
50-60 years	9	18	27
60-70 years	14	37	51
70-80 years	7	11	18
80-90 years	4	4	8
		Total	104

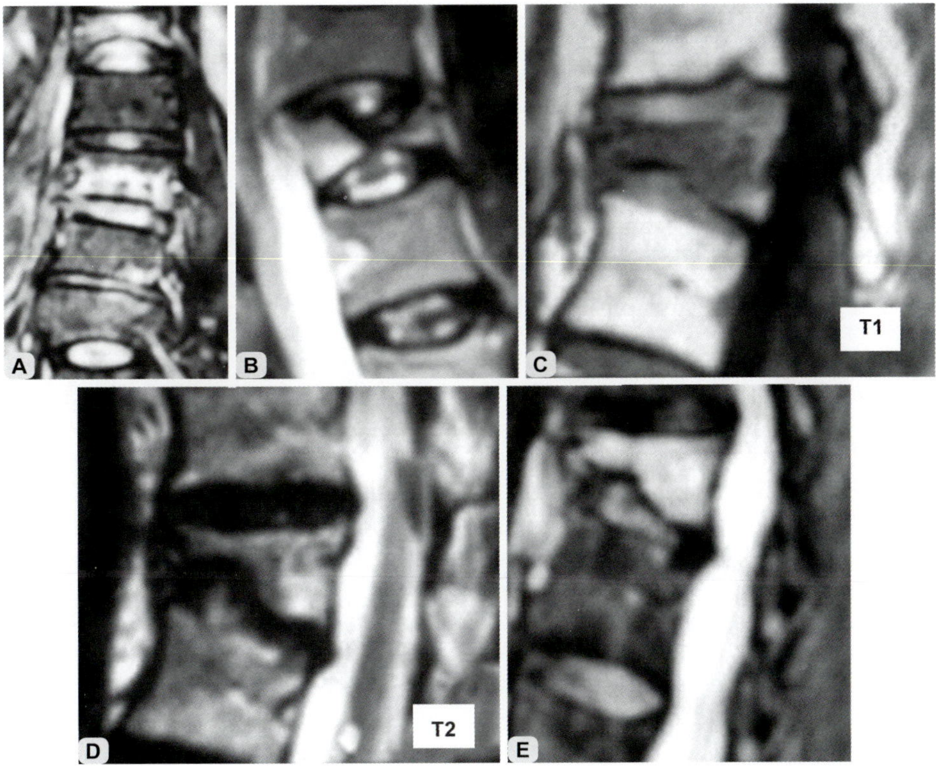

Fig. 12.1 MRI showing high density signals on T2-weighted or short-tau inversion recovery (STIR) sequences signify intraosseous edema

Table 12.2 Distribution of the study population according to the vertebral level at which the vertebroplasty was performed

vertebral level	*total*	*males*	*Female*
D5	2	1	1
D8	2	1	1
D10	6	2	4
D11	2	0	2
D12	41	15	26
L1	51	20	31
L2	14	3	11
L3	14	4	10
L4	5	0	5
	137		

Table 12.3 Pre- and postprocedural VAS pain scores (mean ± sd) among patients

	N	*VAS score*	*P **
Preprocedural	102	7.78 ± 0.64	
Postprocedural 1 hour	102	3.06 ± 1.12	0.000
2 days	102	2.16 ± 0.89	0.000
1 month	102	1.27 ± 0.63	0.000
3 month	100	0.66 ± 0.65	0.000
6 month	97	0.33 ± 0.52	0.000
1 year	97	0.14 ±0.38	0.000

* Significance compared with preprocedural VAS score

In another retrospective study by Uppin et al. the incidence of new vertebral fractures was 12% in 177 vertebroplasties over a 2-year follow-up.[6]

In a prospective study done by Lin et al. out of the total 38 patients who had undergone percutaneous vertebroplasty, the incidence of new vertebral compression fractures was 36% at 1 year of follow-up.[7]

In another prospective study, Voormolen et al. found that the incidence of new vertebral compression fractures at 1 year of follow-up was 24%.[8]

There is always a problem of how much cement to be injected while performing a vertebroplasty. One of the most important postprocedural risks is related to vertebral body over-augmentation. An excessive injection of cement may cause some biomechanical changes, including end-plate necrosis, leakage into the disk space, spinal canal and vascular area, and increased stiffness of the vertebral body leading to an increased stress on the adjacent level vertebrae, which may cause a new fracture. Therefore, some studies have focused on the optimal amount of the cement to be injected into the fractured vertebral body. In procedure-related fractures of adjacent vertebrae, end plates adjacent to the treated vertebra were more commonly found to be involved. Inferior end-plate fractures of the vertebra, rostral to the treated vertebra were commonly observed, in spite of the fact that such fractures were rare in the natural history of osteoporosis.[9]

Chen et al. studied incidence of the new adjacent vertebral fractures in vertebroplasties with and without cement leaks and followed for 24 months postoperatively. The mean cement injected in their series was 6.78 mL (range: 2 to 18 mL). They found adjacent vertebral fractures in 20 (18.9%) of 106 patients and at 22 adjacent vertebral bodies after PV. In the group which had cement leakage in the disk space 42% had new adjacent level fractures.[10]

Biomechanical data that support such a relationship claimed that the local spinal segment surrounding the treated vertebra may be weakened due to several factors. First, vertebroplasty increased the stiffness of the treated vertebra that altered the load transfer to noncemented adjacent vertebrae. Second, intravertebral cement increased the impact on adjacent endplates and disk spaces caused by the resistance of endplates of treated vertebra to inward bowing.[11]

Liebschner et al. reported that vertebral stiffness recovery after vertebroplasty was strongly influenced by the volume fraction of the implanted PMMA. Only a small amount of bone cement (14% fill or 3.5 cm^3) was necessary to restore stiffness of the damaged vertebral body to the predamaged value.[12] Using of a 30% fill increased stiffness by more than 50% compared with the predamaged value. They concluded that only a small amount of PMMA (approximately 15% volume fraction) was needed to restore stiffness to predamage levels and greater filling could result in substantial increase in stiffness well beyond the intact level. Using finite element model techniques, Liebschner et al. studied L1 fractures. They found that small amount of bone cement, 14% fill or about 3.5 mm^3 PMMA, was necessary to restore stiffness of the damaged vertebral body to predamaged value. Using 30% fill increased stiffness by more than 50% as compared to the predamaged value. Vertebral stiffness recovery was strongly influenced by the volume fraction of the implanted cement, and less so by its distribution. The least amount of bone cement, 4% volume fraction, restored stiffness to within 10% of the intact value. 14% volume fill restored the vertebral stiffness to its intact value. The maximum volume of cement increased stiffness to almost 50% above the intact value.[12]

In an interesting article titled 'Volume matters: a review of procedural details of two randomized controlled vertebroplasty trials of 2009' by Bronek **Boszczyk**,[13] quoted reference of the study by Molloy S, Mathis JM, Belkoff SM[14] (Table 12.4).

The first column of numbers provides average vertebral body volume per level in ml as determined by Molloy et al.

Table 12.4 The average vertebral body volumes determined by Molloy et al. at different levels and the estimated 16% of the volume

Vertebral level	*Average volume [mL]*	*16% volume [mL]*
T6	12.3	2
T7	13.9	2.2
T8	19.3	3.1
T9	20.6	3.3
T10	23.4	4.4
T11	27.4	4.4
T12	31.9	5.1
L1	33.9	5.4
L2	40.3	6.5
L3	42	6.7
L4	44	7
L5	44.8	7.2

The second column of numbers provides the calculated minimum required (16%) fill volume per level in mL for restoration of vertebral strength.

Kaufmann et al.[15] retrospectively analyzed 158 cases of percutaneous vertebroplasty and thought of minimum amount of cement injected without leak can give optimum clinical results. Any increase in the cement volume can lead to complications. The PMMA cement volumes injected in their study were 2.5 mL (range, 0.8–6.1 mL) and 3.5 mL (range, 0.5–10.3 mL) for thoracic and lumbar vertebrae, respectively.

Nieuwenhuijse et al.[16] all in the prospective series of 196 vertebroplasties found 24% fraction of vertebral body was found to have optimal cement volume for having good pain relief and less adjacent vertebral fractures. A vertebral body fraction of 24% was identifi ed as the optimal fraction to be cemented. This fraction corresponded to a 93 – 100% specificity for accomplishment of pain relief without being significantly associated with a higher risk of occurrence of cement leakage or new OVCFs. Their results suggest a CVBF [cement vertebral body fraction] of 24% or higher almost guarantees accomplishment of pain relief through PVP and is a safe threshold regarding the occurrence of cement leakage or new OVCFs.

Our series consisting of long-term follow-up of the vertebroplasties with low volume of cement, i.e in the range of 16 – 30% of the prefracture volume of the vertebra .it has good long-term pain relief . Also we had only 2 adjacent vertebral fractures, as it may occur with natural history of osteoporosis. Our clinical studies are in line with the finding that a cement quantity equivalent to about 16 – 30% volume of the intact vertebral body is sufficient to reduce the pain and also reduce long-term adjacent vertebral fractures. The appropriate cement volume also reduces the extravasation of the cement and hence the associated complications.

Figures 12.2 to 12.6 showing the representative preoperative, postoperative, and long-term postoperative pictures of the patients who have undergone low volume vertebroplasty.

Conclusion

In our study, the average cement used was about 2.5 cc in upper thoracic vertebrae. 3 cc-3.5cc in lower thoracic vertebral bodies and about 5 cc in lumbar vertebrae. The long term follow up showed that there were only 2 adjacent fractures in the series. Hence, we conclude that low volume of cement during vertebroplasty, in the range of 16 – 30% of its volume is sufficient to gain vertebral strength to its prefracture status. This does not cause excessive pressure on the adjacent vertebrae and hence reduces the incidence of the new fractures after vertebroplasty.

References

1. Meyers SP, Wiener SN. Magnetic resonance imaging features of fractures using the short tau inversion recovery (STIR) sequence: correlation with radiographic findings. Skeletal Radiol. 1991;20:499–501.
2. Quaiyun M. MRI detection of unsuspected vertebral injury in acute spinal trauma: Insidence and significance. Skeletal radiology. 2001;30:299-304
3. Yamato M, Nishimura G, Kuramochi E, Saiki N, Fujioka M. MR appearance at different ages of osteoporotic compression fractures of the vertebrae. Radiat Med.1998;16:329–34.
4. Gaitanis IN, Hadjipavlou AG, Katonis PG, et al. Balloon kyphoplasty for the treatment of pathological vertebral compression fractures. Eur Spine Journal. 2005;14:250-60.
5. Lindsay R, Silvermann SC, Cooper C. Risk of new vertebral fracture in the year following the fracture. JAMA. 2001; 285:320-3.
6. Uppin AA, Hirsch JA, Centevera LA, Pfiefer BA. Recurrence of new vertebral compression fracture after percutaneous vertebroplasty in patients with osteoporosis. Radiology. 2003; 266:119-24.
7. Lin EP, Ekholm S, Hiwatashi A, Westessen PL. Vertebroplasty: cement leakage into disc increase the risk of new fracture of adjacent vertebral body. Am J Neuroradiol. 2004; 25:175-80.
8. Voormolen MHJ, Lohle PNM, Juttmann JR. The risk of new osteoporotic vertebral compression fracture in year following percutaneous vertebroplasty. J Vasc Interv Radiol. 2006; 17(1):71-6.
9. Melike Mut, Sait Naderi. Risk of Refracture and Adjacent Vertebra Fracture after Vertebroplasty and Kyphoplasty. WSJ. 2006;2(1):1-4.

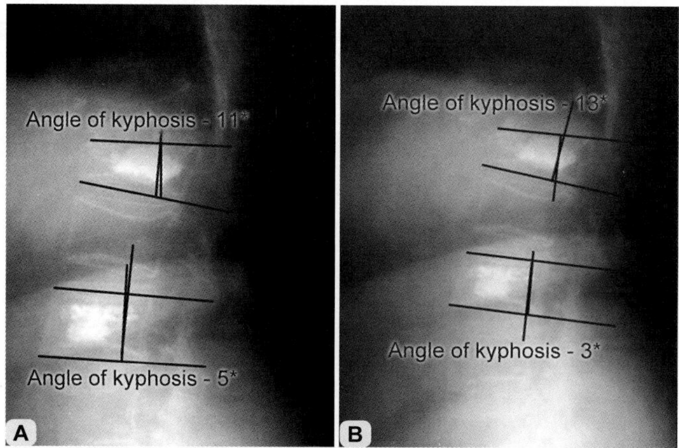

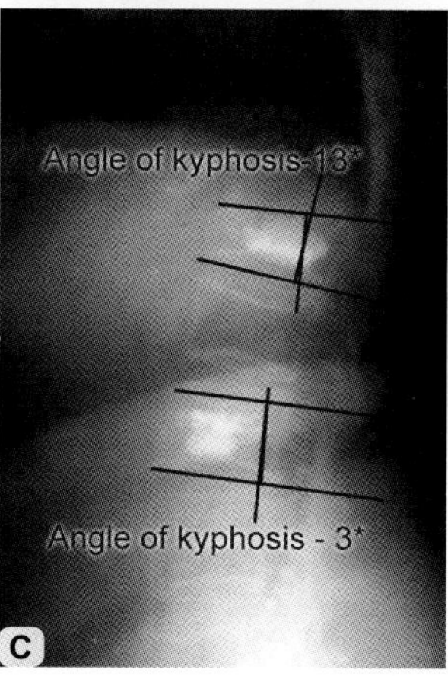

Figs. 12.2 Case 1: (A) Postoperative radiograph after 2 level vertebroplasty; (B) Radiograph of the same patient after 3 years. The angles of kyphosis have remained the same; (C) Radiograph of the same patient after 5 years of vertebroplasty

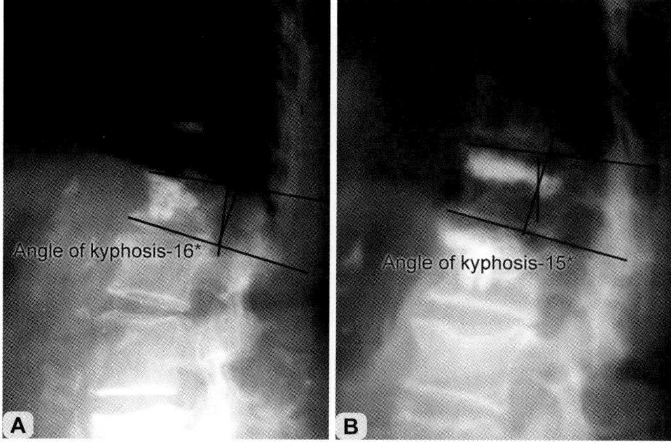

Fig. 12.3 Case 2: (A) Radiograph of another case of single level vertebroplasty; (B) Radiograph of the same patient after 3 years, shows not much collapse

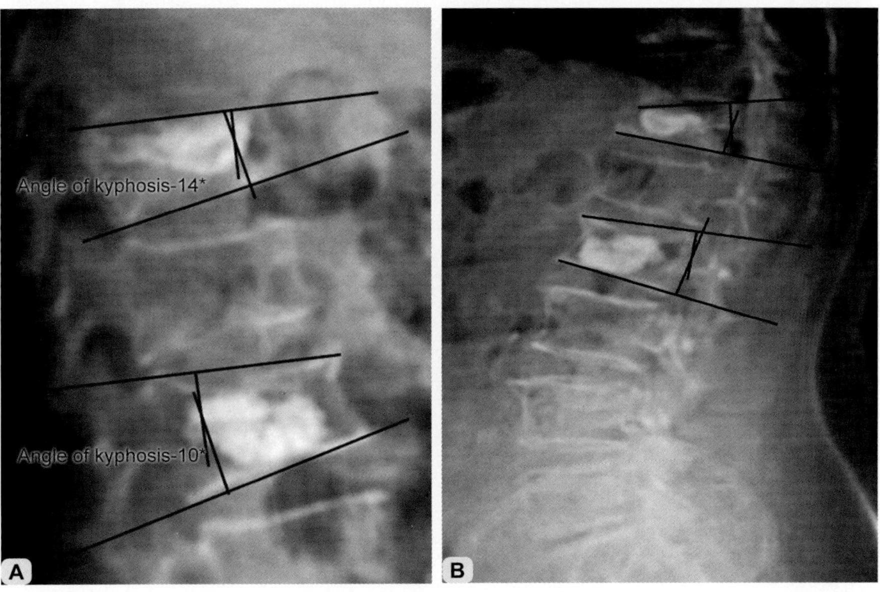

Fig. 12.4 Case 3: Postoperative and 3 year follow-up radiographs of another patient who had undergone 2 level vertebroplasy. The angles of kyphosis show no further change in 14 degrees and 10 degrees kyphosis

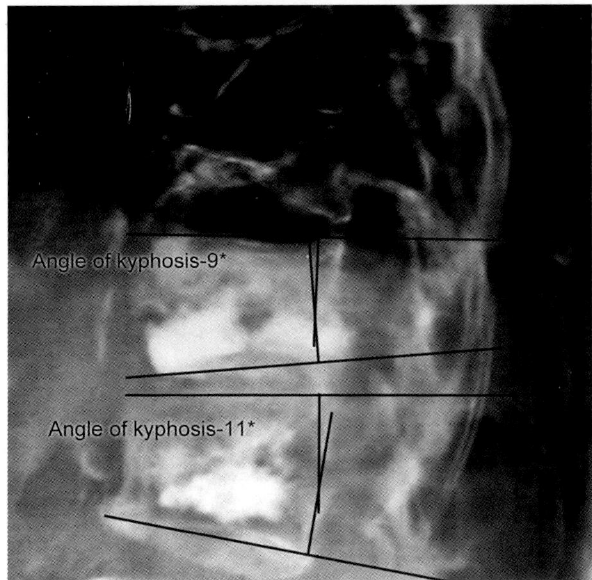

Fig. 12.5 Radiograph showing long-term follow up 8 years after adjacent level vertebroplasty. No further deformity is seen

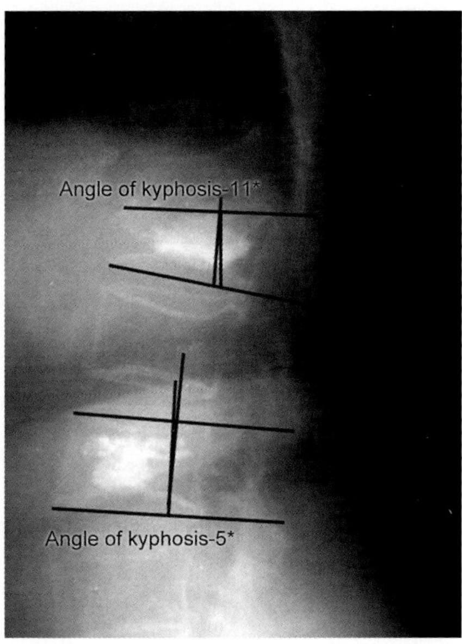

Fig. 12.6 Radiograph 42 months after follow-up shows no evidence of adjacent fracture

10. Impact of Cement Leakage Into Disks on the Development of Adjacent Vertebral Compression Fractures.Wen-Jer Chen, MD,* Yu-Hsien Kao, MD,w Shih-Chieh Yang, MD,w z Shang-Won Yu, MD,wYuan-Kun Tu, MD,w and Kao-Chi Chung, PhD Chen et al J Spinal Disord Tech _ Volume 23, Number 1, February 2010 38 | www.jspinaldisorders.com r 2010 Lippincott Williams & Wilkins
11. Trout AT, Kallmes DF. Does vertebroplasty cause incident vertebral fractures? A review of available data. Am J Neuroradiol. 2006; 27:1397-403.
12. Liebschner MAK, Rosenberg WS, Keaveny TM. Effects of bone cement volume and distribution on vertebral body stiffness recovery after vertebroplasty . Spine(Phila Pa 1976).2001; 26: 1547-54.
13. Boszczyk B. Volume matters: a review of procedural details of two randomized controlled vertebroplasty trials of 2009. Eur Spine J. 2010 Nov;19(11):1837-40.
14. Molloy S, Mathis JM, Belkoff SM. The effect of vertebral body percentage fill on mechanical behaviour during percutaneous vertebroplasty. Spine, 2003; 28:1549–54.
15. Kaufmanna TJ, Trouta AT, Kallmesa DF. American Journal of Neuroradiology. 2006; 27:1933-37. © 2006 American Society of Neuroradiology SPINE The Effects of Cement Volume on Clinical Outcomes of Percutaneous Vertebroplasty From the Department of Radiology, Mayo Clinic, Rochester, Minn Please address correspondence to Timothy J. Kaufmann, MD, Mayo Clinic, Department of Radiology, Mayo Building E2, 200 1st St SW, Rochester, MN 55905; e-mail:kaufmann.timothy@ mayo.edu .
16. Dijkstra PD, Nieuwenhuijse MJ, Bollen L, van Erkel AR Optimal intravertebral cement volume in percutaneous vertebroplasty for painful osteoporotic vertebral compression fractures. Spine (Phila Pa 1976). 2012; 15;37(20): 1747-55.

CHAPTER

13

Key Points in Minimally Invasive Spine Stabilization for Thoracic and Lumbar Lesions with Spine Navigation

Koji Sato

Introduction

Since 2005, several instrument systems used for minimally invasive spine stabilization (MISt) have been introduced in Japan.[1] These systems are mainly used for thoracic and lumbar lesions, via a percutaneous approach (small skin incision) that would allow percutaneous pedicle screws (PPS) and rods to be inserted. Currently, the systems are applied to procedures ranging from monosegmental stabilization for lumbar spinal stenosis to multisegmental stabilization for metastatic spinal tumors or trauma.[2] These systems are often modifications of open instruments used in conventional instrumentation systems (open systems) which unfold the back muscle from the posterior median line to right and left. However, some experience is required before PPS can be inserted with the guidance of guide pins, and to insert rods via a small visual field. Because the spine and the tips of instruments are invisible, extratime may be needed for MISt, and there is the risk of development of the critical complication of anterior wall perforation of the vertebral body. This article describes the key points for safe and quick insertion of these instruments and the pitfalls.

Features and Structures of Percutaneous Instrument Systems

Percutaneous instrument systems differ from the conventional open systems in the following points: cannulated screws are inserted with guide pins, and rods are inserted percutaneously. The percutaneous systems vary in structure depending on the manufacturer. Surgeons should always practice the use of these instrument systems with sawbones before initial use on patients. As animal laboratory sessions and cadaver workshops are offered, it would be preferable to apply for these opportunities.

Preoperative Planning

Preoperative planning is especially important for MISt. As is also true for use of open systems, surgery should never be performed without preparation. Before surgery, images should be examined closely. The lateral curvature, rotation of vertebral bodies, sclerosis, thickening of the facet joint, etc. should be assessed. The diameter and length of the PPS should be determined based on the findings on preoperative computed tomographic (CT) images.

Operating Table

In order to freely use a surgical imaging system, a narrow operating table (such as the Jackson spinal table) is preferable. A radiolucent carbon bed is preferred. The bed posts should be arranged in such a way as not to interfere with the imaging system. If an operating table is equipped with a large 4-poster support system, the space available between the imaging system and the surgical field will be small, and it will be difficult to obtain adequate working space. The use of a roll mat may also be advisable.

Position of the Patient and Installation of the Imaging C-arm System

First, place the patient in a surgical position that would facilitate instrumentation. The intervertebral lesion should be perpendicular to the floor. In a patient with L5 spondylolisthesis at the lumbosacral region (L5/S), for example, PPS need to be very obliquely inserted. Because the head of a patient would be placed upward, strap the hips to the 4-poster support system to prevent the body from slipping caudally and also prevent increase of the abdominal pressure; increased abdominal pressure increases the risk of occurrence of epidural venous hemorrhage.

Set the direction of the imaging C-arm system to show the correct forms of the pedicle and the intervertebral disk. Mark the spinous process of the intervertebral lesion with needle through images obtained with the imaging C-arm system. Before the incision, take anterior-posterior and lateral radiographs and identify the highest point. This point may also be used as a guide during surgery.

Drape the patient 360 degrees. Also cover the imaging system with a plastic cover in order to maintain asepsis and to quickly view the anterior-posterior and lateral images (Fig. 13.1).

Use of the Surgical Imaging C-arm System

In this procedure, an imaging system needs to be used because the instruments are not visible after they are inserted in the body. However, the instruments should also not be inserted by looking at the images alone; instead, the images should be used for confirmation. A knowledge of the risks of radiation exposure is necessary to reduce the exposure. Consider the direction and distance, etc. of the X-rays from the imaging system. First, step away from it. Moreover, take accurate anterior-posterior or lateral images of the spinal lesion in one shot. It would be preferable for a radiation technologist having a knowledge of the surgical procedure to take the images, rather than a resident or nurse who does not have adequate knowledge about the disease or the surgery. Especially in the case of degenerative scoliosis, images should be taken with an adequate knowledge of the direction of the intervertebral lesion and rotation of the vertebral bodies. Our recent mean duration of radiation use has been 0.6 minutes (including 0.4 minutes of CT scanning time).

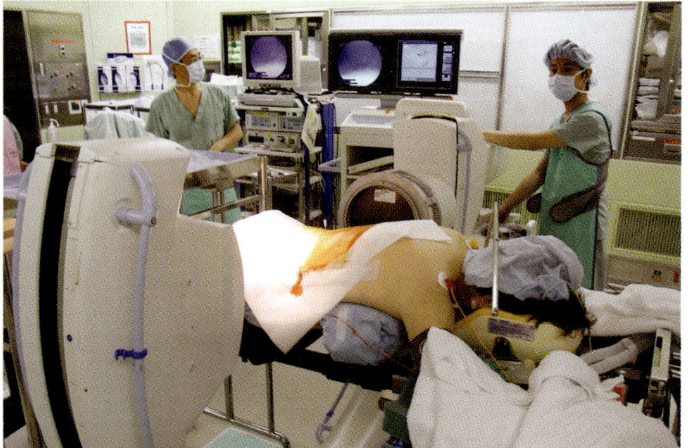

Fig. 13.1 Positioning of a patient, marking, and preparation for the imaging C-arm system

Use of the Spinal Navigation System

Spine navigation is effective for correct placement of the instruments, orientation for the decompression site, training novices to perform MISt, reduction of radiation exposure, and reduction of the operative duration.[3] As the third eye, spine navigation enables surgeons to more safely perform surgery within shorter periods of time. It is better to use spine navigation combined with an imaging system to allow intraoperative CT scanning (Iso-C 3D SIREMOBILE, ARCADIS Orbic 3D, O-arm, Ziehm Vision FD). MISt does not allow registration of many points. It is better to use a system (3rd-generation Spine navigation software) that provides CT images of the spinous processes with reference marks and allows registration-free navigation (Fig. 13.2).

Key Points in the Insertion of Jamshidi or PAK Needles

Use Jamshidi needles to insert guide pins. If fingers can be inserted through the small skin incision, touch the exterior of the facet joint or transverse process with the fingertips (finger navigation). When you get used to the procedure, touch the transverse process with the needle tip and gradually move it toward to the base of the transverse process. Focus your senses on the needle tip.

Once the insertion point is determined, hammer the needle to insert it to a depth of approximately 1 cm. The position of the needle tip should be confirmed by imaging. The needle should be inserted so that it precisely penetrates the pedicle. The medial pedicle in the frontal image of the

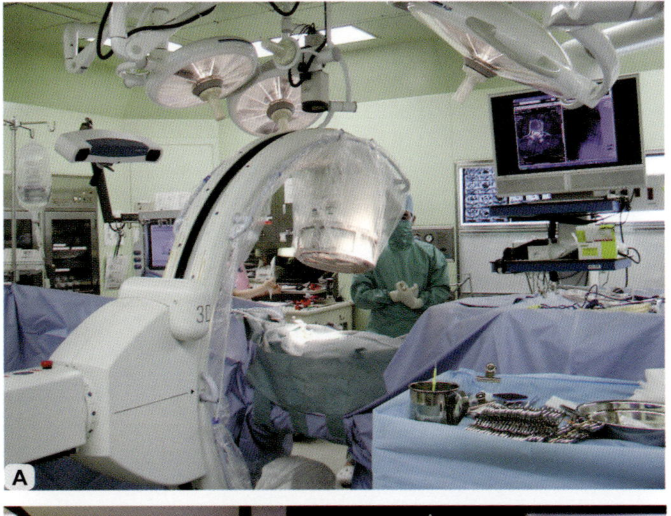

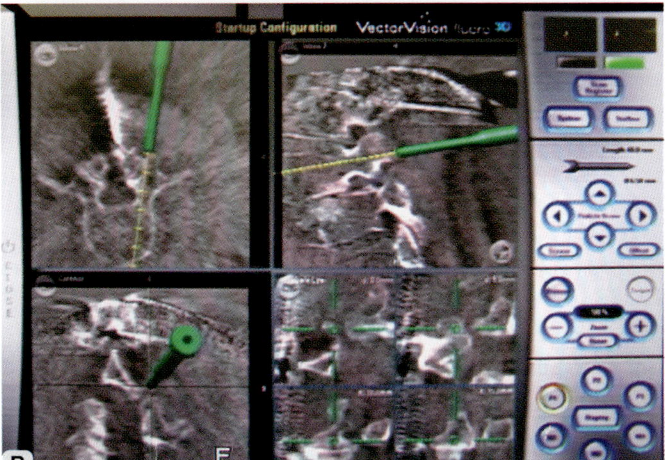

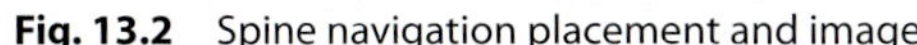

Fig. 13.2 Spine navigation placement and image

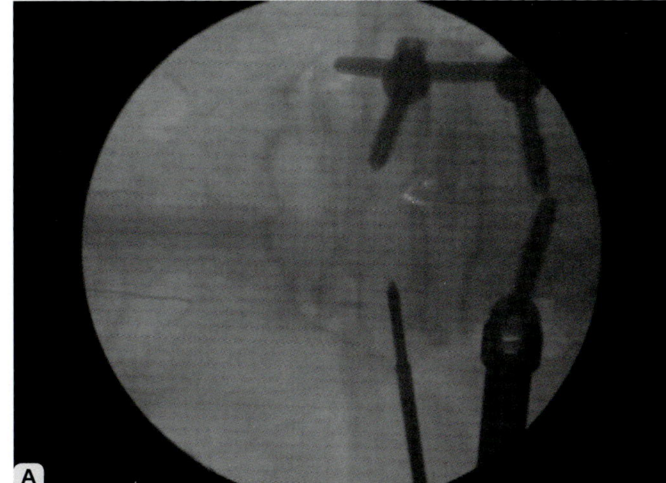

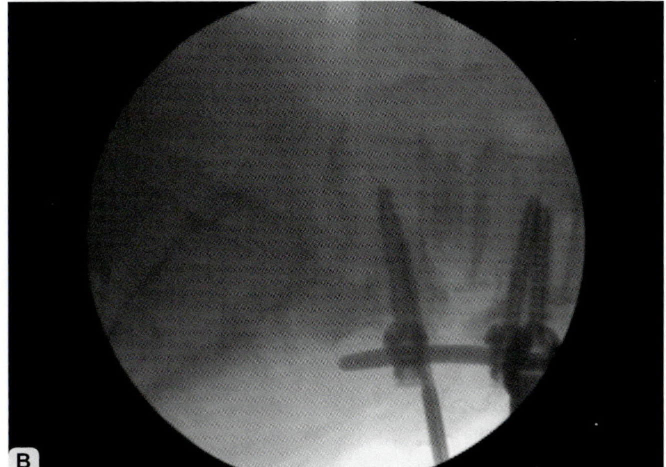

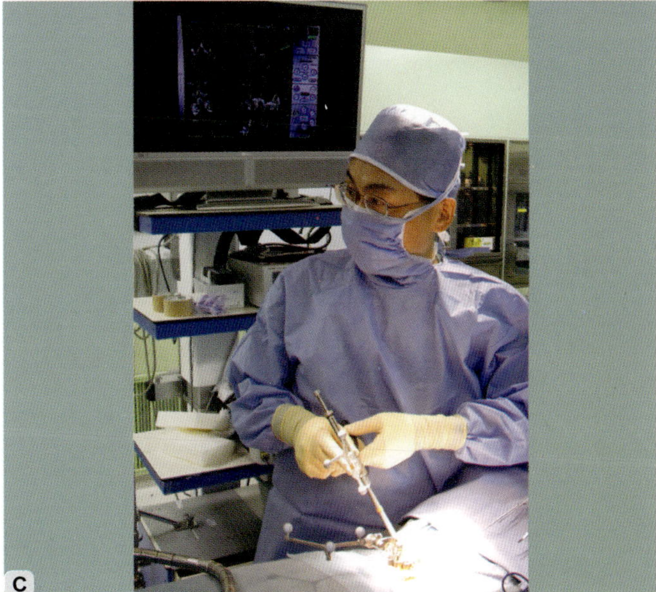

Fig. 13.3 Medial margin of the pedicle and posterior margin of the vertebral body. Images obtained by the imaging system and application of the drill guide

lumbar spine and the posterior margin of the vertebral body in the lateral image should be used as guides (Figs 13.3A and B).

When the transverse process is fractured, make an additional small incision. Touch and move the needle tip with the fingers toward an appropriate site. Open the insertion site and recover the needle with a small surgical retractor (such as Quadrant^{TM}). A cannulated pedicle probe facilitates recovery.

Using the navigation guide, needles can be inserted accurately and quickly. Using a precalibration drill guide (2.6 mm), drill a hole into the bone at an appropriate site with a hand drill. Guide pins can be placed immediately (Fig. 13.3C).

Although a skin incision for PPS is usually made rostrocaudally, a transaxial incision, made after a certain level of skill is acquired, is less likely to leave a surgical scar.

Troubles with Guide Pins

Accurate placement of guide pins is important for accurate placement of PPS. The positions of guide pins should always be confirmed by imaging. When the positions are uncertain, they should be confirmed by imaging. To prevent the guide pin from penetrating through the anterior wall of a vertebral body, the position of the guide pin tip should be clearly identified. Feel the bone with the tip of the guide pin. Insert the guide pin not greater than halfway into the vertebral body.

Guide pins, if bent, cannot be removed after insertion of PPS. Keep the guide pins straight during dilation or tapping. Do not apply excessive force. If you become skillful at inserting guide pins, a single pin can be used 4 times (for 1 session of facet joint stabilization, 1 level fusion).

The guide pins may fall off if the taps are clogged. The pins may also fall off while inserting and removing the instruments, which causes stress to the surgeon. After placement of Jamshidi needles, hold a guide pin with a needle holder and hammer the pin to insert it to a depth of approximately 1 cm.

How to Use a Dilator, Oar, and Taps

The tap-in dilator (Fig. 13.4) is useful for shortcutting the procedure.

If the facet joint is thickened, it will be difficult to insert a tap. Make a dent with a cannulated oar.

In regard to selection of the tap diameter, taking into consideration the possibility of osteoporosis, a tap with a smaller diameter by a rank should be used. When PPS with a diameter of 6.5 mm are used, we generally use taps with a diameter of 5.5 mm. In general, when PPS measuring 45 mm in length are used, we use taps cut to 30 mm length.

With increasing sclerosis of the pedicle in the vertebral body, the size of a tap is increased in a stepwise fashion. After 4.5 mm taps, 6.5 mm taps are used. Moreover, the tap is cut to the same length as the PPS.

Troubles with PPS

When a PPS slips and cannot be inserted, the tap should be tap cut again. Osteosclerosis of the pedicle and upper margin of the vertebral body should be assessed beforehand on CT images (Fig. 13.5). Doubtless, the diameters and lengths of the screws to be used should be calculated on preoperative CT images.

When S1 screws are inserted, it should be borne in mind that L5 and the screw may become close due to lumbar lordosis. For L5/S stabilization, screw extenders with a small diameter should be selected. PPS for S1 should be inserted approximately from the caudal side toward the promontorium. Insertion of PPS through the ilium may also be considered (Fig. 13.6). In this case, curve the ilium with a gouge while using a small dilator as a guide.

Regarding reinforcement of PPS stabilization, augment the vertebral body with hydroxyapatite paste or bone cement. Special PPS are under development. In MISt, short fusion is preferable.

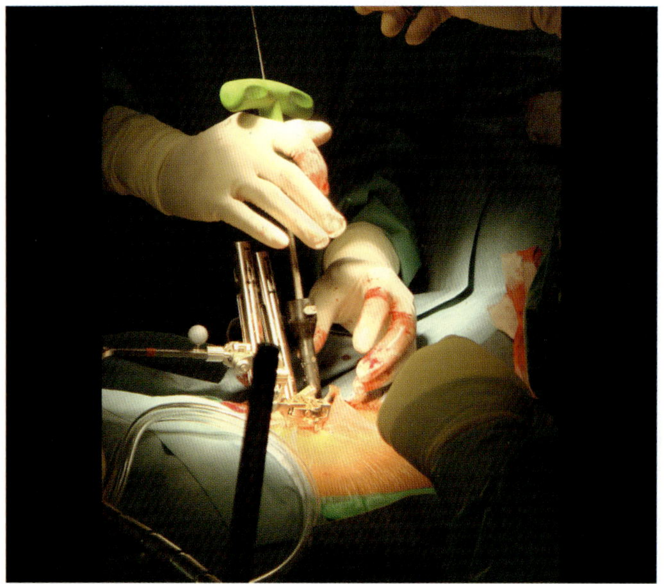

Fig. 13.4 Tap-in dilator

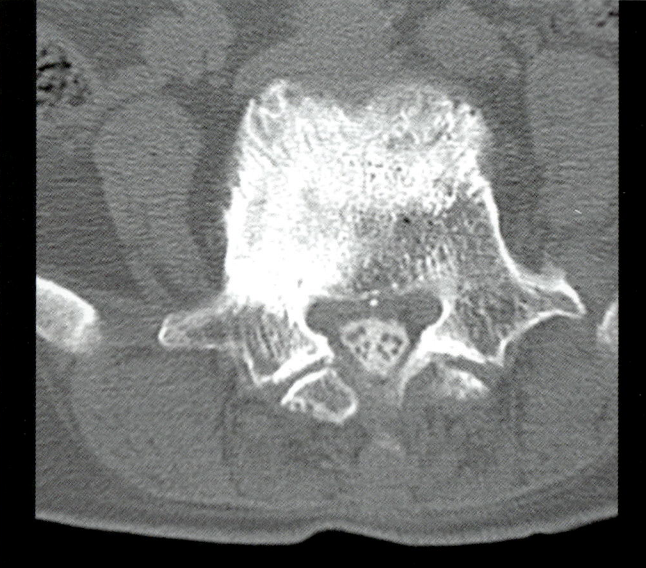

Fig. 13.5 Hard vertebral body difficult for insertion. CT showing sclerosis of the right pedicle and the inside of the vertebral body

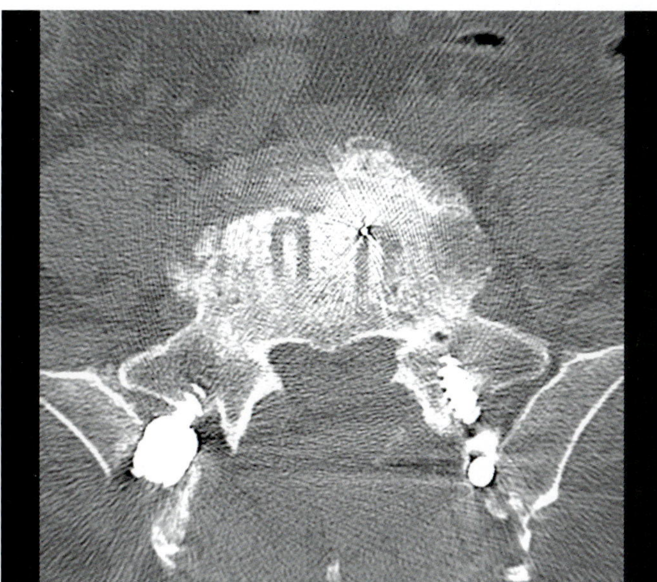

Fig. 13.6 PPS inserted through the ilium. The right PPS penetrating the ilium

Troubles with Rod Insertion

There is a wide choice of rod holders that is available at present (Fig. 13.7). The rod holders are mainly divided into 2 types: a holder for grasping the edge of a rod and that for grasping the center of the rod. The former is easy to use for multisegmental stabilization, and the latter for monosegmental stabilization of the lower lumbar spine in the region of the lordotic curvature.

If a rod cannot be set to PPS, it may be assumed that something is interfering with the rod that the rod is lifted. If set screws (blockers) cannot be inserted into a rod, the persuader should be used. This should be used to align the rod with the PPS rather than reduction. Use of a strong type of persuader at once only causes the PPS to fall off, which is not desirable. Because the alignment between the rod and PPS is invisible, the two should be carefully set according to the resistance felt by the hand.

The curve radii (R) of pre-bent rods vary depending on systems, and cannot be depended upon; rather, they should be bent again before use.

Edges of the rod should be checked for any tucking of the fascia. After insertion of the rod, any tucked in fascia should be gently removed with a mucosal elevator, etc.

Modification of Percutaneous Hooks

Stabilization of pseudarthrosis in cases of osteoporosis, etc., by short fusion requires hooks. Although offset hooks for the open systems can be used for the thoracolumbar junction (Fig. 13.8), their offset is not sufficient for the lumbar region of the spine. Percutaneous hooks are under development, and hook forms and offset degrees are being investigated.

Lumbosacral Stabilization

The report by Ito et al.[4] is useful. It would be easier to insert not only S1, but also S2 or iliac screws, into the appropriate sites with a spine navigation. The percutaneous implanting technique is effective for internal stabilization of AO type-C pelvic fractures. However, because PPS is difficult to link

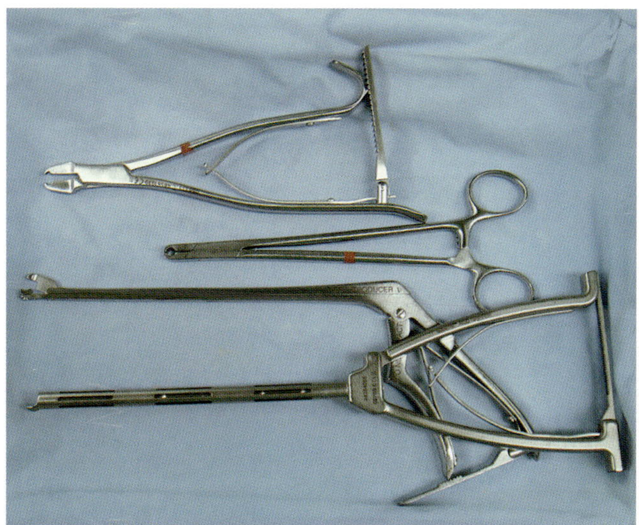

Fig. 13.7 Various rod holders

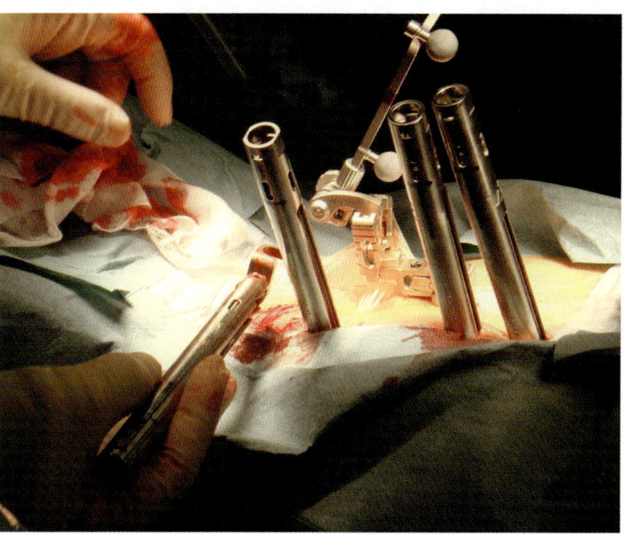

Fig. 13.8 Percutaneous hook

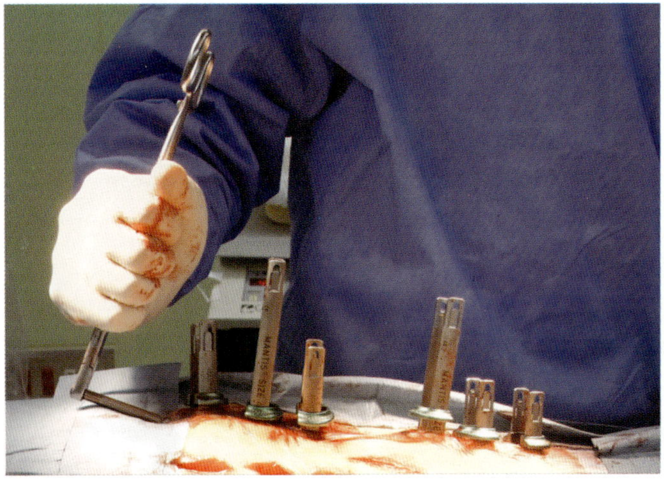

Fig. 13.9 Multisegmental insertion of a rod

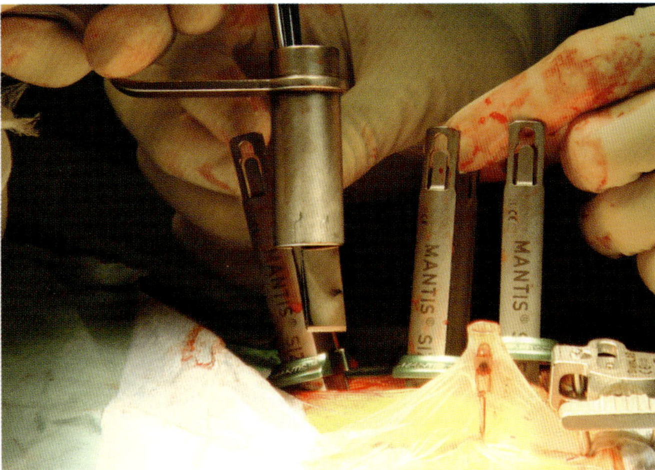

Fig. 13.10 Facet joint stabilization (facet fusion kit by Sato)

with a rod at L5, the modified Galveston technique, which links L3 and L4 to the ilium, is applied.

Key Points in Multisegmental Stabilization

Align the posterior or lateral curvature of the rod to the heights of the screw extenders. Insert a rod from the posterior curvature side while holding its edge (Fig.13.9). While holding the rod with one hand, hold and rotate the screw extender with the other hand. Confirm that the rod has passed through the screw extender, which can be seen from above the screw extenders.

When it is difficult to insert the rod, insert it from a different direction, after checking the height of the PPS again.

In order to extensively correct the alignment, it is necessary to destroy the facet joint and to touch and move the intervertebral disk.

Facet Fusion Technique

In the technique that I developed, the facet joint is destroyed with a 13 mm tube retractor and a chisel (Fig. 13.10). However, blind application of this technique can cause hemorrhage. Hemostasis should be performed with an electrocautery scalpel in the tube. It is advantageous to fill with SURGICEL absorbable hemostat.

Troubles with Damaged Instruments

The tips of cannulated instruments are fragile. We have also experienced damage of the tips of screw extenders, taps, and screw drivers. Because there would be no sign of damage, the tips should be inspected after use. Moreover, it would be desirable to exchange instruments after using them approximately 50 times.

Conclusion

Key points to safely and quickly perform MISt are to understand the structure of the system and to improve skills. Training of the staff is also necessary, in addition to preparation for surgery, such as using an appropriate operating table and placing a patient in an appropriate position. Moreover, the most important key points may be to touch the bone and soft tissue with the instrument tip and to always focus the senses on the tip. Percutaneous instrument systems are still under development. They are expected to be widely applied in the future. We need to make the system for Asian peoples.

References

1. Sato K. Comparison of instruments and implants for minimally invasive spine stabilization. J Spine Res. 2010;1(9): 1669-73.
2. Sato K. Minimally invasive spine stabilization for multiple level lesions: New instrument for less invasive spinal surgery. J Spine Res. 2010;1(8):1475-80.
3. Sato K. Spinal navigation surgery using isocentric C-arm. Journal of Minimally Invasive Orthopaedic Surgery. 2008;49:2-8.
4. Ito Y, Toda K, Yagata Y, et al. Experience with treatment for posterior unstable pelvic fracture using iliosacral-screws combined with C-arm mobile computed tomography and navigation system. Orthopedic Surgery. 2006;57(5):549-53.

CHAPTER

14

Technique of Odontoid Screw Fixation for Type II Odontoid Fractures

Arvind G Kulkarni, Abhilash N Dhruv

Introduction

In the adult population, odontoid fractures account for 9 – 15% of cervical spine fractures.[1-3] These injuries usually result from low-energy impacts such as falls in the elderly or high-energy impacts such as motor vehicle accidents in the young and middle aged. Odontoid fractures are the most common individual cervical spine fractures for persons aged 70 years and are the most common of all spinal fractures for persons aged 80 years, with evidence of increasing incidence in this population, in western literature.[4] There are equal male-to-female distributions in both populations.

The mechanism responsible for odontoid fractures is generally agreed to be hyperextension or hyperflexion of the cervical spine. The identification, classification, and treatment of odontoid fractures remain controversial and are evolving with the advent of new fixation methods.

Classification

The most widely used classification scheme used is described by Anderson and D'Alonzo.[5] According to this, type I fractures are near the tip of the odontoid process, above the transverse ligament. Type II fractures occur at the base of the odontoid, between the level of the transverse ligament and the C2 vertebral body. Type III fractures extend into the vertebral body (Fig. 14.1).

Based on their relative stability, type I and III fractures can often be treated with collar immobilization. However, there is no consensus on type II fracture treatment. Immobilization options may include a collar, halo, or anterior or posterior internal fixation. Increased patient age, extent and direction of fracture displacement, delay in diagnosis, and fracture comminution have all negatively influenced union rates.[1,2,5]

Type II can be further classified using Grauers treatment oriented classification.[6] It classifies type II into type IIA, IIB and IIC fractures. Type IIA was defined as a minimally or nondisplaced type II fracture with no comminution.Type IIB was a displaced fracture extending from anterior-superior to posterior-inferior or a transverse fracture. Type IIC was a fracture line extending from anterior-inferior to posterior superior or a fracture with significant comminution (Fig. 14.2).

Indications/Contraindications

It is indicated in patients with acute type II and high type III with a shallow base odontoid fractures (according

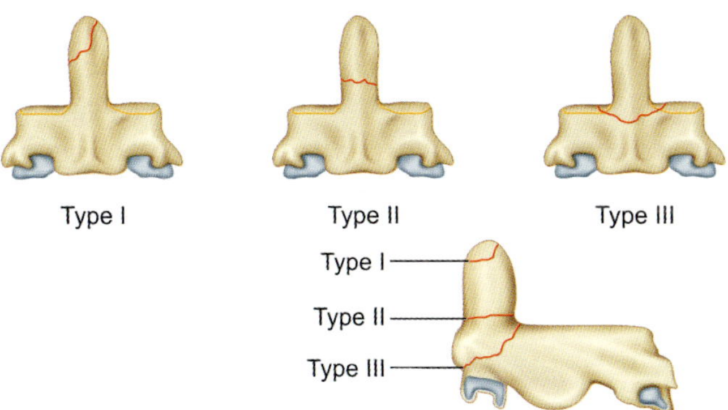

Fig. 14.1 The Anderson and D'Alonzo classification

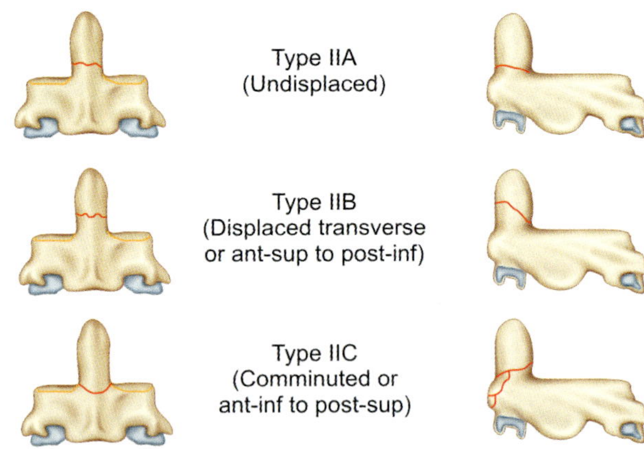

Fig. 14.2 The Grauer modification of type II fractures

to Anderson and D'Alonzo classification); and type IIB (according to Grauer modification) and in patients unable to tolerate a halo. It is an alternative to atlantoaxial arthrodesis for management of odontoid fractures at risk for non-union, with a high healing rate, similar to that of posterior atlantoaxial arthrodesis (92–100%), and a low complication rate.[7-11] Direct osteosynthesis also can be used in patients who refuse halo treatment and in whom fracture reduction can be obtained but not maintained.

Anatomic reduction of the fracture is imperative before this technique is attempted as inability to achieve anatomic reduction is an absolute contraindication. Relative contraindications include transverse atlantal ligament (TAL) disruption, fracture non-union and an oblique fracture in an anteroinferior-to-posterosuperior plane (Grauer type IIC) that can cause the fracture to shear anteriorly at the fracture site during lag compression. Caution should be used in osteopenic patients.

Also ideal drill trajectory can be hindered by a barrel-chest, a short neck, kyphotic thoracic spine and fractures that require flexion for reduction. These are again relative contraindications.

Rationale

The rationale is preservation of C1-C2 rotation while providing rigid internal fixation and avoiding restrictive bracing and the complications associated with bone grafting techniques.[9, 12, 13]

A number of factors appear to be associated with an increased incidence of nonunion for type II odontoid fractures, including posterior fracture displacement, displacement 4–6 mm, 10° of angulation, fracture comminution, fracture malalignment during follow-up, delayed treatment, and patients older than 40–65 years.[14,15] External immobilization, such as a halo vest has its own complications, such as poor reduction maintenance, pneumonia, wound infection, cerebral spinal fluid leakage, and even death. Also,multiple studies have documented higher rates of complications, including unstable pin fixation, bronchopulmonary difficulty, and decreased tolerance in the elderly, as compared to young adults.[16, 17]

Examination and Evaluation/Pathology

The standard, initial cervical spine radiographic series in trauma patients includes a cross table lateral view, AP view, and an open-mouth view, this three-view screening series can be detect 65–95% of axis injuries.[10] Thin-section computed CT is the best study for evaluating C2 bony fractures.[18] Sagittal reconstruction of CT images is important because axial images may not show a transverse odontoid fracture.

Dynamic flexion/extension lateral fluoroscopic evaluation has been advocated for polytrauma patients to identify occult ligamentous instabilities and confirm that the cervical spine is uninjured[19] (Fig. 14.3).

Magnetic resonance imaging (MRI) also is helpful in assessing the spinal cord in patients with neurologic deficit and is becoming increasingly important in evaluating the status of ligamentous structures, such as the transverse atlantal ligament (TAL).

The assessment of TAL integrity in patients with odontoid fractures is an important consideration in selecting appropriate treatment options.[20] Injuries of the TAL can result in atlantoaxial instability after odontoid fracture, healing, and the chance of non-union is increased with TAL disruption.

Surgery

Positioning

Before beginning the operation, the surgeon must ensure that anatomic reduction is possible by simple tong traction or manipulation while the patient is awake, with lateral fluoroscopic imaging (Fig. 14.4). The head is placed in a head ring with a roll under the shoulder between the scapulae to aid in extending the neck to achieve reduction. The head can be fixed by a Mayfield three-point head holder. Alternately, Gardener-Wells tongs may be applied to achieve ideal position for reduction. The tongs or the Mayfield are used only to stabilize the head and not for any kind of traction since traction can distract the fracture. It is important to adjust the position of the neck to bring

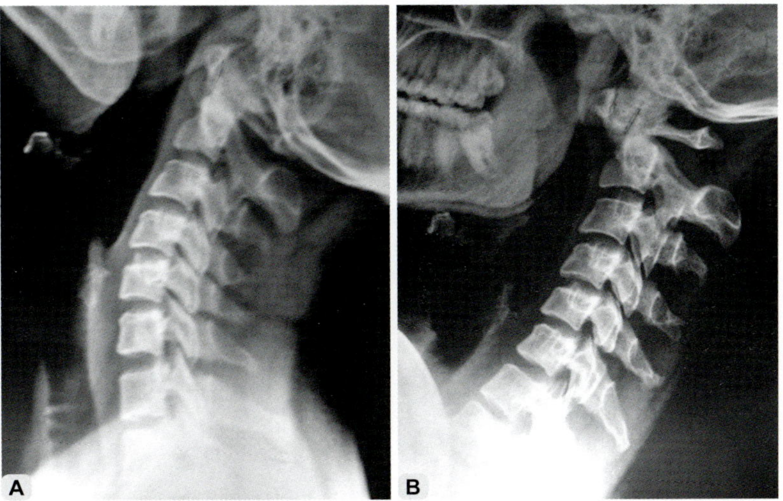

Fig. 14.3 Preoperative flexion and extension radiographs

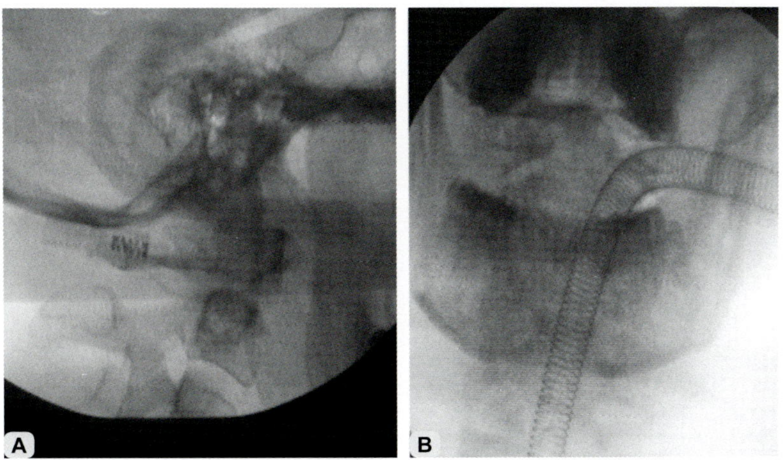

Fig. 14.4 Lateral and anteroposterior views demonstrating reduction of fracture

the entire cervical spine anterior, away from the chest. The shoulders may be pulled down and secured to the edge of the table by adhesive tape, to facilitate a good lateral view.

Biplanar fluoroscopy is used to assess anatomic reduction. It involves placement of two C-arms. One should be placed directly above the patients head perpendicular to the position of the neck. Another C-arm is used for lateral views. Excellent visualization of the odontoid in both planes is mandatory (Fig. 14.5). A wad of gauze in the mouth facilitates the visualization of the odontoid by the open-mouth view.

Before the incision is made, trajectory of the drill is ensured by placing a Steinmann pin or a K-wire along the lateral aspect of the patient's neck while shooting a lateral fluoroscopic image (Fig. 14.6). This also helps in further positioning to take the neck away from the chest and anteriorly.

Under biplanar fluoroscopy, the surgeon obtains anatomic reduction. Depending on the amount of flexion or extension required for reduction, the AP view might be best shot through the mouth.

Procedure

The surgeon makes a transverse skin incision at the C5–C6 level as described by Smith and Robinson and blunt

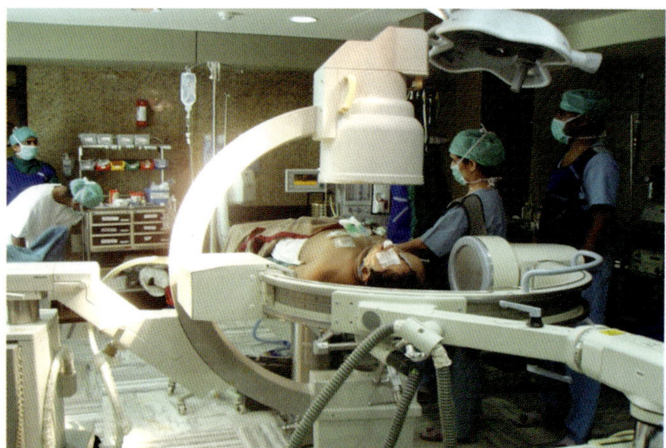

Fig. 14.5 Biplanar radiography in operating room

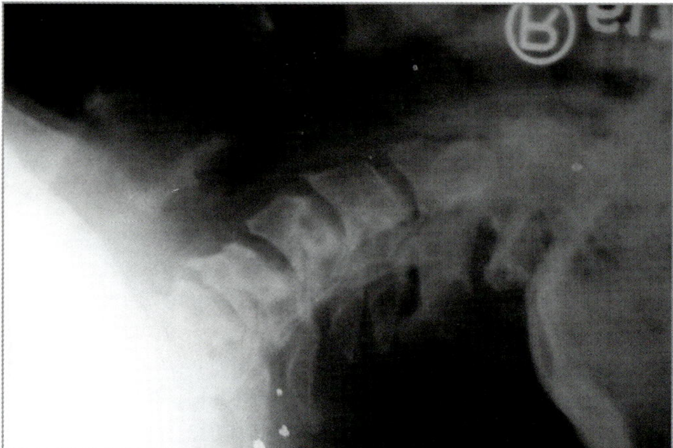

Fig. 14.6 Trajectory of the drill-bit directed towards the center of odontoid through the anterior part of the inferior end-plate of C2

dissection is performed to reach the anterior vertebral bodies. Then the surgeon dissects cephalad to the C2–C3 disk. Dissection can be aided by a large size Penfield dissector which can create a plane required for the drill. It is important to protect the esophagus throughout the procedure. The entry point is in the anterior aspect of the inferior endplate of C2 in the lateral view and centre of the base of C2 body in the AP projection (Figs 14.7 and 14.8). The starting point can be smoothed with a burr for accuracy. Also a cannulated 7 mm drill bit can be used to gain an entry point into the body of C2 at the anteroinferior corner in the midline.

The use of an odontoid fixation set provided by some implant manufacturers aids the procedure. A power drill is used. A 2–mm guide–wire, is passed through a sleeve and directed toward the entry point prepared by the 7 mm drill. It is advanced under fluoroscopic monitoring across the fracture line and into but not across the far cortex of the tip. It should be in the middle of the body of C2 directed towards the centre of odontoid in the AP view and in the lateral view; it should enter the anteroinferior cortex of C2 body, directed towards the center of the odontoid tip. A 2.5 mm drill bit is then threaded over the guidewire and gently advanced under fluoroscopic control. It is stopped just short of the tip of the guidewire. It is then gently withdrawn, taking care that the guidewire does not back out. It is useful to hold the guidewire with a Kocher clamp to prevent this. A depth gauge is used to measure the length of the screw. Alternately, a guidewire of similar length can be used. It is advanced upto the entry point. The length of this guidewire extending beyond the inserted guide wire is the screw length. The appropriate 4 mm partially threaded cancellous screw is then gently advanced, all the while taking care that the guidewire is held firmly with a Kocher clamp. Care is taken not to advance the screw tip beyond the cortex. As the screw head contacts the strong cortical inferior endplate, compression occurs across the fracture. The patient's neck is then flexed and extended to check for stability of the fixation.

Pearls

Hottet et al.[21] have described a unique head-holding device which has an articulating arm that can be placed in a paramedian position, facilitating unobstructed open-mouth view.

Fracture reduction can be aided by direct oropharyngeal pressure by a padded laryngoscope. This maneuver can also be carried out to hold the reduced fragment in place.

The placement of two screws is technically more difficult and often not anatomically possible, and it offers no biomechanical advantage, in comparison with one-screw fixation.[9,22-24] Also, the author has studied the morphometry of the odontoid in in the Indian population and has observed that the odontoid cannot accommodate two 3.5-mm screws in its narrowest diameter.[25]

Alternately a fully threaded screw can be used. It requires drilling across the fracture site by a 2.5 mm drill and overdrilling the near cortex by a 3.5 mm drill to prepare a 'gliding hole'. This is followed by tapping the entire tract with a 3.5 mm tap. A 3.5 or 4 mm fully threaded screw is then inserted gradually. A noncannulated screw can be used as well.

On occasion when the adequate length of the screw is not available, longer length screws can be utilized. In such a situation the distal threaded portion can be appropriately cut with a Harrington rod cutter and the screw can be then advanced.

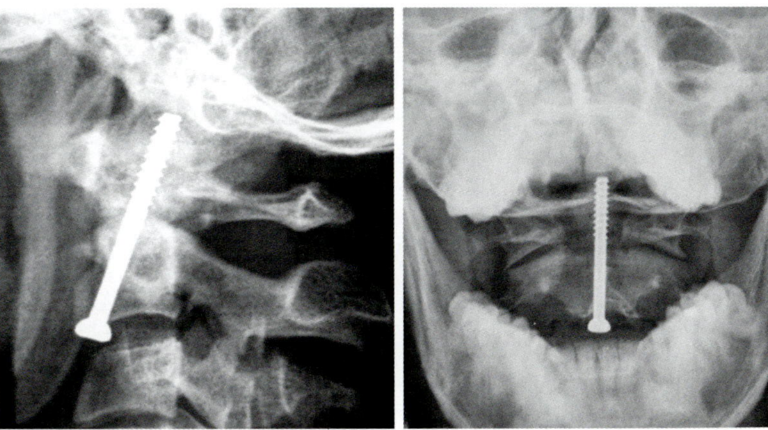

Fig. 14.7 AP open mouth view and lateral view of odontoid fracture fixed with a screw

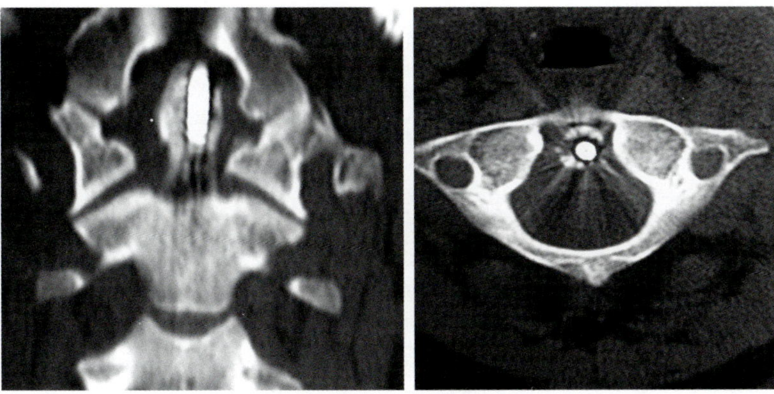

Fig. 14.8 CT sections of odontoid fracture fixed with a screw

Pitfalls

Odontoid screw fixation is a technically demanding procedure that requires thorough preoperative planning and adequate surgical training. Determining the correct entry point is critical. Also, poor proximal fragment purchase with subsequent screw cutout may occur. It is important to engage the far cortex of the odontoid tip to ensure adequate purchase. AP and lateral fluoroscopy is essential for constant monitoring during all stages of the surgery.

Postoperative Management

Progressive ambulation is initiated immediately after surgery, and the simple soft cervical or a Philadelphia collar is kept in place for 6 weeks. A hard cervical collar is worth postoperatively for the first one week.

Complications

Overall, studies reported in the literature have established this technique as an efficacious treatment for odontoid fractures.[26-29] Complications and their incidences, reported in clinical series as results of direct anterior odontoid screw fixation, include screw malpositioning, screw breakout, and neurologic or vascular injury. The procedure in several series has an aggregate fusion rate of 94.5%.

The most common problems are inability to anatomically reduce the fracture, difficulty positioning the surgeon's hand for proper drill trajectory because of interference with the patient's chest, and nonvisualization of the odontoid on fluoroscopy because of osteopenia. If a partially threaded lag screw is used, a high fracture may not allow the threads to be completely contained in the dens fragment. These threads across the fracture site keep the fracture distracted.

Recent Advances

Apfelbaumet al.[30] and Dickman et al.[31] have described the use of tubular retractors for accurate passage of the odontoid screw. They are used in conjunction with the open techniques. Hott et al.[32] described a new table-fixed retractor system. The system is reported by the authors to obviate the need for dissection of the longus colli and excess retraction of the trachea and the esophagus, while allowing fine adjustments for proper trajectory of the screw.

A fully threaded variable pitch screw or a Herbert screw has been used for the fixation of these fractures. Lee and Sung[33] reported the use of a 4.5 mm cannulated Herbert screw in fixation of these fractures. They showed successful clinical results comparable with that of the 4 mm cannulated cancellous screw and distinct advantages over conventional screws in the aspect of biomechanical properties. Magee et al.[34] compared Herbert screw with conventional partially threaded cancellous screws in cadavers and demonstrated that a Herbert screw is a biomechanically favorable alternative to a cannulated lag screw and washer for fixation of type II odontoid fractures. By virtue of its headless design and lack of requirement for bicortical screw purchase, this implant appears to offer increased clinical safety over current implants. As Herbert screws do not require purchase in the far cortex, they obviate the possibility of vascular and neural complications that can occur due to protrusion of the screw tip.

There are few studies comparing the biomechanical properties of cannulated bioabsorbable screw made of polylactide copolymer with titanium screws.[35] These bioabsorbable implants have not yet been utilized clinically.

With the advent of improved imaging techniques and interest in minimally invasive surgery, new techniques are emerging for the fixation of odontoid fractures.

The use of neuronavigation has made life easier for the surgeon. Isocentric 3-dimensional (Iso-C 3D) fluoroscopy machines are now being used for the intraoperative imaging in fixation of these difficult fractures. Yang et al.[36]assessed the value of Iso-C 3D fluoroscopy for the insertion of an anterior odontoid screw. They concluded that this technique can be safely extended to the treatment of technically difficult spinal injuries and at the same time reduce total radiation exposure time both for the patient and the surgeon. Martirosyan et al.[37] compared the results of Iso-C 3D fluoroscopy and traditional biplanar fluoroscopy for the fixation of odontoid fractures. This series represents the largest cohort of patients treated with intraoperative real-time navigation assistance for odontoid fractures. They concluded that Iso-C 3D significantly decreased surgical time and Iso-C 3D assistance was associated with improved rates of radiographic fusion with comparable outcome and complication profiles.

Percutaneous techniques have been developed for fixation. They involve a smaller incision than used in open techniques. They make use of special set of tubular dilators or a trocar and cannula sheath. The dissection up to the area of interest is done bluntly using these devices. The remaining steps remain the same. As a minimally invasive fixation method, percutaneous anterior odontoid screw fixation was described first by Kazan et al.[38]

Yong-Long Chi et al.[39] have described their indigenous percutaneous technique and instrumentation for the same. Wang et al.[40] compared the open and the percutaneous techniques and concluded that in comparison with open fixation group, percutaneous fixation group had significantly less operating time and less blood loss with comparable outcomes. Percutaneous anterior screw fixation is a safe and reliable procedure for treatment of type II fractures.

In severely osteopenic bones the cortex at the entry point of the screw may fail or there may be a failure of achieving good contact between the odontoid and the body. In such cases supplementation of bone defects with Norian SRS, an osteoconductive agent may facilitate successful bone union in selected patients as reported by Harrop and Przybylski.[41] However, further evaluation with this is required.

References

1. Subach BR, Morone MA, Haid RW Jr, et al. Management of acute odontoid fractures with single-screw anterior fixation. Neurosurgery. 1999;45:812-9.
2. Lee PC, Chun SY, Leong JC. Experience of posterior surgery in atlanto-axial instability. Spine. 1984;9:231-9.
3. Vaccaro AR, Madigan L, Ehrler DM. Contemporary management of adult cervical odontoid fractures. Orthopedics. 2000;23:1109-13.
4. Ryan MD, Henderson JJ. The epidemiology of fractures and fracture-dislocations of the cervical spine. Injury. 1992;23:38-40.
5. Anderson LD, D'Alonzo RT. Fractures of the odontoid process of the axis. J Bone Joint Surg Am. 1974;56:1663-74.
6. Grauer JN, Shafi B, Hilibrand AS, et al. Proposal of a modified, treatment oriented classification of odontoid fractures. Spine J. 2005;5:123-9.
7. Aebi M, Etter C, CosciaM. Fractures of the odontoid process : treatment with anterior screw fixation. Spine. 1990;14:1065-70.
8. Bohler J. Anterior stabilization for acute fractures and non unions of the dens. J Bone Joint Surg Am. 1982;64:18-27.
9. Jenkins JD, Coric D, Branch CL. A clinical comparison of one and two screw odontoid fixation. J Neurosurg. 1998;89:366-70.
10. Marchesi DG. Management of odontoid fractures. Orthopaedics. 1997;20:911-6.
11. Montesano PX, Anderson P, Schehr F, et al. Odontoid fractures treated by anterior odontoid screw fixation. Spine. 1991;16:5337.

12. Apfelbaum RI. Screw fixation of the upper cervical spine: Indications and techniques. Contemp Neurosurg. 1994;16:1-8.
13. Lesoin F, Autricque A, Franz K, et al. Transcervical approach and screw fixation for upper cervical spine pathology. SurgNeurol. 1987;27:459-65.
14. Clark CR, White AA III. Fractures of the dens. A multicenter study. J Bone Joint Surg Am. 1985;67:1340-8.
15. Hadley MN, Browner C, Sonntag VK. Axis fractures: A comprehensive review of management and treatment in 107 cases. Neurosurgery. 1985;17:281-90.
16. Garfin SR, Botte MJ, Waters RL, et al. Complications in the use of the halo fixation device. J Bone Joint Surg Am. 1986;68:320-5.
17. Lind B, Nordwall A, Sihlbom H. Odontoid fractures treated with halo-vest. Spine. 1987;12:173-7.
18. Blacksin MF, Lee HJ. Frequency and significance of fractures of the upper cervical spine detected by CT in patients with severe neck trauma. AJR Am J Roentgenol. 1995;165:1201-4.
19. Harris MB, Waguespack AM, Kronlage S. "clearing" cervical spine injuries in polytraumapatients. Is it really safe to remove the collar? Orthopaedics. 1997;20:903-7.
20. Dickman CA, Mamourian A, Sonntag VKH, et al. Magnetic resonance imaging of the transverse atlantalligament for the evaluation of atlantoaxial instability. J Neurosurg. 1991;75(2):221-7.
21. Hott JS, Deshmukh VR, Papadopoulos SM, Spetzler RF. Application of a novel headrest system for odontoid screw fixation. Technical note. J Neurosurg Spine. 2007;6(1):90-1.
22. Doherty BJ, Heggeness MH. Quantitative anatomy of the second cervical vertebra. Spine. 1995;20:513-7.
23. NucciRC, Seigal S, MerolaAA, et al. Computed tomographic evaluation of the normal adult odontoid: Implications for internal fixation. Spine. 1995;20:264-70.
24. Sasso RC, Doherty BJ, Crawford MJ, et al. Biomechanics of odontoid fracture fixation:comparison of the one and two screw techniques. Spine. 1993;18:1950-3.
25. Kulkarni AG, Shah Siddharth. CT-based study of odontoid morphology in the Indian population: Implications in fixation of type 2 odontoid fractures. Paper presented at WIROC 2008, IOACON 2010, MOACON 2010, ASSICON 2012.
26. FujjiE,Kobayashi K, Hirabayashi K. Treatment in fractures of the odontoid process. Spine. 1988;13:604-9.
27. GeislerFH,ChengC,Poka A, et al. Anterior screw fixation of posteriorly displaced type II odontoid fractures. Neurosurgery. 1989;25:30-8.
28. Nakanishi T, Sasaki T,Tokit N, et al: Internal fixation for the odontoid fracture. Orthop Trans. 1982;6:176.
29. Borne GM,Bedou BL, Pinaudeau M,et al: Odontoid process fracture osteosynthesis with a direct screw fixation technique in nine consecutive cases: J Neurosurg. 1988;68:223-6.
30. Apfelbaum RI, Lonser RR, Veres R, Casey A.Direct anterior screw fixation for recent and remote odontoid fractures. J Neurosurg. 2000;93(Suppl):S227-36.
31. Dickman CA, Foley KT, Sonntag VK, Smith MM. Cannulated screws for odontoid screw fixation and atlantoaxial transarticular screw fixation technical note. J Neurosurg. 1995;83:1095-100.
32. Hott JS, Henn JS, Sonntag VK A new table-fixed retractor for anterior odontoid screw fixation: technical note. J Neurosurg. 2003 Apr;98(3) Suppl:294-6.
33. Lee SH, Sung JK. Anterior odontoid fixation using a 4.5-mm Herbert screw: The first report of 20 consecutive cases with odontoid fracture. Surg Neurol. 2006 Oct;66(4):361-6; discussion
34. William Magee et al. Biomechanical Comparison of a Fully Threaded, Variable Pitch Screw and a Partially Threaded Lag Screw for Internal Fixation of Type II Dens Fractures Spine. 2007; 32(7): E475-9.
35. Ames CP, Crawford NR, Chamberlain RH, Deshmukh V, Sadikovic B, Sonntag VK. Biomechanical evaluation of a bioresorbable odontoid screw. J Neurosurg Spine. 2005;Feb;2(2):182-7.
36. Yang YL, Fu BS, Li RW, Smith PN, Mu WD, Li LX, Zhou DS.Anterior single screw fixation of odontoid fracture with intraoperative Iso-C 3-dimensional imaging. Eur Spine J. 2011 Nov;20(11):1899-907.
37. Nikolay L, Martirosyan et al. Comparative Analysis of Isocentric 3-dimensional C-arm Fluoroscopy and Biplanar Fluoroscopy for Anterior Screw Fixation in Odontoid Fractures. J Spinal Disord Tech. 2011.
38. Kazan S, Tuncer R, Sindel M Percutaneous anterior odontoid screw fixation technique. A new instrument and a cadaveric study. Acta Neurochir (Wien). 1999;141:521-4.
39. Yong-Long Chi et al. Management of odontoid fractures with percutaneous anterior odontoid screw fixation. Eur Spine J. 2007;16:1157-64.
40. Jian Wang et al. Comparison of Percutaneous and Open Anterior Screw Fixation in the Treatment of Type II and Rostral Type III Odontoid Fractures. Spine. 2011;36:1459-63.
41. Harrop JS, Przybylski GJ. Use of an osteoconductive agent (Norian) in anterior surgical management of odontoid fractures. Technical note. Neurosurg Focus. 2000; B.A8(6):e8.

CHAPTER

15

Anterior Foraminotomy for Cervical Disk Disease

Janusz Bonkowski

When cervical disk prolapse was first defined as a clinical entity the surgical approach in those patients coming to operation was posteriorly, via a laminectomy or by a more limited posterior fenestration and foraminotomy. Cloward[1,2] and Smith and Robinson[3] independently devised the anterior approach used most often today. Their two approaches gave a more direct access to prolapse or osteophyte without the need to manipulate the nerve root which always lay posterior to the compressive agent. Fusion of the adjacent vertebrae was regarded as an important part of the procedure. Anterior diskectomy without an interpositioning graft has been used and actually gives results comparable with formal fusion but has failed to gain wide acceptance.[4,5] Much of the recent literature revolves around improving the fusion rates, with implants either into the disk space or plating to increase rigidity and bone incorporation and even more recently cervical arthroplasty.

Anterior cervical diskectomy and fusion seems to have been adopted as the "gold standard" in the surgical management of intractable cervical nerve root compression causing brachialgia. I suspect the adoption has been advanced so that cervical arthroplasty can have a legitimate control for randomized trials. However this adoption has arisen by default. Cloward (in 1953) found an anterior approach more satisfactory; and because he had to create a large "burr hole" to obtain access to the disk or osteophyte causing the compression he had to add a bone graft to plug and fill the hole. Smith and Robinson (1953) used fusion as an alternative to removing the compression, arguing that rigidity across the segment would allow the compressing agent to melt away once the movement was abolished. These two approaches and arguments coalesced into the anterior cervical diskectomy and fusion used today without ever being formally trialed against posterior foraminotomy, or indeed again conservative treatment. Therefore, the anterior cervical diskectomy and fusion has become a gold standard without ever passing the rigorous evidence-based approach we adhere to today.

Posterior foraminotomy fell into near obsolescence but has recently been resurrected as it can easily be modified to a minimally invasive approach as a microdiskectomy or endoscopic technique.[6] The arguments in favor of minimal nerve decompression are grounded on the natural history of nerve root compression syndromes, cost advantages, and by using the analogy with lumbar nerve root compression.

The natural history of most disk prolapses in the cervical spine causing brachialgia is very benign[7-10] most cases improve spontaneously and the recurrence rate is relatively low. Therefore, to carry out a major operation to fuse segments is probably over management.

In terms of cost advantages foraminotomy is certainly cheaper than an arthroplasty (and even cheaper than ACDF as the latter is also being backed up with plates and cages which add to costs at probably a fairly marginal benefit in terms of efficiency).

A lumbar nerve root compression due to either disk, or for that matter lateral recess compression by osteophytes, is more than adequately dealt with my simple decompression. Therefore, cervical nerve root compression should be similarly approached.

There is a disadvantage to posterior foraminotomy and that is that the compression is almost invariably anterior to the nerve root, the nerve root is relatively immobile and access anterior to it is limited when approached from behind. Unlike the lumbar situation, where nerve roots can be manipulated and even gently retracted away, the ability to manipulate cervical nerve roots is severely constrained. Therefore, a posterior foraminotomy can really only deal with a very laterally placed disk fragment and osteophytic compression is even less well dealt with usually the procedure then becomes limited to a pure decompression, opening up the channel posteriorly in the hope that the nerve root will also move posteriorly sufficiently to prevent or limit impingement. More medial fragments or large disk bulges would necessitate retraction of the cord with its attendant risks. Indeed the reason surgeons' embraced anterior cervical approaches so readily in the 1950s and 1960s was that many felt that the posterior foraminotomy was a rather "cramped" approach.

Modern microscopes and endoscopic instruments certainly help, but most surgeons still prefer an anterior approach to the cervical spine. The anterior foraminotomy is actually a refinement of Cloward's original technique: his original illustration[1] showed an off-center burr hole drilled directly down onto the obstructing element, whether it be disk or osteophyte. Without magnification, his access hole had to be fairly large, often a minimum of 12–14 mm in diameter in most cases. With microscopic magnification and modern microinstruments Cloward's access port can be made smaller, tilted over the extreme lateral edge of the disk, removing the uncinate process only and maintaining sufficient disk integrity to make fusion unnecessary.[11] However, the advantage of anterior foraminotomy is that it maintains the familiar anterior approach to the spine, attacks the compressive element directly and does not require nerve root or cord manipulation.

History of Anterior Foraminotomy

The initial descriptions of far lateral (transuncal) foraminotomy were by Verbiest[12] and Habuka.[13] They independently suggested a technique of removing the uncinate process to directly access the nerve root foramen for far lateral disks and osteophytes. This was recommended because they thought that accessing these fairly lateral process was difficult from a midline approach and a lateral to medial resection was better than a medial to lateral approach. However, in both of these cases the foraminotomy was then continued to a complete diskectomy and a fusion.

It was left to George[14] to perform an uncinate process resection of the foraminotomy as a stand alone procedure without disk removal. His extensive experience with vertebral artery surgery meant that he felt at ease working around the artery, mobilizing the vessel to improve lateral access to the intervertebral foramen.

Subsequently Jho[15-17] gave a most rigorous description of uncinate process resection and suggested the procedure could be accomplished without necessarily mobilizing or otherwise disturbing the vertebral artery. He became a popularizer of the technique and there has been a subsequent trickle of publications, most of which consist of case series extolling both the ease and efficacy of the technique to deal with nerve root compression[18,19]. There has never been any blinded series of the technique comparing it with other techniques (which is the truism of virtually all cervical surgical procedures prior to cervical arthroplasty).

There was a very adverse series report by Hacker[20] who suggested a higher recurrence in failure rate (50% in 33 three cases) and Savolainen[21] published experiments performed on cadaver spines suggesting the uncinate process resection could lead to some rotational instability of the spine. However, there has never been any clinical evidence that this is a real phenomenon.

Both George[14] and Jho have expanded the technique, utilizing it for more radical spinal canal decompression, suggesting that the foraminal decompression can act as an access port for more extensive removal of the large chronic disk bars causing spinal canal stenosis. These more extensive techniques rely on the undoubted fact that such patients invariably have advanced spondylitic degeneration with disk space collapse, the result of rigidity imparting sufficient stability to allow a rather liberal removal of disk and bone and would be judicious otherwise.

The Operation

The techniques of the operation is largely as described by Jho.[15] It is essentially a standard anterior cervical approach between the carotid sheath and the cervical strap musculature and larynx. A more oblique approach can be achieved by passing behind the sternomastoid and the carotid and jugular complex, but this is usually unnecessary. Therefore, the procedures starts as a conventional anterior cervical approach down to the prevertebral level; once the level to be decompressed has been identified with a marker and image intensifier the technique then diverges from standard midline disk excision. It is only necessary to retract laterally the longus colli muscle on the side to be decompressed. The midline can be retracted with a blade passed under the longus colli on the opposite side but the author has developed a blade which is pinioned into the vertebral body with a Caspar pin, limiting the contralateral resection to the midline only without any pharyngeal retraction necessary. Hence, postoperative hoarseness and swallowing difficulties can be minimized by limiting retraction.

The ipsilateral longus colli can be dissected laterally off the vertebral bodies and the disk as far laterally as the base of the transverse processes. It is often split leaving a medially based strip of muscle which I usually remove (this muscle tissue is then preserved as it can be used as a hemostat in preference to surgical or collagen sponging).

The core part of the operation is to remove the uncinate process of the dorsal vertebral edge. A 3 mm cutting burr creates a central cavity in the bone, slowly enlarging the hole until only a thin core of lateral cortex remains. Dissecting subperiosteally lateral to this, a plane can be created between bone and periosteum which is relatively bloodless and preserves the vertebral complex, which is usually not even visualized. This thin bone, which has been created, is infractured, opening the more lateral portions of the intervertebral foramen. Even a large lateral osteophyte can be readily de-gutted centrally and infractured with a very satisfying "crack" as it teases inwards. Changing to a 2 or 3 mm diamond burr the bone removal can be cautiously continued until the foramen of the nerve root has been opened. At this stage the more medial foramen will usually on probing with a fine curette reveal a fragment of sequestered disk material or further cartilaginous osteophytic tissue, which can be either teased out with micro-rongeurs or with a very fine Kerrison, eventually fully releasing the nerve root. The membrane which represents a lateral extension of the posterior longitudinal ligament can be opened to fully expose the nerve root sheath, but this often not necessary because sufficient disk fragment or osteophyte has been removed.

Hemostasis is readily achieved with bipolar and plugging the bone defect with small tags of the before mentioned muscle removed during longus colli dissection. A routine closure and vacuum drain is then affected.

Postoperative care is as for any anterior cervical approach, the drain can be removed after six to eight hours, the patient's mobilize readily and invariably are discharged home within twenty four hours (Figs 15.1 to 15.9).

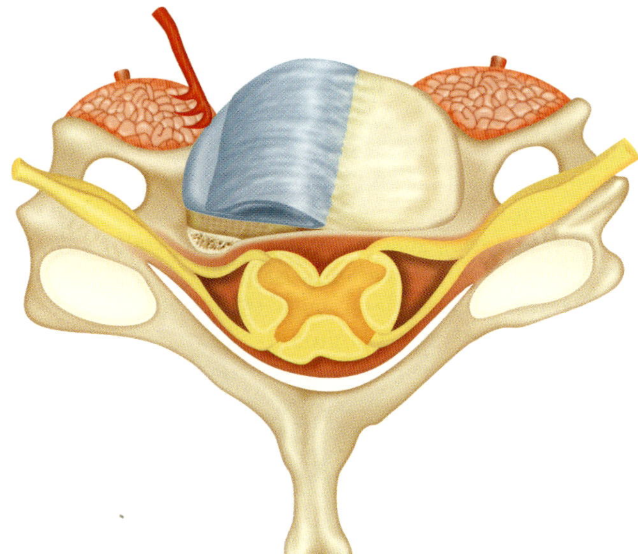

Fig. 15.1 Anterior cervical diskectomy
Source: Cloward RA. J Neurosurg. 1958;15:602-17

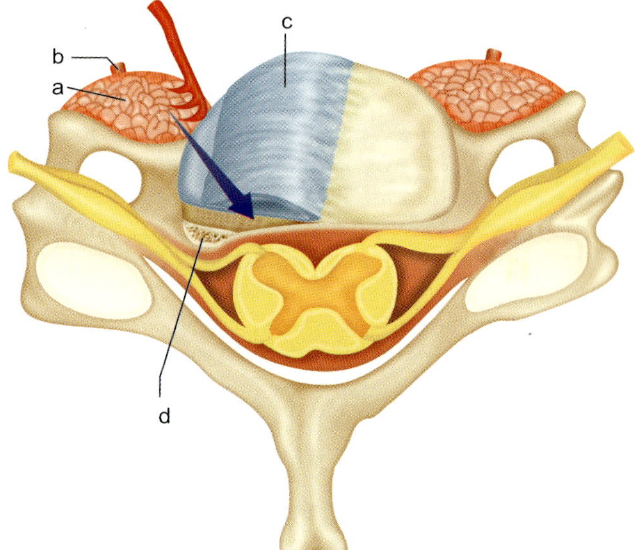

Fig. 15.2 Showing approach for diskectomy

Discussion

When Cloward first described his anterior approach to cervical nerve root compression he stated that fusion by means of an interpositional bone graft was an essential part of the technique. It was mandated because he drilled a large burr hole through the disk and adjacent vertebrae and its considerable caliber necessary to obtain access had to be filled or it might create collapse of the weakened vertebrae. He felt that the distraction used to fit the oversized dowel also provided extrawidening of the nerve root canal for further decompression, but rigidity was also important to protect against nerve irritation. Cloward believed that once a disk had suffered an episode of rupture it was so dysfunctional that complete removal and fusion was necessary in every

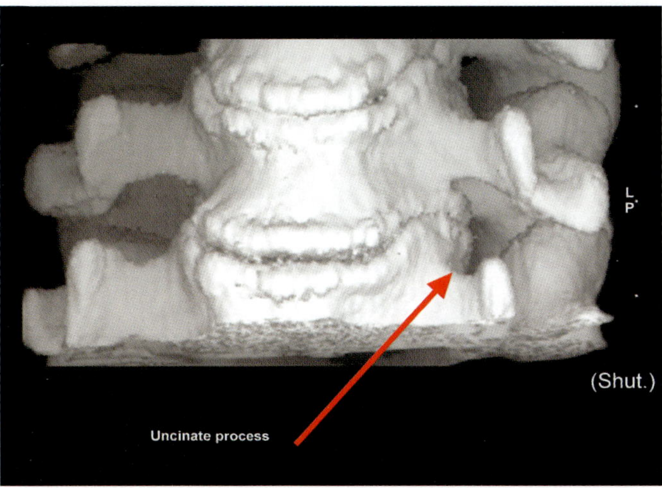

Fig. 15.3 Showing uncinate process

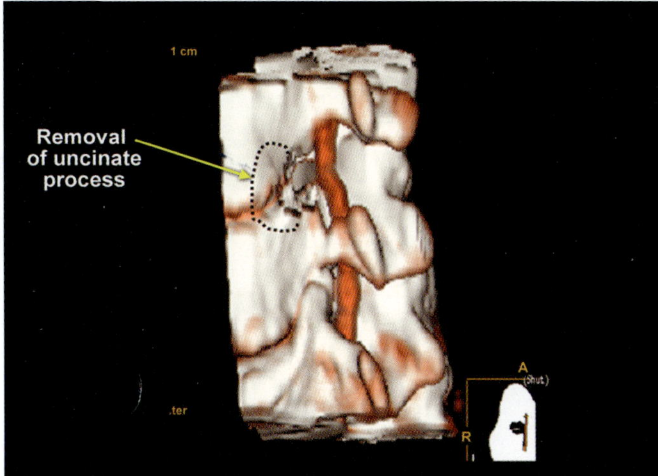

Fig. 15.4 Removal of uncinate process

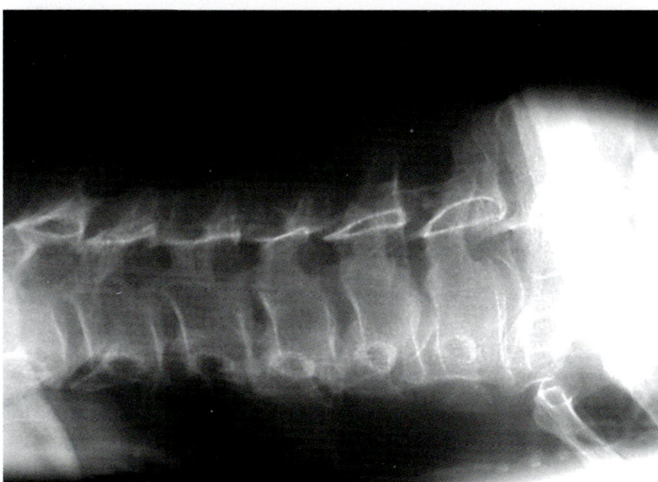

Fig. 15.5 Showing postoperative lateral oblique-left C6–7 transuncal disk approach

case (in the lumbar spine as well). Smith and Robinson also though fusion was necessary as movement encouraged osteophyte growth and mechanical irritation of the nerve by protruding disk, and their technique initially was purely a fusion, without any attempt to directly remove the compressive agent. Prolapses and osteophytes would melt away once rigidity was achieved.

Whilst both of these paradigms are intuitively appealing, the underlying hypothesis has never been subjected to proper empirical scrutiny. Yet, they remain the primary drivers of the belief that fusion is a central part of the surgical strategy in anterior approaches to cervical nerve root compression. It is difficult to design an experiment to evaluate these rationales, but there are clues in nature and the results of nonfusion surgery.

The first line of evidence arises out of the natural history of cervical disk prolapses. Not every episode of neuralgia due to cervical disk prolapse or osteophyte requires surgery. Indeed the majority settles spontaneously over several weeks to months and it is estimated that no more than 20–30% of cases come to operation. Furthermore whilst longitudinal follow-up of conservatively managed cases is not available, the experience of most clinicians is that few of these cases keep representing because of recurrent pain or neurology. Hence, cervical nerve root compression is a benign and usually singular event. It is possible that all of those cases where no recurrence occurs go on to spontaneous fusion or sufficient fibrous bonding to render the level functionally rigid, but I think this is by no means universal. It seems far more likely that the patient will be left with a somewhat spondylitic but mobile motion segment which generates either no or minor local symptoms. Hence, if an operation was available that simply excised the compressive fragment, it should achieve results comparable to those seen in nature, and these are generally highly satisfactory.

There is an operation available to meet some of these requirements, and this is the posterior approach; practiced for sixty years and despite periodic dips in its popularity still being practised with considerable success. It does cause some posterior muscle disruption, though marginal in the more contemporary microforaminotomy, and in most cases only the fragment causing the compression is removed (and in some cases not even that but merely a foraminal widening) leaving most of the disk behind. The reported results, though generally again not long-term, are very good. If there was a considerable cohort of these patients representing late with either further nerve root compression or severe mechanical or diskogenic symptoms I think they would have stimulated some reporting, yet the reports of failed posterior discectomy are not there or little more than occasional anecdotes.

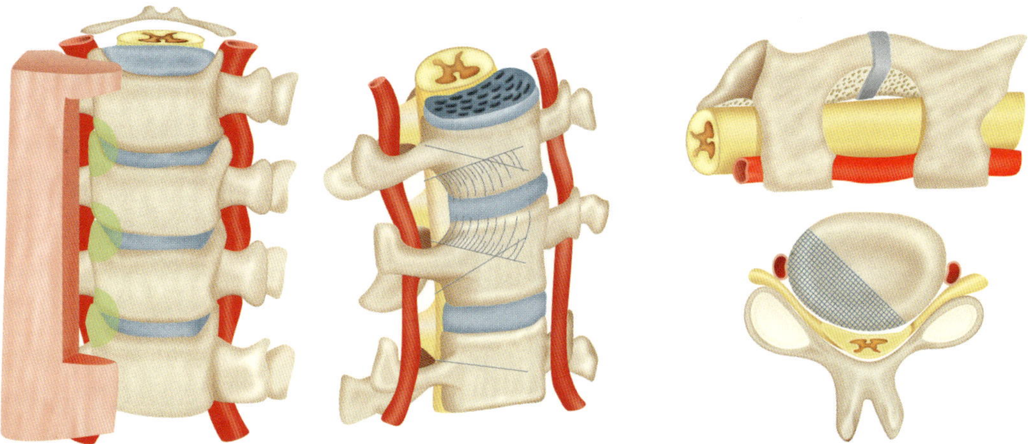

Fig. 15.6 Showing multiple transforaminal decompressions for cervical myelopathy
Source: JHO HD. Multiple transforaminal decompressions for spondylitic myelopathy. J Neurosurg 86:279-302, 1997

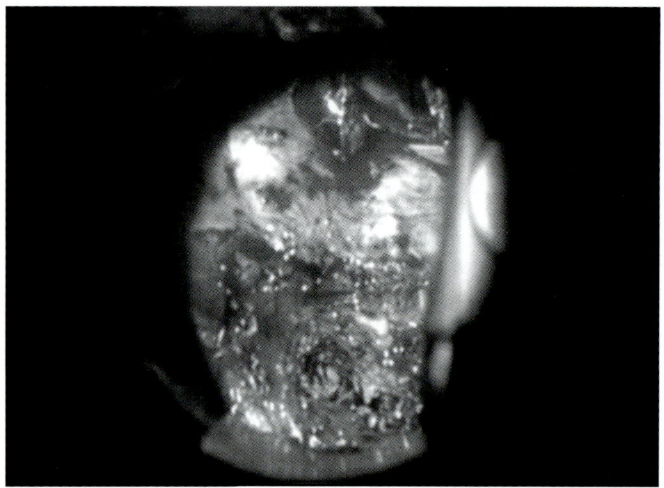

Fig. 15.7 Right-sided C5–6 approach

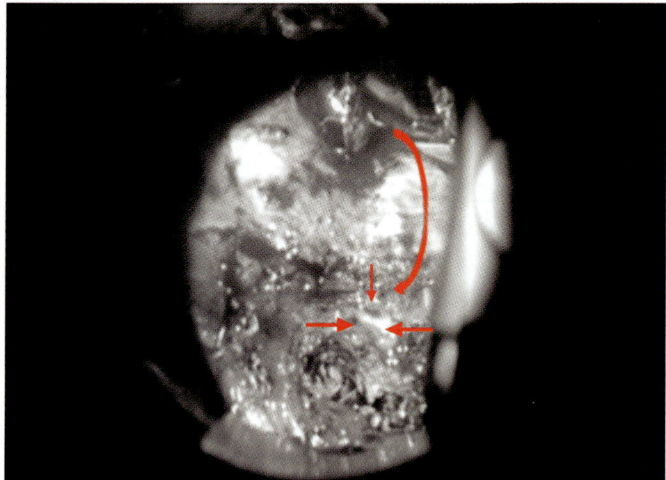

Fig. 15.9 Showing exposure of the disk after burr hole

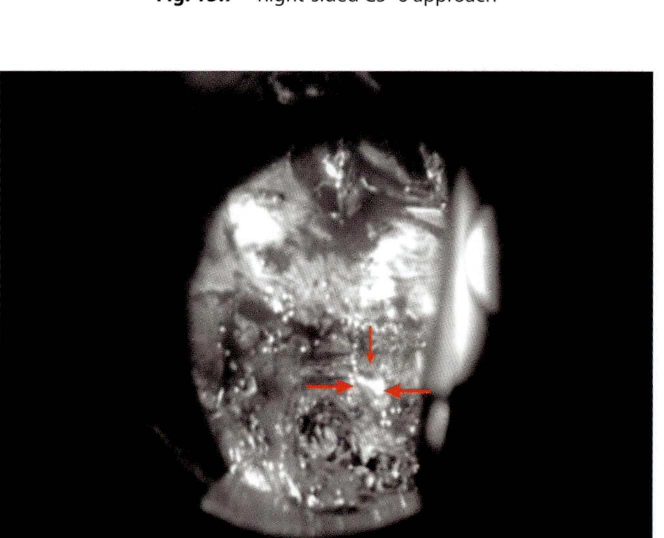

Fig. 15.8 Showing making burr hole

Hence, proponents of minimalist intervention already have an operation available. Why another one? The problems with posterior nerve root decompression are mainly technical, related to a limited view of the compressing agent with the nerve lying between surgeon and pathology, venous bleeding which can be quite troublesome from the epidural space, and a limited ability to remove very hard material or osteophytes without manipulating the nerve and carrying some risk of iatrogenic nerve damage (the "battered nerve syndrome"). Hence, some surgeons find the technique too constricting to be comfortable with it.

Anterior approaches appeal because the compressing agent is viewed directly and lifted away from the nerve with usually minimal or no neural manipulation, and even bone can be removed with little difficulty or risk. The anterior approach via a disk space clearance has been advocated and used with considerable success for forty years. Despite good reported figures in the literature, it has never become the "standard" operation, largely due to occasional anecdotal criticism of postoperative discomfort which has never been statistically scrutinized. However, the literature shows that diskectomy without fusion gives short-term results comparable with fusion. In long-term, there is evidence that the cleared disk space does eventually bond across, so the result is a fusion by default (or semi-intention).

The most minimalist approach, using the anterior planes in the neck with very little muscular disruption and a limited anterior transforaminal access port into the extradural space anterior to the nerve and dura, has been periodically reported by various authors over the years. Initially, these approaches involved mobilizing the vertebral artery and removing variable amounts of bone, including all of the lateral uncinate process and understandably generated little enthusiasm because of concerns about vascular injury and the destabilizing effects of bone dissection. However, Jho and Gill have described refinements in the amount of bone that needs to be resected, to the point where bone removal is limited to only part of the uncinate process and the compressive agent can sometimes be removed with virtually no resection of anatomical structures, apart from osteophytic outgrowths. The adverse results of Hacker are difficult to explain unless the amount of bone or disk resection was virtually tantamount to a subtotal diskectomy and access port of near Cloward proportions. The procedure can on occasions amount to a more substantial diskectomy when a very degenerate and fibrous disk is encountered, and in these case some precipitation of a more acute spondylitic collapse of the disk will occur, possibly with increased local neck pain for a period. The author's experience is that very few patients with increased neck pain require more than conservative treatment with good symptomatic resolution in most cases. In the author's hands, in a series of over 250 anterior foraminotomies there has only been a single case of reprolapse which occurred contralateral to the operative site. The risk of reprolapse, therefore, appears to be slight if the true disk space is not excessively dissected or tampered with.

There is also the problem of patient selection or dealing preemptively with patient expectations: the operation is for nerve compression and brachialgia, not for neck ache, neck stiffness, nor headache. It is dubious whether any surgery at all should be offered patients with predominantly such mechanical or referred symptom are the results are generally poor. However, patients present with a mixture of neuralgic and more nonspecific symptoms, will accept preoperatively explanations to the effect that only nerve pain will be helped by the operation and yet postoperatively express disappointment that the whole cacophony of their cervical symptomatology has not been fully alleviated by the surgery. If this is accompanied by demands for more surgery to correct residual symptoms the whole process can avalanche into unmanageable proportions.

No operation currently makes anatomy normal. The transuncal approach appears to be the closest we can get to a "natural" result with minimal interference with the motion segments of the cervical spine and there is a cohort of patients who are actively seeking, just such an approach to the problem. It is an approach that every spinal surgeon should be aware of and be able to offer these patients who find the concept of artificially stiffening the neck to be unacceptable. They should not be talked into a fusion because the evidence that it gives superior results is simply not present.

There is also a strategic argument for disk preserving surgery: arthrodesis of virtually all extraspinal joints is falling into the end stage "salvage" category of treatment. Surgery is usually replacement with artificial joints. Artificial disk replacement has progressed past the experimental phase and is being actively offered in many centers. It may well become a standard part of surgical treatment in a fairly short time frame. It is unlikely that artificial disks will function or even be implanted into a chronically fused motion unit, so fusing a cervical segment is tantamount to foreclosing the possibility of later restoring movement to that segment. If and disk is left after an operation, the segment may maintain sufficient mobility to be later replaced by an artificial disk. In the author's series of cases six of the original cohort of 250 have proceeded to arthroplasty at the previously operated segment as salvage strategy. Therefore, the foraminotomy has the advantage of being an operation where no bridges are burnt.

References

1. Cloward RB. The anterior approach for removal of ruptured cervical discs. J Neurosurg. 1958;15:602-17.
2. Cloward RB. The anterior surgical approach to the cervical spine. Spine. 1998;13:823-7.
3. Smith GW, Robinson RA The treatment of certain cervical spine disorders by anterior removal of the intervertebral disc and interbody fusion. J Bone Joint Surg AM. 1958;40:607-24.
4. Adamson TE. Microendoscopic posterior cervical laminoforaminotomy for unilateral radiculopathy: results of a new technique in 100 cases. J Neurosurg (Spine 1). 2001;95:51-7.
5. Johnson JP, Filler AG, McBridge DQ, Batzdorf U. Anterior cervical foraminotomy for unilateral radicular disease. Spine. 2000;25:905-9.
6. Tan LC. Medial cervical facetectomy for radiculopathy due to foraminal stenosis: 71 personal consecutive cases. J Clin Neurosc. 1999;6:207-11.

7. Maigne J-Y, Deligne L. Computed tomographic follow-up study of 21 cases of nonoperatively treated cervical intervertebral soft disc herniations Spine. 1994;19(2):189-91.
8. Mochida K, Komor H, Okawa A, Muneta T, Haro H, Shinomiya K. Regression of cervical disc herniation observed on Magnetic Resonance images. Spine. 1998;23(9):990-7.
9. Radhakrishnan K, Litchy WJ, O'Fallon M, Kurkland LT. Epidemiology of cervical radiculopathy. A population-based study from Rochester, Minnesota, 1976 through 1990. Brain. 1994;117:325-35.
10. Saal JS, Saal JA, Yurth EF. Nonoperative management of herniated cervical intervertebral disc with radiculopathy. Spine. 1996;21(16):1877-983.
11. Savolainen S, Rinne J, Hernes-Niemi J. A prospective randomized study of anterior single-level cervical disc operations with long-term follow-up: surgical fusion is unnecessary. Neurosurg. 1998;43:51-5.
12. Verbiest H. A lateral approach to the cervical spine: technique and indications. J Neurosurg. 1968;28:
13. Hakuba A. Trans-unco-discal approach. A combined anterior and lateral approach to cervical discs. J Neurosurg. 1976;45:284-91.
14. George B, Gauthier N, Lot G. Multisegmental cervical spondylitic myelopathy and radiculopathy treated by multilevel oblique corpectomies without fusion. Neurosurgery. 1999;44:81-90.
15. Jho HD. Microsurgical anterior cervical foraminotomy for radiculopathy: a new approach to cervical disc herniation. J Neurosurg. 1996;84:155-60.
16. Jho HD. Decompression via microsurgical anterior foraminotomy for cervical spondylitic myelopathy. Technical note. J Neurosurg. 1997;86:297-302.
17. Jho HD. Failed anterior cervical foraminotomy: Editorial. J Neurosurg (Spine 2). 2003;98:121-5.
18. Grundy PL, Germon TJ, Gill S S. Transpedicular approaches to cervical uncovertebral osteophytes causing radiculopathy. J Neurosurg (Spine 1). 2000;93:21-7.
19. Snyder GM, Bernhardt M. Anterior cervical fractional interspace decompression for treatment of cervical radiculopathy. A review of the first 66 cases. Clinical Orthop. 1989;246:92-9.
20. Hacker RJ, Miller C G. Failed anterior cervical foraminotomy. J Neurosurg (Spine 2). 2003;98:126-30.
21. Schmieder K, Kettner A, Brenke C, Harders A, Pechlivanis I, Wilke H. In vitro flexibility of the cervical spine after ventral uncoforaminotomy. J Neurosurg. 2007;7:537-41.

CHAPTER

16

Anterior Cervical Corpectomy for Cervical Spondylotic Myelopathy

Ajoy P Shetty, Vishnu Prasad, Rishi M Kanna, S Rajasekaran

Introduction

Cervical spondylotic myelopathy (CSM) has been first defined by Brain et al. in the year 1952.[1] CSM is defined as spinal cord dysfunction secondary to extrinsic compression of the cord and its vascular supply or both that is caused by degenerative disease of cervical spine. CSM has been observed in two age groups: (i) age <55 years, where a soft disc herniation is the most likely cause (Fig. 16.1) and (ii) age >55 years, where the most likely etiology of stenosis are osteophytes, calcification of posterior disk, annulus buckling, and hypertrophy of ligamentum flavum[2] (Fig. 16.2).

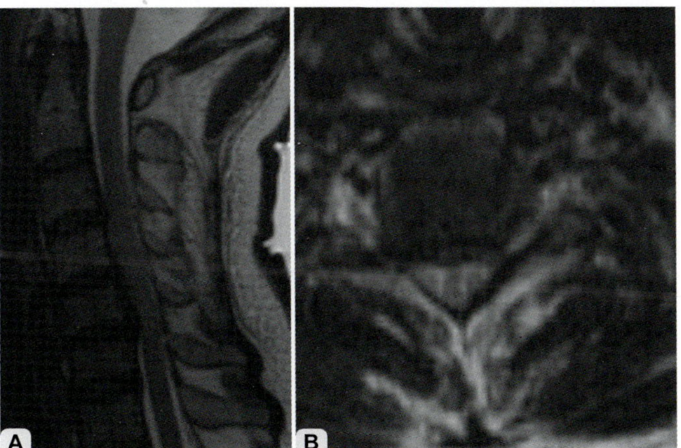

Fig. 16.1 Sagittal and axial T2 MRI images showing soft disk herniation at C5–6 level causing cord compression

The direct compression of the arteries and impairment of the venous flow leading to venous congestion also contributes to spinal cord ischemia.

The natural history of CSM has not been clearly defined despite extensive clinical studies in this area. There is evidence that the natural history of CSM may be mixed with many patients experiencing a slow, stepwise decline. Long periods of quiescence are not uncommon, however, and a subgroup of patients may improve. Severe stenosis may ultimately result in necrosis of both gray and white matter. So early surgery is a key point in the natural history of CSM and can potentially improve neurological prognosis. In fact, there is strong evidence showing that surgery within one year from onset of symptoms strongly improves outcomes in CSM.[1,3-5]

Surgical Treatment for Cervical Spondylotic Myelopathy

The main aims of the surgical procedure are decompression of the spinal cord, achieving proper cervical alignment, and restoring or maintaining stability. Surgical techniques can be broadly divided into anterior, posterior, or combined surgical approaches. Anterior approach includes anterior cervical diskectomy and anterior cervical corpectomy. Posterior approaches include laminectomy with or without fusion, laminoplasty, and their modifications. The selection of an appropriate surgical procedure for CSM is complex and depends on several factors mentioned in Table 16.1.

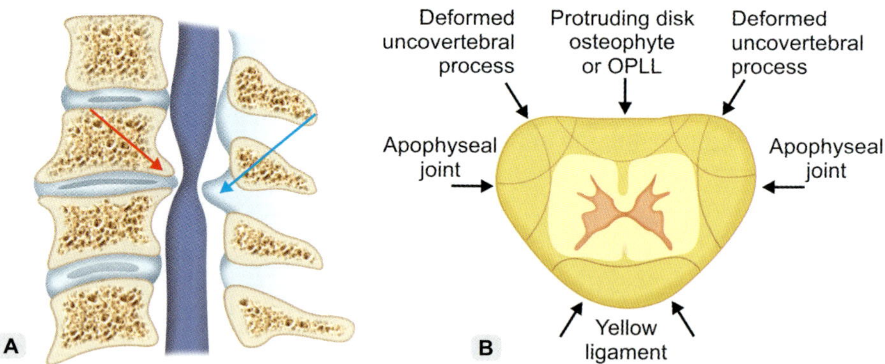

Fig. 16.2 Pathophysiology of cervical spondylotic myelopathy. (A) The posterior disk osteophytes complex (red arrow) and the buckled ligamentum flavum (blue arrow) circumferentially compress the spinal cord; (B) Osteophytes from the apophyseal joints and uncovertebral process lead to a combination of myelopathic and radicular symptoms

Table 16.1 Factors influencing the choice of CSM surgery

- Location of primary compression
- Number of levels of compression
- Alignment of cervical spine
- Presence of instability
- Previous surgeries
- Presence of tandem stenosis
- Axial neck pain
- Surgeon's preference

Location of Primary Compression

When the compression of the spinal cord is predominantly anterior due to disk protrusions or osteophytes, anterior approach is preferred (Fig. 16.3). Posterior approaches are considered in cases of hypertrophied ligamentum flavum where the compression is predominantly from posterior aspect. Posterior decompression also addresses anterior com-pression, because it indirectly decompresses the spinal cord by enlarging the spinal canal.

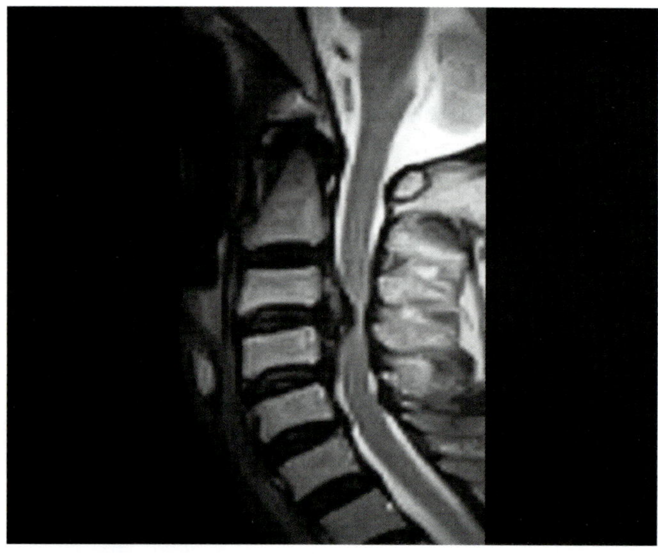

Fig. 16.3 MRI showing predominantly anterior compression

Levels of Compression

One or two level compressions are preferably treated by anterior techniques whereas multilevel (≥3) compressions require posterior surgeries. Anterior cervical discectomy and fusion (ACDF) up to 1–3 levels have been reported to be safe and effective in decompressing ventral pathology. Early complications due to duration of surgery, blood loss, prolonged anesthesia and chronic graft related complications increase with the number of levels of ACDF. Multilevel ACDF is associated with an increased risk of pseudoarthrosis, as high as 54% in three-level fusions[6] with a significant potential for plate failure and graft extrusion.[7] Yonenobu et al. recommended anterior procedure for no more than three levels and posterior procedure for four levels or more.[8]

Alignment of Cervical Spine

The cervical spine has a normal physiologic lordosis of 30–50 degrees. A minimum of 10 degrees of cervical lordosis is mandatory to contemplate posterior decompression surgeries in CSM so that the spinal cord can "fall back". In cases of kyphotic cervical spine, either an anterior procedure or a posterior procedure with instrumentation is needed (Figs 16.4 to 16.6).

Presence of Instability and Axial Neck Pain

CSM patients with instability or axial neck pain should be considered for instrumentation and fusion through an anterior or posterior approach. Posterior surgeries, especially laminoplasty have a higher incidence of postoperative axial neck pain.

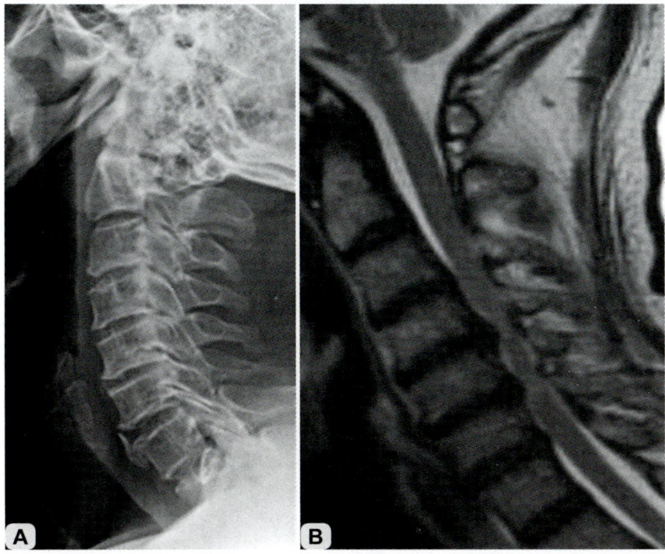

Fig. 16.4 (A) Lateral radiograph and (B) sagittal MRI demonstrating multiple level cervical cord compression with lordotic alignment

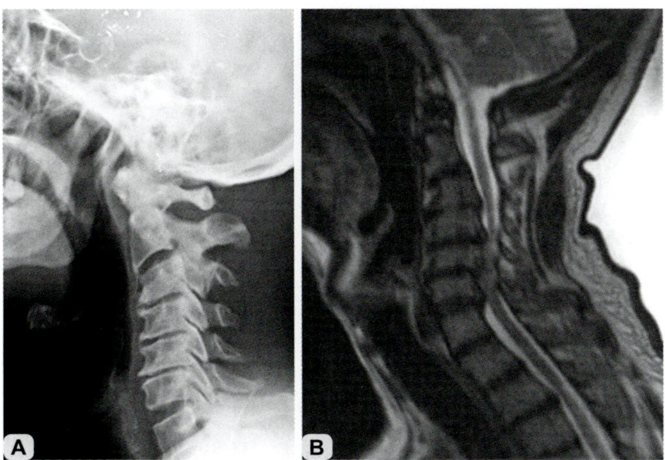

Fig. 16.5 (A) Lateral radiograph and (B) sagittal MRI showing kyphotic alignment of cervical spine in a patient with multilevel cervical spondylotic compression

Previous Surgeries

Patients who have had previous anterior surgeries will need either an anterior approach from the other side (right or left) or a posterior approach.

Presence of Tandem Stenosis

Coexistence of thoracic or lumbar canal stenosis should also be considered while planning the approach. Elderly patients with multilevel tandem stenosis are preferably treated by posterior decompression surgeries, either in a single stage or two stages.

Anterior Cervical Corpectomy and Fusion (ACCF)

1. *What is anterior cervical corpectomy with reference to treatment of CSM?:* In patients with ventral cervical cord compression at more than one level, the need for a corpectomy versus multilevel diskectomy should be considered. Patients with significant stenosis behind the body, ossified posterior longitudinal ligament (OPLL), soft disk migrations behind the vertebral body, posterior osteophytes extending behind the vertebral body and those with a kyphotic cervical alignment would benefit from corpectomy (Fig. 16.7). To decompress the spinal cord, subtotal corpectomy is performed by removing a central trough of vertebral body. The trough is centered between the uncovertebral joints, which helps to orient

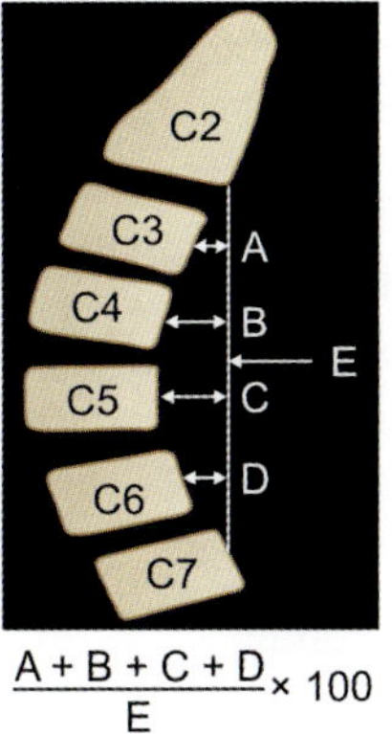

$$\frac{A + B + C + D}{E} \times 100$$

Fig. 16.6 Measurement of cervical sagittal alignment using Ishiharas curvature index. A straight line is drawn from the posterior inferior corner of the C2 vertebral body to the posterior superior corner of the C7 body (E). The transverse distance of this line from the posterior surfaces of the vertebral bodies of C3 to C6 are measured and added together (A + B + C + D). This value is divided by "E" and multiplied by 100. The normal value ranges from - 10 to 11. Lesser values indicate kyphotic alignment

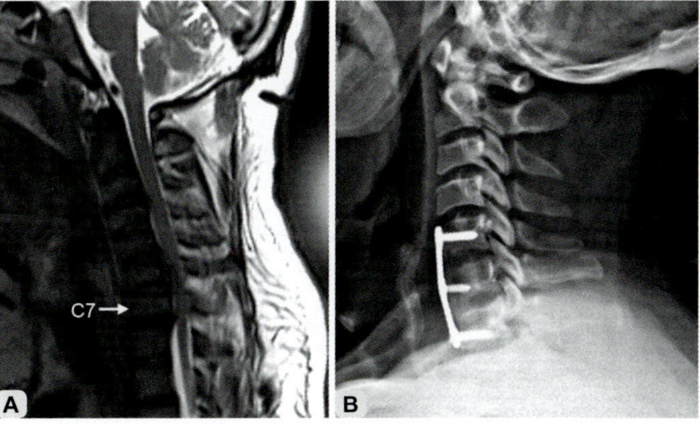

Fig. 16.7 Extruded disk fragment behind C6 body with kyphotic alignment which was treated with ACCF

the trough over the spinal cord and ensure complete decompression.

2. *What is the specific advantage of an anterior approach?:* Advantages of anterior approach include direct decompression of offending structures and the anterior spinal artery, restoration of the cervical lordosis, and reduction in axial neck pain. In other words, it addresses the axial, radicular, and myelopathic symptoms of cervical spondylosis.
3. *What are the clinical indications for corpectomy?:* Other indications of anterior cervical corpectomy are trauma, infection, tumor and correction of kyphotic deformity.
4. *ACDF vs ACCF in multiple level compressions:* Multilevel ACDF is preferred in certain situations over ACCF where the compression is confined to the level of the disc spaces[9] (Fig. 16.8). Also, it is associated with a less blood loss and has a lower risk of graft kick out and catastrophic failures.[10] However multilevel ACDF is associated with an increased risk of pseudarthrosis, as high as 54% in three-level fusions.[11] A potential benefit of ACCF is that fewer graft surfaces are required to fuse than multilevel ACDF (i.e. for a decompression at C4–5/C5–6, ACDF would require 4 surfaces to fuse versus 2 surfaces if treated with ACCF). With modern plating techniques, it appears that fusion rates are similar between the two techniques.
5. *Contraindication to anterior approach:* Contraindications are very rarely encountered which includes previous irradiation to the anterior neck, aberrant vertebral artery (Fig. 16.9) and chin on chest deformity where anterior approach becomes impossible.

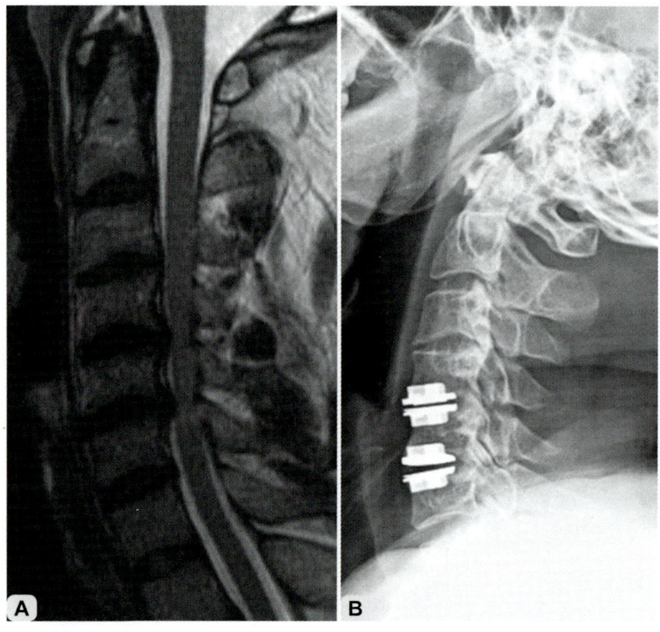

Fig. 16.8 Multiple level compressions at C4–5 and C5–6 confined to the disk spaces treated with anterior diskectomy and disk replacement

Radiological Investigations and Preoperative Evaluation

All patients require anteroposterior and lateral X-rays of the cervical spine. The sagittal curvature of the cervical spine, the disk height, presence of osteophytes and the degree of degenerative changes, and any ossification of posterior longitudinal ligament (OPLL) are evaluated in the X-rays (Fig. 16.10). Adequacy of visualization of the lower cervical spine in X-ray is also evaluated. Dynamic flexion extension X-rays are necessary to see for any dynamic instability (Fig. 16.11).

MRI is the gold standard investigation for evaluating a cervical myelopathy. The things to look in MRI are given in Table 16.2 (Fig. 16.12). All these factors aid in surgical decision making. The vertebral artery should be carefully assessed in the axial cuts for any anomalies like unilateral agenesis, dilatation and the presence of an intracorporeal aberrant course, which are all contraindications for anterior cervical corpectomy. If there are any contraindications for an MRI, a CT myelogram is performed.

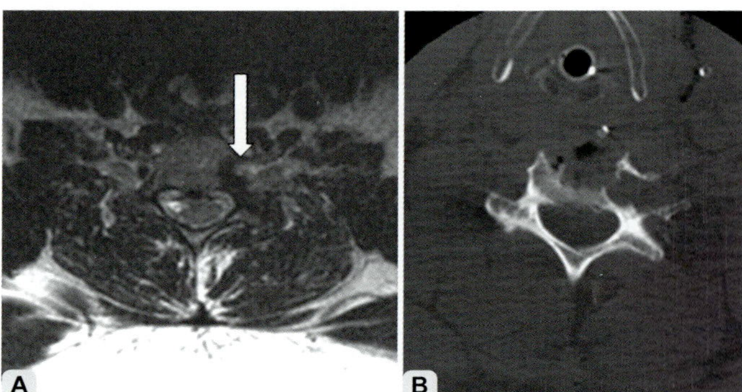

Fig. 16.9 Abberent vertebral artery course into the vertebral body. (A) MRI; (B) CT

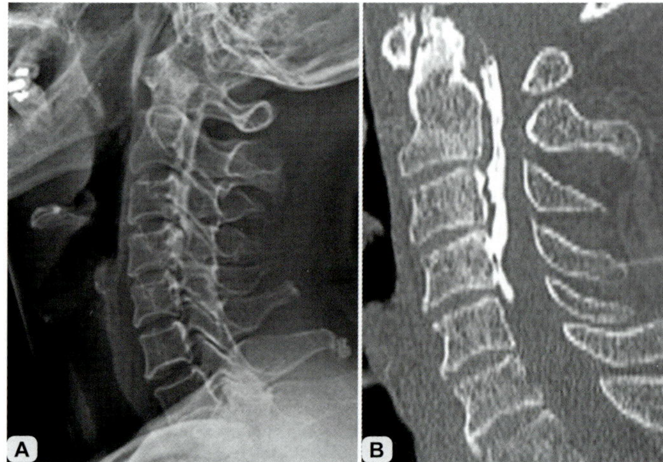

Fig. 16.10 Lateral radiograph and sagittal CT image of a patient with continuous type OPLL extending from C2 to C4

Table 16.2 Features to look for in a MRI of a patient with CSM

- Levels of compression
- Predominant anterior or posterior compression
- Compression at the level of disks or behind the vertebral body
- T2 hyperintense signal, which represent inflammation and edema of cord
- T1 hypointense signal, which represents gliosis, myelomalacia or ischemia
- Other regions of the spine

CT scan is not routinely performed but can clearly demonstrate the bony anatomy, the size and dimensions of OPLL, extent of compression in central canal and neural foramen and the extent of decompression required (Fig. 16.10 and 16.13). It also gives the relationship between vertebral artery and spinal canal as rarely vertebral foramina can be situated medially limiting the decompression laterally.

Clinical Evaluation

Clear documentation of the neurological status including exact motor power, sensory impairment, deep tendon reflexes, special hand signs of myelopathy, bladder–bowel disabilities are essential for comparing postoperative changes (improvement/deterioration). The presence of radiculopathy along with myelopathy features mandates special attention to the involved nerve root during the decompression, and hence, its preoperative documentation is crucial for better postoperative outcomes.

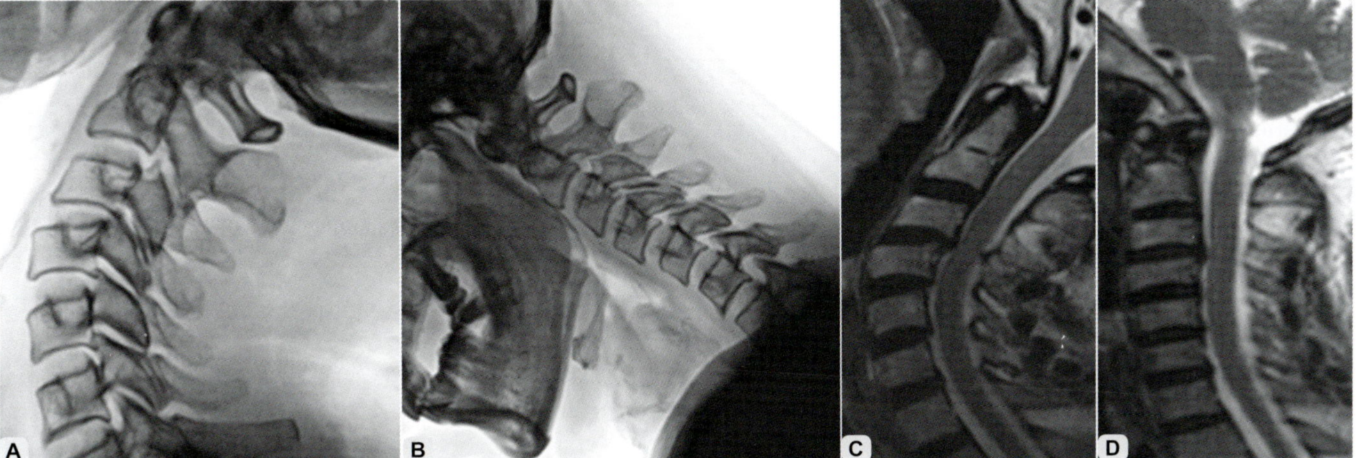

Fig. 16.11 Dynamic flexion-extension radiographs showing instability at C3–C4 level (retrolisthesis), which is also reflected in the dynamic MRI

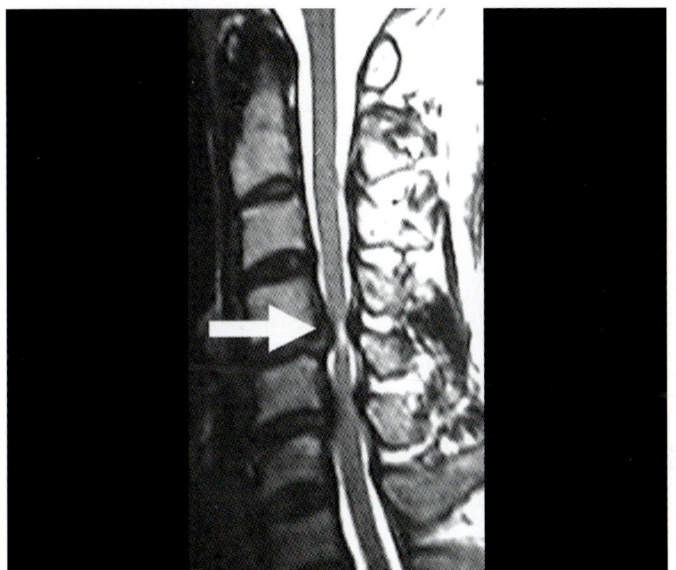

Fig. 16.12 T2 sagittal MRI showing CSM with hyperintense signal intensity changes at C4–C5 level

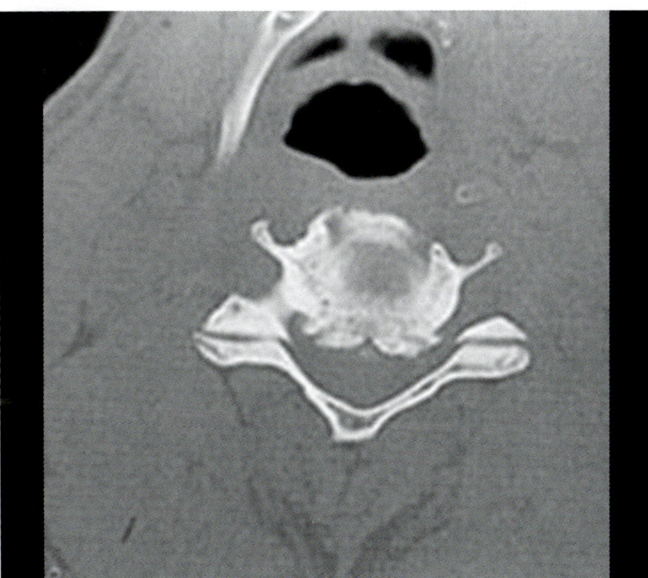

Fig. 16.13 CT axial image showing posterior osteophytes compressing the cord and the foramen

Preoperative discussion with the patient is mandatory and should include about the need and the goals of the surgery, its limitations, and the possible complications. It should be explained that the main aim of the surgery is to halt the progression of the disease and the prognosis for neurological improvement is variable. Postoperative course, wound care, physical therapy, and follow-up should also be explained.

Operative Techniques

The critical issues while executing the surgical management (anterior cervical decompression) of patients with CSM can be clearly explained by discussing the different stages of the surgery as depicted in Table 16.3.

Anesthesia

The preoperative range of motion determines the intubation techniques and guides the positioning of patient. In patients where the myeloradiculopathy symptoms are worsened by neck extension, fiberoptic intubation is recommended. In upper cervical procedures (above C4), nasotracheal intubation is preferred, as it helps to push the mandible away from operative area. In the author's hospital, RAE North Pole$^{(R)}$ tube is used for intubation which prevents kinking of the tube while positioning. After intubation, the neck should be positioned in neutral position during the surgery. Patients with prior history of cervical spine surgery should be evaluated for vocal cord dysfunction. If vocal cord dysfunction is present, then the ipsilateral approach has to be used to avoid bilateral vocal cord dysfunction.

Instruments Needed for Performing ACCF

The instruments needed are tabulated Table 16.4 (in the order of usage during surgery):

Table 16.4 Instruments for ACCF

- Operative microscope
- Long handed retractors/self retractor
- Self retaining retractors
- Cloward lamina spreader
- Caspar retractor and retractor pins
- Different sized straight and angled currettes
- Pituitary and Kerrison rongeurs
- High speed burr/ultrasonic bone cutter
- Rongeurs
- Blunt hooks
- Hemostatic aids—thrombin, gel foam, patties, surgical and bone wax
- Instruments for bone graft harvesting-osteotomes and oscillating saw
- Cervical plate/cage systems

Positioning of the Patient

Under general anesthesia, the patient is positioned supine over the operating table. A rolled sheet is placed beneath the scapula to allow the shoulders to drop back. A sand bag should be placed under the iliac crest for harvesting the bone graft. The cervical spine is positioned in neutral or in mild extension. Excessive extension of the cervical spine should be avoided which might cause cord compression and deteriorating neurology. The occiput is stabilized with a bean bag placed around the head and behind the cervical spine. The shoulders are secured using tapes with mild traction distally allowing for radiographic imaging of the lower cervical spine (Fig. 16.14). The table is positioned with head end elevated to minimize the venous engorgement and bleeding. Various anatomical land marks give us an approximate guide to the level of cervical spine. The hyoid bone corresponds to the C3 vertebra, the thyroid cartilage to the C4 and C5 vertebrae and the cricoid cartilage to the C6 vertebra (Fig. 16.15). Alternatively, the cervical vertebra planned for corpectomy is marked using a fluoroscope.

Once the level is identified, infiltration of the skin and subcutaneous tissue is performed with a 1:500,000 epinephrine solution to aid in hemostasis. For correction of kyphosis and to achieve distraction, Gardner-Well tongs can also be applied with approximately 4–5 kg weight. Neurophysiologic monitoring can be used to monitor spinal cord function (SSEP & MEP). MEP is preferred in myelopathic

Table 16.3 Stages of surgery

1. Anesthesia
2. Instruments needed for performing ACCF
3. Positioning
4. Operative steps
    i. Step 1: Approach
    ii. Step 2: Diskectomy
    iii. Step 3: Corpectomy
    iv. Step 4: Reconstruction of defect
    v. Step 5: Plating
5. Postoperative care

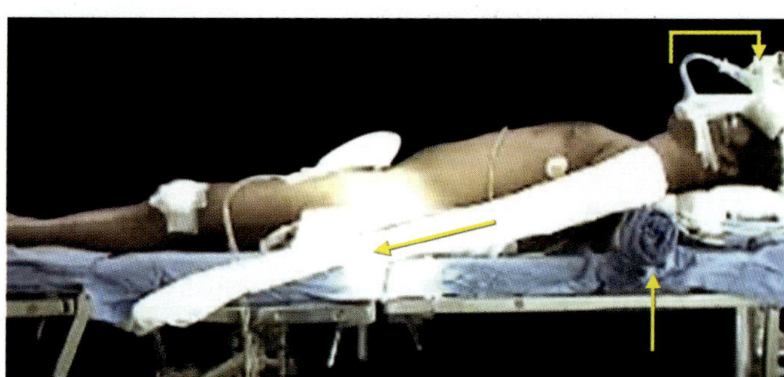

Fig. 16.14 Patient positioning for an anterior cervical surgery. A North pole endotracheal tube has been used. A rolled towel is placed between the scapula to provide hyperextension. Both the upper limbs are pulled down and strapped to the table to enable visualization of the lower cervical spine

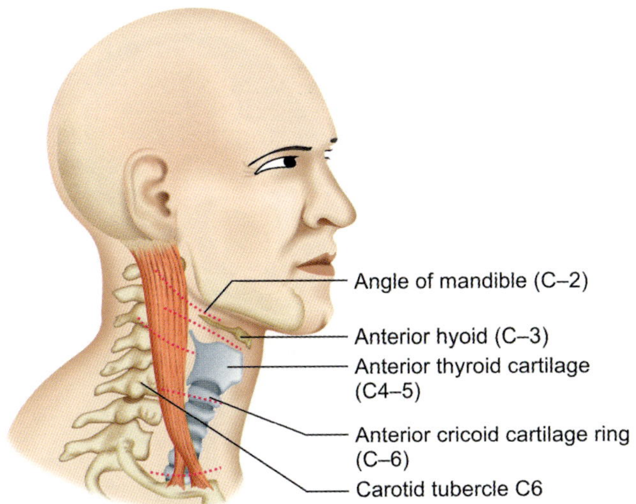

Fig. 16.15 Surface anatomical landmarks for cervical spine

patients and base-line values should be obtained before the start of the procedure.

Operative Steps (Figs 16.16 and 16.17)

Step 1: Exposure

The approach to the anterior cervical region is through a Southwick and Robinson (Smith– Robinson) approach (Fig. 16.18). Although the literature indicates that the injury to recurrent laryngeal nerve (RLN) is less with left-sided approach, the author routinely uses the right-sided approach without any increased incidence of injury to RLN. Left-sided approach is preferred for cervicothoracic junction where the right-sided approach might easily injure RLN. The author insists for intermittent release of traction to relieve the pressure to RLN which is situated medially in the tracheoesophageal groove.

A transverse incision is adequate for one or two level corpectomy. A transverse incision offers better cosmesis. Extending the incision across the midline, undermining the platysma, release of mid cervical fascia proximally and distally facilitates exposure of up to three levels. A longitudinal incision should be considered for 2 or 3 level corpectomy.

A transverse incision is made from just across over the midline to the medial border of the sternocleidomastoid muscle. The incision is carried through the skin and subcutaneous fat. The platysma muscle is also cut in line with the skin incision. The anterior border of the sternocleidomastoid muscle is identified by palpation and the direction of muscle fibres towards the mastoid process. Just medial to the sternomastoid muscle, the superficial layer of the deep cervical fascia is identified and cut longitudinally using a scissor. Beware of large branches of external jugular veins in this layer. They can be ligated without serious consequences.

The next step is to identify the plane between the carotid sheath and the "tubes" (trachea and esophagus). The carotid pulse is felt by palpation with the left index and middle finger. By blunt dissection, the middle layer of deep cervical fascia that encloses the omohyoid medial to the carotid sheath is dissected. Long artery forceps with cotton pledgets or the surgeon's finger can be used for blunt dissection. As the sternomastoid and carotid sheath are retracted laterally with blunt hand-held retractors, the anterior aspect of the cervical spine can be palpated. The trachea, esophagus, and thyroid gland are retracted medially exposing the anterior cervical spine. The deep layers of the deep cervical fascia, consisting of the pretracheal and prevertebral fascia overlying the longus colli muscles are divided with a scissor. Now the appropriate surgical level is identified at this point using a bent spinal needle placed in the disk space. The needle is bent like a double L to prevent inadvertent plunging of needle into the spinal canal (Fig. 16.19). Fluoroscopy is used to confirm the position of the needle in the appropriate disk space. In view of recent concerns about potential disk degeneration following needle placement into a normal disk, the authors prefer to place the needle on the vertebral body. The confirmed level can then marked with electrocautery. The longus colli muscles are elevated subperiosteally from the vertebral body up to the uncovertebral joints. This serves three purposes: (a) helps identify the uncovertebral joint and hence the lateral extent of decompression is defined, (b) identification of midline, which then can be marked with cautery or burr, and (c) placement of retractors underneath the longus colli, protecting the vital structures (Fig. 16.20A). Either hand-held or self-retaining retractors can be used to keep the cervical spine exposed. If self-retaining retractor is used, it is advisable to deflate and reinflate the endotracheal cuff after applying the retractors, to decrease the incidence of recurrent laryngeal nerve palsy.

Step 2: Diskectomy

Further steps of the procedure are performed under operative microscope. The advantages of using operative microscope are better illumination and magnification and teaching of the assistant and residents. Operative microscope should be oriented perpendicular to the vertebral bodies. Angular orientation can possibly lead to an oblique corpectomy leading towards the pedicle and vertebral artery injuries (Fig. 16.20B).

The next part is decompression. Single-level corpectomy is explained here and multiple level corpectomies can be done in a similar manner. A diskectomy is performed above

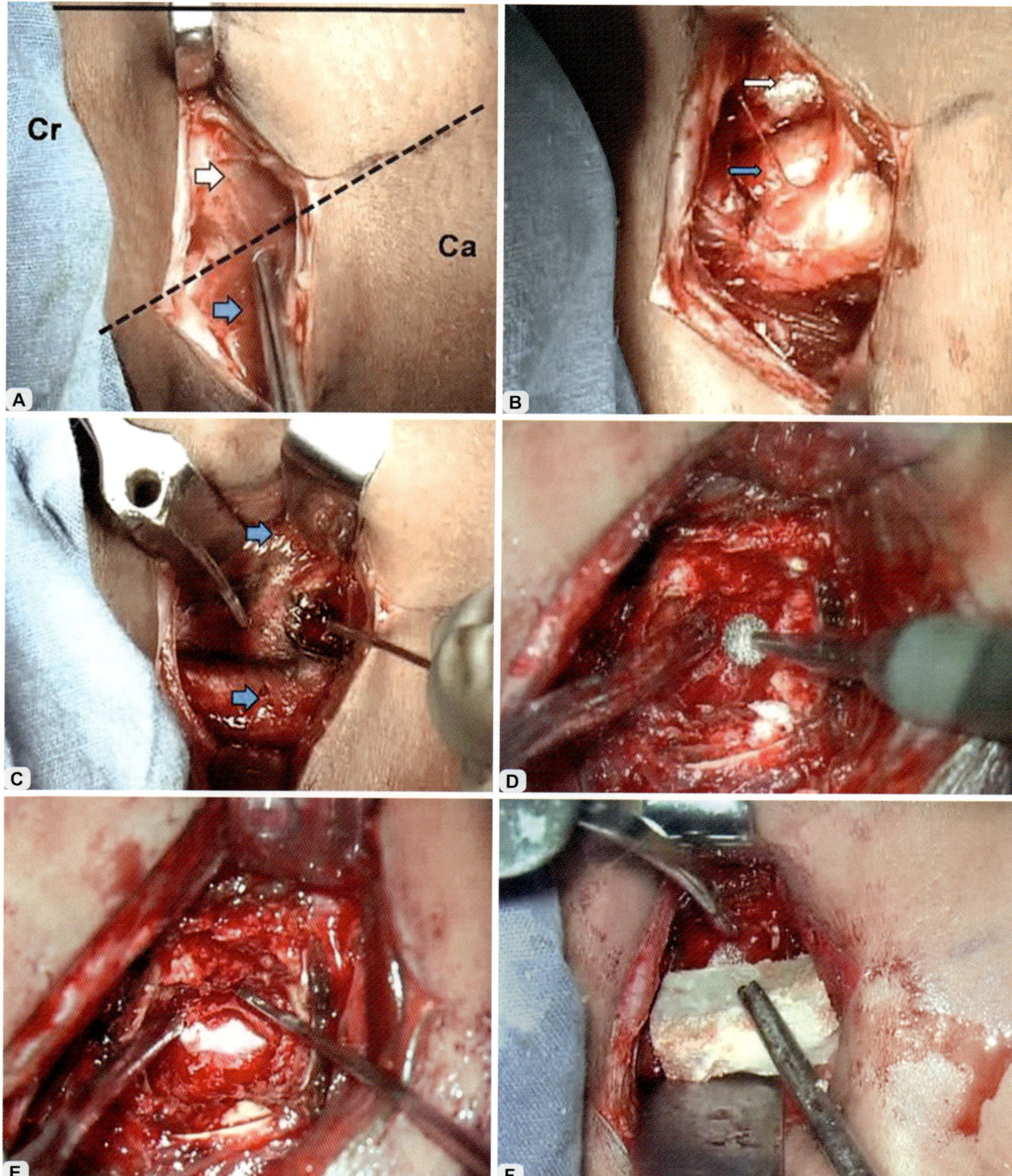

Fig. 16.16 Anterior cervical dissection for a corpectomy. (A) The midline is indicated by the solid black line. The dotted line indicates the anterior border of sternomastoid along which a vertical incision is made. The plane between sternomastoid (blue arrow) and the strap muscles (white arrow) is identified; (B) The next plane is developed between the carotid sheath (blue arrows) and the esophagus (white arrow); (C) The prevertebral fascia is opened between the two longis colli muscles (blue arrows) to expose the vertebra; (D) The corpectomy is performed with burr and rongeurs to decompress the spinal cord; (E and F) An appropriate sized tricortical iliac crest graft is harvested to reconstruct the defect (Cr-cranial, Ca-caudal)

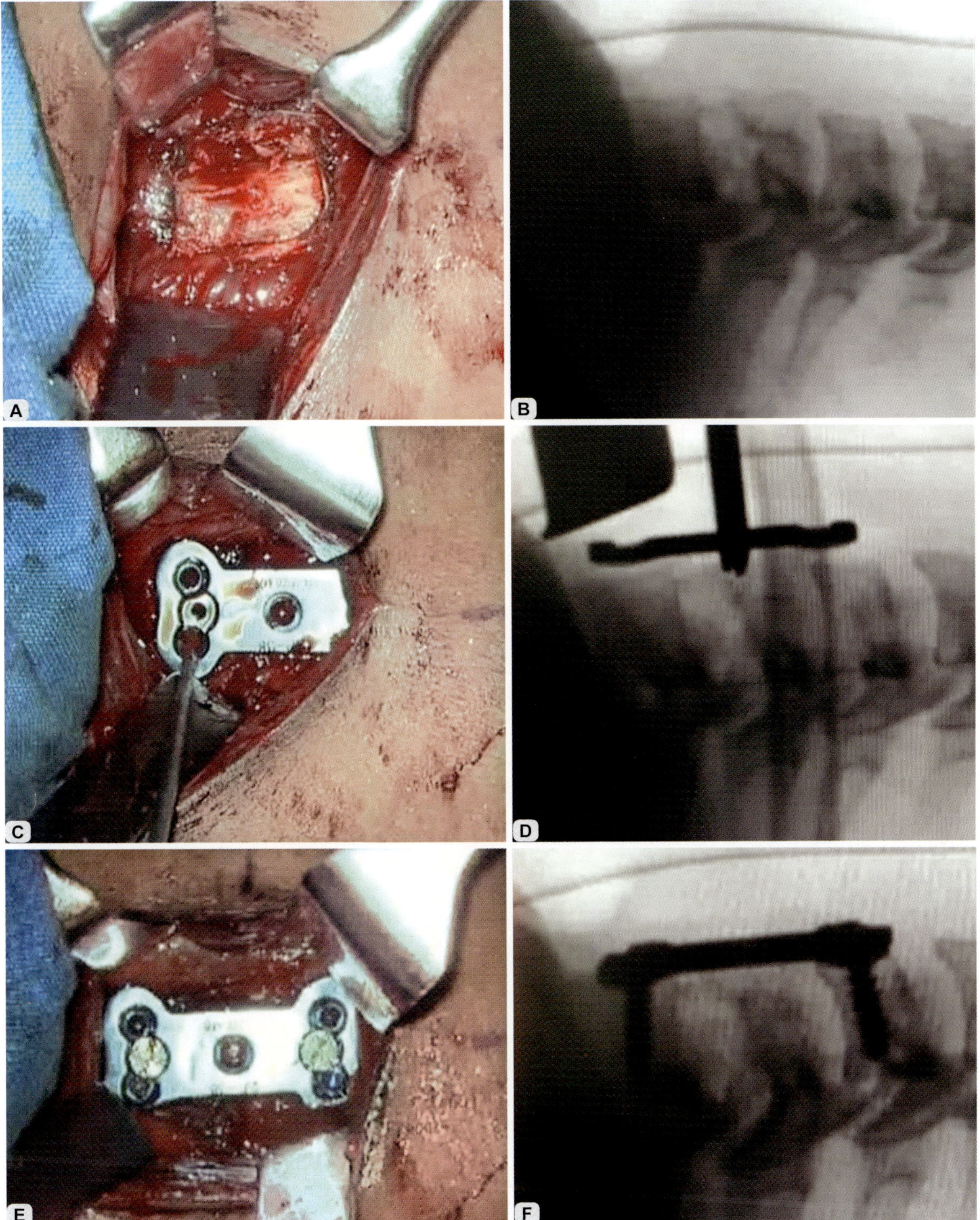

Fig. 16.17 (A and B) The graft has been used to reconstruct the anterior column defect; (C and D) An appropriate sized locking plate is placed to check the length of the plate and screw dimensions; (E and F) The unicortical locking screws have been inserted into the superior and inferior vertebral bodies through the plate holding the graft in place

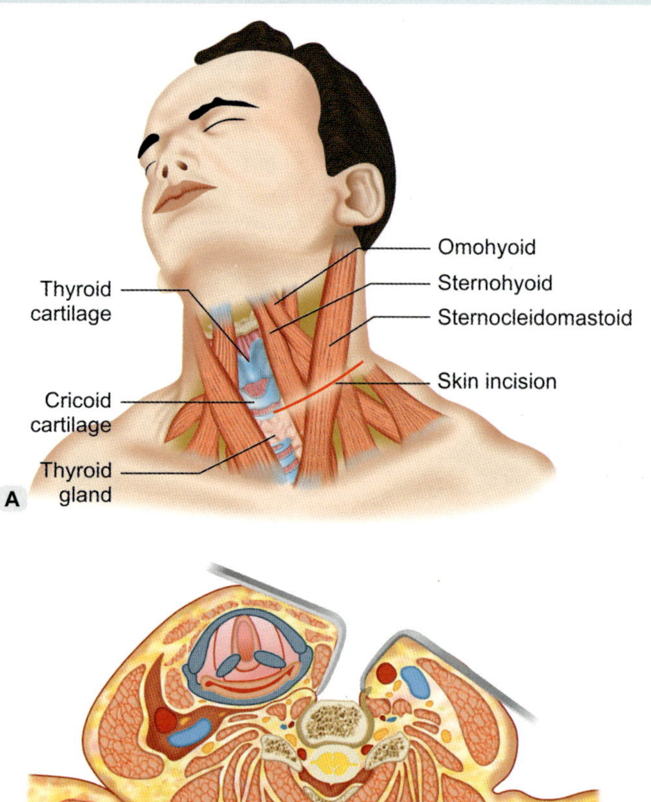

Fig. 16.18 The classical anterior Smith Robinson approach. The incision is placed from the midline across the neck till the anterior border of sternomastoid (A). The plane of dissection is medial to the carotid sheath (B)

and below the level of vertebra to be removed. The annulus is incised with a number 11 blade knife. Pituitary rongeurs and small size curettes are used to loosen and remove the disk and cartilaginous end plate. The direction of curetting should preferably from posterior to anterior and from inside to outside to prevent accidental injury to the cord. The anterior two-third of the disk is removed using the curettes. The uncovertebral joints at each level are identified laterally. The disk space is then distracted using Cloward lamina spreader or a Caspar screw-postdistractor. Using a high-speed burr and small currettes, the remaining disk material is removed up to the posterior longitudinal ligament at each disk level. Posteriorly, the posterior longitudinal ligament should be visible and laterally the uncovertebral joint should be visible to give a three-dimensional orientation regarding the midline, spinal canal, neural foramina, and the vertebral arteries.

Step 3: Corpectomy

Appropriate length Caspar screw-post are inserted above and below the level of corpectomy and gently distracted. Aggressive distraction should not be applied as it might lead to spinal cord impingement. The lateral limits of the corpectomy are marked first by making drill holes with high speed burr centered on the uncovertebral joint bilaterally (Fig. 16.20B). The line connecting these points determines the lateral extent of the corpectomy. The anterior half of vertebral body can be removed with Leksell rongeur. This bone should be used for arthrodesis if cages are used to reconstruct the defect.

The posterior part of vertebral body can be removed safely with high speed burr with constant visualization of the

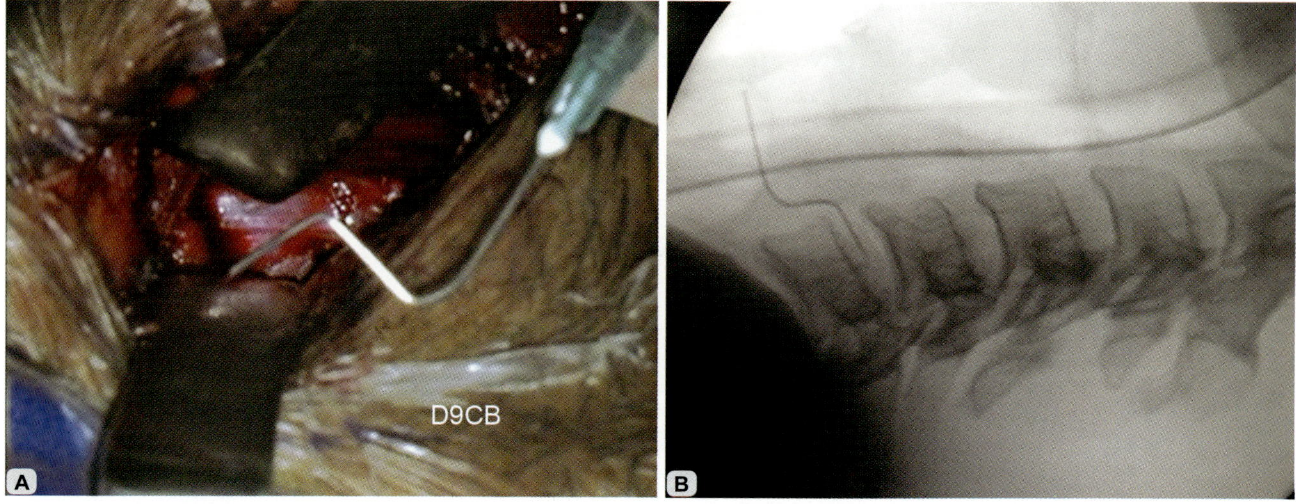

Fig. 16.19 A double bent needle is used for level identification which prevents inadvertent plunging

posterior limit of the discectomy. A 3 mm cutting burr is used initially (Fig. 16.20C). The sinosidal bleeders from the bone can be plugged with bone wax. Once the posterior most part is reached, it is thinned with a diamond tip burr (Fig. 16.20D). The advantages of using a diamond tip are that it causes less bone bleeding and there are lesser chances of dural injury. The bleeding pattern of bone changes from a cancellous pattern to a cortical pattern at this point. Now a small currette or 1 mm Kerrison ronguer can be used to pull the remaining thin wafer of bone anteriorly detaching it from the posterior longitudinal ligament. It is important to elevate the bone away from the dura anteriorly (Fig. 16.20E and F). The width of decompression at this point should be not more than 16 mm with the uncovertebral joint determining the widest safe extent of bony resection. The width can be measured either by a special scale or by using 15 mm osteotome which is readily available in the tray. Studies have shown that a 19 mm wide central decompression can be carried out at C6 with a 5 mm safety margin to the vertebral artery. The posterior longitudinal ligament should be removed if any disk material is found to be extruding posteriorly between dura and PLL. Otherwise routine removal of PLL is not indicated (Fig. 16.20G). If PLL is adherent to the dura, small islands of PLL can be left floating. The neural foramina should be decompressed using curettes or 1mm pituitary rongeurs. Using a blunt hook, the neural foramina should be probed for any loose disc fragments or osteophytes.

How to address bleeding?

- Bleeding from the bone can be packed with the bone wax
- Bleeding from veins of the anterior aspect of dura can be controlled by using nonstick bipolar cautery or gentle packing with surgicel.

Step 4: Reconstruction of the Defect

The corpectomy defect can be reconstructed with autograft – iliac crest or fibula, allograft or titanium cages – mesh cages or expandable cages. Once the decompression has been completed, the next step is to insert the graft. The end plates are prepared using burr such that bleeding bone is visible and the surface should be made flat to maximize the contact area between graft and the endplate. Leaving a 2–3 mm posterior lip in the end plate would minimize

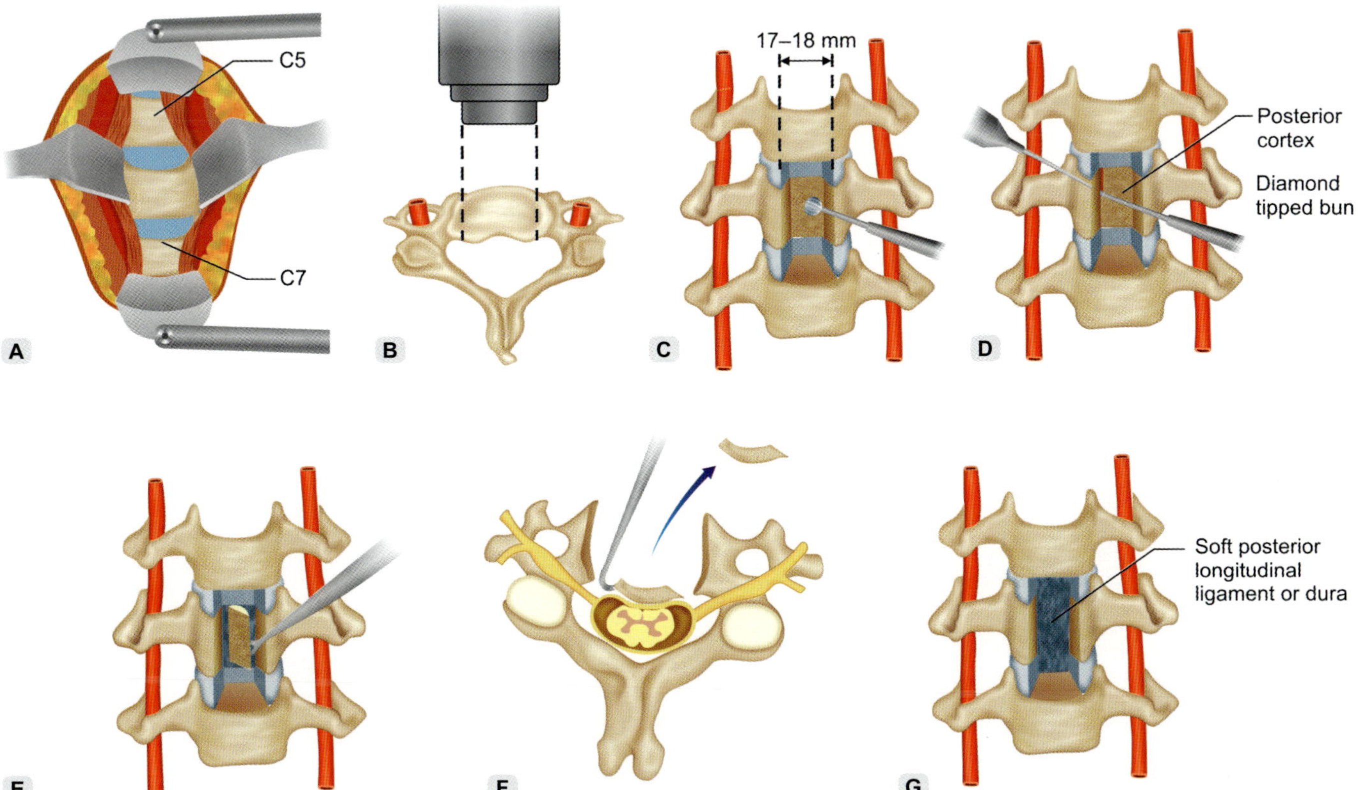

Fig.16.20 (A) Retractors are placed underneath the longus colli muscle; (B) The microscope should be oriented perpendicular to the vertebral body to prevent an oblique corpectomy; (C) Following the diskectomy, the body is removed with a nibbler and carbide tipped burr; (D) Posterior half of the vertebral body is thinned using a diamond tip burr; (E and F) the thinned out posterior cortex is removed using thin curettes; (G) The PLL is now exposed which need not be removed routinely unless the disk fragment has extruded posterior to PLL

posterior extrusion of graft. Both iliac crest and fibular graft are ideal options for one or two level corpectomy. The curved anatomy of iliac crest limits its fusion in a 3 level corpectomy. For one level corpectomy, tricortical iliac crest graft can be used and for more than one level, fibular graft can be used. Being a cortical bone, the fibular graft takes longer time for incorporation. Autografts have significant donor site morbidity and hence its use is on the decline.

Cages packed with autogenous cancellous graft are ideal choices. The bone from the corpectomy can also be used to pack the cage. There are various type cages available ranging from Harms cage to expendable cage which can be used with allograft instead of iliac crest or fibular graft. The author prefers to use iliac crest bone for a single level corpectomy. Appropriate size graft is harvested and prepared. It is always better to harvest a few mm longer graft than a shorter one since the shorter one is more difficult to deal with and a second graft might be needed. Distraction is applied using the Caspar retractor. Some authors prefer traction using skull tongs for more than one level corpectomy. The proximal part of the graft is inserted first and the distal part is gently tamped in so that graft fits in snugly (Fig. 16.21). For uninstrumented fusion, a good graft-endplate interface is necessary for stability. The distraction is released once the graft is placed. The position of the graft is confirmed under fluoroscope. The Caspar pin retractors are removed and the holes sealed with bone wax to prevent bleeding.

Step 5: Plating

Anterior cervical plates prevent graft dislodgement, provide graft stability and obviate the need for external immobilization. Stand alone anterior fusion and instrumentation is ideal for one or two level corpectomy. It is advisable to perform additional posterior instrumentation whenever 2 or 3 level corpectomy is performed as this has been associated with high rates of failure. The author prefers to augment the graft with plate in all cases of corpectomy (Fig. 16.22). Care should be exercised in selecting the proper plate length so that the screws are not too close to the graft-recipient site interface. Anterior cervical plate is placed in the center and secured with locking screws after confirming under fluoroscope. The graft can be secured to the plate with a screw to prevent graft migration and graft settling. The hole for the screw in the graft should be made with a K-wire followed by the drill to prevent excessive force while drilling which would push the graft in. Not more than one screw is needed as more screws would weaken the graft. An excellent graft end plate interface is a prerequisite for fixing the graft. After grafting, the position of the plate is confirmed with lateral fluoroscopy. The wound is closed with a deep drain. The platysma is sutured back and the skin is closed with subcuticular stitches.

Anterior corpectomy in ossified posterior longitudinal ligament (OPLL)

OPLL compresses the cord from anterior direction. Posterior decompression gives a satisfactory result in most cases of OPLL, and it works by cord "falling back" into the enlarged spinal canal. But it is argued that the anchoring effect of the dentate ligaments, nerve roots and root sleeves exerted over the spinal cord prevents the cord to fall back and the possible anterior adhesion to dural tube argues against the validity of posterior decompression. Corpectomy and anteriorly floating the OPLL enlarges the narrow spinal canal and restores the spinal cord to its original place. The anterior approach is limited to C2–T3, and it is advocated when there is high ratio of canal narrowing exceeding 60–70%.

During surgery, after the corpectomy is performed, breaking the ossification at its proximal and distal part is done first followed by lateral release of bony spur and

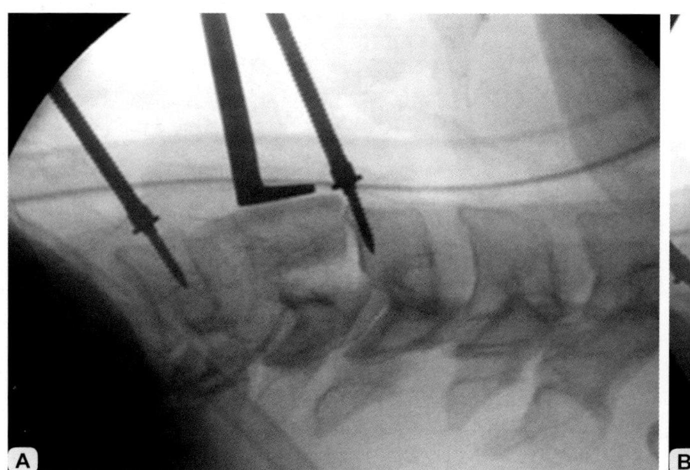

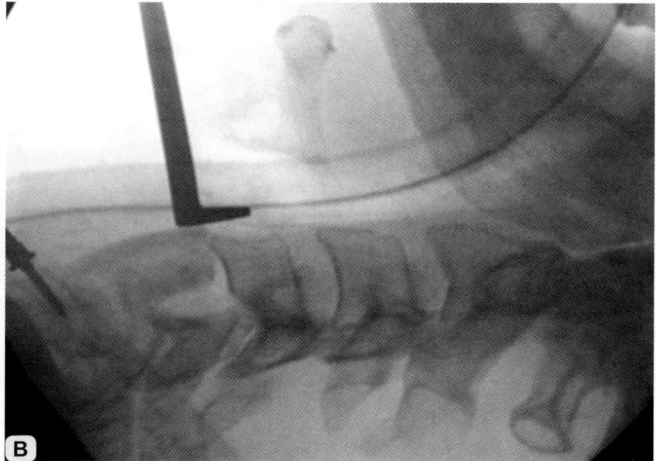

Fig. 16.21 (A) Wrong way of tamping the graft which might lead to cord injury; (B) Correct way of graft tamping. Part of the "L" of the punch is over the graft and part over the adjacent intact body

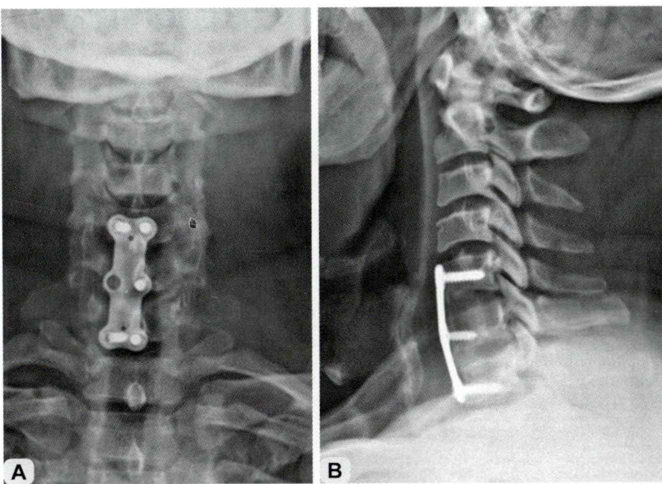

Fig. 16.22 Postoperative X-rays after corpectomy and plating for the patient showed in Figure 16.7

lateral decompression extending to the joints of Lushka. This allows proper floatation of OPLL. The choice of graft and instrumentation are same as that of conventional corpectomy. The difficulties encountered are excessive bleeding from anterior internal vertebral venous plexus, increased risk of damage to spinal cord and dural tear compared to conventional corpectomy procedure. Insufficient anterior flotation is noted if there is inadequate decompression, inadequate thinning of OPLL, and insufficient space for flotation after bone grafting, elongation of spine column during fusion and presence of matured ossification, which does not float as easily as immature OPLL.

Postoperative Protocol

After extubation, the patient is allowed to talk to observe for hoarsness of voice (indicating RLN Palsy). Look for drooping of eyelid which would indicate Horners syndrome. Overnight ventilation is advised in multilevel corpectomy, duration of surgery >4 hours, excessive bleeding and revision surgery. Patient is provided a rigid collar post operatively and mobilized on the 2nd postoperative day. Duration of immobilization would depend on the levels of corpectomy, quality of bone and the stability of construct.

Complications

Peroperative and Immediate Postoperative Complications

Injury to the Recurrent Laryngeal Nerve

In about 50% of patients, minor hoarseness of voice can occur postsurgically which resolves spontaneously. This is caused by edema due to intubation and excessive retraction. The incidence of true recurrent laryngeal nerve palsy varies between 2% and 11%.[11,12] Direct trauma or an indirect pressure or stretch injury caused by a hematoma or by prolonged retractor placement, bipolar cauterization are the other causes and can cause permanent laryngeal dysfunction. Though there are reports of higher incidence of recurrent laryngeal nerve palsy with right sided approach because of its variation in its course (Fig. 16.23), Beutler et al. found no difference in the rate of postoperative dysphonia between the two sides.[13]

Following true nerve palsy, the patients usually have recurrent cough and hoarseness of voice. Major steps in prevention of recurrent laryngeal nerve palsy are gentle dissection with minimal use of bipolar cautery and deflating and reinflating of endotracheal cuff after placement of the self-retaining retractor. Decrease in the rate of this complication from 6.8 % to 1.7% by this maneuver which decreases the pressure on the nerve has been reported.[14]

In majority of patients, recurrent laryngeal nerve palsy is temporary and usually resolves in a week. Immediate measures include ENT consultation, steroid and phonation exercise. If symptom persists even after two months, then injection of collagen or Teflon in to vocal cord should be considered.

Injury to Esophagus and Pharynx

Swallowing difficulties are the most common postoperative problems encountered which arises out of oesophageal

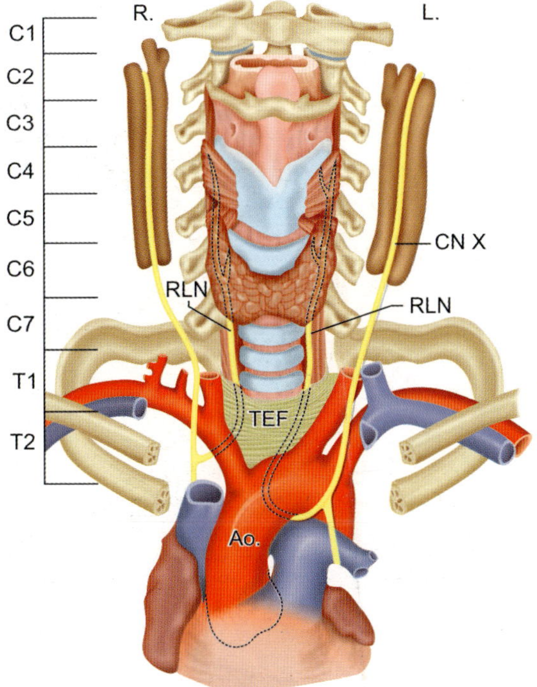

Fig. 16.23 Course of the recurrent laryngeal nerve

dysmotility resulting from excessive traction. This usually follows a transient course. There have been reports of use of thin layer of collagen with Depomedrol to decrease the severity and duration of this symptom with good success.

Esophageal injury, a serious complication can occur secondary to excessive retraction, electrocautery, or perforation from sharp instruments. The incidence of esophageal perforation has been reported to be approximately 0.25%.[15] The longus colli muscle has to be retracted from the vertebral body both proximally and distally and, the blades of the retractor should be placed under them. If diagnosed during the procedure, the tear has to be repaired and patient should be fed through a nasogastric tube for 7–10 days to allow healing.

Late presentation is however more common. Patient presents with fever, pharyngeal crepitus and an enlarging neck mass. Diagnosis is made by high index of suspicion and confirmed by esophagogram or esophagoscopy. Treatment consists of re-exploration of wound and repair of defect, followed by nasogastric tube and antibiotics. In the event of spread to mediastinum leading to mediastinitis, the prognosis is poor and can be associated with high mortality.

Vascular Injuries

Vascular injuries, though rare have devastating sequelae. The carotid sheath contents, superior and inferior thyroid arteries, and the vertebral artery are the structures at risk while performing an anterior corpectomy. Using blunt-edged retractors and avoiding overzealous retraction reduces the risk of injuries to these vessels.

Injury to vertebral artery, which has a reported incidence of 0.3–0.5% occurs[16] if the decompression is continued too laterally breaching the uncovertebral joint (Fig. 16.24) and rarely due to aberrant vertebral artery course into the vertebral body (Fig. 16.9). An abnormal course of the vertebral artery should always be looked for in the preoperative axial MRI images. Intraoperatively, the midline should be identified by exposing both the uncovertebral joints and the microscope has to be oriented perpendicular to the vertebral body.

Hemorrhage arising out of vertebral artery injury is difficult to control and if not controlled by hemostatic efforts, vascular surgeons' help is sought for repair or ligation. The vertebral artery should be isolated and clamped temporarily both proximally and distally. If there is retrograde flow from proximal end, it indicates that blood flow in the opposite vertebral artery is normal and adequate. In the absence of retrograde flow, an intraoperative arteriogram will help decide whether to repair or to ligate the vertebral artery. In the event of injury to the dominant vertebral artery, it should be repaired. Ligation of dominant vertebral artery has got potential for permanent neurological injury to the patient.

Injury to the Sympathetic Nervous System

Injury to the cervical sympathetic ganglion can result in Horner syndrome, characterized by ipsilateral ptosis, miosis, and anhidrosis. Incidence of 1.1% has been reported in literature.[17] To prevent this complication, the dissection should be kept medial to the carotid and the longus colli muscles should be dissected of the anterior vertebral body in a subperiosteal fashion, and retractors should be placed deep to the longus colli muscles.

Spinal Cord Injury

Apart from direct injury to the spinal cord due to slippage of instruments and high speed burr, direct manipulation of spinal cord, too much distraction of the spine and vigorous manipulation of vertebra can lead to cord injury with neurological deficit .The reported incidence is around 0.1– 0.64%.[18] Any distraction or manipulation

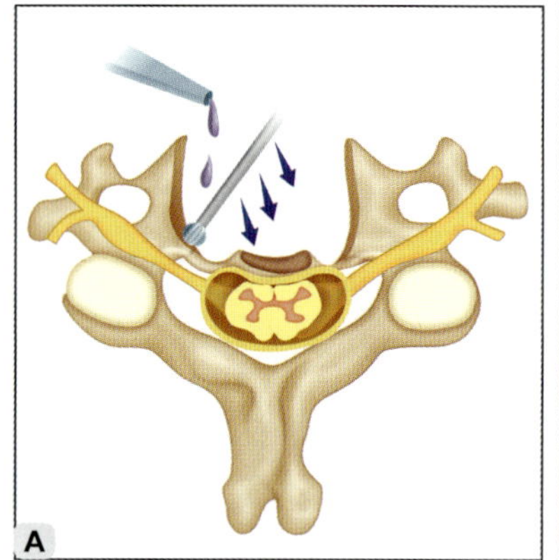

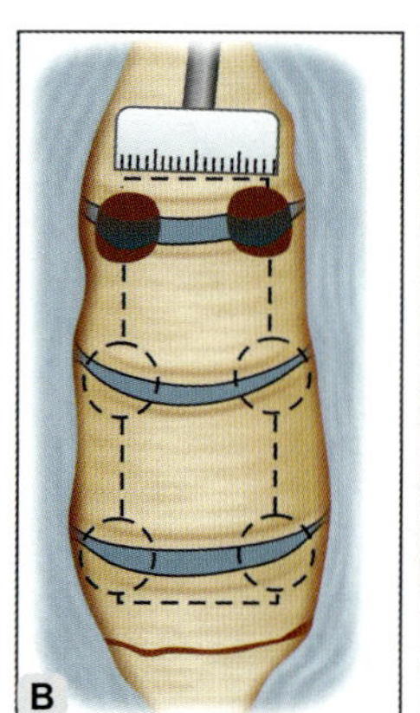

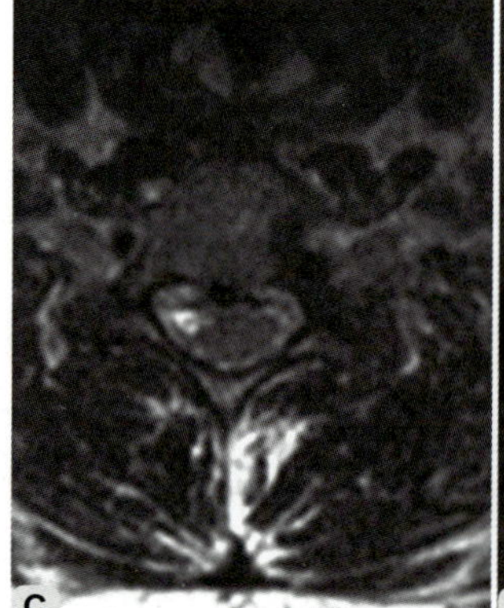

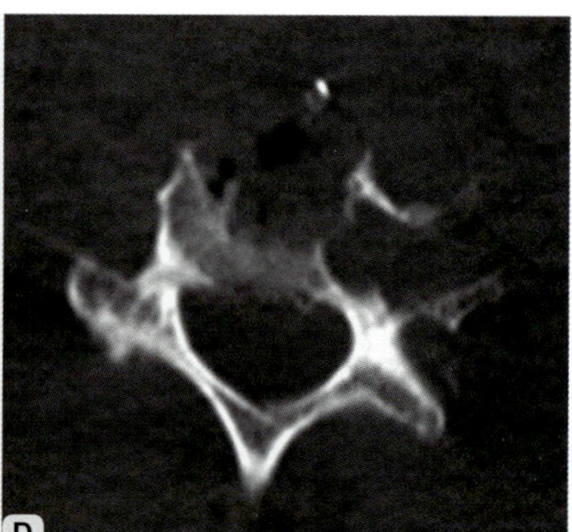

Fig. 16.24 The lateral decompression should not extend beyond the uncovertebral joint which risks the vertebral artery; Aberrant and enlarged vertebral artery course into the vertebral body demonstrated in sagittal MRI and CT in Figure 16.9

should be attempted only after decompression of the cord. Neuromonitoring is of great help in detecting these injuries peroperatively. In addition, neck manipulation (hyperextension) during intubation, intraoperative hypotension, cervical malalignment after decompression and grafting, and postoperative epidural hematoma must all be considered in the evaluation of the patient with postoperative neurologic deterioration.

Prevention of neurological deficit starts during induction of anesthesia itself. Hyperextension of cervical spine should be avoided during intubation and positioning. The mean aterial pressure should be kept above 80 mm Hg to prevent ischemic insult to the cord. The localizing needle used to mark the level, should be bent so as to prevent needle advancement into spinal canal (Fig. 16.19). Complete and through decompression of the cord should be performed before graft placement. The posterior vertebral osteophytes should be symmetrically thinned out before an attempt is made to release it from the vertebral body. The osteophyte should be pulled away from the vertebral body using a hook or thin currette. The graft dimensions should be planned by measuring the required length of graft on preoperative imaging and measuring intraoperatively after the corpectomy. Most commonly used length of graft is about 14 mm. While introducing the graft, an L-shaped punch with part lying on vertebral body below prevents inadvertent advancement of graft into the spinal canal (Fig. 16.21).

Once postoperative neurological deficit is identified, management should include maintenance of normotensive blood pressure, administration of steroids, and imaging studies to assess for possible graft dislodgment.[16] If compressive pathology is identified, then rapid re-exploration and decompression is indicated.

Delayed neurological deficit which occurs after few hours of surgery is usually due to epidural hematoma and should be explored immediately. Rarely, epidural abscess can cause late onset deficit, which usually presents a week after surgery. This has to be treated as an emergency after confirming the diagnosis by MRI.

Dural Tear

Anterior dural tear, which is not so common, might be problematic in patients with long-standing ossification of posterior longitudinal ligament. Small, angled curettes and Kerrison rongeurs should be sharp so that excessive force is not needed which might lead to loss of control of the instruments. Extreme caution is needed in removing the posterior disk fragments and osteophytes during which the occurrence of dural tear is high (Fig. 16.25). Although repairing the tear is ideal, the limited working space available makes it difficult. The defect can be covered

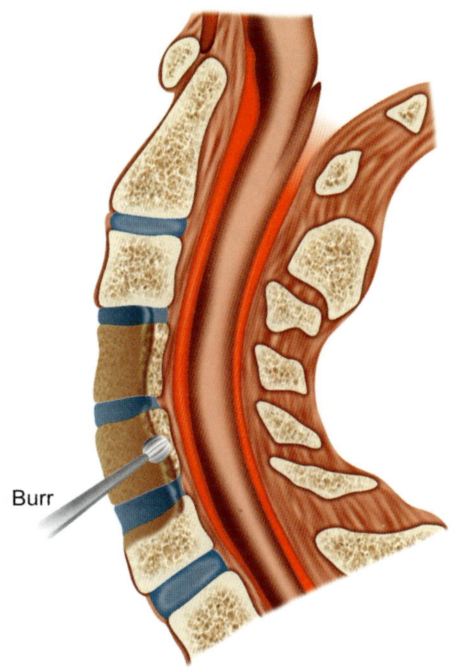

Figs 16.25 Once the posterior vertebral cortex is reached, a diamond burr is used to thin the cortex. The burr is used in continous, side to side, "brushing" strokes so that it does not plunge into the dura

with dural patch *(Duragen)* and sealed with dural sealants *(Tissel)*. Postoperative lumbar subarachnoid drain should be inserted and approximately 200–250 mL of CSF should be drained every day. This reduces the CSF pressure, helps to keep the cervical wound dry and should be continued for about 5 days. The author prefers to use fibrin glue after sealing the defect with surgicel and had not encountered any postoperative CSF leaks.

Postoperative Radiculopathy

Secondary to an impingement of the ventral aspect of the spinal cord against the edges of the corpectomy trough, postoperative radiculopathy can occur in anterior corpectomy surgeries. The reported incidence in the literature ranges from 3.9 to 20%.[19,20] Limiting the ventral trough to 14 or 15 mm might help in reducing the incidence of radiculopathy.[19]

Airway Obstruction

Although injury to trachea is very rare, airway obstruction due to other causes can occur and typically occurs 12–36 hours postoperatively. The patient in the immediate postoperative period might land up in respiratory difficulty either due to airway edema occurring as a result of prolonged retraction of trachea or due to postoperative retropharyngeal hematoma, which can produce obstruction of the airway with its subsequent complications. All anterior surgical wounds are best drained to decrease the risk of retropharyngeal hematoma and delay in extubation should be considered if airway edema is anticipated.

Delayed and Late Complications

Graft-related Complications

In ACCF without instrumentation, the initial stability of the graft depends on the snug fit of the graft. The incidence of graft migration reported is 6.2%[21] and was most commonly noted in inferior end of longer fusions ending in C7 vertebra (Fig. 16.26). None of the patients had respiratory or neurological problems as a result of graft migration. Adding anterior plate fixation has been shown to improve the rate of fusion, reduce the risks of graft related complications and the incidence of segmental kyphosis.[22,23] The author who uses anterior plating routinely with anterior corpectomy has not faced the problem of graft extrusion. But there are reports that 50% of patients with more three-level corpectomies and long anterior cervical plating end up in failure.[24-26] Augmentation with posterior instrumentation is advisable in these cases.

Pseudoarthrosis

The reported rate of fusion for one level corpectomy is 90% and for two level corpectomy is 56%.[27] Augmenting with an anterior plate in patients with 2 level corpectomies and additional posterior instrumentation in patients undergoing 3 or more levels of corpectomy increases the rate of fusion. The previous reports[28,29] of increased rates of nonunion with allograft have been contradicted by recent reports[30,31] which claim that the results are comparable between autograft and allograft. Nonunion rates are higher in osteoporosis, tobacco use and rheumatoid arthritis patients. Although asymptomatic in most of the patients, psudoarthrosis may lead to construct failure, loss of sagittal alignment, and late onset deterioration of neurology.

Inadequate Restoration of Sagittal Alignment

Usually the anterior strut graft inserted after anterior corpectomy is supported by tensile force generated by posterior ligaments, lateral part of annulus and soft tissue structures remaining after decompression. In cases of previous laminectomy with kyphotic deformity (Fig. 16.27), the posterior ligamentous support is lost, increasing the chances of graft extrusion and loss of lordodic alignment. To restore the sagittal balance adding posterior instrumentation is necessary in these cases.

Adjacent Segment Degeneration (ASD)

Although it is stated that fusing a segment increases the stress on the adjacent segments leading to accelerated degeneration, other factors that would increase the chances of ASD are oversized grafts, damaging the adjacent disk during surgery, extension of the plate to the adjacent disk space (Fig. 16.28). Hilibrand et al.[32] reported that in 10 years, 25% of patients developed adjacent segment disease. They also concluded that the degeneration occurring in adjacent segment was more likely a manifestation of the natural aging process rather than a consequence of the fusion.

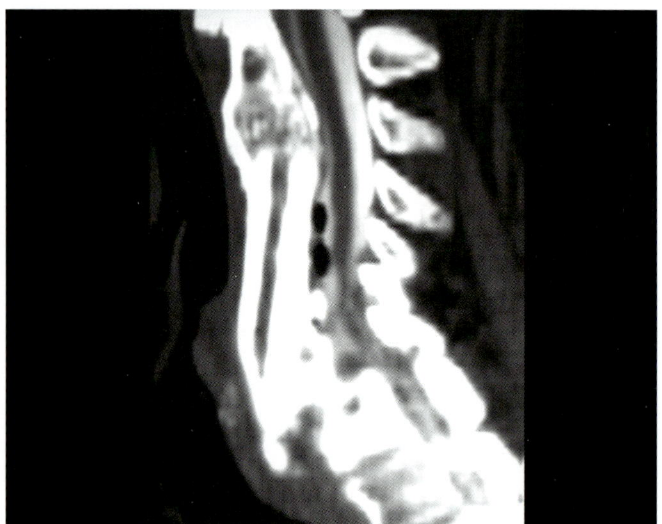

Fig. 16.26 Sagittal CT image showing graft extrusion at its inferior margin

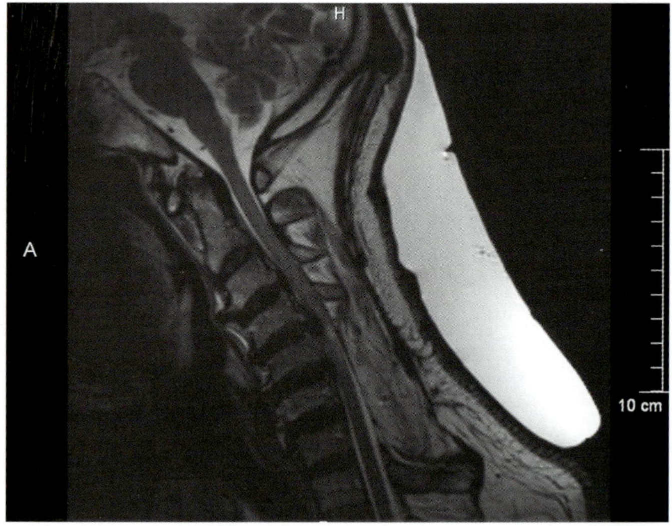

Fig. 16.27 MRI of post laminectomy kyphosis compression at C4-C5 levels

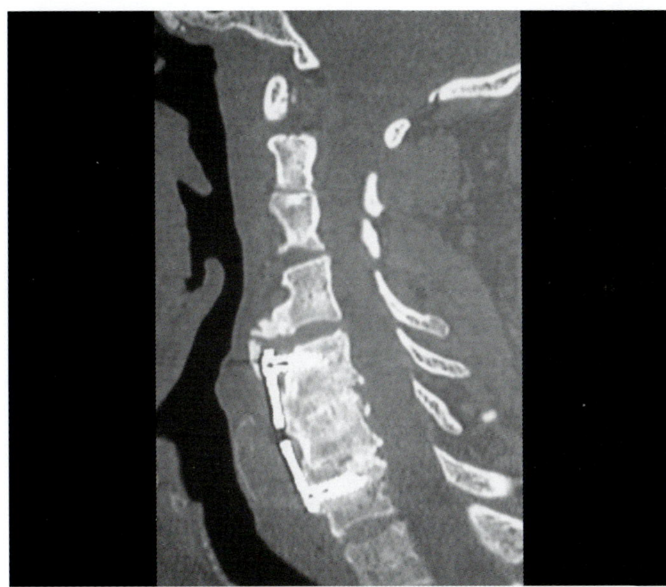

Fig. 16.28 CT scan showing ossification of adjacent disk due to long plate

Graft Site-related Complications

Iliac crest[33] bone graft site complications have a prevalence of 20%. Persistent pain and numbness resulting from injury to superficial nerves is most common followed by iliac crest fracture, cosmetic deformity, injury to superior gluteal artery and infection. While harvesting fibula, injury to the peroneal nerve, contracture of the flexor hallucis longus and flexor digitorum longus tendons, development of lower extremity deep venous thrombosis and stress fractures of the tibia have also been reported.[34-37]

Summary

ACCF should be considered for patients with kyphotic spine and compressions that extend behind the vertebral body. ACCF provides a direct approach to the anterior cord compression and the uncovertebral spurs, thus decompressing the cord and the nerve roots. It also allows prevention and correction of kyphosis. Proper patient selection, meticulous planning and understanding of anatomy are essential to prevent and reduce the complications associated with the procedure.

References

1. Brain WR, Northfield D, Wilkinson M. The neurological manifestations of cervical spondylosis. Brain. 1952;75(2): 187-225.
2. Tobias A Mattei et al. Cervical spondylotic myelopathy: pathophysiology, diagnosis, and surgical techniques. ISRN Neurol. 2011;2011:463729.
3. Baron EM, Young WF. Cervical spondylotic myelopathy: a brief review of its pathophysiology, clinical course, and diagnosis. Neurosurgery. 2007;60(supplement 1):S35-S41.
4. Ferguson RJL, Caplan LR. Cervical spondylitic myelopathy. Neurologic Clinics. 1985;3(2):373-82.
5. Furlan JC, Kalsi-Ryan S, Kailaya-Vasan A, Massicotte EM, Fehlings MG. Functional and clinical outcomes following surgical treatment in patients with cervical spondylotic myelopathy: a prospective study of 81 cases. J Neurosurgery. 2011;14(3):348-55.
6. Swank ML, Lowery GL, Bhat AL, McDonough RF, "Anterior cervical allograft arthrodesis and instrumentation: multilevel interbody grafting or strut graft reconstruction," Euro. Spine J. 1997;6(2):138-43.
7. Vaccaro AR, Falatyn SP, Scuderi GJ et al. "Early failure of long segment anterior cervical plate fixation." J Spinal Disord. 1998;11(5):410-5.
8. Yonenobu K, Fuji T, Ono K, et al. Choice of surgical treatment for multisegmental cervical spondylotic myelopathy. Spine (Phila Pa 1976). 1985;10:710-6.
9. Praveen K Yalamanchili, Michael J Vives, Saad B. Chaudhary. Cervical spondylotic myelopathy: factors in choosing the surgical approach. Advances in Orthopedics. 2012;2012, Article ID 783762.
10. Wang JC, Hart RA, Emery SE, Bohlman HH. "Graft migration or displacement after multilevel cervical corpectomy and strut grafting," Spine 2003;20(10):1016-21.
11. Yue WM, Brodner W, Highland TR. Persistent swallowing and voice problems after anterior cervical discectomy and fusion with allograft and plating: A 5 to 11 year follow-up study. Eur Spine J. 2005;14:677-82.
12. Frempong-Boadu A, Houten JK, Osbom B, et al. Swallowing and speech dysfunction in patients undergoing anterior cervical discectomy and fusion: A prospective, objective preoperative and postoperative assessment. J Spinal Disord Tech. 2002;15:362-8.
13. Beutler WJ, Sweeney CA, Connolly PJ: Recurrent laryngeal nerve injury with anterior cervical spine surgery risk with laterality of surgical approach. Spine (Phila Pa 1976). 2001;26:1337-42.
14. Apfelbaum TI, Kriskovich MD, Haller JR. On the incidence, cause, and prevention of recurrent laryngeal nerve palsies during anterior cervical spine surgery. Spine (Phila Pa 1976). 2000;25:2906-12.
15. Newhouse KE, Lindsey RW, Clark CR, et al. Esophageal perforation following anterior cervical spine surgery. Spine (Phila pa 1976). 1989;14:1051-3.
16. Smith M, Emery S, Dudley A, et al. Vertebral artery injury during anterior decompression of the cervical spine'a retrospective review of ten patients. J Bone Joint Surg 1993;75B:410-5.
17. Bertalanffy H, Eggert HR. Complications of anterior cervical discectomy without fusion in 450 consecutive patients. Acta Neurochir (Wien). 1989;99:41-50.

18. Flynn T. Neurologic complications of anterior cervical interbody fusion. Spine 1982;7:536-9.
19. Saunders RL, Pikus HJ, Ball P. Four-level cervical corpectomy. Spine (Phila Pa 1976). 1998;23:2455-61.
20. Yonenobu K, Hosono N, Iwasaki M, et al. Neurologic complications of surgery for cervical compression myelopathy. Spine (Phila Pa 1976). 1991;13:1277-82.
21. Wang JC, Hart RA, Emery SE, et al. Graft migration or displacement after multilevel cervical corpectomy and strut grafting.Spine (Phila Pa 1976). 2003;28:1016-21.
22. Wang JC, McDononugh PW, Endow K, et al. The effect of cervical plating on single level anterior cervical discectomy and fusion. J Spinal Disord. 1999;12:467-71.
23. Kaiser MG, Haid RW Jr, Subach BR, et al. Anterior cervical plating enhances arthrodesis after discectomy and fusion with cortical allograft. Neurosurgery. 2002;50:229-38.
24. DiAngelo DJ, Foley KT, Vossel KA, et al. Anterior cervical plating reverses load transfer through multilevel strut-grafts. Spine (Phila Pa 1976). 2000;25:783-95.
25. Foley KT, DiAngelo DJ, Rampersaud YR. The in vitro effects of instrumentation on multilevel cervical strut-graft mechanics. Spine (Phila Pa 1976). 1999;24:2366-76
26. Vaccaro AR, Falatyn SP, Scuderi GJ, et al. Early failure of long segment anterior cervical plate fixation. J Spinal Disord. 1998;11:410-5.
27. Swank ML, Lowery GL, Bhat AL, et al. Anterior cervical allograft arthrodesis and instrumentation: Multilevel interbody grafting or strut graft reconstruction. Eur Spine J. 1997;6:138-43.
28. Zdeblick TA, Ducker TB: The use of freeze-dried allograft bone for anterior cervical fusions. Spine (Phila Pa 1976). 1991;16:726-9.
29. Fernyhough JC, White JI, LaRocca H. Fusion rates in multilevelcervical spondylosis comparing allograft fibula with autograft fibula in 126 patients. Spine (Phila Pa 1976). 1991;16(10Suppl):S561-4.
30. MacDonald RL, Fehlings MG, Tator CH, et al. Multilevel anteriorcervical corpectomy and fibular allograft fusion for cervicalmyelopathy. J Neurosurg. 1997;86:990-7.
31. Samartzis D, Shen FH, Matthews DK, et al. Comparison ofallograft to autograft in multilevel anterior cervical discectomy and fusion with rigid plate fixation. Spine J. 2003;3:451-9.
32. Hilibrand AS, Carlson GD, Palumbo MA, et al. Radiculopathy and myelopathy at segments adjacent to the site of a previous anterior cervical arthrodesis. J Bone Joint Surg Am. 1999;81:519-28.
33. Whitecloud T. Complications of anterior cervical fusion. In: American Academy of Orthopaedic Surgeons, Instructional course lectures. 1978;vol.30.
34. Bohay DR, Manoli A 2nd. Clawtoe deformity following vascularised fibula graft. Foot Ankle Int. 1995;16:607-9.
35. Bodde EW, de Visser E, Duysens JE, et al. Donor-site morbidity after free vascularized autogenous fibular transfer: Subjective and quantitative analyses. Plast Reconstr Surg. 2003;111:2237-42.
36. Emery SE, Heller JG, Petersilge CA. Tibial stress fracture after a graft has been obtained from the fibula: A report of five cases. J Bone Joint Surg Am. 1996;78:1248-51.
37. Vail TP, Urbaniak JR. Donor-site morbidity with use of vascularised autogenous fibular grafts. J Bone Joint Surg Am. 1996;78:204-11.

CHAPTER

17

Acute Management of Patients with Spinal Cord Injury and Rehabilitation

HS Chhabra, Rajat Mahajan, Shipra Chaudhary, Mohit Arora

Introduction

Spinal cord injury (SCI) refers to any injury to the spinal cord that is caused by trauma instead of disease.[1] Depending on where the spinal cord and nerve roots are damaged, the symptoms can vary widely, from pain to paralysis to incontinence.

Injury to the spinal column can be devastating. Some degree of neurologic deficit occurs in 10–25% of patients at all levels of injury, in 40% at cervical spine levels, and in 15–20% at thoracolumbar levels.[2,3] Even with the development of specialized spinal injury centers, the cost to society per patient remains staggering.[4] The ultimate solution rests in prevention of the original injury, but in the meantime, those managing a spine injury can minimize the risk of further damage by using accepted techniques of initial transportation and treatment. A thorough understanding of the demography, anatomy, and pathophysiology of spinal cord injury, use of logical algorithms for initial evaluation and treatment, and knowledge of the potential complications seen with specific patient populations are critical for optimal patient treatment.

The most significant cause of spinal column injury is motor vehicle accidents (45%), followed by falls (20%), sports-related accidents (15%), acts of violence (15%), and miscellaneous causes (5%) in developed nations[2,3,5,6] (Fig. 17.1). However, in developing countries, falls are the leading cause of spinal cord injury.[7] At the extremes of age, the role of falls increases from 9% in the 0–15-year-old group to 60% in those older than 75 years. The male-to-female ratio is 4:1. When a neurologic deficit is associated with spinal column injury, the overall survival rate for all levels of injury is 86% at 10 years. The survival rate drops off for patients injured after age 29 to about 50% at 10 years. Accidents and suicides are most common in those younger than 55 years of age, in nonwhites, and in paraplegics.[8]

Fractures and dislocations of the spine are serious injuries that most commonly occur in young people. Nearly 43% of patients with spinal cord injuries sustain multiple injuries. Kraus et al. estimated that each year 50 people in 1 million sustain a spinal cord injury.[9] Of individuals who die within 1 year of their accidents, 90% die en route to the hospital. With the development of regional trauma centers and increased training of paramedics and emergency medical technicians, the chances of survival after serious spinal cord injury have increased. The initial appraisal of spinal injuries carries particular importance because of the potential for catastrophic and permanent neurologic impairment.

According to the National Spinal Cord Injury Association, the most common cause of death is respiratory failure,

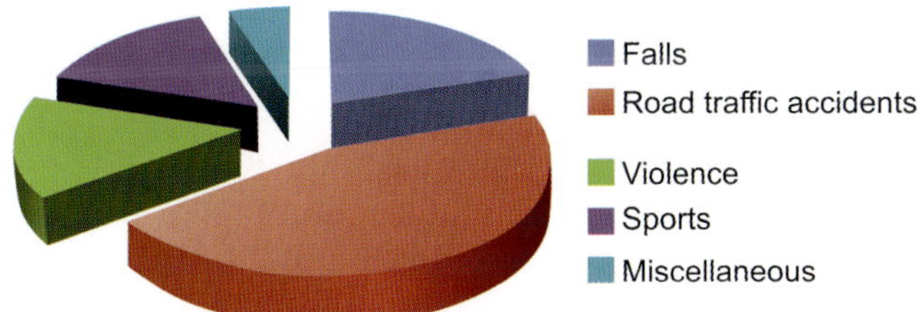

Fig. 17.1 Showing causes of spinal cord injuries in developed nations. In developing nations like India falls are the leading cause of spinal cord injuries

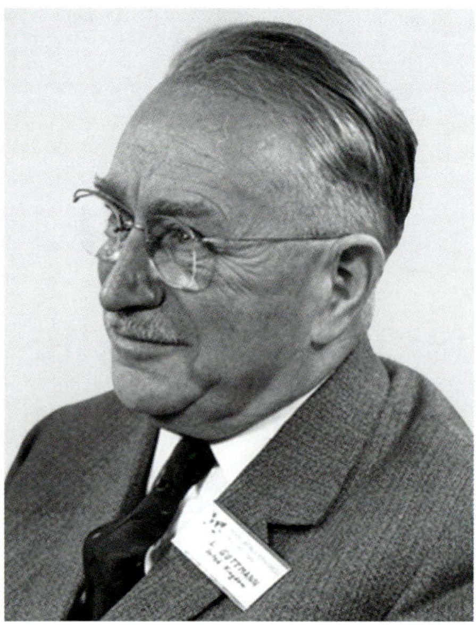

Fig. 17.2 Sir Ludwig Guttmann (1899 – 1980): Accredited with creation and development of the National Spinal Injuries Centre at Stoke Mandeville Hospital after World War II

whereas in the past it was renal failure. An increasing number of individuals with spinal cord injury die of unrelated causes, such as cancer or cardiovascular disease, similar to that of the general population.[10] Mortality rates are significantly higher during the first year after injury than during subsequent years.

The establishment of spinal cord injury centers and the improvement in prehospital management of spinal cord injuries has been of significant benefit in the overall outcome for such patients. The concept of a spinal cord injury center as a separate unit began at the Ministry of Pensions Hospital, Stoke Mandeville, England, under the supervision of Sir Ludwig Guttman in 1943 (Fig. 17.2).

Founding of this unit was followed by the establishment in 1945 of a unit in Toronto, Canada, and later by the creation of eight units in Veterans Affairs Hospitals in the United States. When compared with the outcomes in other centers, such specialized facilities in the United States are credited with a shorter length of hospitalization, a lower rate of complications (e.g. urinary tract infection, pulmonary complications, decubitus ulcers), and therefore, an overall lower cost of patient care. In addition, these centers have greatly lowered the percentage of complete versus incomplete injuries, with a decrease of 65–46% in one study and 20–9% in another.[11,12]

Recognition of Injury

Spinal column and spinal cord injuries are typically associated with high-energy mechanisms, such as motor vehicle accidents and the inherently risky pursuits of youth. A second peak is seen in older age, resulting from lower-energy injuries in persons prone to fragility fractures or those with a preexisting ankylosed spine.[13] It is imperative that both the physician and the patient be aware that concomitant injuries may potentially distract from the presence of a spinal injury. Closed head injuries and facial trauma should heighten clinical suspicion because they imply that the cervical spine was likely subjected to a great deal of force. Additionally, the identification of a single spinal fracture should prompt the physician to rule out other spinal injuries: a recent evaluation of 492 patients with CT-identified cervical spine injuries revealed noncontiguous spinal injuries in 19% of cases.[14]

Prehospital Care and Management

The protection of the injured spine and spinal cord begins at the accident scene. In as many as 25% of patients, poor immobilization and improper handling have been implicated in causing further neurologic injury after the initial accident.[15] The initial evaluation of any trauma patient begins at the scene of the accident with the time-honored ABCs of resuscitation, such as the advanced trauma life support[16] (ATLS) method described by the American College of Surgeons. The ABC (airway, breathing, and circulation) method can be described more accurately as A (airway), B (breathing), and C (circulation and cervical spine). All patients with potential spine injuries arriving at the emergency department should be on a backboard with the cervical spine immobilized. A spinal column injury should be considered in all polytrauma patients, especially those who are unconscious or intoxicated and those who have head and neck injuries. Suspicion of a spine injury must begin at the accident scene so that an organized extrication and transport plan can be developed to minimize further injury to neural tissue.

Systems and protocols to immobilize and protect the spine during extrication and transport to the emergency department have likely contributed to the increased survival of spine injured patients and to the overall reduction in the neurologic sequelae of their injuries. Current recommendations for patient immobilization during transport consist of a rigid cervical collar, lateral supports, and tape and body straps to secure the patient to a backboard to protect the entire spine.[17] Any patient wearing a helmet at the time of injury should arrive at the emergency department with it still in place unless a face shield that cannot be removed separately from the helmet is obstructing ventilation, a loose-fitting helmet is preventing adequate cervical spine immobilization, or the paramedic has been trained in helmet removal. A scoop-style stretcher is now recommended for transfer; previously recommended maneuvers, such as the four-man lift and the log roll have been shown to cause an excessive amount of motion at thoracolumbar fracture sites.[17] In young children, because the head is disproportionately larger than the body, positioning on a flat surface can result in anterior translation and flexion of a cervical injury.[18] Therefore, to maintain the pediatric cervical spine in a neutral position, either an occipital recess or a mattress placed under the torso needs to be added to the standard backboard (Fig. 17.3).

When one suspects or detects a fracture in a patient with ankylosing spondylitis, it is essential to remember that the underlying disease has likely given the patient a preexisting kyphotic deformity. Immobilization, involving propping up the head with padding when necessary, should aim to respect this posture. Forcing a patient who is ankylosed in kyphosis into a cervical orthosis and then taping the forehead down to the spine board could further displace an extension–distraction injury, with potentially catastrophic consequences.

Indiscriminate, prolonged, and unmonitored immobilization of patients also can lead to significant morbidity. Cervical collars can elevate intracranial pressure and cerebrospinal fluid pressure, and they may increase the risk of aspiration by altering swallowing mechanics, particularly in elderly patients.[19] Ruling out cervical injuries quickly so that such collars can be removed is, therefore, extremely important.[20,21] Spine boards are often mistakenly viewed as measures for providing spine stability; in fact, their purpose is to aid extrication and transfer. Because these boards can also reduce respiratory function and cause severe pressure sores, particularly in patients who lack protective sensation, orthopedic surgeons should advocate that patients be removed from spine boards as soon as possible.

Initial Emergency Evaluation

Emergency medical service (EMS) providers should use the following five clinical criteria to determine the potential risk of spinal injury in a trauma patient:[17]

- Altered mental status.
- Evidence of intoxication.

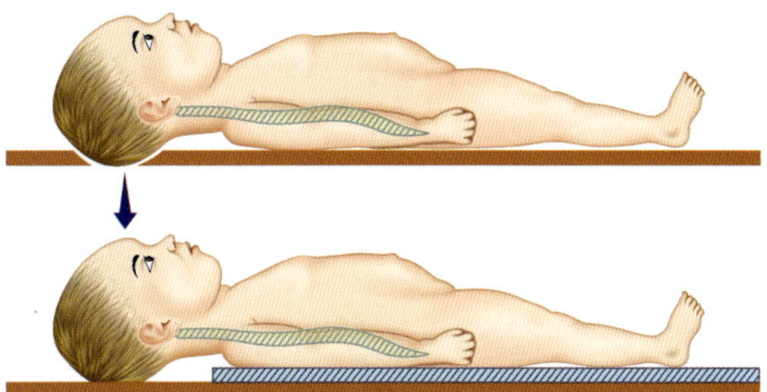

Fig. 17.3 Showing position of immobilization of children with spinal cord injury

- Suspected extremity fracture or distracting injury.
- Focal neurological deficit.
- Spinal pain or tenderness.

The initial evaluation and resuscitation of the injured patient adheres to the advanced trauma life support protocols, with assessment of the airway (A), breathing (B), and circulation (C) taking precedence (Fig. 17.4). During each of these critical evaluations, the presence of a spinal column or spinal cord injury raises important considerations.

A: Airway

Airway management in the setting of spinal cord injury, with or without a cervical spine injury, is complex and difficult. The cervical spine must be maintained in neutral alignment at all times. Clearing of oral secretions and/or debris is essential to maintain airway patency and to prevent aspiration. The modified jaw thrust and insertion of an oral airway may be all that is required to maintain an airway in some cases. However, intubation may be required in others. Failure to intubate emergently when indicated because of concerns regarding the instability of the patient's cervical spine is a potential pitfall.

B: Breathing

Patients with motor-complete injury at a level rostral to C5 will almost invariably require ventilatory support. Intense monitoring for respiratory failure is warranted in all patients

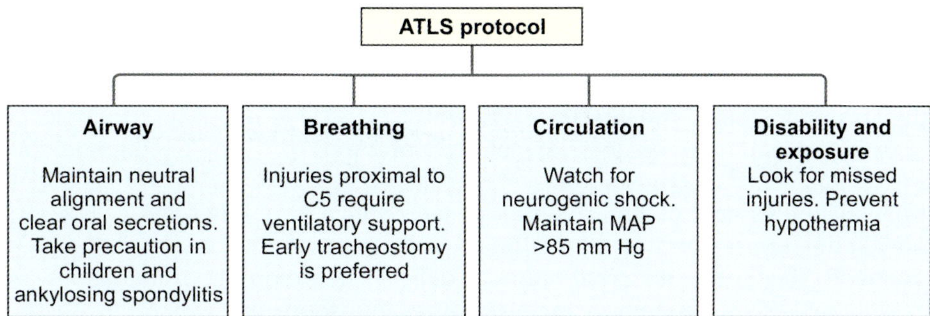

Fig. 17.4 Showing components of ATLS protocol

with cervical spine injury.[17] A variety of management options may be employed for support of ventilation and endotracheal intubation (Consortium for Spinal Cord Medicine, 2005). Endotracheal intubation can be particularly difficult in the patient with SCI, especially if the lesion is in the cervical spine. In addition, intubation frequently needs to be accomplished before the presence or location of an injury can be confirmed. As a result, everyone who needs urgent endotracheal intubation following trauma should be treated as if he or she has a cervical spine injury. The goal of intubation is to secure the airway with as little movement of the cervical spine as possible. The standard urgent or emergent intubating technique for someone with a presumed or known cervical spine injury is a rapid sequence induction with cricoid pressure and manual inline stabilization.

C: Circulation

Hypotension may be hemorrhagic and/or neurogenic in acute spinal cord injury. Because of the high incidence of associated injuries, a diligent search for occult sources of hemorrhage must be made. Seat-belted individuals with a thoracolumbar flexion–distraction injury are at risk for significant intraabdominal trauma, including blunt aortic injuries. Neurogenic shock, which occurs in approximately 20% of patients with cervical spinal cord injury, results when a spinal cord injury disrupts the sympathetic tone on the peripheral vasculature and heart.[22] This is classically characterized as hypotension in association with bradycardia, and it is most typical in spinal cord injury rostral to T4. To minimize secondary ischemic damage to the injured cord, hypotension (of whatever etiology) must be aggressively corrected. Invasive monitoring from arterial and central venous access is imperative to guide interventions. Initial treatment involves fluid resuscitation. Once the patient is volume replete, ongoing hypotension can be managed with vasopressors, such as dopamine and norepinephrine, whose α-agonist activity raises the systemic vascular resistance. Low cardiac output resulting from persistent bradycardia can be treated with atropine; if recalcitrant, temporary pacing may be required.

D and E: Disability and Exposure

During the secondary survey, a log roll allows inspection and palpation of the posterior spine. The presence of tenderness, swelling, or a step deformity can be signs of disruption to the posterior ligamentous complex.

In the tetraplegic patient, the absence of thoracolumbar tenderness will be difficult to interpret, because of the loss of sensation. In these patients, noncontiguous spinal injuries need to be excluded radiographically. It is imperative to cover the patient with warm blankets to prevent hypothermia in the emergency department. Intravenous fluids should be warmed and a warm environment maintained.

Neurologic Assessment

A careful neurologic examination is critical to the spinal evaluation. However, such an examination often is not possible in a polytrauma patient or one who is intoxicated, sedated, or intubated and pharmacologically paralyzed. Within the context of acute spinal trauma, the neurologic examination is performed in accordance with the International Standards for the Neurologic Classification of Spinal Cord Injury, formerly the ASIA (American Spinal Injury Association) standards (Fig. 17.5).[23]

Motor Examination

The motor examination measures the strength of five key upper and five lower extremity myotomes according to the Medical Research Council grading scheme of 0–5. In the upper extremity, these include C5, elbow flexion; C6, wrist extension; C7, elbow extension; C8, long finger flexion; and T1, finger abductors. In the lower extremity, these include L2, hip flexion; L3, knee extension; L4, ankle dorsiflexion; L5, great toe extension; and S1, ankle plantar flexion. The final but most important motor function to be tested is voluntary anal contraction, which should be documented as being present or absent.

Sensory Examination

The sensory examination is performed by assessing light touch and pinprick sensation along 28 dermatomes (with S4–S5 being one). The sensation is documented as either absent, impaired, or normal and is scored 0, 1, or 2, respectively. Again, most importantly, one should carefully assess the sensation in the lowest sacral segments and document, from the digital rectal examination, whether anal sensation is preserved. Testing of the S4–S5 dermatome is performed at the anal mucocutaneous junction. The most common mistake made during sensory testing is misinterpretation of the dermatomal distribution in the upper thorax. The C4 dermatome extends downward in a cape-like distribution along the upper chest and shoulders and ends just rostral to the nipple line. Because most physicians associate the nipple line with a T4 sensory distribution, it is not uncommon for the inexperienced examiner to document a "T4 sensory level" when, in fact, sensation in the C4 dermatome is being observed.

Because of the progressive evolution of neurological deficits, neurological examinations should be repeated after transport and following such procedures as the

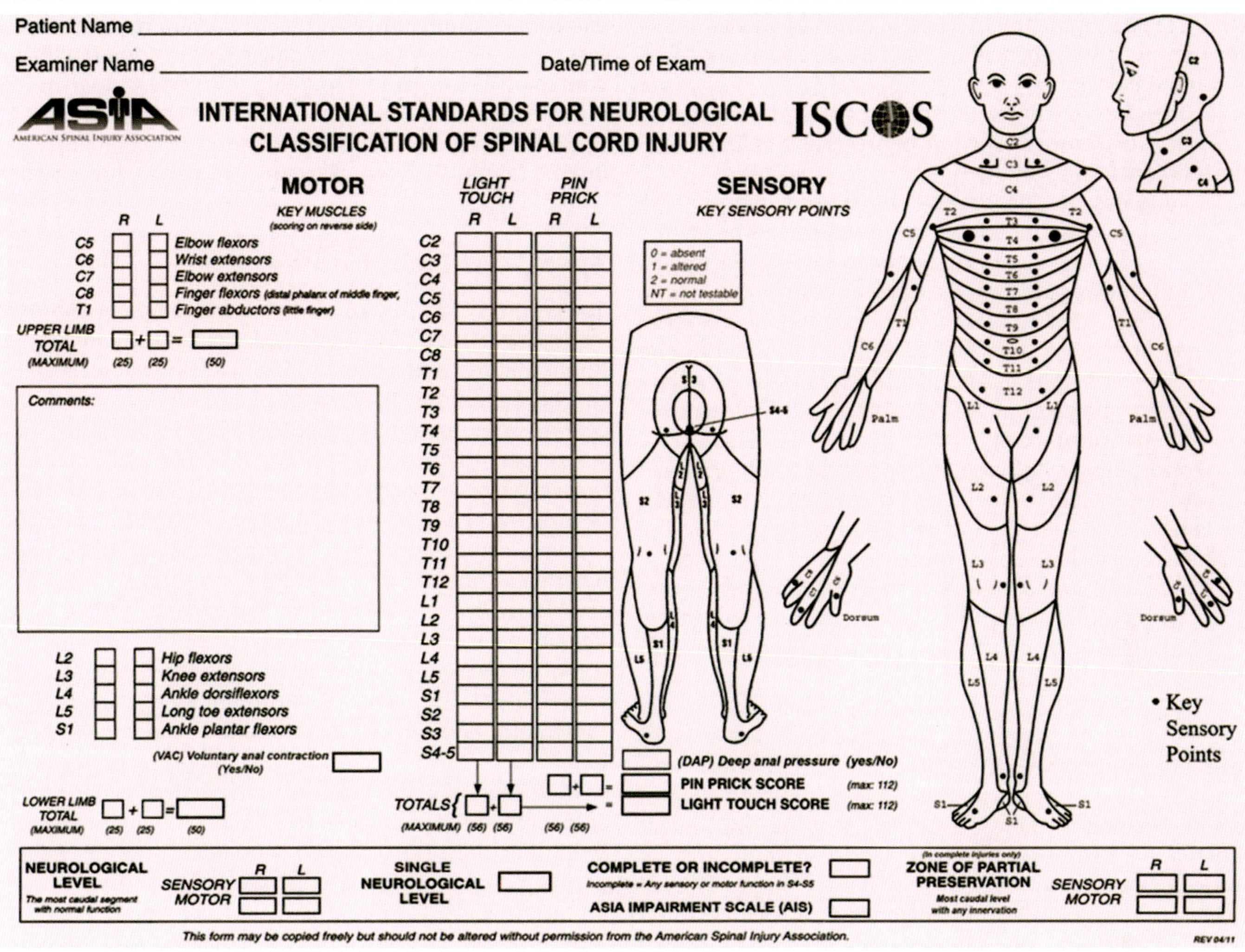

Patient Name ____________

Examiner Name ____________ Date/Time of Exam ____________

ASIA — American Spinal Injury Association

INTERNATIONAL STANDARDS FOR NEUROLOGICAL CLASSIFICATION OF SPINAL CORD INJURY

ISCoS

MOTOR — KEY MUSCLES (scoring on reverse side)

	R	L	
C5			Elbow flexors
C6			Wrist extensors
C7			Elbow extensors
C8			Finger flexors (distal phalanx of middle finger)
T1			Finger abductors (little finger)

UPPER LIMB TOTAL (MAXIMUM) ☐+☐=☐ (25) (25) (50)

Comments:

	R	L	
L2			Hip flexors
L3			Knee extensors
L4			Ankle dorsiflexors
L5			Long toe extensors
S1			Ankle plantar flexors

(VAC) Voluntary anal contraction (Yes/No) ☐

LOWER LIMB TOTAL (MAXIMUM) ☐+☐=☐ (25) (25) (50)

SENSORY — KEY SENSORY POINTS

LIGHT TOUCH R L; PIN PRICK R L

C2, C3, C4, C5, C6, C7, C8, T1, T2, T3, T4, T5, T6, T7, T8, T9, T10, T11, T12, L1, L2, L3, L4, L5, S1, S2, S3, S4-5

0 = absent
1 = altered
2 = normal
NT = not testable

TOTALS (MAXIMUM) (56) (56) (56) (56)

(DAP) Deep anal pressure (yes/No)

PIN PRICK SCORE (max: 112)

LIGHT TOUCH SCORE (max: 112)

NEUROLOGICAL LEVEL (The most caudal segment with normal function) — SENSORY R L; MOTOR R L

SINGLE NEUROLOGICAL LEVEL ☐

COMPLETE OR INCOMPLETE? ☐ Incomplete = Any sensory or motor function in S4-S5

ASIA IMPAIRMENT SCALE (AIS) ☐

ZONE OF PARTIAL PRESERVATION (In complete injuries only) Most caudal level with any innervation — SENSORY R L; MOTOR R L

This form may be copied freely but should not be altered without permission from the American Spinal Injury Association.

REV 04/11

Fig. 17.5 Showing ASIA assessment chart

application of traction or reduction maneuvers to monitor for deterioration or improvement. The frequency of repeat neurological examinations must be individualized, based on the clinical status of the patient and on the protocols of the institution, but in the first 3 days the exam will be performed at least once daily.

Spinal Shock

After a severe spinal cord injury, a state of complete spinal areflexia can develop and last for a varying length of time. This state, conventionally termed spinal shock, is classically evaluated by testing the bulbocavernosus reflex, a spinal reflex mediated by the S3–S4 region of the conus medullaris.[17] This reflex is frequently absent for the first 4–6 hours after injury but usually returns within 24 hours. If no evidence of spinal cord function is noted below the level of the injury, including sacral sparing, and the bulbocavernosus reflex has not returned, no determination can be made regarding the completeness of the lesion. After 24 hours, 99% of patients emerge from spinal shock, as heralded by the return of sacral reflexes. If no sacral function exists at this point, the injury is termed *complete,* and 99% of patients with complete injuries will have no functional recovery.[17] One exception to this dictum is an injury to the distal end of the spinal cord itself. A direct injury to the conus medullaris can disrupt the bulbocavernosus reflex arc and thus make its absence an unreliable indicator of spinal shock.

Severity of Neurologic Injury: ASIA Impairment Scale

The American Spinal Injury Association (ASIA) first published an international classification of spinal cord injury in 1982, called the International Standards for Neurological and Functional Classification of Spinal Cord Injury, also now called as ASIA impairment scale (Fig. 6). Traumatic spinal cord injury is classified into five categories on the ASIA Impairment Scale:

- **A** indicates a "complete" spinal cord injury where no motor or sensory function is preserved in the sacral segments S4–S5
- **B** indicates an "incomplete" spinal cord injury where sensory but not motor function is preserved below the neurological level and includes the sacral segments S4–S5
- **C** indicates an "incomplete" spinal cord injury where motor function is preserved below the neurological level and more than half of key muscles below the neurological level have a muscle grade of less than 3, which indicates active movement with full range of motion against gravity
- **D** indicates an "incomplete" spinal cord injury where motor function is preserved below the neurological level and at least half of the key muscles below the neurological level have a muscle grade of 3 or more
- **E** indicates "normal" where motor and sensory scores are normal. Note that it is possible to have spinal cord injury and neurological deficits with completely normal motor and sensory scores.

The neurologic level describes the remaining sensory and motor functions on each side of the body. The sensory level is defined as the most caudal dermatome in which both pinprick and light touch sensation are normal. The motor level is defined as the most caudal myotome with intact innervation, below which motor deficits exist. Because of muscle poly-innervation, the most caudal muscle to have at least grade 3 power is considered to be fully innervated provided there is grade 5 power in the immediate proximal myotome. For example, if a quadriplegic patient has grade 5 biceps (C5), grade 3 wrist extensors (C6), grade 2 triceps (C7), and grade 1 finger flexors and abductors (C8,T1), the patient is considered to have a C6 motor level. The grade 3 wrist extensor strength is a reflection of intact C6 innervation but loss of C7, T1 innervation. In patients with complete spinal cord injuries, the "zone of partial preservation" refers to the most caudal dermatome and myotome beyond the motor and sensory level that has some limited preserved function. In the example above, the zone of partial preservation would be T1.

ASIA IMPAIRMENT SCALE
♦ A = **Complete:** No motor or sensory functionis preserved in the sacral segments S4-S5.
♦ B = **Incomplete:** Sensory but not motor function is preserved below the neurological level and includes the sacral segments S4-S5
♦ C = **Incomplete:** Motor function is preserved below the neurolgical level, and more than half of key muscles below the neurological level have a muscle grade less than 3.
♦ D = **Incomplete:** Motor function is preserved below the neurological level, and at least half of key muscles below the neurological level have a muscle grade of 3 or more.
♦ E = **Normal:** Motor and sensory function are normal

Fig. 17.6 Showing ASIA impairment scale grading

Spinal Cord Syndromes

Spinal cord syndromes resulting from incomplete traumatic lesions have been described by Schneider and Kahn and by Bosch, Stauffer, and Nickel.[24,25] The following generalizations can be made from their investigations: (i) the greater the sparing of motor and sensory functions distal to the injury, the greater the expected recovery; (ii) the more rapid the recovery, the greater the amount of recovery; and (iii) when new recovery ceases and a plateau is reached, no further recovery can be expected. The importance of determining whether a patient has a complete or incomplete cord injury cannot be overemphasized in the overall prognosis. By definition, an incomplete spinal cord injury is one in which some motor or sensory function is spared distal to the cord injury. A complete spinal cord injury is manifested by total motor and sensory loss distal to the injury. When the bulbocavernosus reflex is positive, and no sacral sensation or motor function has returned, the paralysis is permanent and complete in most patients. An incomplete spinal cord syndrome may be a Brown-Séquard syndrome, central cord syndrome, anterior cord syndrome, posterior cord syndrome, or rarely monoparesis of the upper extremity. Ninety percent of incomplete lesions produce a central cord syndrome, a Brown-Séquard syndrome, or an anterior cervical cord syndrome.

Central cord syndrome: It is a form of incomplete spinal cord injury characterized by impairment in the arms and hands and, to a lesser extent, in the legs. This is also referred to as inverse paraplegia, because the hands and arms are paralyzed while the legs and lower extremities work correctly (Fig 17.7).

Most often the damage is to the cervical or upper thoracic regions of the spinal cord, and characterized by weakness in the arms with relative sparing of the legs with variable sensory loss.

This condition is associated with ischemia, hemorrhage, or necrosis involving the central portions of the spinal cord (the large nerve fibers that carry information directly from the cerebral cortex). Corticospinal fibers destined for the legs are spared due to their more external location in the spinal cord. Prognosis varies, but more than 50% of patients have return of bowel and bladder control, become ambulatory, and have improved hand function. This syndrome usually

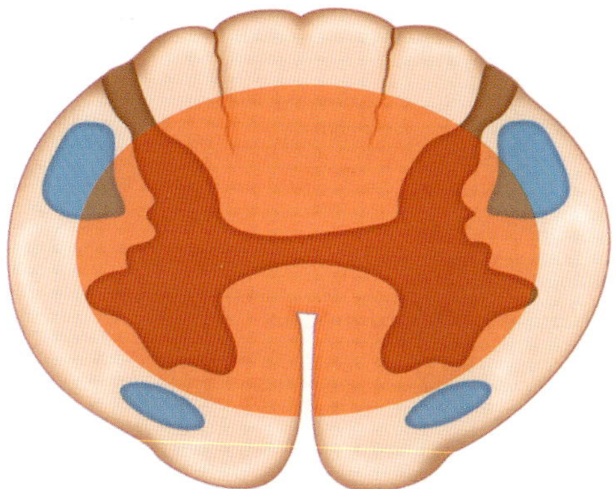

Fig. 17.7 Showing central cord syndrome

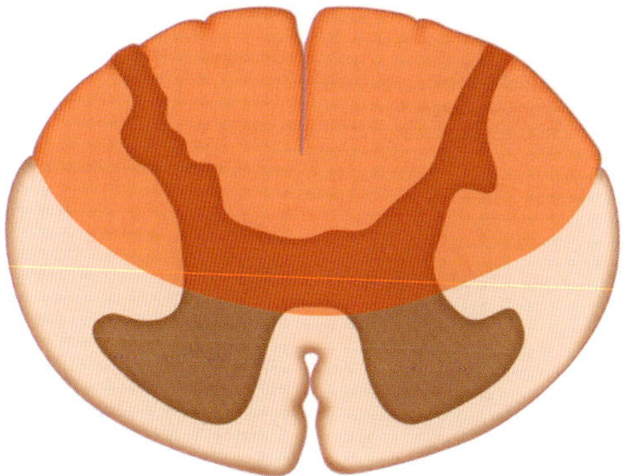

Fig. 17.8 Showing anterior cord syndrome

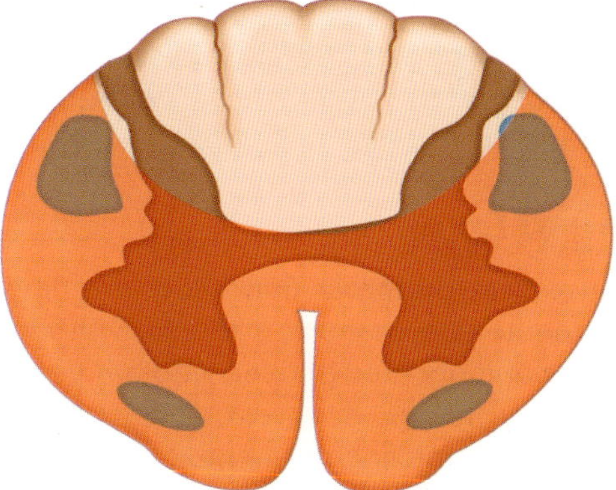

Fig. 17.9 Showing posterior cord syndrome

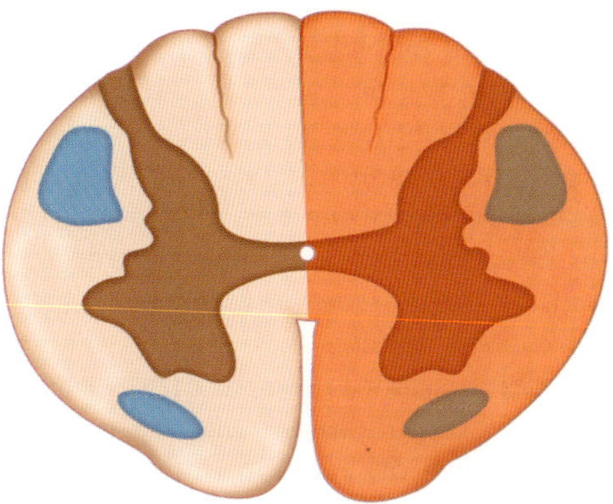

Fig. 17.10 Showing Brown Sequard syndrome

results from a hyperextension injury in an older individual with preexisting osteoarthritis of the spine. The spinal cord is pinched between the vertebral body anteriorly and the buckling ligamentum flavum posteriorly. It also may occur in younger patients with flexion injuries.

Anterior cord syndrome: It is often associated with flexion type injuries to the cervical spine, causing damage to the anterior portion of the spinal cord and/or the blood supply from the anterior spinal artery. Below the level of injury motor function, pain sensation, and temperature sensation are lost. While touch, proprioception (sense of position in space), and sense of vibration remain intact. Prognosis for significant recovery in this injury is poor (Fig. 17.8).

Posterior cord syndrome: It can also occur, but is very rare. Damage to the posterior portion of the spinal cord and/or interruption to the posterior spinal artery causes the loss of proprioception and epicritic sensation (e.g. stereognosis, graphesthesia) below the level of injury. Motor function, sense of pain, and sensitivity to light touch remain intact. (Fig. 17.9).

Brown-Séquard syndrome: It usually occurs when the spinal cord is hemisectioned or injured on the lateral side. True hemisections of the spinal cord are rare, while partial lesions due to penetrating wounds (e.g. gunshot wounds or knife penetrations) are more common. On the ipsilateral side of the injury (same side), there is a loss of motor function, proprioception, vibration, and light touch. Contralaterally (opposite side of injury), there is a loss of pain, temperature, and crude touch sensations (Fig. 17.10).

Conus medullaris syndrome: It is an injury of the sacral cord (conus) and lumbar nerve roots within the spinal canal. It usually results in areflexic bladder, bowel, and lower extremities. Most of these injuries occur between T11 and L2 and result in flaccid paralysis in the perineum and loss of all bladder and perianal muscle control. The irreversible nature of this injury to the sacral segments is evidenced by the absence of the bulbocavernosus reflex and the perianal wink. Motor function in the lower extremities between L1 and L4 may be present if nerve root sparing occurs.

Cauda equina syndrome: It is an injury between the conus and the lumbosacral nerve roots within the spinal canal. It also results in areflexic bladder, bowel, and lower limbs. With a complete cauda equina injury, all peripheral nerves to the bowel, bladder, perianal area, and lower extremities are lost, and the bulbocavernosus reflex, anal wink, and all reflex activity in the lower extremities are absent, indicating absence of any function in the cauda equina. The cauda equina functions as the peripheral nervous system, and there is a possibility of return of function of the nerve rootlets if they have not been completely transected or destroyed. Most often, cauda equina syndrome manifests as a neurologically incomplete lesion.

Imaging of Spine

There are clinical protocols that allow clearance of the cervical spine in asymptomatic patients without imaging. In a fully alert and oriented patient, who has been involved in a low-energy trauma, is devoid of neurologic signs or symptoms, has no midline tenderness, can actively rotate the head 45° in both directions, and lacks distracting injuries that might divert his or her attention away from a severe neck injury, the NEXUS[26] (Fig. 17.11) and Canadian C-spine[27] (Fig. 17.12) rules are highly sensitive in ruling out clinically significant cervical injuries without radiographs. Patients with neck pain, tenderness, or neurologic symptoms and obtunded patients require radiologic evaluation. Patients with distracting injuries or short-term cognitive dysfunction can either be protected with spinal precautions until management of these issues is completed and definitive clinical examination possible or, if urgency dictates, can be examined under the same criteria as the obtunded patient.

In patients who do require radiographic investigation, the optimal choice of imaging modality is changing because modern helical CT has been found to be more sensitive, specific, and efficient than conventional radiography.[28] In addition to providing better resolution of the bony elements, CT overcomes the difficulties that often arise in adequately visualizing the occipitocervical and cervicothoracic junctions. CT also provides the option of delineating the surrounding vasculature.The drawback of CT is its limited soft-tissue definition.

MRI is unequivocally superior at identifying ligamentous injury, intervertebral disk extrusions, and neural element trauma and compression. MRI may be the only modality able to detect this pathology in cases of transient dislocation-subluxation followed by spontaneous reduction and bony realignment.[29,30]

However, not all abnormal findings on MRI are necessarily clinically significant; recent studies correlating

Cervical-spine radiography is indicated for patients with trauma unless they meet all of the following criteria:
No posterior midline cervical-spine tenderness,
No evidence of intoxication
A normal level of alertness
No focal neurologic deficit, and
No painful distracting injuries

Fig. 17.11 Showing NEXUS low risk criteria

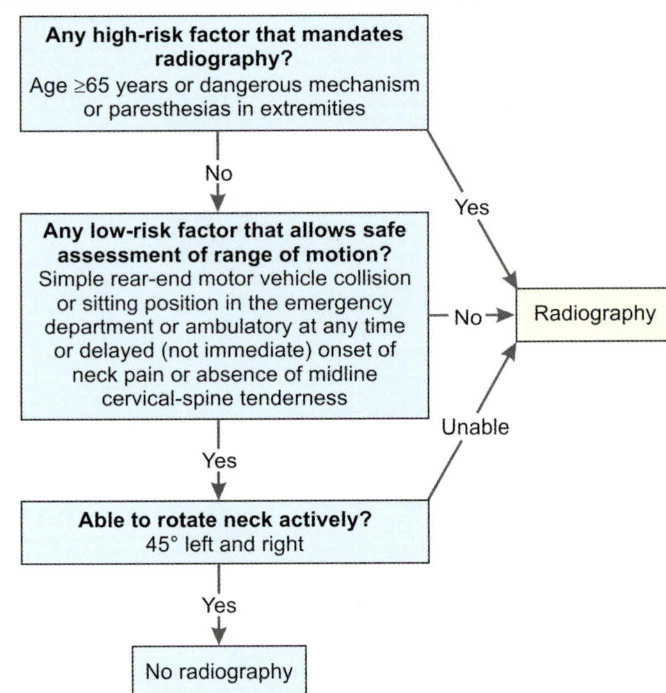

Fig. 17.12 Showing Canadian C spine criteria to rule out cervical spine injury

MRI findings with direct surgical inspection illustrate the tendency of MRI to "over-read" injury to the cervical and thoracolumbar posterior ligamentous complex. How MRI should be incorporated into the evaluation of the obtunded patient remains a contentious issue. Some suggest that a negative helical CT alone can clear an unexaminable patient of clinically meaningful injuries; others state that both CT and MRI are necessary for definitive clearance.

Spinal cord injuries without radiographic abnormalities (SCIWORA) were first described by Pang and Wilberger in 1982.[31] Spinal cord injuries in children frequently occur without fracture-dislocation. Because of the inherent elasticity of the juvenile spine, the spinal cord is vulnerable to injury even though the vertebral column is not disrupted. SCIWORA is most common in children younger than 8 years old. In a review of 159 pediatric patients with cervical spine injuries, Dickman et al. reported that 16% had sustained SCIWORA. More recently, Chiu et al. reviewed the outcome of ligamentous injuries in unreliable patients (patients with a Glasgow Coma Scale score <15) and concluded that in this adult group the incidence of ligamentous injury without radiographic evidence of injury was low. Tewari et al. suggested, however, that SCIWORA may constitute 12% of spinal cord injuries. In their 40 adult patients with SCIWORA, patients with parenchymatous hemorrhage and contusion, as shown on MRI, had the worst results.

Clinical Management

The Edwin Smith papyrus, the world's oldest surgical document, states that an injury of the spinal cord that renders the patient "unconscious of his two legs and his two arms" is "an ailment not to be treated".[32] Although outcomes from spinal cord injuries are still usually poor, our understanding of these injuries and potential treatments has advanced considerably in the 5000 years since this document was written.

The two main confounding clinical scenarios in acute spinal cord injury are hypotension and hypoxemia. The presence of these conditions is highly variable, depending on the presence of concomitant injuries and level of spinal cord injury. Hypoxemia in spinal cord injury can be caused by many factors. The two most common causes are decreased respiratory drive due to unconsciousness and decreased mechanics of ventilation due to a cervical spinal cord injury. In each case, early intubation and aggressive oxygenation should be implemented. Some authors recommend oxygenation to a PaO_2 of more than 100 mm Hg,[33] at least for an initial period. Patients with a complete injury above C5 should seriously be considered for prophylactic intubation, because of the high rate of ventilatory decompensation in these patients. The authors also recommend other measures such as early nasogastric decompression, head-of-bed elevation if possible, and early start of a bowel regimen to assist with respiratory effort by decreasing the work of breathing. If ventilatory decompensation begins, prophylactic intubation should be undertaken to prevent hypoxemia and its additive effect on the secondary injury cascade.

Hypotension can be related to the spinal cord injury itself or to hypovolemia from another traumatic injury. When sympathetic outflow is disrupted in the cervical or upper thoracic spinal cord, peripheral vascular resistance decreases profoundly, leading to hypotension. This is the primary mechanism underlying neurogenic shock and can usually be differentiated from hypovolemic shock by the relative lack of a tachycardia response. Based on the extensive experimental evidence and prospective clinical data, systemic blood pressure should be maintained above a mean of 85–90 mm Hg immediately after injury and for at least 1 week thereafter.

Neuroprotection in Patients with Spinal Cord Injury

A recent explosion in basic research has focused on attenuating the secondary injury cascade in spinal cord injury. The cascade is a promising target for acute treatment of spinal cord injury because it develops hours to weeks after injury. In various experimental animal models of spinal cord injury, neuroprotective agents that limit excitotoxicity and membrane breakdown have been studied extensively. Significant neurologic improvement has followed treatment with sodium channel modulators, glutamate-receptor blockers, glucocorticoids,and gangliosides. Only a few treatments, however, have been tested in human trials of acute spinal cord injury.

A controversial treatment for spinal cord injury is the use of high-dose steroids. Glucocorticoids, such as methylprednisolone stabilize cellular membranes, reduce vasogenic edema, enhance spinal cord blood flow, alter the concentration of electrolytes at the site of injury, inhibit endorphin release, scavenge damaging free radicals, and limit the inflammatory response after injury. Based on these basic properties of methylprednisolone and on the promising results from animal trials, the first randomized trial in humans was reported as the National Acute Spinal Cord Injury Study (NASCIS) in 1984.[34] One year after injury, however, this study showed no differences in the neurologic outcomes of patients receiving low and high doses of methylprednisolone. Subsequent animal studies, however, showed that the dose used in the trial was too low to produce significant differences in long-term functional outcomes.

To address the issue of underdosing with methylprednisolone in the first trial, a second trial (NASCIS 2)[35] was undertaken with a high dose of methylprednisolone to assess neurologic improvement after acute spinal cord injury. This trial demonstrated a small but significant improvement in motor scores 1 year after injury compared with a placebo group. However, several aspects of the study have been criticized strongly. The primary complaints were the lack of a standardized assessment of functional outcome (as opposed to basic motor scores) and the use of post hoc analysis to determine statistical significance. A third trial (NASCIS 3)[36] was then undertaken and showed that methylprednisolone had a greater benefit if given within 3 hours rather than within 8 hours.

Nowadays, the use of methylprednisolone in patients with acute spinal cord injury should be regarded as a treatment option only and not a standard of care. Central to the criticism of methylprednisolone is the fact that the neurologic benefit reported in National Acute Spinal Cord Injury Studies (NASCIS II and III) was extremely modest, whereas the complications associated with prolonged infusion (eg, sepsis, pneumonia, prolonged stay in the intensive care unit) were substantial.[37] Many centers have subsequently abandoned the use of methylprednisolone for acute spinal cord injury.

Two randomized clinical trials have analyzed the effectiveness of the ganglioside GM1 on neurologic improvement after spinal cord injury. The first, smaller study showed a marked improvement in functional neurologic outcome in the GM1 group compared with controls. This improvement failed to materialize in the larger study. This treatment is only considered an option for acute spinal cord injury and is not used in routine clinical practice.

Acute Management of Dislocations

Acute management of dislocations in cervical spine has been a controversial topic for long being. Flexion–distraction injuries in cervical spine can result in facetal subluxations and dislocations and can result in permanent neural deficit. Most of these facetal jumps are reducible by applying close reduction in awake patients. Controversy exists however with few reports in literature which show deterioration of neurology after applying close reduction with herniation of disk in the canal. However the risk associated is very small (<1%) and can result in significant improvement in some patients with in complete deficit. Controversy also exists whether prereduction MRI should be done in these patients. Author feels that in patients with neural deficit valuable time should not be lost in getting MRI done in these patients and reduction should be done as soon as possible in these patients. However if neurology is intact with facetal subluxation then MRI can be done in these patients as there is no emergency in them and risk of disk herniation associated with closed reduction can be avoided in them.

If MRI shows minimal or no disk herniation, patients should undergo gradual reduction in a monitored setting. After reduction, they can undergo fixation and fusion. If closed reduction is unsuccessful, open reduction can be performed in the operating room with neurophysiologic monitoring. If MRI shows a worrisome disk herniation, a diskectomy, followed by an open reduction, can be performed.[38–40]

Timing of Surgery

A critical factor in the decision to operate emergently in patients with a spinal cord injury is the severity of injury. Most clinicians consider an incomplete injury to be a more urgent priority for decompression than a complete injury. The rationale for early decompression of incomplete injuries is that continued compression will lead to further tissue injury and loss of neurologic function.

In complete injuries, there are a lot of debates in literature regarding the timing of surgery in spine trauma patients. A recent multicentre prospective trial, the Surgical Treatment of Acute Spinal Cord Injury Study recently reported that following cervical injuries, patients who received surgical or closed decompression within 24 hours had a higher rate of significant neurologic recovery (defined as at least a 2 grade AIS improvement) at 6-month follow-up compared with those receiving delayed (>24 hours) decompression (19.8% versus 8.8%).[41]

Spinal Cord Injury—Rehabilitation

The main goal of rehabilitation is to make the individual as independent as possible in his/her activities of daily living and to get him/her back to a near normal lifestyle. Rehabilitation requires specially trained staff and team effort. The rehabilitation team includes spinal injury consultant, rehabilitation physician, nurse, physiotherapist, occupational therapist, orthotist, psychologist, peer counselor, social worker, and vocational counselor.

The rehabilitation team should plan the goals in consultation with the patient and the family and regularly monitor the achievement of goals. It should start on day one of injury and should be implemented according to the environment in which the patient has to return, e.g. village or an urban setting.

The goals of rehabilitation include prevention of secondary complication like pressure ulcers, beginning bowel and bladder programs, maintenance of joint range of motion, beginning sitting program and instituting self care and activities of daily living appropriate to medical conditions and level of injury.

Neurogenic bladder is one of the most common causes of morbidity and mortality, hence, it is appropriate management plays a vital part in spinal injury management. Neurogenic bladder could be evaluated by simple clinical tests and investigations like ultrasound KUB and urodynamics.

The bladder could be managed by indwelling catheter, in spinal shock phase clean intermittent catheterization (CIC) after spinal shock and self-CIC at varying period before discharge and at home. The goal is to have a balanced bladder that is maintaining low bladder pressure and continence with minimal risk of infection and deterioration of upper tract.[42,43] In tetraplegic and female patients an indwelling supra pubic catheter may be an option. In patients with upper motor neuron bladder who do not want to do CIC and with no detrusor sphincter dyssynergia or hyperreflexic detrusor, reflex voiding could be an option. Catheter clamping has no role in management of neurogenic bladder. Crede's maneuver can lead to upper tract changes and hence is not advisable bladder wash could be reserved for refractory cases of urinary tract infection resistant to antibiotics.

Indications for concomitant medications for bladder management include detrusor hyperreflexia, detrusor external sphincter dyssynergia, chronically contracted bladder and all patients on reflex voiding.

Complications of Neurogenic bladder are lower urinary tract complications like urinary tract infection, bladder calculi, orchitis/epidydmitis and urethral fistulae/ false passage; upper urinary tract complications like vesicoureteral reflux, hydronephrosis, pyelocaliectasis, renal calculi, renal/perirenal infection, renal insufficiency and failure; and contracted bladder.

A lifelong regular urological follow-up is required. Urine routine and culture is done monthly initially and then on signs/symptoms suggestive of infection. Renal function test is done yearly or more frequently if they are deranged. Urodynamics is done only if there are repeated infections. Ultrasound KUB is done yearly. Cystoscopy is done yearly for patients on indwelling catheter.

Sacral anterior root stimulator and artificial bladder sphincter are advanced surgical techniques for continence. Bladder augmentation could be done for contracted bladder.

An effective bowel management program is important to both the physical and psychological wellbeing of the SCI patient. Stool incontinence may leads to embarrassment, social isolation, work absenteeism and decrease quality of life.[44–46] In bowel training a fixed time pattern takes the place of cerebrally monitored urge. The goal is to provide an effective bowel program with consistent and complete evacuation of bowel and continence inbetween. For most patients, a complete bowel evacuation every other day is satisfactory.[47] This is preceded by night before laxatives or stool softeners and triggered by suppositories or rectal touch technique. Advantage is also taken of gastro colic reflex. A good diet with sufficient bulk (fiber) and adequate fluid intake are essential for a good bowel program. Sitting upright on padded commode could facilitate bowel evacuation.

Pressure ulcers (PU) are one of the most common and potentially serious complications of SCI. More than 24% SCI patients develop PU in initial rehabilitation.[48] The longer the time since injury, the greater is the risk involved with 80% developing pressure ulcer at some point of time in their lifetime.[49] Pressure ulcer can be classified according to NPUAP[50] staging into four categories as under:

Stage I: Nonblanchable erythema of intact skin even after 1 hour of pressure relief. Reactive hyperemia is usually misinterpreted as grade 1 ulcer. However this usually disappears after pressure relief within an hour.

Stage II: Partial thickness skin loss involving the epidermis and dermis. The ulcer is superficial and presents clinically as an abrasion, blisters or shallow craters.

Stage III: Full thickness skin loss involving damage or necrosis of subcutaneous tissue that may extend down to, but not through, underlying fascia. The ulcer presents clinically as a deep crater with or without undermining of adjacent tissue.

Stage IV: Full thickness skin loss with extensive destruction, tissue necrosis or damage to muscles, bone, and other supporting structures.

PU develop at the bony prominence. The most common location is sacrum followed by ischium, heel and trochanter.[48] The most common risk factor for developing PU are shear and pressure. Other risk factor are moisture, level of injury, immobility, nutritional status, etc. Prevention of pressure ulcer is important and education regarding it is important and should start early in rehabilitation. Education includes inspection of skin (use of mirror), two to three hourly turning in bed, regular weight relief when seated, proper equipment and early recognition and treatment of PU.

The treatment of PU involves appropriate seating so that appropriate pressure redistribution occurs while sitting. Various gels, dressing and ointments are available for treatment of PU. Debridement and surgical options are also available for grades 3 and 4 pressure ulcers.

Some other medical condition that needs attention are autonomic dysreflexia, orthostatic hypotension, DVT, spasticity, osteoporosis, prevention of fracture, and neuropathic pain.

Once the patient's motor level of injury, AIS and prognosis for neurological recovery are determined, the short and long-term functional goals are worked out by the team in consultation with the patient and the family. The projected long-term goals are the starting point of rehabilitation. The rehabilitation goals are determined keeping in mind the strength and weaknesses and individual circumstances.

Rehabilitation begins in the acute care and includes SCI specific needs to help the individual to meet their potential in terms of medical, physical, social, emotional, recreational and vocational aspects.[51]

Role of every team member is important. The physiotherapist along with occupation therapist should work together to achieve optimum level of self care skills and mobility. The physiotherapy training includes positioning, respiratory care (breathing exercises, postural drainage and assisted cough), functional ranges of movement, bed mobility skills, increasing sitting tolerance, trunk balance, and strengthening program. As the spine is stabilized and patient is mobilized, vertical mobilization should be done on a tilt table. After overcoming postural hypotension, patient should be made to stand on a frame and mat activities like rolling, side sitting, prone pushups and coming to quadruped are started for functional independence. Simultaneously upper limb strengthening program is also carried out.

The occupational therapists should work towards making an individual indepenedent in self care and ADL activities. OT activities include mat exercises and activities like rolling, sitting, balance training, wheel chair transfer, wheelchair propulsion, hand functions and ADL training. The responsibilities include prescription for appropriate splint, adopted devices, sensory reeducation, activity analysis, dress modification, vocational and prevocational assessment, community outing, home medication and workplace modification.

The rehabilitation nurse has the added responsibility of serving as educator, motivator and listener and should assist in discharge planning. They should help patient and family recognize the medical issues and focus on preventing complications which include bladder and bowel care, maintaining nutrition and skin care and enforcing ROM and transfer techniques. They encourage the patient to actively participate in the rehabilitation program and this subsequently ensures better participation and outcome of the patient.

Wheelchair clinic, use of assistive technology devices and educational classes for patient and care giver are important components of rehabilitation as are issues of fertility, sexual counseling, peer counseling, psychosocial counselling and sports and recreational therapy.

In the wheelchair clinic an appropriate wheelchair and cushion is prescribed to each patient. In the pressure clinic pressure mapping of the ischial tuberosity region is performed and appropriate changes in the wheelchair/cushion are suggested in order to avoid excessive pressure in this region thus reducing the chances of pressure sores.

Assistive technology devices (ATDs) helps the patient become independent as far as possible in his/her activities of daily living. The correct ATDs can enhance a person's life by giving them a sense of control and security. A range of products are available in the developed countries in this regard.

Sexual rehabilitation is a very important but often a neglected field. The importance of non-penetrative and emotional part of sex should be emphasized. Most men with complete and incomplete UMN achieve reflexogenic erection.[52] However, these are often poorly sustained. Several options are available for erectile dysfunction that includes oral sildenafil which is effective for achieving erection in majority of patients.[53] Other options include vacuum constriction device, surface application of nitroglycerin, intracavernous injections of papaverine, and penile prosthesis. In females, lubricating jellies may be required. Counseling of both partners is required. The able partner could play the more active part and after adequate time, trials and privacy to both partners a normal sexual life can be achieved.

Upto 50–60% success rate is possible in the field of fertility for spinal cord injured.[54] After ejaculation (pro or retrograde) by vibrator or electroejaculation by transrectal electrical stimulation, the semen is collected from urethra or bladder and artificial insemination, in vitro fertilization or embryo transfer is carried out. A cesarean section or vaccum delivery is more common.

A peer counselor is a very important member of the team. The spinal injured tends to be more receptive to counselling by an individual who himself/herself has had a spinal injury and has since been successfully rehabilitated into a normal lifestyle.

Spinal injury is a life altering event and it has major consequences psychologically not only for the patient but also for the whole family. Hence psychosocial counseling is important for the patient as well as the whole family. Depressive disorder are the most common form of psychological distress after SCI, usually occur within first months.[55] Anxiety and post traumatic stress disorder have been reported.[56] Treatment includes psychiatric counseling and medications.

Sports and recreational therapy are important not only as a form of exercise and to stimulate the creative mind of the individual but also to encourage them to incorporate these important activities in their lifestyle subsequently but also to break the monotony of the prolonged treatment

Social workers plays a very important role in spinal cord injury rehabilitation. They are the intermediaries between the patient and the entire team. Their other role include imparting knowledge for financial aid matters (government finances, pension plans, disability allowances, etc.), litigation matters, family issues, employment planning and home, and workplace modifications.

Rehabilitation process is not complete unless the individual is made economically productive members of the society through vocational counseling and training. This is importance especially since most of the spinal injured are the sole or important bread earners for the family and are not able to go back to the same vocation after spinal injury. Vocational rehabilitation begins typically begins with an evaluation of the person's functional limitations, barriers to employments, transfer skills, career interests, and prior achievements. Evaluation was followed by counseling and vocational retraining. Efficient vocational rehabilitation involves couseling, job accommodation and supported employment. This is facilitated by rehabilitation counselor who could liaise with the employer as most of the employer have little knowledge and experience in interacting with the person with disability.

A predischarge home visit to suggest home modifications is an important aspect of rehabilitation process. A number of general guidelines and recommendations are available for making the home accessible. The main areas to be evaluated include the entrances, bedroom, bathroom, kitchen and general safety issues ensuring safe space for wheelchair access and maneuverability.[57] A followup home care services to nip any complications at inception and to help the patient in coming back to a normal life style and reintegration back into the community is important.

Patient and care giver education is important as it helps them understand the ailment, participate better in the rehabilitation process and manage any complications/problems themselves once they go back home. A properly designed education program helps the SCI individual and care givers not only to gain knowledge, but also to get emotionally adjusted and prepare for successful community integration. Though learning can occur through group discussion, reading educational material but one-to-one discussion with the healthcare professional is the most effective way to address individual need and concern.[58]

Although not the exclusive determinant, functional independence is closely correlated with motor level.[59] Patients with C2–C4 lesions are the most profoundly injured SCI patients. They have no significant strength in any limb. Many are ventilator dependent and have long-term tracheostomies. These patients require assistance for all self care and activities of daily living (ADL). Mobility requires a powered wheelchair. Most require an indwelling urinary catheter for bladder management. Technological advances like talking tracheotomy tube and computer driven environmental control systems can improve the quality of these patients' lives.

C5 tetraplegic patients have some preserved biceps function. They are able to assist in their self-care activities. They require adaptive devices to feed independently Most require an indwelling urinary catheter for bladder management. They require assistance for transfer. Mobility is with a powered wheelchair.

In a C6 tetraplegic the tenodesis effect increases functional independence. They may be able to achieve modified independence in dressing and bathing. Bowel care on the commode may be performed with modified independence. Males may be able to perform self-catheterization. Transfers may be completed without the assistance of a caregiver with a sliding board. Manual wheelchair may suffice for mobility and they may be able to drive a modified vehicle.

In C7 and C8 tetraplegics transfers should be independent. Patients should be independent in most functional tasks at a modified level. They should be able to perform self-intermittent catheterization. A manual wheelchair should suffice and some may be able to drive a modified vehicle.

Splints, tender transfer surgery and functional electrical stimulation (FES) could be used for management of Tetraplegic hand.

As the level lowers thoracic paraplegics have more truncal stability in a wheelchair. Patients at level below T6 are not at risk for autonomic dysreflexia. They should achieve modified independent selfcare and transfer, as well as bowel and bladder management. Mobility is with a manual wheelchair. Most should be able to drive a modified vehicle.

Lumbar paraplegics are independent in self-care and transfer, as well as bowel and bladder management. They may be able to ambulate with bilateral ankle foot orthosis (AFO) (L3) or knee ankle foot orthosis (KAFO) (L2). However most people with L2 injuries will find a wheelchair more practical for community mobility. Individuals with neurological level above L2 may walk with hip knee ankle foot orthosis (HKAFO) in the gymnasium.

Special Considerations

Women with Spinal Cord Injury

Women comprise a smaller proportion of people living with SCI. The male: female ratio is approximately 5:1. Secondary health issues related to sex and gender differences, and management options are different for women. Some of the important areas which need attention are menstruation, gynecological and menopausal, pregnancy and delivery, parenting and care giver issues. After SCI, amenorrhea occurs which could extend for a period of six months.[60] Women with SCI have normal reproductive potential, hence appropriate birth control measures should be advocated when sexually active. During mensturation there is increased difficulty in maintaining perineal hygiene, bladder and bowel care and increased bladder complications. Frequent pelvic examinations may be necessary for detection of pelvic inflammatory disease as symptoms are masked due to loss of sensation, which could increase morbidity Autonomic dysreflexia could occur during mensturation, labor and delivery. Prescription of NSAIDs for menstruation cramps and routine use of epidural analgesia during delivery in women with SCI above T6 level decreases the incidence of autonomic dysreflexia. Other complication which could increase during pregnancy are deep vein thrombosis, pressure ulcer, pneumonia, lower extremity edema, constipation (bowel routines need to be modified), urinary tract infection, urinary incontinence, severe spasticity, loss of prepregnancy independence.[61] There is increase incidence of preterm delivery, caesarian section and vaccum-assisted delivery. In acute SCI increased resorption of bone occurs and results in increased fracture risk. The postmenopausal bone loss can increase risk of fracture.

Women have historically been responsible for the care of family members. When the woman is affected with the injury the traditional caregiver roles might need to be reversed. There are various negative consequences and many care giver issues need to be addressed on personal basis.[62,63] There have been concerns about the increased demand for caring for an infant. It was found that mothers with SCI are well adjusted with a well functioning social network. Being mothers provide the motivation to stay healthy and improve the quality of life. Rehabilitation team should identify strategies and provide adaptive equipment to facilitate independent parenting.

Pediatric Spinal Cord Injury

SCI in children is relatively uncommon. Pediatric and adult with SCI experience same clinical manifestations and management is essentially in the same manner. However SCIWORA, high cervical injury, delayed onset of neurological deficits, scoliosis, hip subluxation and psychological development during childhood and adolescence are certain aspects that are different from adult due to anatomic, physiological and developmental differences.

Reflex bladder is managed with diaper in infant and CIC is started at the age of 3-4 years of age.

Various orthopedic problems are experienced during growing stage, most significant being scoliosis and hip instability.[64] Treatment of scoliosis includes closed observation with radiograph, prophylactic TLSO although controversial and spinal surgery if the curve increases beyond 40 degrees.[64] Treatment of hip instability includes application of hip abduction orthosis and prevention of contracture.[64] Main areas of concern in pediatric SCI include social and cognitive development , emotional support and family dynamics, transition to adulthood and sexuality.[65]

Geriatric Spinal Cord Injury

SCI in older age group is relatively rare and is often related to cervical spinal stenosis which is caused by relatively minor trauma. They are more likely to have incomplete lesions.[66,67] Older people with SCI have higher prevalence of preexisting medical conditions and subsequently higher complications. They reach low level of independence in terms of walking and selfcare activities as compared to adults with SCI. There is a significant increase in fatigue, increasing dependence and assistance for participation in work and community activity.[68] Regular aerobic exercises, counseling and smoking cessation improves the cardiovascular status of the individual and imparts a sense of wellbeing.

As the survival after SCI improves aging with SCI become one of the important issues. SCI accelerates the process of aging.[68] There are increased complications with advancing age like increased incidence of renal stones, development of pressure ulcers, gastrointestinal complaints, neurological decline, entrapment neuropathies, pneumonia etc. Influenza and pneumococcal vaccine is recommended in all person with SCI above 60 years.[69] To manage aging with SCI effectively, strategies to minimize conditions and complications which occur with aging need to be identified and implemented.[70] Education pertaining to psychological, social and environmental factors in context with aging and stressing the need of equipments and medication is important.

People with SCI require regular and comprehensive care through out their lifetime. Yearly follow-up includes patients current medical condition, medications, review of systems and age appropriate screening. Recommendations for the general medical screening should be followed. Counseling is important aspect of follow up visits both for medical as well as physical and social issues.

The dictum "Prevention is better than cure" is very relevant in spinal injuries and a very strong focus should be given on it. Legislation for implementing seat belt use, safety precautions while working on a height/construction site etc and public awareness program would go a long way in preventing this devastating ailment.

Key Points

1. Motor vehicle accidents are the most common cause of spinal cord injuries in developed nations while fall from height is most common in developing nations.
2. Respiratory failure due to pneumonia is now the most common cause of death in spinal cord injured patients while earlier it was renal failure.
3. Any patient who presents with the symptoms of altered mental status, evidence of intoxication, suspected extremity fracture or any other distracting injury with focal neurological deficit or with spinal pain or tenderness should be immobilized and should be worked to rule out spinal injury.

4. Immediate spinal immobilization should be started at the accident scene and continued until no evidence of a spinal fracture or instability is found.
5. Hypoxemia and hypotension should be avoided in spinal injured patients as it can cause secondary damage to cord. Mean arterial pressure should be kept above 85 mm Hg.
6. Role of steroids is yet not proven in spinal cord injured patients although adverse effects of steroids, including gastrointestinal bleed and infection are well known.
7. In patient with facetal dislocation with neural deficit close reduction can be attempted before getting MRI done, if getting MRI can delay the treatment. Chances of a prolapsed disk causing deficit after reduction are very minimal.
8. Early decompression or realignment of the spinal column is safe and may improve neurologic outcome.
9. Main goal of the rehabilitation is to make the individual as independent as possible. Goals are planned in consultation with the patient and family.
10. Neurogenic bladder is one of the most common causes of mortality and morbidity. Hence its appropriate evaluation and management is important.
11. Bowel care and management of complications like pressure ulcer autonomic dysreflexia, orthostatic hypotension, deep vein thrombosis, spasticity, osteoporosis, prevention of fracture and neuropathic pain are other important areas which needs attention.
12. Expected level of outcome is determined according to the neurological level of injury of an individual. The rehabilitation should be focused to achieve independence accordingly.
13. Special considerations are required in pediatric, women and geriatric SCI keeping in mind the issues specific to age and gender.

References

1. Taber, Clarence Wilbur; Venes, Donald (2009). Taber's cyclopedic medical dictionary. F.A. Davis. pp. 2173-4. ISBN 0-8036-1559-0.
2. Benson DR, Keenen TL, Antony J. Unsuspected associated findings in spinal fractures. J Orthop Trauma. 1989;3:160.
3. Riggins RS, Kraus JF. The risk of neurologic damage with fractures of the vertebrae. J Trauma. 1977;7:126-33.
4. Devivo MJ, Kartus PL, Stover SL, et al. Benefits of early admission to an organised spinal cord injury care system. Paraplegia. 1990;28:545-55.
5. Bohlman HH. Acute fractures and dislocations of the cervical spine. J Bone Joint Surg [Am]. 1979;61:1119-42.
6. Bosch A, Stauffer ES, Nickel VL. Incomplete traumatic quadriplegia: A ten year review. JAMA. 1971;216:473-8.
7. Wen-Ta Chiu, et al. Review paper: Epidemiology of traumatic spinal cord injury: Comparisons between developed and developing countries. Asia. Pac J Public Health. 2010;22(9):9-18.
8. Stover SL, Fine PR. The epidemiology and economics of spinal cord injury. Paraplegia. 1987;25:225-8.
9. Jess F, Kraus, et al. Incidence of traumatic spinal cord lesions. Journal of Chronic Diseases. 1975;28(9):471-92.
10. Frankel HL, Coll JR, Charlifue SW, et al: Long term survival in spinal cord injury: A fifty-year investigation. Spinal Cord. 1998;36:266-74.
11. Tator CH, Duncan EG, Edmonds VE, et al. Demographic analysis of 552 patients with acute spinal cord injury in Ontario, Canada, 1947–1981. Paraplegia. 1988;26:112-3.
12. Midwestern Regional Spinal Cord Injury Care System: Northwestern University and Rehabilitation Institute of Chicago Progress Report No. 9, Chicago: Northwestern University; 1980.
13. Schouten R, Albert T, Kwon B. Review article-The spine injured patient initial assessment and emergency treatment. JAAOS. 2012;20:336-46.
14. Miller CP, Brubacher JW, Biswas D, Lawrence BD, Whang PG, Grauer JN. The incidence of noncontiguous spinal fractures and other traumatic injuries associated with cervical spine fractures: A 10-year experience at an academic medical center. Spine (Phila Pa 1976). 2011;36(19):1532-40.
15. Toscano J. Prevention of neurological deterioration before admission to a spinal cord injury unit. Paraplegia. 1988;26(3):143-50.
16. American College of Surgeons Committee on Trauma. Advanced Trauma Life Support for Doctors: ATLS Student Course Manual, ed 8. Chicago,IL, American College of Surgeon; 2008.
17. Paralyzed Veterans of America. Early Acute Management in Adults with Spinal Cord Injury: A Clinical Practice Guideline for Health-Care Professionals.Washington, DC, Consortium for Spinal Cord Medicine, 2008. Guidelines_and_Publications.htm
18. Herzenberg JE, Hensinger RN, Dedrick DK, Phillips WA. Emergency transport and positioning of young children who have an injury of the cervical spine: The standard backboard may be hazardous. J Bone Joint Surg Am. 1989;71(1):15-2.
19. Davies G, Deakin C, Wilson A. The effect of a rigid collar on intracranial pressure. Injury. 1996;27:6479.
20. Como JJ, Diaz JJ, Dunham CM, et al. Practice management guidelines for identification of cervical spine injuries following trauma: Update from the eastern association for the surgery of trauma practice management guidelines committee. J Trauma. 2009;67(3):651-9.
21. Morris CG, McCoy E: Clearing the cervical spine in unconscious polytrauma victims, balancing risks and effective screening. Anaesthesia. 2004;59(5):464-82.
22. Guly HR, Bouamra O, Lecky FE. Trauma Audit and Research Network:The incidence of neurogenic shock in patients with isolated spinal cord injury in the emergency department. Resuscitation. 2008;76(1):57-62.

23. Waring WP III, Biering-Sorensen F, Burns S, et al. 2009 review and revisions of the international standards for the neurological classification of spinal cord injury. J Spinal Cord Med. 2010;33(4):346-52.
24. Stauffer ES. Neurologic recovery following injuries to the cervical spinal cord and nerve roots. Spine. 1984;9:532-4.
25. Stauffer ES. A quantitative evaluation of neurologic recovery following cervical spinal cord injuries. Atlanta: Georgia; 1988.
26. Hoffman JR, Mower WR, Wolfson AB, Todd KH, Zucker MI. National Emergency X-Radiography Utilization Study Group: Validity of a set of clinical criteria to rule out injury to the cervical spine in patients with blunt trauma. N Engl J Med. 2000;343(2):94-9.
27. Stiell IG, Wells GA, Vandemheen KL, et al. The Canadian C-spine rule for radiography in alert and stable trauma patients. JAMA. 2001;286(15):1841-8.
28. Brown CV, Antevil JL, Sise MJ, Sack DI. Spiral computed tomography for the diagnosis of cervical, thoracic, and lumbar spine fractures: Its time has come. J Trauma. 2005;58(5):890-6.
29. Vaccaro AR, Rihn JA, Saravanja D, et al. Injury of the posterior ligamentous complex of the thoracolumbar spine: A prospective evaluation of the diagnostic accuracy of magnetic resonance imaging. Spine (Phila Pa 1976). 2009;34(23):E841-7.
30. Rihn JA, Yang N, Fisher C, et al. Using magnetic resonance imaging to accurately assess injury to the posterior ligamentous complex of the spine: A prospective comparison of the surgeon and radiologist. J Neurosurg Spine. 2010;12(4):391-6.
31. Pang D, Wilberger JEJ. Spinal cord injury without radiographic abnormalities in children. J Neurosurg. 1982;57:114-29.
32. Breasted J. The Edwin Smith surgical papyrus. In Wilkins R (ed): Neurosurgical Classics. New York, Johnson Reprint Corp; 1965;pp1-5.
33. Dyson-Hudson TA, Stein AB: Acute management of traumatic cervical spinal cord injuries. Mt Sinai J Med. 1999;66:170-8.
34. Bracken MB, et al. Efficacy of methylprednisolone in acute spinal cord injury. Journal of the American Medical Association. 1984;251:45-52.
35. Bracken MB, Shepard MJ, Collins WF Jr, et al. Methylprednisolone or naloxone treatment after acute spinal cord injury: 1-year follow-up data. Results of the second National Acute Spinal Cord Injury Study. J Neurosurg. 1992;76(1):23-31.
36. Bracken MB, et al. Methylprednisolone or tirilazad mesylate administration after acute spinal cord injury: 1-year follow up. Results of the third National Acute Spinal Cord Injury randomized controlled trial. J Neurosurg. 1998;89:699-706.
37. Sayer FT, Kronvall E, Nilsson OG. Methylprednisolone treatment in acute spinal cord injury: The myth challenged through a structured analysis of published literature. Spine J. 2006;6(3):335-43.
38. Doran SE, Papadopoulos SM, Ducker TB, et al. Magnetic resonance imaging documentation of coexistent traumatic locked facets of the cervical spine and disk herniation. J Neurosurg. 1993;79:341-5.
39. Vaccaro AR, Falatyn SP, Flanders AE, et al: Magnetic resonance evaluation of the intervertebral disk, spinal ligaments, and spinal cord before and after closed traction reduction of cervical spine dislocations. Spine. 1999;24:1210-7.
40. Rizzolo SJ, Piazza MR, Cotler JM, et al: Intervertebral disk injury complicating cervical spine trauma. Spine. 1991;16:S187-9.
41. Fehlings MG, Vaccaro A, Wilson JR, et al. Early versus delayed decompression for traumatic cervical spinal cord injury: Results of the Surgical Timing in Acute Spinal Cord Injury Study (STASCIS). PLoS One. 2012;7(2);e32037.
42. Consortium for Spinal Cord Medicine. Bladder management for adults with spinal cord injury: a clinical practice guideline for health care providers. J Spinal Cord Med. 2006;29:527-73.
43. Samson G, Cardenas DD. Neurogenic bladder in spinal cord injury. Phys Med Rehabil Clin N Am. 2007;18:255-74
44. Steins SA, Bergman SB, Goetz LL. Neurogenic Bowel management after Spinal Cord injury: Clinical coorelation and rehabilitative management. Arch Phys Med Rehabil. 1997;76:S80-102.
45. Paralyzed Veteran of America. Neurogenic Bowel management in Adults with Spinal Cord injury: A Clinical Practice Guidelines. Washington DC. Paralyzed Veteran of America; 1998.
46. Roach MJ, Fros FS, Greasy G. Social and personel consequences of acquired bowel dysfunction for person with spinal cord injury. J Spinal cord Med. 2000;23:263-9.
47. Spinal Cord Medicine Consortium: A Clinal Practice Guidelines for Neurogenic Bowel management in Adults with Spinal Cord injury. J Spinal Cord Med. 1998;21:248-93.
48. Chen D, Apple DF Jr, Hudson LM, et al. Medical Complication during acute rehabilitation following traumatic spinal cord injury - current experience of the model systems. Arch Phys Med Rehabil. 1999;80:1397-401.
49. Furher MJ, Garber SL, Rintala DH, et al. Pressure ulcer in community resident persons with spinal cord injury :prevalence and risk factor. Arch Phys Med Rehabil. 1993;74:1172-7.
50. International pressure Ulcer Guidelines for prevention: The International Pressure Ulcer Advisory Panel. www.npuap.org
51. Whiteneck G, Adler C, Biddle A K et al. Consortium for Spinal Cord Medicine. Outcomes following Spinal Cord injury: A Clinical Practice Guidelines for Health Care Professional. Washington DC. Paralyzed Veteran of America; 1999.
52. Comarr AE. Sexual functions among patients with spinal cord injury. Urol Int. 1970;25:134-68.
53. Dery F A, Dinsmore WW, Fraser M, et al. Efficacy and safety of all oral sildenaphil Viagra) in treatment in men with erectile dysfunctions caused by spinal cord injury. Neurology. 1988;58:1629-33.
54. Rutkowski SB, Gerahty TJ, Hagen DL, et al. A comprehensive approach to the management of male infertility following spinal cord injury. Spinal Cord. 1999;37:508-14.
55. Dryden DM, Saunders LD, Rowe BH, et al. Depression following traumatic spinal cord injury. Neuroepidemiology. 2005;25:55-61.

56. Nielsen MS. Post traumatic stress disorder and emotion distress in persons with spinal cord lesion. Spinal Cord. 2003;41:296-302.
57. Eberhardt K. Home modificationfor person with spinal cord injury. Occup Ther Pract. 1998;3:24-7.
58. Hammond MC, Burns SC. Yes you can! A guide to self care for persons with spinal cord injury. Washington: Paralyzed Veterans of America; 2000.
59. Ho CH, Wuermser LA, Priebe MM, et al. Spinal Cord injury Medicine: epidemiology and classification. Arch Phys Med Rehabil. 2007;S88:S49-54.
60. Menarch; Jackson AB, Wadley VA. A multicentric study of women, self –reported reproductive healthafter spinal cord injury. Arch Phys Med Rehabil. 1999;80:1420-8.
61. Pregnancy _ Burns AS, Jackson AB. Gynaecological and reproductive issues in women with spinal cord injury. Phys Med Rehabil. Clin N Am. 2001;12:183-7.
62. O'Brien MT. Multiple sclerosis: stressors and coping strategies inspousal caregivers. J Commun Health Nursing.1993;10:123-35.
63. Allen SM, Goldscheiider F, Ciambrone DA. Gender, roles, marital intimacy and nomination of spouse as primary care giver. Gerantologist.1999;39:150-8.
64. Betz RR. Ortheopedic problem of the child with spinal cord injury. Top Spinal Cord Inj Rehbil. 1984;3:9-19.
65. Anderson CJ. Psychological and sexuality issues in pediatric spinal cord injury. Top Spinal Cord Inj Rehbil. 1997;3:70-8.
66. DeVivo MJ, Kartus PL, Rutt RD, et al. The influence of age at the time of spinal cord injury on rehabilitation outcome. Arch Neurol. 1990;47:687-91.
67. Scivoletto G, Morganti B, Ditunno P, et al. Effects on age on spinal cord lesion patients' rehabilitation. Spinal Cord. 2003;41:457-64.
68. Lammertse DP. Maintaining health long term with spinal cord injury. Top Spinal Cord Inj Rehbil. 2001;6:1-21.
69. Mckenly WO, Jackson AB, Cardenas, et al. Long term medical complications after traumatic spinal cord injury: a regional model systems analysis. Arch Phys Med Reabil. 1999;80:1402-10.
70. Whitneck GG, Menter RR. Where do we go from here? In:Whiteneck GG, Charlifue SW, Gerhart KA, et al. (eds): Aging with Spinal Cord Injury. New York Demos;1993. pp 361-9.

CHAPTER

18

Laminoplasty with Suture Anchor Fixation

Lance K Mitsunaga, Eric O Klineberg, Munish Gupta

Introduction

Laminoplasty was initially developed by the Japanese in the early 1970s to treat patients with ossification of the posterior longitudinal ligament (OPLL).[1] OPLL and cervical spondylosis are the most common causes of multilevel cervical stenosis and myelopathy. Anterior and posterior approaches can be used to achieve decompression of the canal in these cases, but for multilevel cervical decompression, a posterior approach is usually preferred because it allows for decompression at multiple levels via a single incision. Potential complications and morbidities associated with laminectomy alone include instability and kyphosis or, if performed in association with a fusion procedure, loss of motion and adjacent segment disease.[2,3] Laminoplasty was designed to indirectly decompress the spinal canal without disrupting the dorsal elements, thereby maintaining cervical stability and obviating the need for a fusion procedure and its associated problems. Hinging the laminae open unilaterally or bilaterally allows the spinal cord to drift posteriorly, away from pathologic anterior structures. This chapter will review the indications and contraindications for laminoplasty, the advantages and disadvantages of the procedure, the authors' preferred technique for performing a laminoplasty with suture anchor fixation, and the potential complications of this procedure.

Indications

The indication for laminoplasty is multilevel cervical cord compression at more than three intervertebral disc spaces due to OPLL, cervical spondylosis, multilevel disk herniations, central cord syndrome, spinal cord tumors, or developmental spinal stenosis.

Contraindications

In patients with kyphotic deformities of the cervical spine, laminoplasty results in decreased posterior migration of the cord and decreased expansion of the canal.[4] The anterior cord compression seen in these patients is not improved with laminoplasty. Further, laminoplasty can introduce some instability and worsen kyphotic deformity.[5-21] Thus, kyphotic deformity is one contraindication to laminoplasty. Laminoplasty is also contraindicated in patients with cervical instability. To prevent progression of this instability, spinal fusion should be performed in any patient with instability undergoing laminoplasty. Rheumatoid arthritis, which has been associated with instability following laminoplasty, is a relative contraindication to laminoplasty.[22]

Advantages of Laminoplasty

By avoiding disruption of the posterior bony-ligamentous structures that contribute to stability, laminoplasty decreases the risk of kyphosis and instability compared to laminectomy.[2,5, 6, 23-38] By retaining the lamina, revision procedures following laminoplasty via posterior approaches are safer. In addition, the retained lamina can also provide some protection against the epidural scar that has been associated with post-laminectomy pain and neurologic deficits.[39-41] By avoiding a fusion procedure, laminoplasty can avoid the problems associated with fusion, such as loss of motion, pseudarthrosis, adjacent segment disease, and the need for prolonged postoperative immobilization. In addition, decompressing the spinal cord without actually removing anterior pathologic structures is possible with laminoplasty procedures, thus avoiding the potential morbidity that can accompany anterior approaches, such as dysphagia, recurrent laryngeal nerve injury, dysphonia, and injury to the esophagus or carotid sheath contents.

Disadvantages of Laminoplasty

Some range of motion is usually lost following laminoplasty.[6-8,23,27,35,42-48] Laminoplasty may also cause or worsen neck pain. Finally, patients may find the longitudinal incision that is made during laminoplasty less cosmetically appealing than anterior incisions.

Preoperative Workup/Planning

Patients who are considered candidates for laminoplasty should be evaluated for neck pain or radicular symptoms, the presence of which would warrant consideration of supplementing the laminoplasty with fusion or foraminotomies, respectively. Upright plain films of the cervical spine, including flexion–extension views, should be obtained to assess preoperative alignment and stability. We also obtain advanced imaging, such as MRI or CT myelogram, which can be used to correlate with clinical findings and to plan where foraminotomies may be necessary.

Patient Positioning, Preparation, and Draping

General endotracheal anesthesia is necessary but special attention should be paid to cervical alignment during intubation. Awake fiberoptic intubation is preferable in patients with severe myelopathy to prevent spinal cord injury due to excessive neck extension and to assess neurologic status following intubation. Following intubation, neuromonitoring electrodes are placed and baseline transcranial motor evoked potentials and somatosensory potentials are recorded prior to positioning the patient prone. We then apply Mayfield tong retractors and the patient is ready for positioning.

We prefer the 180° operating room setup for our laminoplasty procedures. The patient is positioned prone on a standard table with gelfoam bolster pads and a Mayfield tong attachment. The Mayfield tongs are useful to control alignment of the cervical spine while the patient is being positioned.

In general, we position the patient's head in maximum capital flexion and neutral cervical spine alignment. This widens the interspinous and interlaminar intervals and also opens the facet joints which facilitates neuroforaminal decompression. If, however, we anticipate performing a fusion procedure, it is necessary to extend the neck slightly. Taping the shoulders down allows complete radiographic visualization of the lower cervical spine. In addition, placing the table in reverse Trendelenburg position at about 20–30 degrees helps with venous bleeding and visualization. Our typical patient positioning setup is shown in Figure 18.1.

Once the patient is properly positioned, MEP and SSEP signals should be rechecked. Any changes compared to baseline measurements may indicate the need for repositioning. The posterior cervical spine is then prepped and draped in the standard sterile fashion from the occipital protuberance superiorly down to the T3 spinous process inferiorly.

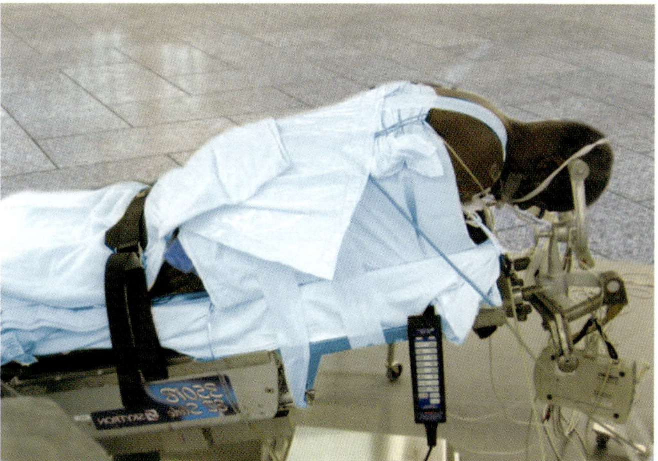

Fig. 18.1 Image demonstrating preferred patient positioning. Patient is placed prone. Mayfield tongs are applied without traction to stabilize the head and neck. The head is in maximum capital flexion and the neck is neutral. The shoulders are taped down and the table is placed in reverse Trendelenburg

Key Procedural Steps

Cervical laminoplasty was initially described by Oyama in 1973 as a treatment for OPLL.[1] Since that time, various modifications of the laminoplasty procedure have been developed in terms of how and where the hinge is made to reposition the laminae and how the expanded canal is maintained in an open position. In general, all of these technical modifications yield similar results. This chapter will provide a detailed description of our preferred laminoplasty technique, a modification of Hirabayashi's unilateral expansive open door laminoplasty using suture anchors to stabilize the lamina in an open position (Figs 18.2 to 18.6).[23,45] With this procedure, a unilateral hinge is made on one side of the lamina–spinous process–ligamentum flavum complex. The roof of the canal can then be repositioned on the contralateral side in such a way that the canal is decompressed.

Usually, we perform a laminoplasty from C3 to C6 with undercutting of the superior half of the C7 lamina. The surgical exposure should include all of these levels. We make a standard posterior longitudinal midline incision that starts superiorly at the occipital protuberance and continues inferiorly to the spinous process of C7. Electrocautery is used to split the midline fascia and ligamentum nuchae to expose the spinous processes from C2 to C7. The interspinous and supraspinous ligaments can be released at the levels that will be included in the laminoplasty but they should be preserved at the rostral and caudal extents of the exposure. Disruption of the muscular attachments to C2 should also be minimized as much as possible to decrease the risk of postoperative kyphosis between C2 and C3. Proceed with a midline, subperiosteal elevation of the paravertebral muscles which can be retracted laterally off the spinous processes of C3 to C7, the laminae, and the medial aspect of the facets. The avascular, subperiosteal plane should be identified during dissection in order to minimize trauma to the paraspinal muscles and blood loss. Carry the dissection out laterally to the lateral masses but avoid disruption of the facet capsules (unless a fusion procedure is anticipated). Meticulous hemostasis with monopolar or bipolar electrocautery is imperative at all times. Once the spinous processes and laminae are completely free of soft tissue, retractors are placed on both sides of the wound and, if necessary, superiorly and inferiorly, as well (Fig. 18.2).

Once we have completed the posterior midline exposure, we prefer to immediately drill the hole at the base of the spinous process that will eventually be used to stabilize the laminar door in an open, expanded position with a suture anchor. A right-angle dental drill with a 2 mm burr tip is used to create a hole at the base of the spinous process. The rest of our suture anchor fixation technique will be described in a subsequent section of this chapter. The hole in the spinous process should be the first step after completing the exposure because if this is done after destabilizing the lamina with a laminoplasty, one risks complete detachment of the lamina.

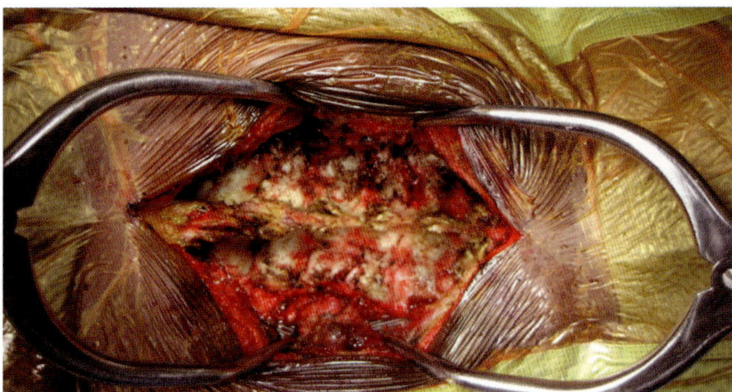

Fig. 18.2 Intraoperative photo following posterior midline dissection and lateral retraction of paraspinal muscles. Note how the spinous processes, lamina, and medial aspect of the facets are completely clear of soft tissue

We prefer to make the cut on the hinged side of the lamina first, followed by the cut on the opening side. Then, if the lamina do not move sufficiently when the door is opened, the cut on the hinged side can be deepened and the dorsal elements can be released further. We generally choose the opening side of the laminoplasty to be on the side on which the patient has more severe stenosis or radiculopathy. This is because it is technically more straightforward to perform a neuroforaminal decompression on the opening side.

For the hinged side of the laminoplasty, a trough is created at the lamina–lateral mass junction. Care should be taken to preserve the facet capsules to maintain postoperative stability. We prefer to make the troughs on the hinged side with a 6 mm diamond burr. A burr of this large caliber makes it possible to cut the outer cortex of the lamina to create a greenstick fracture on the hinged side while minimizing the risk of completely fracturing through the inner laminar cortex. The large tip of this burr also results in a comparatively wider trough on the hinged side. In this way, the walls of the trough do not abut when the door is opened, which would limit the amount of canal expansion possible. Thin the lamina by burring down the outer cortex and approximately half of the cancellous bone using a side to side brushing motion. The burr should be oriented perpendicular to the lamina. These troughs should be made from superior to inferior, from one level above to one level below the stenotic levels. Leave the inner cortex intact, as this will serve as the hinge on which the door opens.

For the opening side of the laminoplasty, we use a 2 or 3 mm cutting burr to decorticate the posterior aspect of the lamina and create a trough at the junction of the lamina and lateral mass. This should be done with particular care at the superior portion of the lamina, as the dura is unprotected by ligamentum flavum in this region. Again, special attention should also be paid to preserving the facet joints. Once the lamina are burred down to a thin cortical layer, a 2 or 3 mm kerrison punch is used to finalize the laminar cut by removing the thin rim of residual lamina and associated ligamentum flavum just medial to the pedicles from inferior to superior. At this stage, bipolar electrocautery and thrombin gel are useful to stop epidural venous bleeding.

A Kerrison rongeur is then used to cut the lamina and attached ligamentum flavum to free up the superior and inferior-most lamina included in the laminoplasty on the open side from adjacent levels. Thus, three free borders are created on which the "door" can now hinge open. If the laminae are thinned sufficiently, the dorsal elements should be more compliant. It should now be possible to open the lamina gradually and cautiously by pulling the spinous processes towards the hinged side and lifting the lamina off the spinal cord with a curette on the opening side. If necessary, additional thinning of the trough on the hinged side can be performed. To minimize the risk of excessively thinning the lamina on the hinged side and completely detaching the entire lamina, periodically assess the degree of "give" in the spinous process. In addition, a curette can be placed on the open side and, when pulled upwards, motion in the lamina suggests that the lamina on the hinged side has been thinned sufficiently. We also find it helpful to gauge how deep the trough should be on the hinged side by using the depth of the lamina on the opening side as a reference.

We use a Kocher grasped onto the spinous process to rotate the lamina towards the hinged side and a curette or penfield dissector to expand the opening (Fig. 18.3). Adhesions between the dura and the ventral lamina on the opening side can be freed up with a Woodsen probe. Opening all of the laminae together as a single unit helps preserve the intraspinous ligaments and dorsal structures that provide stability to the cervical spine. This is best accomplished by hinging the lamina open at each level gradually and to the same extent. Doing so will create a greenstick fracture on the hinged side at the trough and an increasingly larger gap between the lamina and facet on the on the open side. This portion of the procedure must be carried out slowly and gently to prevent complete fracture of the inner cortex on the hinged side. If this does occur, the hinged side must be stabilized or a laminectomy and fusion procedure must be performed. Further, spinal cord injury is another potential risk during this portion of the surgery if

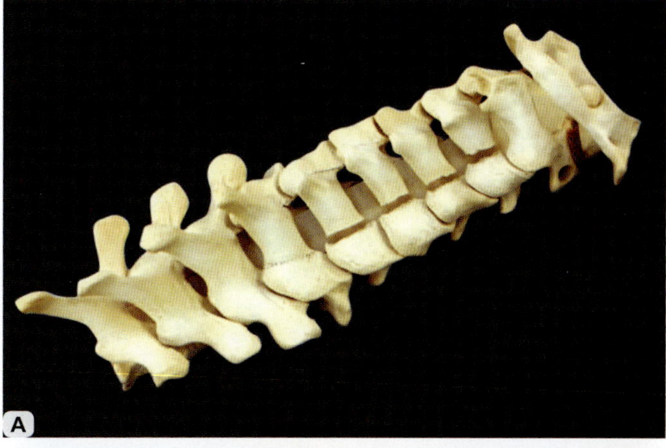

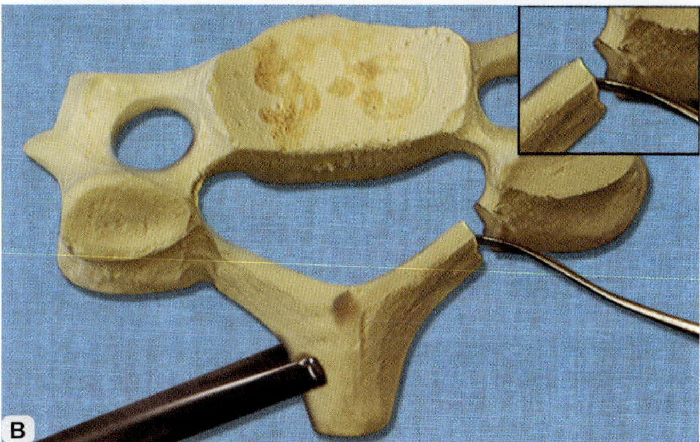

Fig. 18.3 Image depicting an expansive open door laminoplasty. An incomplete trough is drilled on the hinged side of the laminplasty (not shown). Then, for the opening side of the laminoplasty, after drilling a trough at the junction of the lamina and lateral mass with a burr, the thin layer of residual cortical bone is cut with a Kerrison punch. (A) A curette is used to elevate the lamina off the spinal cord on the opening side while using a Kocher attached to the spinous process to reposition the lamina towards the hinged side. This maneuver. (B) functions to expand the canal

one loses control of the lamina and the door unintentionally snaps shut. Once pulsatile flow in the dura is observed, which usually occurs at approximately 8–10 mm of opening, the canal has been expanded sufficiently. Surgicel or gelfoam is used for hemostasis, bone wax on a kittner can control bony bleeding, and bipolar electrocautery is helpful to address any epidural bleeders.

When he first described the laminoplasty procedure, Hirabayashi used sutures through the facet capsule and spinous process on the hinged side to stabilize the laminae in an open position. Since then, numerous methods have been developed to keep the door propped open and to prevent the laminar door from closing including facet cables, ceramic implants, various structural wedge allografts and autografts, bone anchors through the lateral mass, titanium miniplates with or without autograft or allograft, allograft stabilized with CG clips, facet cables, stainless steel wiring, and various suture techniques.[25, 49-56]

We prefer using suture anchors to maintain the expanded position because they are a simple, safe, and time-efficient technique to achieve that goal. Our suture anchor technique requires no grafting or fixation of the lamina to the lateral mass. In addition, the risk of injuring nerve roots or disrupting the facet joints are minimized with this method of laminar stabilization.

First, suture anchors are placed into the lateral masses on the hinged side (as shown in Figure 18.4A and B. The laminae are hinged open and a Keith needle can be used to bring the nonabsorbable suture from the suture anchor in the lateral mass through the drill hole that was created at the base of the spinous process at the beginning of the case right after the exposure was completed (Fig. 18.4C). Tie a slip knot to tension the suture appropriately and then square knots are tied under tension (Fig. 18.4D).

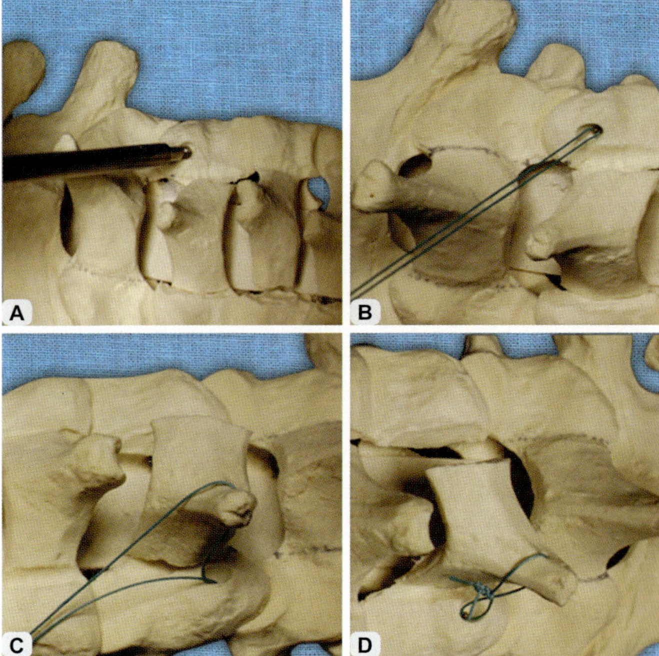

Fig. 18.4 Once the laminar door is hinged open, suture anchors can be used to stabilize the expanded position and to maintain the open hinge. Place suture anchors into the lateral masses on the hinged side, as shown in Figures A and B. Bring the suture through the hole at the base of the spinous process that was initially drilled right after the exposure was completed (C) Tie the suture securely to maintain the expanded laminar position (D).

Foraminotomy

Foraminotomy should be performed in conjunction with laminoplasty in patients with radicular symptoms. Foraminotomy is also indicated in patients with imaging studies that suggest neuroforaminal stenosis regardless of symptoms. Foraminotomy in these patients helps minimize the risk of postoperative neck pain due to intraoperative nerve root compression and stretch and also to prevent symptoms due to the development of nerve root compression following laminoplasty.

Foraminotomy is technically easier on the opening side of the laminoplasty so the side of the patient's radicular symptoms should be the side designated as the opening side. Foraminotomy is performed after all the bony cuts are made, the lamina is elevated, the ligamentum flavum is excised, and the laminoplasty is complete. This makes it easier to check the foraminal opening to confirm adequate decompression. Foraminotomy involves removing the roof of the foramen, or the superior articular facet of the inferior segment that covers the foramen. This generally involves the medial third of the facet.

With a high-speed burr, remove about half of the inferior articular facet, medial to lateral, that overlies the superior articular facet dorsally. This will bring the articular surface of the superior articular facet into view. We then use a cutting burr to thin the facet before using a 1 mm Kerrison punch to deroof the foramen and expose the exiting nerve root. Care must be taken to resect only the superior articular facet overlying the inferior pedicle but not lateral to it, as this may destabilize that level. A nerve hook can be used to probe the neuroforamen and verify a complete decompression. Gelfoam and thrombin can help achieve hemostasis at this stage of the procedure.

Arthrodesis

Patients with radiographic evidence of instability, significant axial neck pain, or bilateral radicular symptoms in addition to myelopathy are indicated for fusion in addition to laminoplasty. If a fusion procedure is anticipated, the exposure should be carried out laterally to the lateral aspect of the facets and the facet capsules should be excised. Once the laminoplasty is performed, lateral mass screws are placed at the levels included in the laminoplasty/fusion procedure. The start point is 1 mm medial to the center of the lateral mass and the trajectory is 15 degrees rostral and 30 degrees lateral.[57] The lateral masses are decorticated and the fusion bed is packed with iliac crest autograft or allograft.

Wound Closure

Irrigate the wound copiously and remove the retractors. Achieve meticulous hemostasis, debride the wound of

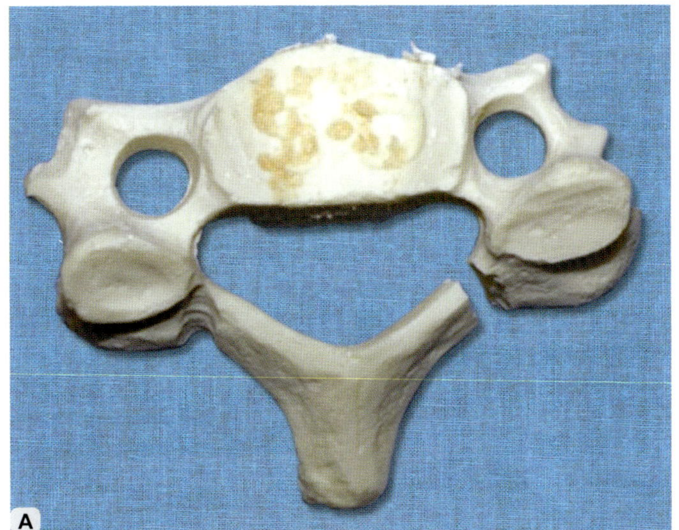

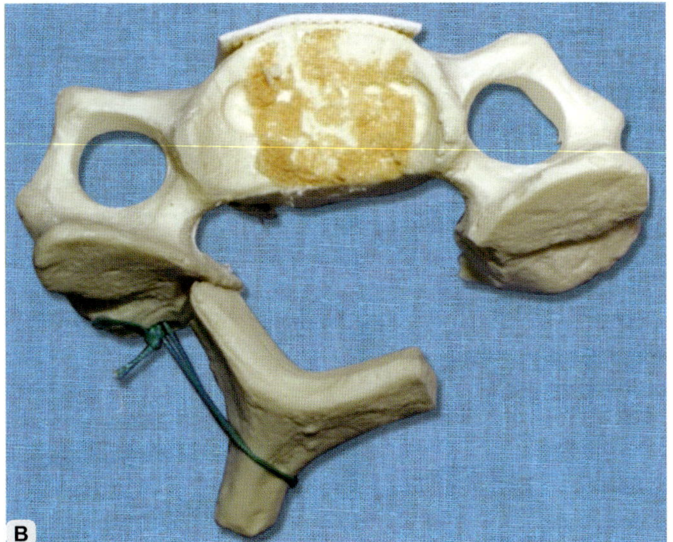

Fig. 18.5 Sawbones depiction of the increase in A-P diameter of the canal from the preoperative state (A) to the postoperative state (B) following laminoplasty with suture anchor fixation

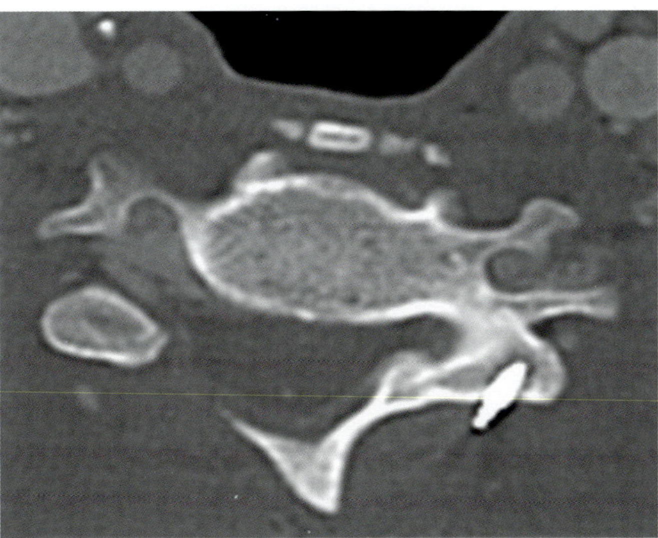

Fig. 18.6 Axial cut of a CT scan of a patient following expansive open door laminoplasty with suture anchor fixation.

any necrotic soft tissue, and place a deep drain. We close the fascia covering the paravertebral musculature with a No. 0 vicryl suture in a figure-of-eight fashion. This layer is then reinforced by a no. 0 PDS running stitch. A no. 2-0 vicryl suture is used to close the subcutaneous layer in an interrupted, buried fashion. We close the skin with a no. 3-0 monocryl suture using a running subcuticular technique.

Postoperative Management

During the first couple of days following surgery, maintain the head of the bed at greater than 45° to minimize venous bleeding. We immobilize our laminoplasty patients in rigid cervical collars for about 3–4 weeks. Patients start mobilizing with the assistance of physical therapists on postoperative day one, focusing on ambulation and bed transfers. AP and lateral plain films of the cervical spine are obtained prior to discharge from the hospital. Generally, patients are hospitalized for 24–48 hours after surgery. We see them for their first follow-up visit about 3–4 weeks later. We get repeat AP and lateral cervical spine films at this first follow-up visit. Also at this first postop appointment, we discontinue the use of the rigid cervical collar and have patients start working on isometric neck exercises. Patients are encouraged to resume their day-to-day activities as soon as possible.

Complications

Wound complications

It has been suggested that wound complications, such as infection and wound deshiscence, are more likely with laminoplasty compared to laminectomy since the former involves rotating the lamina into a more superficial position.[58] In our experience with laminoplasty, however, the rate of infection and dehiscence has been extremely low. The risk of soft tissue problems can be minimized by atraumatic soft tissue handling, thorough irrigation and hemostasis, debridement of necrotic soft tissue prior to closure, placement of a deep drain, achieving a watertight closure, and administering perioperative antibiotics.

Neurologic Complications

Neurologic injury is a potential risk of laminoplasty and it may occur as a result of various factors, including direct mechanical injury to nerve roots intraop, incomplete decompression, hematoma, restenosis or persistent stenosis due to insufficient elevation of the lamina, dislodgement or closure of the laminar opening, and fracture of the hinged lamina.[16, 21] Closure of the laminar opening may be due to hardware failure, such as fracture of a miniplate, or inadequate stabilization of the opening.

Isolated nerve root injury is a well-described complication of laminoplasty, occurring in five to 11% of cases.[6, 23, 59, 60] Patients with nerve root injuries usually present primarily with motor deficits and C5 is the most commonly affected nerve root. C5 nerve root palsies generally present 1–3 days postop with shoulder pain and deltoid weakness, but C5 palsies presenting as late as 20 days postop have been reported.[61] It is thought that post-laminoplasty C5 palsies are due to a traction injury to the C5 nerve root which is shorter and less forgiving to traction injuries compared to other nerve roots. In addition, C5 is at the apex of the cervical spine lordosis and it is, generally, at the center of the laminoplasty.[6, 48, 60-62]. For this reason, during laminoplasty, the C5 nerve root is preferentially stretched as the spinal cord migrates posteriorly at C5 more dramatically compared to other levels.

Management of postop nerve root palsies includes nonsteroidal anti-inflammatory medication and physical therapy. Recovery from nerve root palsies following laminoplasty spontaneously occurs within one year, in general, though it can take up to six years.[48]

Loss of Cervical Alignment

No laminoplasty technique can completely avoid the development of some loss of cervical lordosis in the postoperative period. The range of worsening cervical alignment following laminoplasty varies from 22-53% in the literature, even when it is performed in conjunction with arthrodesis.[5-8, 10-21, 63] In terms of the clinical significance of the loss of cervical alignment following laminoplasty, the literature is scant and controversial.[18, 21, 47, 63]

Postoperative Axial Pain

The literature is inconsistent when it comes to the true incidence of axial neck pain following laminoplasty. Some series have found no association between laminoplasty and neck pain, while others have shown that up to 60% of patients undergoing laminoplasty have some element of axial neck pain postoperatively.[20,64,65] Postoperative neck pain is hypothesized to be due to facet dissection and soft tissue retraction, necrosis, and scarring.[58, 65] Neck pain following laminoplasty usually presents itself in the early postop period and it usually resolves within a year. We encourage physical therapy and early neck range of motion in our laminoplasty patients to minimize the risk of postoperative neck stiffness and pain.

Diminished Cervical Motion

Although laminoplasty preserves some cervical range of motion since it allows for decompression without arthrodesis, cervical range of motion has been shown to decrease following laminoplasty. This loss of motion is in the range of 17–75% but, usually, a global loss of cervical motion of approximately 50% is seen.[7,11,16,18,19,23,44-48,51,53,66-68] The clinical significance of this loss of cervical motion is debatable. Some have suggested that post-laminoplasty stiffness is helpful for the resolution of OPLL, to minimize dynamic motion and protect the spinal cord, and to maximize the potential for neurologic recovery.[11,21,63] Others, however, propose that preserving as much range of motion as possible following laminoplasty helps minimize mechanical stress, the risk of adjacent segment disease, and postop neck pain.[17]

Conclusion

Numerous studies have demonstrated reliable neurologic recovery rates following laminoplasty of at least 50–70% and as high as 90%.[6, 7, 14, 16, 17, 27, 35, 47, 48, 59, 67, 69-72] These favorable outcomes that can be achieved with laminoplasty appear to be maintained in the long-term[13, 47] In addition, laminoplasty has been shown to potentially be safer and at least as effective as other surgical options, including laminectomy, anterior decompression and fusion, and subtotal corpectomy.[14,18, 73-75] With the right indications and meticulous surgical technique, relief of myelopathy can be expected with laminoplasty using suture anchor fixation in patients with multilevel cervical compression.

References

1. Oyama M, Hattori S, Moriwaki N. A New method of cervical laminoplasty. Cent Jpn J Orthop Trauma Surg. 1973;16:792-4.
2. Lonstein J, Winter R, Moe J, et al. Post laminectomy spine deformity. J Bone Joint Surg Proc. 1976;58-A(5):727.
3. Houten JK, Cooper PR. Laminectomy and posterior cervical plating for multilevel cervical spondylotic myelopathy and ossification of the posterior longitudinal ligament: effects on cervical alignment, spinal cord compression, and neurological outcome. Neurosurgery. 2003;52:1081-7.

4. Baba H, Uchida K, Maezawa Y, Furusawa N, Wada M, Imura S. Three-dimensional computed tomography for evaluation of cervical spinal canal enlargement after en bloc open-door laminoplasty. Spinal Cord. 1997;35:674-9.
5. Hukuda S, Ogata M, Mochizuki T, Shichikawa K. Laminectomy versus laminoplasty for cervical myelopathy: Brief Report. J Bone Joint Surg Br. 1988;70:325-6.
6. Hirabayashi K, Toyama Y, Chiba K. Expansive laminoplasty for myelopathy in ossification of the longitudinal ligament. Clin Orthop. 1999;359:35-48.
7. Edwards CC, Heller JG, Silcox DH. T-Saw laminoplasty for the management of cervical spondylotic myelopathy: Clinical and radiographic outcome. Spine. 2000;25:1788-94.
8. Herkowitz HN. A comparison of anterior cervical fusion, cervical laminectomy, cervical laminoplasty for the surgical management of multiple level spondylotic radiculopathy. Spine. 1988;13:774-80.
9. Kawai S, Sunago K, Doi K, Saka M, Taguchi T. Cervical laminoplasty (Hattori's method), procedure and follow-up results. Spine. 1988;13:1245-50.
10. Sasai K, Saito T, Akagi S, Kato I, Ogawa R. Cervical curvature after laminoplasty for spondylotic myelopathy—involvement of yellow ligament, semispinalis cervicis muscle, and nuchal ligament. J Spinal Disord. 2000;13:26-30.
11. Kimura I, Shingu H, Nasu Y. Long-term follow-up of cervical spondylotic myelopathy treated by canal-expansive laminoplasty. J Bone Joint Surg Br. 1995;77:956-61.
12. Lee T, Manazano GR, Green BA. Modified open-door cervical expansive laminoplasty for spondylotic myelopathy: operative technique, outcome, and predictors for gait improvement. J Neurosurg. 1997;86:64-8.
13. Kawaguchi Y, Kanamori M, Ishihara H, Ohmori K, Nakamura H, Kimura T. Minimum 10-year followup after en bloc cervical laminoplasty. Clin Orthop. 2003;411:129-39.
14. Yonenobu K, Hosono N, Iwasaki M, Asano M, Ono K. Laminoplasty versus subtotal corpectomy: a comparative study of results in multisegmental cervical spondylotic myelopathy. Spine. 1992;17:1281-4.
15. Matsunaga S, Sakouo T, Nakanishi K. Analysis of the cervical spine alignment following laminoplasty and laminectomy. Spinal Cord. 1999;37:20-4.
16. Mochida J, Nomura T, Chiba M, Nishimura K, Toh E. Modified expansive open-door laminoplasty in cervical myelopathy. J Spinal Disord. 1999;12:386-91.
17. Shaffrey CI, Wiggins GS, Piccirilli CB, Young JN, Lovell LR. Modified open-door laminoplasty for treatment of neurological deficits in younger patients with congenital spinal stenosis: analysis of clinical and radiographic data. J Neurosurg Spine. 1999;90:170-7.
18. Wada E, Suzuki S, Kanazawa A, Matsuoka T, Miyamoto S, Yonenobu K. Subtotal corpectomy versus laminoplasty for multi-level cervical spondylotic myelopathy: a long-term follow-up study over 10 years. Spine. 2001;26:1443-8.
19. Kawai S, Sunago K, Doi K, Saka M, Taguchi T. Cervical laminoplasty (Hattori's method), procedure and follow-up results. Spine. 1988;13:1245-50.
20. Sani S, Ratliff JK, Cooper PR. A critical review of cervical laminoplasty. Neurosurg Quart. 2004;14:5-16.
21. Morio Y, Yamamoto K, Teshima R, Nagashima H, Hagino H. Clinicoradiologic study of cervical laminoplasty with posterolateral fusion or bone graft. 2000;25:190-6.
22. Mukai Y, Hosono N, Sakaura H, Ishii T, Fuchiya T, Fijiwara K, Fuji T, Yoshikawa H. Laminoplasty for cervical myelopathy caused by subaxial lesions in rheumatoid arthritis. J Neurosurg. 2004;100:7-12.
23. Hirabayashi K, Watanabe K, Wakano K, Suzuki N, Satomi K, Ishii Y. Expansive open-door laminoplasty for cervical spinal stenotic myelopathy. Spine. 1983;8:693-9.
24. Epstein JA. The surgical management of cervical spinal stenosis, spondylosis, and myeloradiculopathy by means of the posterior approach. Spine. 1988;13:864-9.
25. O'Brien M, Peterson D, Casey ATH, Crockard HA. A novel technique for laminoplasty augmentation of spinal canal area using titanium miniplate stabilization: a computerized morphometric analysis. Spine. 1996;21:474-8.
26. Kaptain GJ, Simmons NE, Replogle RE, Pobereskin L. Incidence and outcome of kyphotic deformity following laminectomy for cervical spondylotic myelopathy. J Neurosurg. 2000;93:199-204.
27. Herkowitz HN. Cervical laminoplasty: Its role in the treatment of cervical radiculopathy. J Spinal Disord. 1988;1(3):179-88.
28. Yasuoka S, Peterson HA, McCarty CS. Incidence of spinal column deformity after multilevel laminectomy in children and adults. J Neurosurg. 1982;57:441-5.
29. Crandell M, Gregorious FK. Long term follow-up of surgical treatment of cervical spondylotic myelopathy. Spine. 1977;2:139-46.
30. Mikawa Y, Shikata J, Yamamuro T. Spinal deformity and instability after multilevel cervical laminectomy. Spine. 1987;12:6-11.
31. Baba H, Imura S, Kawahara N, et al. Osteoplastic laminoplasty for cervical myeloradiculopathy secondary to ossification of the posterior longitudinal ligament. Int Orthop. 1995;19(1):40-5.
32. Jenkins DH. Extensive cervical laminectomy: Long-term results. Br J Surg. 1973;60:852-4.
33. Kato Y, Iwasaki M, Fuji T, et al. Long-term follow-up results of laminectomy for cervical myelopathy caused by ossification of the posterior longitudinal ligament. J Neurosurg. 1998;89:217-23.
34. Rogers L. The surgical treatment of cervical spondylotic myelopathy: Mobilization of the complete cervical cord into an enlarged canal. J Bone Joint Surg Br. 1961;43:3-6.
35. Hirabayashi K, Satomi K. Operative procedure and results of expansive open-door laminoplasty. Spine. 1988;13:870-6.
36. Inoue A, Ikata T, Katoh S. Spinal deformity following surgery for spinal cord tumors and tumorous lesions: Analysis based on an assessment of the spinal functional curve. Spinal Cord. 1996;34:536-42.
37. Narayan P, Haid RW. Neurologic treatment: treatment of degenerative cervical disk disease. Neurol Clin. 2001;19:217-29.

38. Albert TJ, Vacarro A. Postlaminectomy kyphosis. Spine. 1998;23:2738-45.
39. Ishida Y, Suzuki K, Ohmori K, Kikata Y, Hattori Y. Critical analysis of extensive cervical laminectomy. Neurosurgery. 1989;24:215-22.
40. Guigui P, Benoist M, Deburge A. Spinal Deformity and Instability After Multilevel Cervical Laminectomy for Spondylotic Myelopathy. Spine. 1998;23:440-7.
41. Steinmetz MP, Resnick DK. Cervical laminoplasty. Spine J. 2006;6:274S-81S.
42. Hirabayashi K, Bohlman HH. Multilevel cervical spondylosis: Laminoplasty versus anterior decompression. Spine. 1995;20:1732-4.
43. Inoue A, Ikata T, Katoh S. Spinal deformity following surgery for spinal cord tumors and tumorous lesions: Analysis based on an assessment of the spinal functional curve. Spinal Cord. 1996;34:536-42.
44. Kawaguchi Y, Matsui H, Ishihara H, Gejo R, Yoshino O. Axial symptoms after en bloc cervical laminoplasty. J Spinal Disord. 1999;12:392-5.
45. Hirabayashi K, Miyagawa J, Satomi K, Maruyama T, Wakano K. Operative results and postoperative progression of ossification among patients with ossification of cervical posterior longitudinal ligament. Spine. 1981;6:354-64.
46. Kohno K, Kumon Y, Oka Y, Matsui S, Ohue S, Sakaki S. Evaluation of prognostic factors following expansive laminoplasty for cervical spinal stenotic myelopathy. Surg Neurol. 1997;48:237-45.
47. Seichi A, Takeshita K, Ohishi I, Kawaguchi H, Akune T, Anamizu Y, Kitagawa T, Nakamura AK. Long-term results of double-door laminoplasty for cervical stenotic myelopathy. Spine. 2001;26:479-87.
48. Satomi K, Nishu Y, Kohno T, Hirabayashi K. Long-term follow-up studies of open-door expansive laminoplasty for cervical stenotic myelopathy. Spine. 1994;19:507-10.
49. Mochida J, Nomura T, Chiba M, Nishimura K, Toh E. Modified expansive open-door laminoplasty in cervical myelopathy. J Spinal Disord. 1999;12:386-91.
50. Shaffrey CI, Wiggins GS, Piccirilli CB, Young JN, Lovell LR. Modified open-door laminoplasty for treatment of neurological deficits in younger patients with congenital spinal stenosis: analysis of clinical and radiographic data. J Neurosurg Spine. 1999;90:170-7.
51. Morimoto T, Matsuyama T, Hirabayashi H, Sakaki T, Yabuno T. Expansive laminoplasty for multilevel cervical OPLL. J Spinal Disord. 1997;10:286-98.
52. Billett GR, Erasmus AM, Lind CR. CG-clip expansive open door laminoplasty: A technical note. Br J Neurosurg. 1999;13:405-8.
53. Itoh T, Tsuji H. Technical improvements and results of laminoplasty for compressive myelopathy in the cervical spine. Spine. 1985;10:729-36.
54. Nakano N, Nakano T, Nakano K. Comparison of the results of laminectomy and open-door laminoplasty for cervical spondylotic myeloradiculopathy and ossification of the posterior longitudinal ligament. Spine. 1988;13:792-4.
55. Baba H, Furusawa N, Chen Q, Imura S. Cervical laminoplasty patients with ossification of the posterior longitudinal ligaments. Paraplegia. 1995;33:25-9.
56. Kihara: Kihara S, Umebayashi T, Hoshimaru M. Technical improvement and results of open-door expansive laminoplasty with hydroxyapatite implants for cervical myelopathy. Neurosurgery. 2005;57:348-56.
57. An HS, Gordin R, Renner K. Anatomic considerations for plate-screw fixation of the cervical spine. Spine. 1991;16:S548-51.
58. Yonenobu K, Wada E, Ono K. Laminoplasty. In: Clark CR, editor. The cervical spine. Philadelphia: Lippincott Williams and Wilkins. 2005;1057-71.
59. Satomi K, Ogawa J, Ishii Y, Hirabayashi K. Short-term complications and long-term results of expansive open-door laminoplasty for cervical stenotic myelopathy. Spine. 2001;1:26-30.
60. Yonenobu K, Hosono N, Iwasaki M, Asano M, Ono K. Neurologic complications of surgery for cervical compression myelopathy. Spine. 1991;16:1277-82.
61. Uematsu Y, Tokuhashi Y, Matsuzaki H. Radiculopathy after laminoplasty of the cervical spine. Spine. 1998;23:2057-62.
62. Tsuzuki N, Abe R, Saiki K, Zhongshi L. Extradural tethering effect as one mechanism of radiculopathy complicating posterior decompression of the cervical spinal cord. Spine. 1996;21:203-11.
63. Miyazaki K, Tada K, Matsuda Y, Okuno M, Yasuda T, Murakami H. Posterior extensive simultaneous multisegment decompression with posterolateral fusion for cervical myelopathy with cervical instability and kyphotic and/or S-shaped deformities. Spine. 1989;14:1160-70.
64. Yoshida M, Tamaki T, Kawakami M, Nakatani N, Ando M, Yamada H, Hayashi N. Does reconstruction of posterior ligamentous complex with extensor musculature decrease axial symptoms after cervical laminoplasty? Spine. 2002;27:1414-8.
65. Hosono N, Yonenobu K, Ono K. Neck and shoulder pain after laminoplasty: A noticeable complication. Spine. 1996;21:1969-73.
66. Saruhashi Y, Hukuda S, Katsuura A, Miyahara K, Asajima S, Omura K. A long-term follow-up study of cervical spondylotic myelopathy treated by "French Window" laminoplasty. J spinal Disord. 1999;12:99-101.
67. Yoshida M, Otani K, Shibasaki K, Ueda S. Expansive laminoplasty with reattachment of spinous process and extensor musculature for cervical myelopathy. Spine. 1992;17:491-7.
68. Takayasu M, Takagi T, Nishizawa T, Otsuka K, Nakajima T, Yoshia J. Bilateral open-door cervical expansive laminoplasty with hydroxyapatite spacers and titanium screws. J Neurosurg (Spine 1). 2001;96:22-8.
69. Kokubun S, Sato T, Ishii Y, Tanaka Y. Cervical myelopathy in the Japanese. Clin Ortho Relat Res. 1996;323:129-38.
70. Kawakami M, Tamaki T, Iwasaki H, Yoshida M, Ando M, Yamada H. A comparative study of surgical approaches for cervical compressive myelopathy. Clin Orthop. 2000;381:129-36.
71. Hukuda S, Mochizuki T, Ogata M, Shichikawa K, Shimomura Y. Operations for cervical spondylotic myelopathy: A comparison of the results of anterior and posterior procedures. J Bone Joint Surg Br. 1985;67:609-15.

72. Yue WM, Tan CT, Tan SB, Tan SK, Tay BK. Results of cervical laminoplasty and a comparison between single and double trap-door techniques. J spinal Disord. 2000;13:329-35.
73. Kaminsky SB, Clark CR, Traynelis VC. Operative treatment of cervical spondylotic myelopathy and radiculopathy: A comparison of laminectomy and laminoplasty at five year average follow-up. Iowa Orthop J. 2004;24:95-105.
74. Heller JG, Edwards CC 2nd, Murakami H, Rodts GE. Laminoplasty versus laminectomy and fusion for multilevel cervical myelopathy: an independent matched cohort analysis. Spine. 2001;26:1330-6.
75. Edwards CC 2nd, Heller JG, Murakami H. Corpectomy versus laminoplasty for multilevel cervical myelopathy: an independent matched-cohort analysis. Spine. 2002;27:1168-75.

CHAPTER

19

Motion Preservation Surgery in the Cervical Spine

Kim-Soon OH

Introduction

The human spine is a wondrous structure, a mobile column of individual vertebral bones linked together via multiple dynamic articulations. This moving construct flexes and extends, with a slight hint of twisting motion occasionally, all the while enclosing within its central canal its most precious content --- the spinal neural elements.

As a requisite for guarding the integrity of the neural elements and for providing a skeletal axis of the human body, the spinal column needs stability. As a requirement for the physical function of the human body, the spine needs mobility. These two properties, stability and mobility, appear at first hand an oxymoron but it is evident in modern spine treatment that for optimal function of the spine, these two states must be provided for.

In diseases of the cervical spine intervertebral disks, the time-honored method was to excise the offending disc via an anterior technique and replace it with a fusion block which may be either autograft bone, allograft bone or a synthetic mesh or cage. In some cases where an anterior approach is not feasible, a posterior decompressive procedure may be performed to relieve pressure off the compressed nerve root.[1]

Much has been written on the issue of adjacent segment disease after cervical spine fusion.[2-4] With such a body of evidence, the advent of artificial total disk replacement (TDR) offers a possibility that these complications may be reduced through motion preservation of the affected segment.

Relevant Anatomy

The articulations of the cervical spine are multiple (Fig. 19.1):

1. In the anterior part, firm but mildly yielding disks in between vertebrae that are interlaced with bony trabeculae to support loading, shearing and twisting forces.

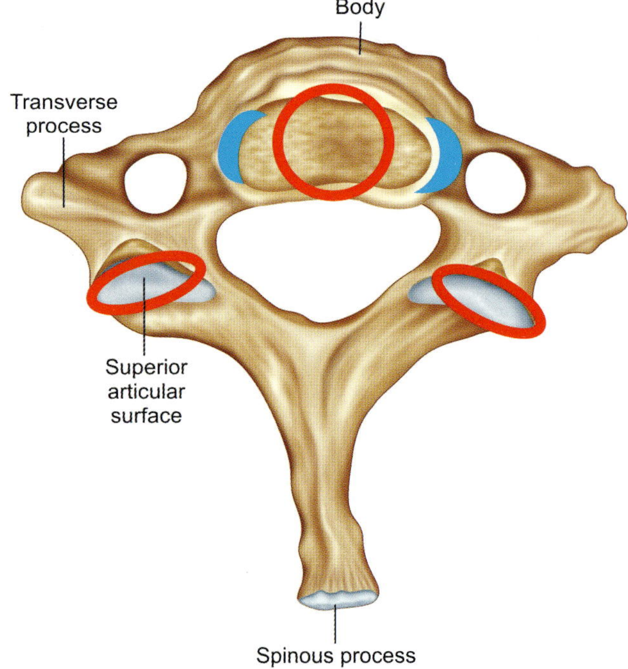

Fig. 19.1 Concept of the tripod joint (shown in red), with additional articulation at the uncovertebral joints (shown in blue)

2. In the middle region, facet joints provide bilateral support, thus along with the anterior disk, completing the basic "tripod joint" concept which was first advocated for the lumbar segments.[5]
3. In the lateral zones, uncovertebral joints.
4. In the posterior part, interspinous and supraspinous ligaments.

The cervical spine's total range of motion is approximately 80°–90° of flexion, 70° of extension, 20°–45° of lateral flexion, and up to 90° of rotation to both sides. These movements are not pure planar motions, though, but are complex movements with mixed multiplanar elements.[6] During flexion and extension, the two principal actions of the spinal column, the intervertebral disk maintains its integrity through the resilience of the annulus fibrosus which ring the rim of the disk in lamellar style. Fibrocartilage makes up most of the annulus, which is innervated and pain-sensitive. The nucleus is composed mainly of loose fibres within a mucoprotein gel (Fig. 19.2).

The facet joints are synovial joints, possessing articular cartilage on opposing surfaces, joint capsule, nerve supply and synovial fluid. Nerve supply comes from a branch from the nerve root that exits the neural foramen of that facet joint level and another from the level above (Fig. 19.3).[7]

Relevant Biomechanics

While it would not be possible to faithfully reproduce all natural motions of the spinal motion segment via an artificial device, such implants are capable of ensuring that the following biomechanical properties are maintained:

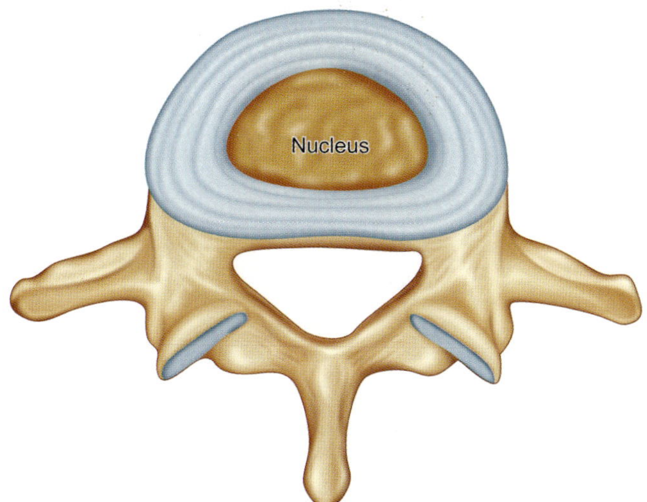

Fig. 19.2 Central nucleus pulposus and peripheral annulus fibrosus

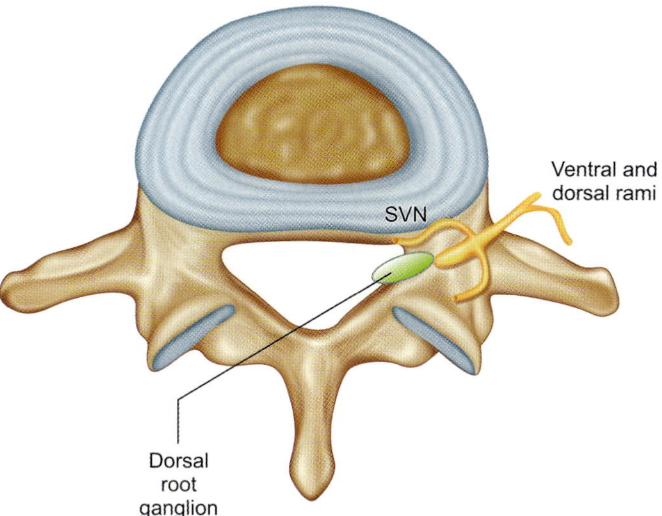

Fig. 19.3 Sinuvertebral nerve (SVN) and the territory supplied, which includes the disk annulus, posterior longitudinal ligament, duramater and the facet joint capsule. It is obvious from both anatomic and clinical observations that the annulus receives nociceptive fibers extensively

1. Intersegment stability, such that movements beyond those imposed by physiological limits do not occur and such that while physiological movements are occurring, no physical instability ensues which may cause neurological injury
2. Flexion-extension, lateral bending, rotation and translational movements are freely exhibited by the cervical spine. Normally, it is a combination of such movements that make up most of our daily physical neck activity --- a term known as *coupling*, where there is consistent association of one motion (like rotation or translation) about or along one axis or plane, with another motion about or along another axis or plane. The vertebra has 6 degrees of freedom; 3 translations and 3 rotations respectively along and about the axes of a coordinate system (Fig. 19.4).[8, 9]
3. Facet orientation in the cervical spine is generally 45 degrees up from horizontal in the typical cervical vertebra, with 5–17 degrees of flexion-extension and 5 –17 degrees of lateral flexion and 8–10 degrees of rotation.
4. The functional spinal unit (FSU) is the term devised by White and Panjabi to describe the smallest physiological motion unit of the spine.[8] Such a unit should possess biomechanical properties akin to that of the entire spine. Such a unit is made up of two adjacent vertebrae, their endplates, adjoining ligaments and the intervertebral disk (Fig. 19.5). In this chapter, I have described the FSU as the motion segment.

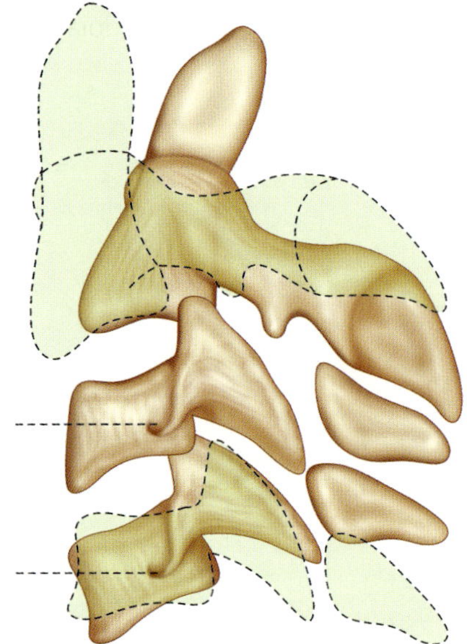

Fig. 19.4 Composite movement studies are used to calculate the individual axes of rotation

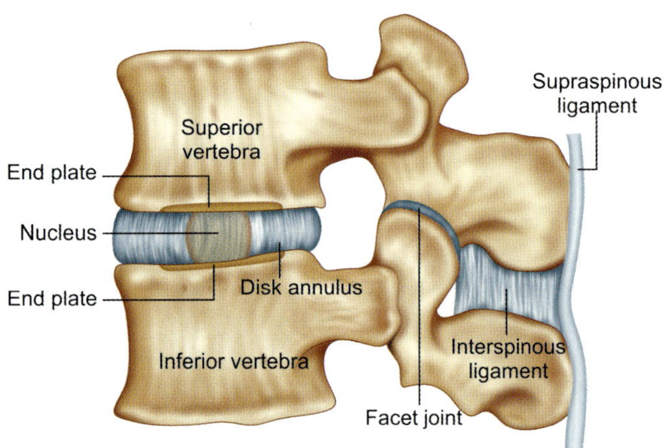

Fig. 19.5 Functional spinal unit

Ideals of Motion Preservation

Motion preservation surgery of the spine certainly was inspired by the success of implants in the large joints, namely the hip and the knee. Early attempts in disc replacement surgery were crude by modern comparison, both in terms of technique used and of materials available at that time and age.

In 1959, Paul Harmon used vitallium balls as a stabilizing augmentation to fusion, and serendipitously discovered that these work well even without the fusion element.[10] Such attempts were repeated by Al MacKenzie in 1971, using steel balls and reporting good results after 25 years.[11]

The ideal total disk prosthesis therefore should have the following properties

- Sound physical construct to provide physiological FSU mobility while maintaining physiological stability and anatomical intervertebral distance
- Inert and indestructible *in vivo*
- Minimal wear and tear properties such that attritional debris is avoided
- Simple, practical insertional technique
- Made of material that creates minimal artefact distortion during postoperative imaging.

We are certainly not capable yet of fully realising such a device, but current technology has provided implants that are usable and practical, while ongoing research promises to deliver enhancements in each of the properties listed above.

The Food and Drug Administration of the United States approved the Prestige® Cervical Disc System on Dec. 16, 2007 and the ProDisc C® artificial disk on Dec. 17, 2007 for use in skeletally mature patients for single-level disk disease in the region C3 till C7. On May 12, 2009, it approved the Bryan® cervical disk, the last such device granted this far. Sensing potentially high economical returns, a flock of new devices from competing companies has come into play, as illustrated in Figure 19.6.

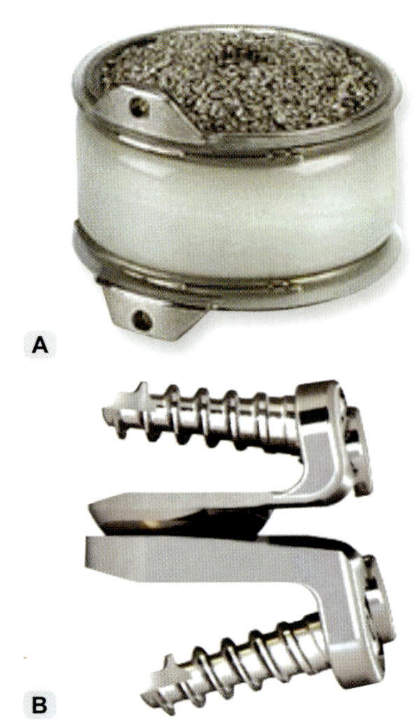

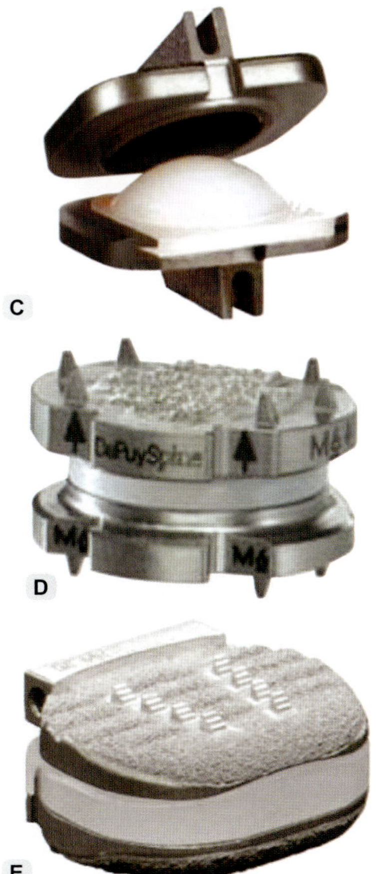

Fig. 19.6 (Composite) Various popular makes of cervical spine artificial disks. (A) Prestige ST disk (Medtronic Sofamor Danek). (B) Bryan disk (Medtronic Sofamor Danek). (C) Prodisc C disk (Synthes). (D) Discover disk (Johnson & Johnson DePuy). (E) Porous-coated motion (PCM) disk (Nuvasive Cervitech)

There is presently no uniform way to classify artificial disc devices. Various attempts to delineate them have been used based on:

1. The spinal region treated and the part of the disk replaced.
2. The material from which the device was made.
3. The type of mechanical construction, including the anatomical description.
4. The biomechanical nature of mobility.

Regionally, there are lumbar and cervical disk prostheses. Lumbar disks were in the forefront of development and usage, including FDA approval earlier in 2004 before cervical devices found wide use. They are characterized by a surgical approach that is more complex than that of cervical implants. There have been forays into zone replacement wherein devices are created to replace that zone of the disc deemed damaged, e.g. nuclear replacement devices or annular support devices. These have not been found to have reproducible reliability and total disk implants are still the common form used.

Metal, ceramic, polyethylene and polyurethane have been some of the material used in constructing such devices. Certain devices have metal-on-metal articulations while others, metal-on-polymer. Lately, fabric has been investigated as a potential material.

Many of the devices are saddle-jointed devices, replacing the ball articulations of before.

Devices may be unconstrained, semiconstrained or fully constrained in their biomechanical mobility. Constrained devices restrict motion to less than that seen physiologically. Devices are considered semiconstrained in certain planes if they allow motion similar to that seen physiologically. Devices are considered nonconstrained if there is no mechanical block to the motion and are dependent on the surrounding perispinal soft tissue, and the inherent soft-tissue hydraulics plus compression across the disk space to provide restraint to extremes of motion.

Adverse Results from Cervical Spine Artificial Disk Replacement

Five years after FDA approval of the artificial cervical intervertebral disk, we have got a better understanding of the device and how it has worked out based on current techniques. While there have been evidence supporting a diminished incidence of adjacent segment disease in the use of such devices and thus fulfilling its primary objective, a slew of reports have emerged describing adverse results and complications.

The complications with an artificial device are at least potentially similar to those of a formal anterior cervical discectomy and fusion. These, although rare, may include the following:

General risks:

- Nerve injury
- Hemorrhage
- Infection
- Risks related to anesthesia.

Risks related to the surgery:

- Injury to surrounding structures—the esophagus, the pharynx
- Injury to nearby nerves—the recurrent laryngeal
- Dural breach
- Nerve root injury
- Spinal cord injury.

Risks related to the device[12-14]

- Facet strain, annular abrasion or ligament stretch—all causing neck pain
- Improper device placement—causing loss of physiological alignment or risk to neural structures
- Implant migration, subsidence or dislodgement—again causing the above complications
- Heterotopic ossification or even spontaneous fusion
- Wear and tear debris.

The hazards of such adverse events are usually not severe ones like mortality or spinal cord injury leading to permanent paralysis but are often troubling symptoms like persistent neck ache, sensory disturbances and reduced range of motion. To the surgeon, adverse events are part and parcel of our surgical practice and are certainly expected of when seen against the context of a relatively new surgical technique—in this case, disk replacement, where the global spine community itself is ascending on a learning curve.

To the patient, however, morbidity after disk replacement surgery leads to frank disappointment and rapidly escalates into negative feelings toward the procedure and toward the surgeon. This is especially so after all the media hype surrounding the introduction of these devices into the market. Some of this hype is industry-driven, but often is propagated further by doctors wishing to offer services that are premium compared to peers doing only "classical spine surgery".

Minimizing Complications and Adverse Results

Artificial disk devices differ in their technical properties. All makes of artificial disks have their own idiosyncrasies, based upon the concept they were made on and upon their creators' design basis. Thus we have the requirement for bone milling in the Bryan disk, the need to make cuts into the corpus of the vertebra to accommodate the keels of the ProDisc C and the requirement for cutting a 7-degree endplate yaw in the case of the Discover disc, to name a few.

Regardless of the make, there are factors common to all devices that must be taken into account to ensure a good outcome. This is the focus of this chapter and shall be discussed piecemeal.

Selecting the Right Patient

The indications for cervical disk replacement are for skeletally mature adults with single level disk degenerative disk disease at any level from C3 till C7. These patients must have been treated without success using conservative measures for at least 6 months. Contraindications recommended by most centers would include post-traumatic spine conditions, osteoporotic patients, the presence of infection or malignancy, any ossifying or ankylosing axial disease, segmental instability of the spine and advanced degenerative disease of the cervical spine.

Patients with Significant Degenerative Spine Disease

A large number of patients in the midlife already have significant facet joint degeneration.[15] Many of them are in the age group of only 35–40 years old, far earlier than the population in which we would come to expect "advanced degenerative spine disease". Their radiographs show mild vertebral endplate lipping, osteophyte-ridden Luschka joints, and facet sclerosis. Choosing this cohort for artificial replacement runs the risk of creating further facet stress and strain, possibly causing chronic pain (Fig. 19.7).

While age is a guiding point, it would be important to peruse the plain lateral and anteroposterior radiographs carefully to ascertain the patient's degree of degeneration. MRI scans show facet degeneration very well and may be correlated with clinical findings of neckache worse on extension.

Disk Replacement in Myelopathy

The use of artificial disk replacement in patients with myelopathy has always been tempered by the fear that motion preservation would maintain unnecessary micro-motion and cause further injury to the already-injured spinal cord. Furthermore, the additional steps taken during preparation for TDR involve prolonged distracting

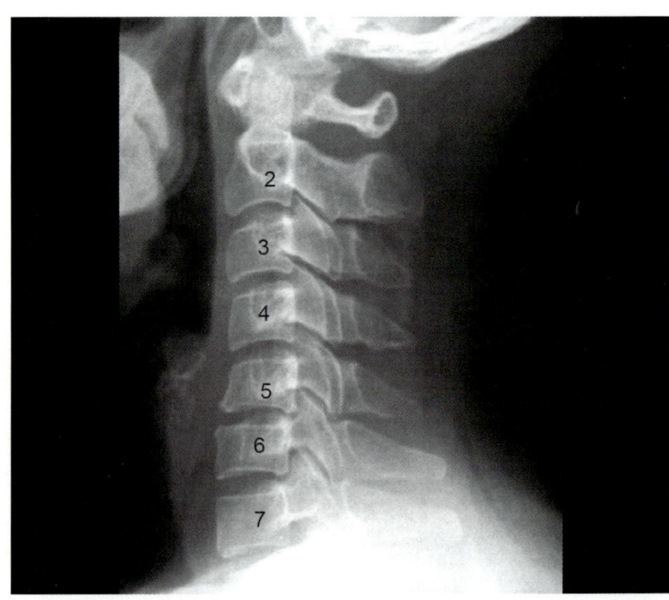

Fig. 19.7 Lateral radiograph of C1–C7 of a 35-year old woman showing lipping, facet degeneration, and abnormal sagittal balance

and multiple sizing trials of the interspace—manoeuvres which may also injure the cord. Lastly, many patients with cervical myelopathy have multiple-level disk disease, thus presenting a different challenge to the single-level norm that characterizes the FDA endorsement for TDR.

Some surgeons have used artificial disk devices in mild grades of myelopathy and have reported of good results equal to that of fusion, with the added advantage of reducing adjacent segment disease. One of the better designed studies was performed by Riew who obtained good preservation of motion in his patients while not worsening their neurological status.[16, 17]

In my practice, prior consultation with the patient is obtained before considering TDR for mild grades of myelopathy (Nurick grade 0, I and II) while higher grades of myelopathy are treated with fusion.

Multiple Levels of Involvement

The FDA approval for TDR involves single-level cervical spine disk disease. Frequently, we face patients with multiple levels of involvement (Fig. 19.8).

Replacing the disk with a motion device preserves an axis of rotation which does not replicate the original axis faithfully. In addition, interspace height and posterior column tension are all altered. While axial kinematic compensation may be realized in a single-level replacement, multiple level surgery would be less forgiving. The benefit of preventing adjacent level disease also decreases in multiple level surgery, as illustrated by Hilibrand et al. in his 1999 study which logically pointed out that multiple-level disease would already have involved the most mobile, and therefore most vulnerable, segments of C5–C7.[18, 19] Lastly, the caudal section of the C6–C7 interspace may not be well visualized intraoperatively on a lateral image intensifier projection, thus making fusion a more likely choice in that segment.

Intraoperative Considerations

Iatrogenic Needle Injury to Adjacent Disk during X-ray Localization

Spine surgeons take AP and lateral radiographs in the initial stage of surgical exposure to ascertain the level of vertebra. This is commonly done using a 24 G needle bent to fit into the interspace held at the crook of the bend by the rim of the vertebral body. There has been some evidence that this innocent puncture, when inadvertently done to the adjacent disk not for surgery, penetrates the annulus and frequently reaches the nucleus pulposus and may possibly hasten disk degeneration.[20]

Knowing our surface anatomy landmarks and using slender identifying pins on the vertebral corpus during radiography would be useful to avoid such an outcome.

Meticulous Endplate Preparation

The removal of endplate cartilage would be desirable in TDR surgery, as all devices have end plates which bear surfaces sintered with absorptive materials like hydroxy-apatite coating that allow bone-implant incorporation. Removal is done using curettes that scrape away cartilage, exposing subchondral bone (Fig. 19.9).

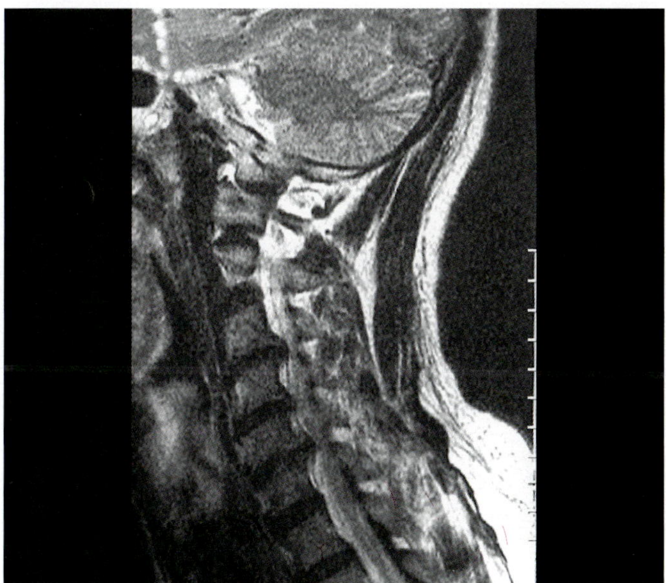

Fig. 19.8 Multiple-level disk involvement on MRI could also be in actual fact the discrete type of ossified posterior longitudinal ligament

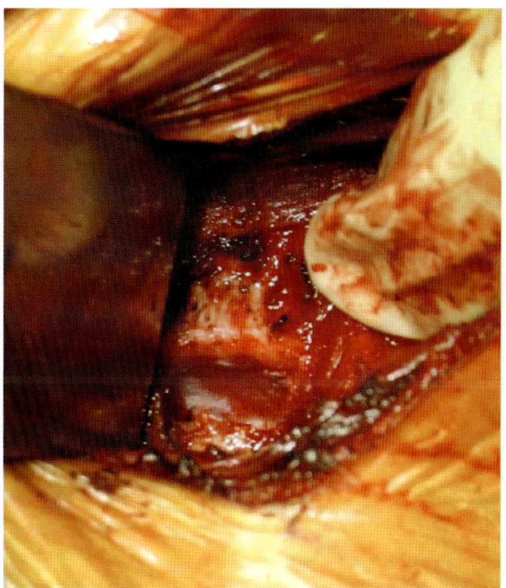

Fig. 19.9 Photograph showing the inferior end plate of the cephalad vertebra, well denuded of cartilage and showing healthy subchondral bone

Overzealous removal injures subchondral bone, yielding fragile cancellous bone that does not provide firm support to the device. End plates in the cervical spine are frequently concave in shape; thus, visual parallax errors are common when performing the curetting action. Another place of contention is at the anterior and posterior rim of the endplate where excessive clearance using Kerrison rongeurs can create defects along the rim.

Damage to the end plate increases the likelihood of implant subsidence, which occurs upon vertical loading when the patient is upright and mobilizing in the postoperative period. The rim of the vertebral body is cortical, but as we advance centrally, soft cancellous bone lie beneath the thin subchondral cortex (Fig. 19.10).

Adequate Clearance of the Uncinate Processes

In performing TDR, it is desirable to achieve the widest possible implant footprint on the vertebral end plate. Frequently, the uncovertebral joints on both lateral sides of the vertebral body are hypertrophied, making partial resection of the uncinate processes necessary (Fig. 19.11).

Inadequate resection crowds the coronal diameter and causes downsizing of implant choice, which may lead to instability or subsidence due to lack of cortical rim purchase. Inadequate resection also results in upward sloping lateral edges, curving the endplate and rocking the implant (Fig. 19.12). The extent of resection may be checked with passing a slim Penfield probe to the lateral wall of the process, and seeing the remaining thickness. Not more than 1/3 of the coronal thickness of the process may be resected without causing instability.

Adequate Clearance of Osteophytes along the Posterior Rim

It is always essential to clear the posterior rim of projecting osteophytes before knocking the implant in. Residual osteophytes may be fractured by the advancing implant and displace into the spinal canal, causing cord injury. Safe clearance can always be checked in direct vision and also on lateral radiography.

Avoid Heterotopic Ossification

Exposure of large areas of raw bone releases osteoprogenitor material into the interspace. In TDR surgery, endplate preparation involves extensive working on bone while many devices require further bone cuts to accommodate keels and fins. Because of the high incidence of osteophytic lipping and concave end plates, the anterior rim is frequently

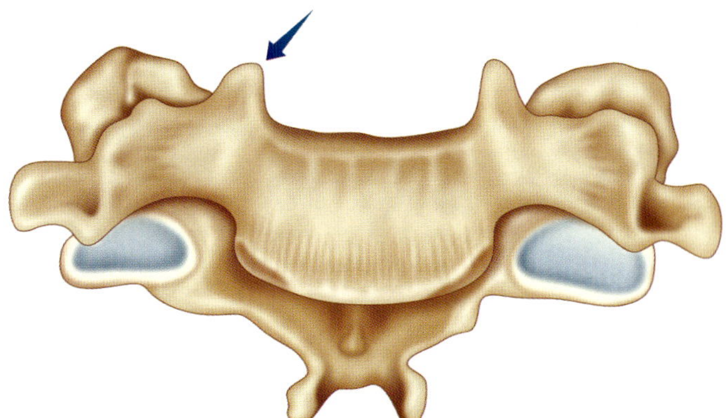

Fig. 19.11 Uncinate processes are best viewed anterior-posteriorly or obliquely

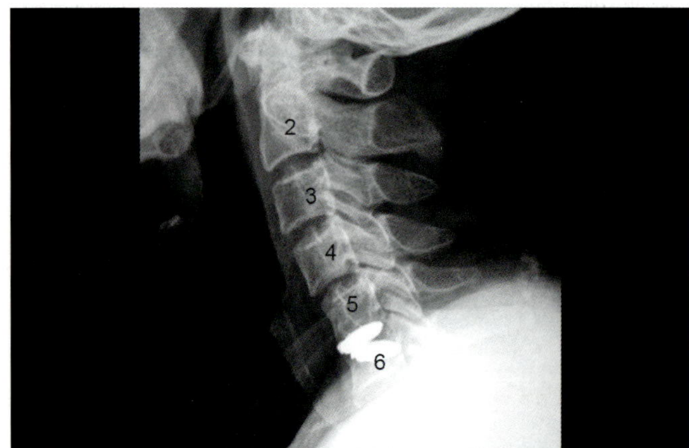

Fig. 19.10 Lateral radiograph depicting postoperative implant subsidence due to insufficiency of the superior end plate of the caudal vertebra

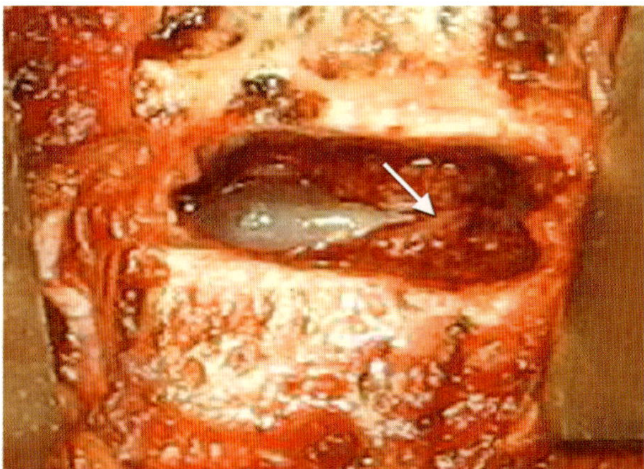

Fig. 19.12 Lateral flare leading to the left uncinate process. If not levelled, it creates a concave end plate and rocks the implanted device

nibbled and shaped by rongeurs. Such bone shaping work increases the chances of heterotopic ossification. Preventive steps are to

- Minimize raw bone surface area, including the end plates and rims of body
- Where this is not possible, cover the areas with a bone wax overlay

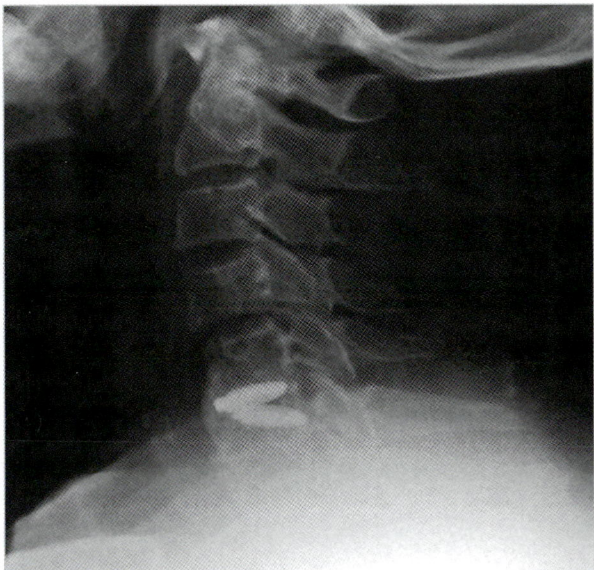

Fig. 19.13 Spontaneous fusion occurring serendipitously a year later in the afore-illustrated patient with subsidence of the implant through an incompetent -- and therefore raw -- end plate

- Irrigate the surgery site copiously with normal saline before the final implantation and again before closing. Remember to avoid direct hydraulic pressure on the cord
- Excise the posterior longitudinal ligament, which may be a conduit for ossification and which may itself liberate osteopotent signals.

Postoperative spontaneous fusion is an established complication that is being discovered at alarmingly increasing frequency (Figs 19.13 and 19.14).[21-24]

Resecting or Keeping the Posterior Longitudinal Ligament

Paul McAfee brought attention to the role of the posterior longitudinal ligament (PLL) during TDR surgery. He felt that the PLL acted much like the cruciate ligaments of the knee in stabilizing the spinal interspace and acting as a restraint.[25] His point was supported by data from other studies showing postoperative changes in sagittal spinal balance.[26, 27]

Resection of the PLL

- Accounts for "completion" of the decompressive procedure
- Allows us to manipulate disk space, achieve parallel distraction and restore height
- Removes any later potential for ossification that may develop along the retained ligament.

However, removing the PLL may also cause instability and possible postoperative kyphosis of that segment especially when an unconstrained device is used (Fig. 19.15).

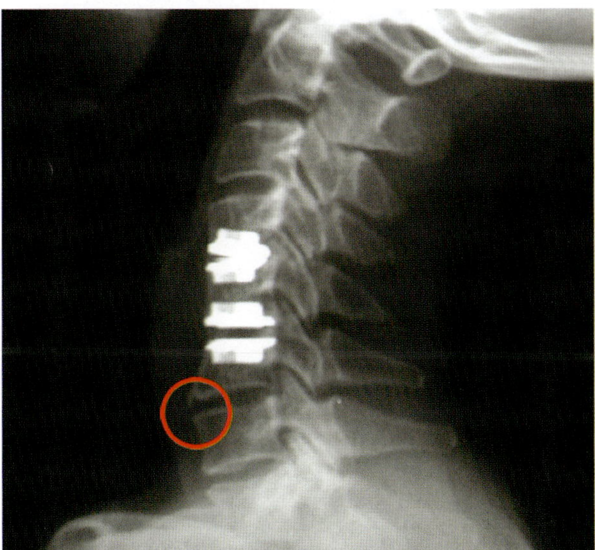

Fig. 19.14 Heterotopic ossification and adjacent segment disease caudal to a 2-level TDR after 2 years of surgery

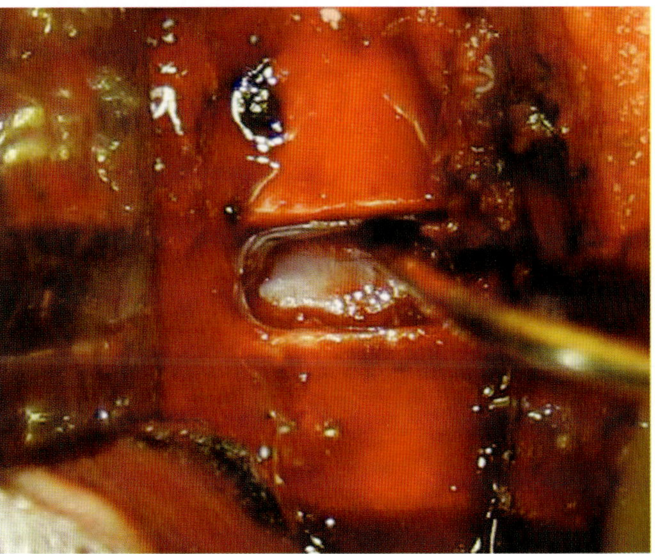

Fig. 19.15 Intraoperative photograph showing the PLL excised

This point becomes even more relevant when multiple-level TDR is considered.

McAfee reasoned that the type of implant used should be chosen based upon whether one retains the PLL or not. In my practice of using semiconstrained implants, I routinely excise the PLL.

Avoid Abnormal Facet Loading

In the functional spine unit, the tripod joint concept is understood better when one considers that increasing or decreasing the intervertebral height loads the posteriorly-sited facets abnormally. These richly innervated joints then become potent pain generators either via undue compression or through unphysiological stretching.

- Unconstrained devices increase eccentric loading on the facets
- Semiconstrained devices allow sharing of translational stresses to the facets
- Constrained devices shield the facets at the expense of increasing stress at the boneimplant interface

To prevent abnormal loading, the device must possess an axis of rotation similar to that of the normal FSU.[28] This is, of course, not achievable but the surgeon is able to diminish eccentric loading by:

- Preparing and positioning the implant as per its technical idiosyncrasy
- Choosing an appropriate interspace height.

The interspace height may be gleaned by studying the preoperative static upright AP and lateral films followed by a series of dynamic spine radiographs in flexion and in extension. During surgery, while distracting the space, care is taken to compare the relationship of the space under surgery with the adjoining levels in terms of interspinous distance and endplate orientation (Fig. 19.16).

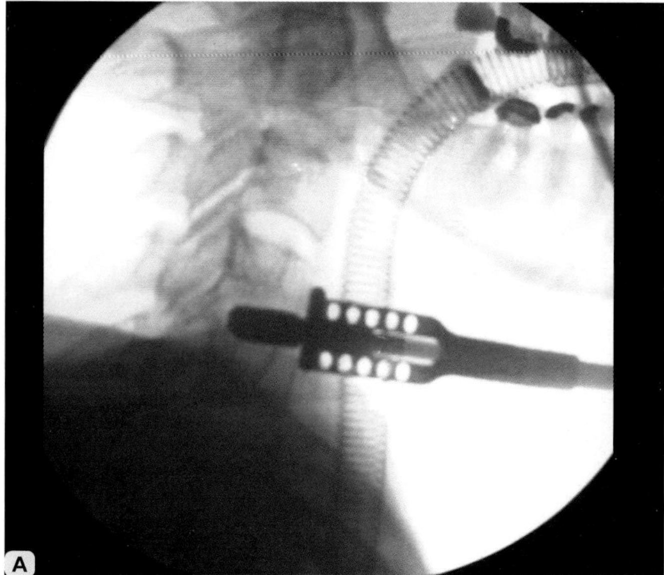

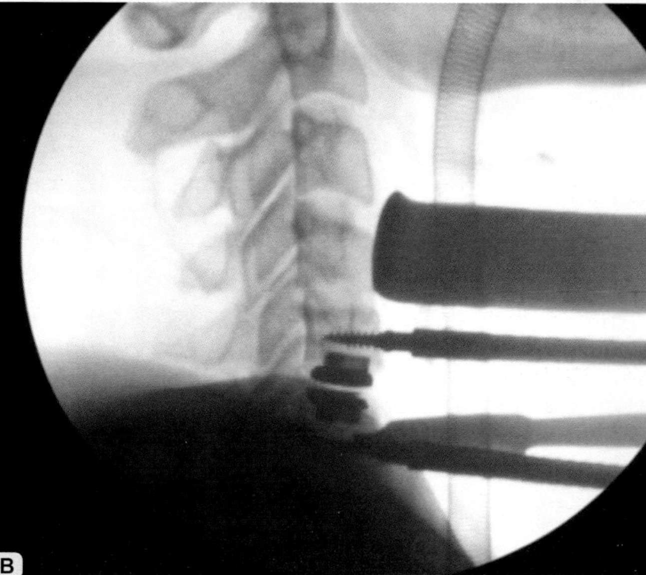

Fig. 19.16 A trial distractor proves too narrow and causes a kyphosis, with adjacent and simultaneous level widened interspinous distance in Figure A. Changing over to a thicker implant in Figure B restores the lordosis as well as the posterior inter-spinous distances

Multiple-level TDR

Many patients presenting to the spine clinic demonstrate multiple levels of cervical spine involvement in their MR scans. Since the FDA currently approves TDR only for single-level use, any usage exceeding one level would be deemed "off-label" by the medical industry, with potential medicolegal ramifications.

Regardless, many surgeons have reported of favorable results with multilevel arthroplasty in the cervical spine.[29-31] Important technical points are relevant in muliple level surgery

- Device placement must be accurate and physio-anatomical symmetry must be observed. Technical skill is required to correctly identify the midline in contiguous levels and insert devices accordingly
- It may be advantageous to retain the PLL for reasons of preserving posterior restraint and thus preventing postoperative kyphosis
- I begin instrumentation by sizing the tightest interspace first, followed by the second tightest. This sequence ensures that I am not finally faced with an already-tight interspace that has been further narrowed by slight over-distraction of its adjacent space (Fig. 19.17).

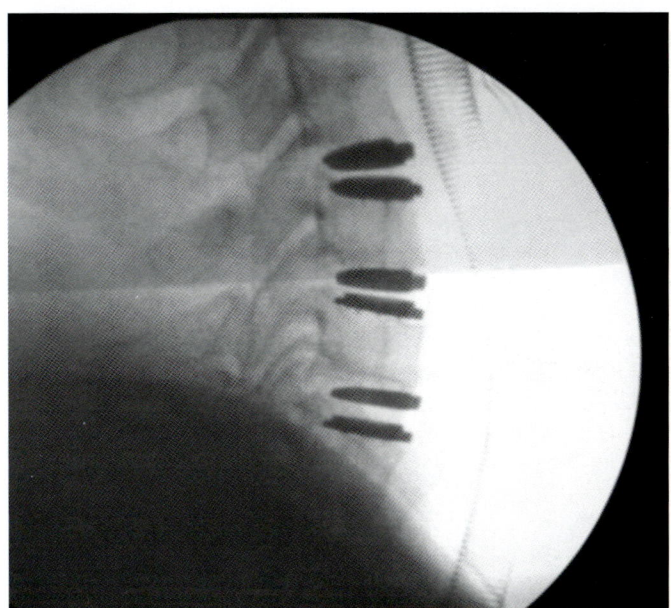

Fig. 19.17 Multiple level TDR of the cervical spine on lateral projection, with preservation of the sagittal axis

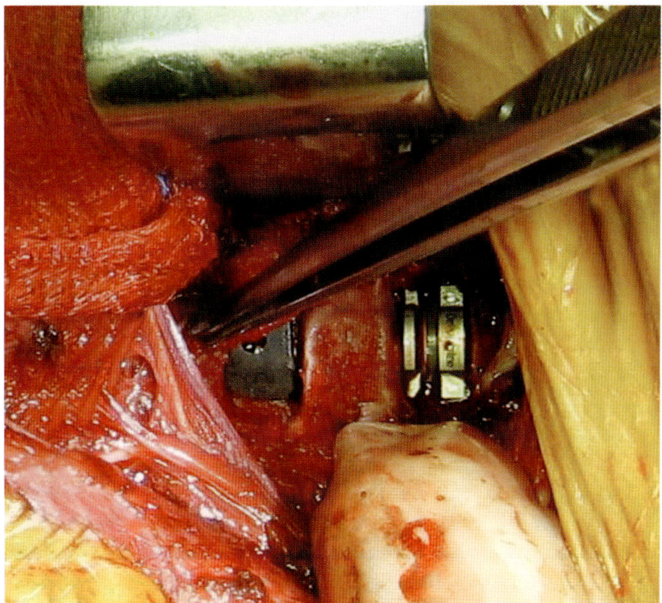

Fig. 19.18 A two-level hybrid construct using a stand-alone resorbable fusion cage caudally and an unconstrained artificial disk device in the cephalad level

Considering Hybrid Constructs

Where multiple-level disk replacement is not feasible, some surgeons have begun hybrid constructs mixing fusion with TDR. Many have reported good results, with some cadaveric studies showing better range of motion and lesser stress in hybrid compared to fusion, and some in vivo data demonstrating superior adjacent segment prevention compared to all-fusion cases.[32-34] In my practice, hybrid constructs may be called into use when:

- Endplate integrity of the segment is compromised during the denudation process
- In a multiple level disk disease, one segment is deemed too spondylotic for TDR
- One or more of the caudal segments originally planned to undergo TDR is/are found to be poorly visualized on lateral image intensifier projection, commonly due to shoulder block.

Technically, it is prudent that

- The fused level be done first such that we may instrument the TDR level while working on a stable base
- Ideally, the chosen mobile segment to be cephalad to the fused, to avoid stressing the device at the bottom end of a long fused moment arm (Fig. 19.18).

Afterword

Cervical spine disk arthroplasty has enjoyed a popularity curve more than that of its lumbar counterpart. It has an easily accessible surgical approach, experiences less demanding physical stress forces, presents more reliable results and is less demanding when revision surgery is called for. Regardless of these, cervical spine TDR surgery is still in its early stages of development and the veracity of current concepts will surely be subjected to states of flux.

This chapter is directed technically to the spine surgeon who, before embarking on cervical spine arthroplasty, has experienced the requisite amount of fusions. It is hoped that this chapter has served as a source of useful knowledge, and that this knowledge has spurred on the tradition of inquiry that is inherent to medicine.

References

1. Smith GW, Robinson RA. The treatment of certain cervical spine disorders by anterior removal of the intervertebral disc and interbody fusion. J Bone Joint Surg Am. 1958; 40-A:607-24.

2. Hilibrand AS, Robbins M. Adjacent segment degeneration and adjacent segment disease: the consequence of spinal fusion? Spine J. 2004; 4(6Suppl): 190-4S
3. Hilibrand AS, Carlson GD, Palumbo MA, Jones PK, Bohlman HH. Radiculopathy and myelopathy at segments adjacent to the site of a previous anterior cervical arthrodesis. J Bone Joint Surg Am. 1999; 81(4): 519-28.
4. Cheng JS, Liu F, Komistek RD, Mahfouz MR, Sharma A, Glaser D. Comparison of cervical spine kinematics using a fluoroscopic model for adjacent segment degeneration. J Neurosurg Spine 2007 Nov;7(5): 509-13.
5. Arbit E, Pannullo S. Lumbar stenosis: a clinical review. Clin Orthop 2001;384:137-43.
6. Swartz E, Floyd RT, Cendoma M. Cervical Spine Functional Anatomy and the Biomechanics of Injury Due to Compressive Loading. J Athletic Training 2005;40(3):1-7.
7. Cloward RB. The Clinical Significance of the sinuvertebral nerve of the cervical spine in relation with the cervical disk syndrome. J Neurol Neurosurg Psychiat. 1960; 23:321.
8. White AA, Panjabi MM. Clinical Biomechanics of the Spine, (2nd ed). Philadelphia: JB Lippincott Company; 1990.
9. Penning L. Normal Movements of the Cervical Spine. Am J Roentgenol. 1978; 130:317-6.
10. McKenzie AH. The Basis for Motion Preservation Surgery: Lessons learnt from the past, in Motion Preservation Surgery of the Spine, Yue JL, Bertagnoli R, McAfee PC, An HS (eds). Philadelphia: Saunders Elsevier; 2008.
11. MacKenzie AH. Fernstrom intervertebral disc arthroplasty: Long term evaluation. Orthopaedics Intl. 1995; 3:313-4.
12. Neil Duggal. Cervical Disc Arthroplasty: A Practical Overview, in Current Orthopaedic Practice. 2009; 20(3): 216-21.
13. Cao JM, Zhang YZ, Shen Y, Ding WY. Complications of Bryan cervical disc replacement. Orthopaedic Surgery. 2010; 2(2): 86-92.
14. The Burton Report on Artificial Discs, an Internet online document at http://www.burtonreport.com/infspine/Surg ArtificialDiscEditorial.htm 2008
15. Okada E, Matsumoto M, Ichihara D, Chiba K, Toyama Y, Fujiwara H, Momoshima S. Ageing of the Cervical Spine in Healthy Volunteers. Spine. 2009; 34:7: 706-12.
16. Buchowski JM, Anderson PA, Sekhon L, Riew DK. Cervical Disc Arthroplasty compared with Arthrodesis for the Treatment of Myelopathy: Surgical Technique. J Bone Joint Surg. 2009; 91, (Suppl 2): 223-32.
17. Riew KD, Sekhon L, Metcalf N, et al. Cervical disc arthroplasty for myelopathy. Spine J. 2006;6(Suppl):57.
18. Hilibrand AS, Carlson GD, Palumbo MA, Jones PK, Bohlman HH. Radiculopathy and myelopathy at segments adjacent to the site of a previous anterior cervical arthrodesis. J Bone Joint Surg Am. 1999; 81(4): 519-28.
19. Albert TJ, direct communication, Kobe CSRS 2010.
20. Nassr A, Lee JY, Bashir RS, Rihn JA, Eck JC, Lim MR. Does incorrect level needle localization during anterior cervical discectomy and fusion lead to accelerated disc degeneration? Spine. 2009; 34(2):189-92.
21. Mehren C, Suchomel P, Grochulla F, Barsa P, Sourkova P, Hradil J, Korge A, Mayer MH. Heterotopic ossification in total cervical artificial disc replacement. Spine. 2006; 31;24: 2802- 6.
22. Leung C, Casey AT, Goffin J, Kehr P, Liebig K, Lind B, Logroscino C, Pointillart V. Clinical significance of heterotopic ossification in cervical disc replacement: a prospective multicentre clinical trial. Neurosurgery. 2005; 57(4): 759-63.
23. Yi S, Kim K, Yang M, et al. Difference in occurrence of heterotopic ossification according to prosthesis type in the cervical artificial disc replacement. Spine. 2010;35(16):1556-61.
24. Lee JH, Jung TG, Kim HS, Jang JS, Lee SH. Analysis of the incidence and clinical effect of the heterotopic ossification in a single-level cervical artificial disc replacement. Spine. J 2010; 10(8): 676-82.
25. McAfee PC, Cunningham B, Dmitriev A, Woo KS, Cappuccino A, Pimenta L. Cervical disc replacement: a comparative biomechanical analysis showing the key role of the posterior longitudinal ligament. Spine. 2003; 15; 28(20):S176-8.
26. Sears W, Sekhon L, Duggal N, McCombe P, Williamson O. Postoperative Kyphosis with the Bryan Cervical Disc Prosthesis -- contributing factors and the Influence of change in Disc Space height. J Bone Joint Surg (Br). 2005; 87-B, Suppl III:411.
27. Yoon DH, Yi S, Shin C, Kim KN, Kim SH. Clinical and radiological results following cervical arthroplasty. Acta Neurochir (Wien). 2006, 148: 943–50.
28. Phillips FM, Garfin SR. Cervical disc replacement. Spine. 30: S27-S33.
29. Cardoso MJ, Rosner MK. Multilevel cervical arthroplasty with artificial disc replacement. Neurosurg Focus. 2010; 28(5):E19.
30. Pimenta L, McAfee PC, Cappuccino A, et al. Superiority of multilevel cervical arthroplasty outcomes versus single-level outcomes: 229 consecutive PCM prostheses. Spine. 2007; 32(12):1337-44.
31. Phillips FM, Tzermiadianos MN, Voronov LI, Havey RM, Carandang G, Dooris A, Patwardhan AG. Effect of two-level total disc replacement on cervical spine kinematics. Spine 2009; 34(22):E794-9.
32. Barrey C, Campana S, Persohn S, Perrin G, Skalli W. Cervical disc prosthesis versus arthrodesis using one-level, hybrid and two-level constructs: an in vitro investigation. Eur Spine J. 2011.
33. Cardoso MJ, Mendelsohn A, Rosner MK. Cervical hybrid arthroplasty with 2 unique fusion techniques. J Neurosurg Spine. 2011; (1):48-54.
34. Lee MJ, Dumonski M, Phillips FM, Voronov LI, Renner SM, Carandang G, Havey RM, Patwardhan AG. Disc replacement adjacent to cervical fusion: a biomechanical comparison of hybrid construct versus two-level fusion. Spine. 2011; 36(23): 1932-9.

CHAPTER

20

Idiopathic Scoliosis: Principles of Surgical Management

A Mezentsev, D Petrenko, Radchenko Vladimir A

Introduction

Idiopathic scoliosis is the most common spinal deformity in children and adolescents. It is divided into three age-related groups: infantile, juvenile, and adolescent. Infantile scoliosis occurs from birth to 3 years old, juvenile scoliosis diagnosed between 3 and 10 years old, and adolescent idiopathic scoliosis occurs after 10 years old. Adults scoliosis appears after the age of 18 years, and it is not being discussed in this chapter.

Adolescent idiopathic scoliosis is the most common form, and girls are mainly affected with right thoracic curve and hypokyphosis. Rare forms are infantile and juvenile deformities. Infantile scoliosis occurs more frequently in boys than in girls. Such deformities are previously left-sided with thoracic hyperkyphosis and about 80% of infantile curves resolve spontaneously.[1,2] Juvenile scoliosis, affects girls more than boys and can be thoracic, lumbar and S-shaped. It has characteristic features of adolescent idiopathic scoliosis. It is important to understand that all these deformities have different natural history and must be managed properly.

There are many articles in orthopedic literature about scoliosis surgical treatment. Modern spinal techniques are extensive and allow to get very good correction in the severe deformity. In spite of this, every case is the great challenge for the treating physician as well as for the patient and his family. All treatments, alternatives and final outcomes should be discussed with the family. When medical staff and patient's relatives understand all possible issues it is the key factor for the successful treatment.

The primary goal of the surgical treatment for the infantile and juvenile idiopathic scoliosis referred as early onset scoliosis is to achieve deformity correction, to spare spinal and lung growth with good pulmonary function. Spinal fusion in skeletal immature patients results in severe trunk asymmetry, crankshaft phenomenon and impacts pulmonary function. New nonfusion methods use anterior convex staples, vertical expandable prosthesic titanium rib (VEPTR), growing rods and growing transpedicular system. All these constructs have defined advantages and drawbacks that will be discussed later.

Surgical management of adolescent idiopathic scoliosis has different directions and depends on the curve severity and patient's wishes. It has been proved that mild and moderate curves occurred beyond the age 10 years old do not lead to severe cardiopulmonary compromise and spinal cord compression. But this spinal deformity severely affects patient's quality of life creating huge psychological problem during all their life and causes disability due to severe back pain. That is why early recognition and curve correction with Cobb angle over 40° is strongly recommended.

Trunk distortion, medical comorbidities and aesthetic state of mind burden medical management and complicate treatment decision. In every case risk to benefit ratio should be weighed. The cornerstone for the severe adolescent idiopathic scoliosis treatment is to improve cardiopulmonary function and at least to prevent further deformity progression.

Indications for Surgical Treatment of Idiopathic Scoliosis

General indications for the surgical treatment of idiopathic scoliosis include following:

- Conservative treatment failure
- Curve progression
- Cosmesis
- Pain
- Scoliotic curve beyond 50° in skeletal immature and 40° in skeletal mature patients
- Cardiopulmonary compromise.

Preoperative Evaluation

The goals of preoperative medical assessment are to define this deformity truly idiopathic, to reveal comorbidities which may affect clinical outcome, and to perform adequate preoperative planning. Patient's history should include age when spinal deformity was diagnosed, family history, associated complaints, neurological disorders and other medical conditions. Onset of the menarche in girls and secondary puberty signs in boys are obligatory. Complete physical examination must be thorough and one should assess anterior and posterior trunk asymmetry, cutaneous lesions (café au lait spots, hairy patches, skin dimples etc.), general morphology (cavus foot, toe clawing, limb discrepancy). Neurological evaluation includes cranial nerves examinations, reflexes, and strength testing, abnormal reflexes.

Standing anteposterior and lateral X-rays, including spine and pelvis for a proper assessment of the entire spinal deformity. Cobb angle, spinal rotation, skeletal age, sagittal profile and structure of the curve can be taken from the radiographs. Functional X-rays (anteposterior projection) with maximal right and left inclination (bending tests), frontal and sagittal fulcrum tests, stretch films views show correctability of the primary and secondary curves.

CT is suitable for the accurate definition of the spinal anatomy and checking in rotation. It is not widely used in idiopathic scoliosis, but this method is valuable for the differentional diagnosis between idiopathic and congenital deformities.

MRI is a noninvasive method and can be used for the determination of intraspinal abnormalities and tumors. It is indicated in patients with neurological deficits, hyperkyphosis, left-sided scoliosis, and in all patients with infantile and juvenile idiopathic scoliosis.

Using of other visualization methods, such as bone scanning, moire topography, discography depends on clinical situation and doctor's preferences.

Surgical Management of Infantile Idiopathic Scoliosis

Progressive infantile idiopathic scoliosis is fatal condition if left untreated. Increased morbidity and mortality are the consequences of poor thoracic and lung growth. This condition termed "thoracic insufficiency syndrome"[3] Progressive infantile scoliosis >40° with rib–vertebral angle difference over 20° should be managed surgically. Ultimate goal for the surgical treatment of infantile curves is to preserve spinal growth and normal chest and lung development. Principle options for the surgical treatment are in situ fusion, convex hemiepiphyseodesis, VEPTR and growing rods.

Surgical decision depends on the patient's age. *In situ* spinal fusion as the method of choice to halt curve progression is not relevant now. Posterior fusion only in skeletal immature children results in curve progression due to anterior spine growth. This situation is known as "crankshaft phenomenon". It has been proved that early fusion in children with Risser 0 and open triradiate cartilage have a high likelihood of curve progression.[4] Anterior and posterior spinal fusion prevents "crankshaft phenomenon" but if this surgery is performed before the age 5 years old chest and spinal growth are seriously affected.

Convex growth retardation by anterior hemiepiphyseodesis for the surgical treatment of infantile idiopathic scoliosis has proponents. Minimally invasive convex side stapling through thoracoscopic approach is an attractive idea for the surgical management of infantile idiopathic scoliosis. It was presented study with thirty-nine patients with adolescent idiopathic scoliosis who have had vertebral body stapling (26 patients with one curve stapling and 13 with two). There were greater or equal to 10° deformity progression in growing children. Major complications occurred in one patient and minor complications occurred in 5 patients.[5] Authors did not attempt to use this technique for the early onset scoliosis patients.

Campbell presented conception of the thoracic deformity correction and lung hypoplasia treatment. VEPTR implantation is predominately used in patients with exotic scoliosis and congenital rib abnormalities.[3] It is limited data regarding usage of this procedure in children with infantile idiopathic scoliosis. This method may be used in infantile curves with the great caution of potentional complications.

The most popular fusionless method is posterior spinal instrumentation with dual growing rod. Akbarnia et al. developed and described the procedure of dual rod spinal instrumentation.[6] Subperiostal dissection is performed only at upper and lower instrumentation zones and where hooks and screws will be inserted. At the upper level hooks or screw are implanted in a claw pattern. Lower end of the implant is anchored by screws as well as by hooks. These sites are termed by authors as "foundations" of the construct. Prebended rods are inserted on each site submuscelary or subcutaneously and linked by connector at the thoracolumbar level. Limited fusion is done at the "foundation" zones. Postoperative bracing is mandatory. Every six month lengthening of the device is performed with distractor fitted inside to the connector.

Growing Study Group presented minimum two years follow-up data in 23 patients with infantile idiopathic scoliosis treated at the mean age of 5,4 years. Preoperative major Cobb angle was 82° on the average, after surgery it was 38° and at the end of follow-up it was 36°. There were on average of 6,6 lengthening with mean growth 1,21 cm per year in this group of patients. Seven patients after definite fusion had on the average of 11,8 cm of total spinal growth during the treatment. Eleven patients had thirteen complications during the follow-up.[7]

In 2006, Growing Study Group presented complications of dual-rod technique in 48 patients with early onset scoliosis managed for two years after the index surgery.[8] Twenty-nine patients had fifty-five complications and twenty-three of them were underwent unplanned revision surgery. Complications were wound related, implant related, poor alignment and general. The most common reason of revision surgery were wound problems required extensive and aggressive treatment. Implant related problems were addressed during the lengthening. Obviously, patients with longer treatment period had more complications then patients with shorter treatment interval. Authors concluded that dual rod technique has high complication rate but all of them are manageable.

In a recent paper Flynn et al. performed a multicenter study of 58 patients who reached skeletal maturity treated with growing rods and younger patients who had final fusion. Of the 58 patients 53 were finally fused, 3 were observed with growing rods in a place, 1 had hardware removal and in 1 patient final fusion was aborted because of neurological problem. Most patients (60%) were fused more levels then the number of levels spanned by growing rods. At the end of treatment, the vast majority of patients had rods removal and final instrumented fusion with less then 50% correction of the deformity remaining at the end of growing rod management.[9]

Surgical treatment of the infantile idiopathic scoliosis remains challenging problem requiring further development. New procedure should be less invasive with good spinal correction, chest and lung growth, and minimal complication rate.

Surgical Management of Juvenile Idiopathic Scoliosis

Juvenile idiopathic scoliosis has high likelihood of progression and surgical treatment is common in these patients. Brace treatment failure, rapid deformity progression and Cobb angle >50° are main indications for the surgical treatment. Making treatment decision one should remember two the most important considerations. The first is that the goal of surgical management in growing children is continued spinal and chest growth with normal pulmonary function. Early fusion results in short spine and thorax with lung hypoplasia. Winter proposed a formula for the determination of the potentional shortening of spinal column. Number of fusion vertebras multiplied 0,7 mm and then product multiplied by number of years of predicted spinal growth.[10] This point is mandatory to discuss with family for better understanding of the treatment protocol.

The second, posterior spinal fusion in skeletal immature children tethers spine while anterior parts of the vertebral column continue to grow (crankshaft phenomenon). A concomitant anterior fusion[11] or segmental pedicle screw fixation[12] can prevent this situation.

Present standard of the medical care in patients with juvenile scoliosis are non-fusion techniques. The most common surgical method is posterior spinal instrumentation with growing-rod system combined with anterior release and convex growth arrest to avoid "crankshaft phenomenon". Standard growing rod technique as well as in the treatment for infantile idiopathic scoliosis includes proximal and distal foundations. Gradual lengthening every 6–12 months is a standard approach in growing patients. Problems associated with this technique are flattening of the spine due to distraction, necessity for frequent surgeries and implant failures.

Dual rod technique is the last generation of growing rod systems. Using of pedicular screws, apical fusion and good understanding natural history of the scoliosis makes improved clinical outcomes, but results are still less then ideal.[13]

Luque et al. proposed polysegmental trolley-like growing construct.[14] This was a first polysegmental growing system with no need of the lengthening procedures. Spine was fixed by sublaminar wires and rods. The risk of passing subluminar wires, frequent spontaneous fusion, wires breakage were reported as major complications in this procedure.[15]

McCarthy developed Shilla technique.[16] This method provides posterior apical transpedicular spinal fusion with other implanted screws that are not locked to the rod.

General idea of this method is to control apical part of the deformity with axial lengthening of adjacent levels. In the recent study of 40 patients cohort McCarthy reported 2–6 years follow-up results. According to this results 18 patients had different complications requiring revision surgery. Author concluded that Shilla is an effective growth guiding technique.[17]

In our current practice we use growing transpedicular polysegmental system developed since 2000 by first author of this chapter. This technique is indicated in skeletal immature patient with Risser 0 at the age before 10 years old and Cobb angle up to 90º. Method provides two stages surgery. The first stage is an anterior convex growth arrest for avoiding crankshaft phenomenon and anterior spinal release. The second stage performed usually at the same day is posterior spinal instrumentation with transpedicular construct (Figs 20.1A to L). For the correction of the deformity we use derotational maneuver. We used basal and medial fixation patterns depending on remaining spinal growth. Two medial screws and crosslinks are locked if predicted growth is more then 4 cm and other anchors are loose allowing the rods to slide during patient's growth. Basal fixation is used if anticipated growth is less then 4 cm. This pattern provides four screws are locked to the rod in the lower part of the instrumentation zone. Reserve length on the rods is left for the future spine growth. Postoperative rigid brace is recommended. After skeletal maturity we lock the screw and perform posterior fusion with the rib bone graft obtained after thoracoplasty (Fig. 20.1).

Clinical results in 33 juvenile scoliosis patients with more then 4 years follow-up were studied. All of them were operated using above described technique. Before the surgery mean Cobb angle was 69°, immediately after surgery 21° and after 4 years follow-up it was 23°. Mean growth of the instrumented spine during the follow-up was 32 mm. There were pull-outs in 2 patients, adding-on in 2 patients, screw breakage in 1 patient, correction loss over 10º in 1 patient and 1 rod exchange because of its length insufficiency. There are no neurological complications or wound infections.[18]

In case of severe deformity with curve angle beyond 90° and severe kyphosis halo-gravity traction is utilized. Six to eight pins are placed under general anesthesia and halo ring is applied. Everyday patient is underwent axial traction of the spine through the halo.[19] This is very useful tool for the gradual correction of the deformity, it makes surgical correction of the deformity more safe because of lower neurological complication rate and improves pulmonary function during the treatment. Pin site problems and possible cranial neuropathy demands careful patient monitoring during the treatment. Our institution approach is using of halo–pelvic or halo–femoral traction after or before anterior release. When planned correction is achieved posterior spinal fixation and fusion are performed (Fig. 20.2).[20]

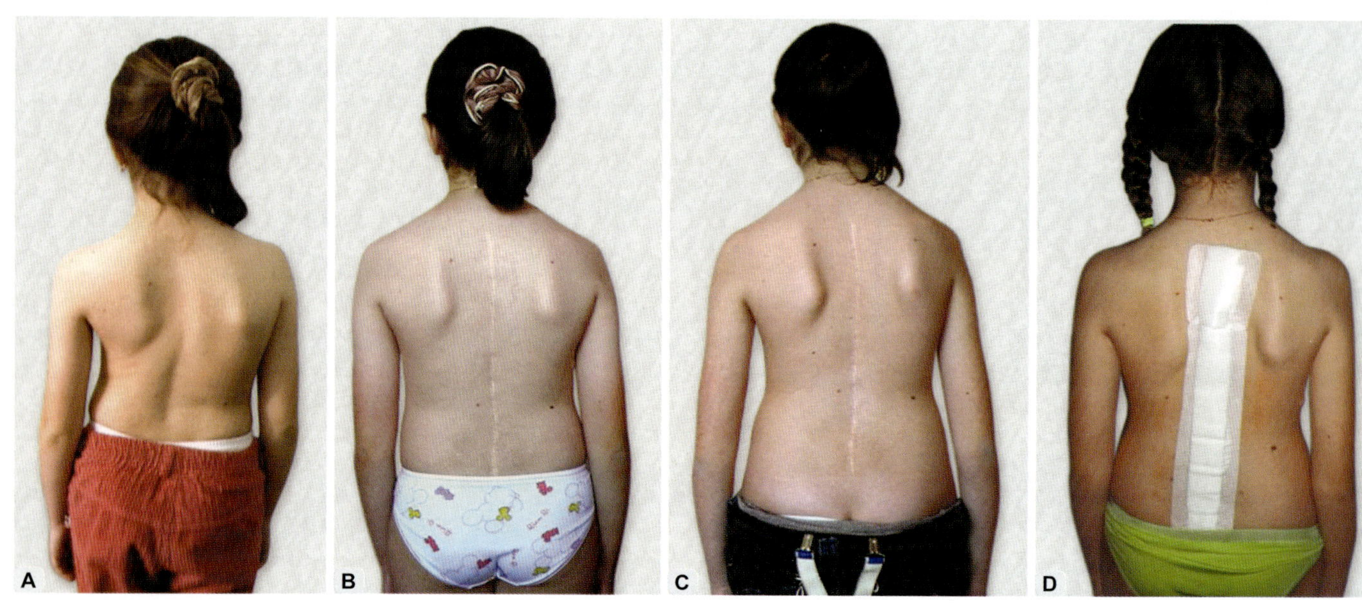

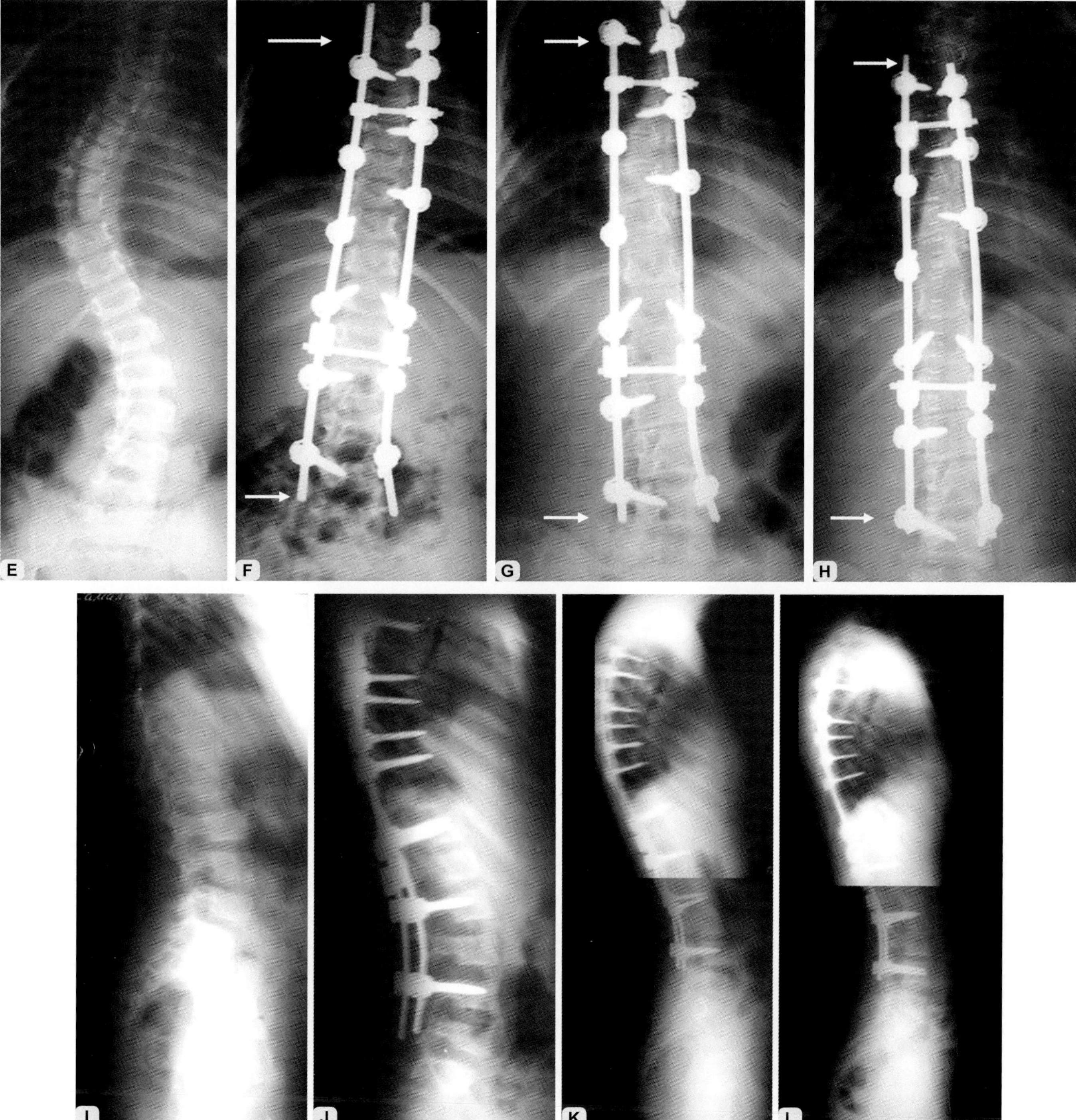

Fig. 20.1 Photographs demonstrates the patient with juvenile idiopathic scoliosis; (A) Preoperative appearance; (B) 1 year after anterior convex growth arrest and posterior spinal instrumentation with growing transpedicular system; (C) 5 years after index surgery; (D) 5 years postoperative, she was underwent final fusion and convex thorakoplasty; (E) Preoperative AP rentgenograms; (F) Growing spinal instrumentation T4–L4; (G) 5 years after the surgical correction. Because of rapid spinal growth concave rod is out of upper screw; (H) 5 years after the index surgery rod exchange and final fusion were performed. White arrow shows the difference of the rod length before and after treatment; I–L Sagittal spinal profile during the follow-up. Preoperative hypokyphosis was reduced due to derotational maneuver and transpedicular spinal fixation

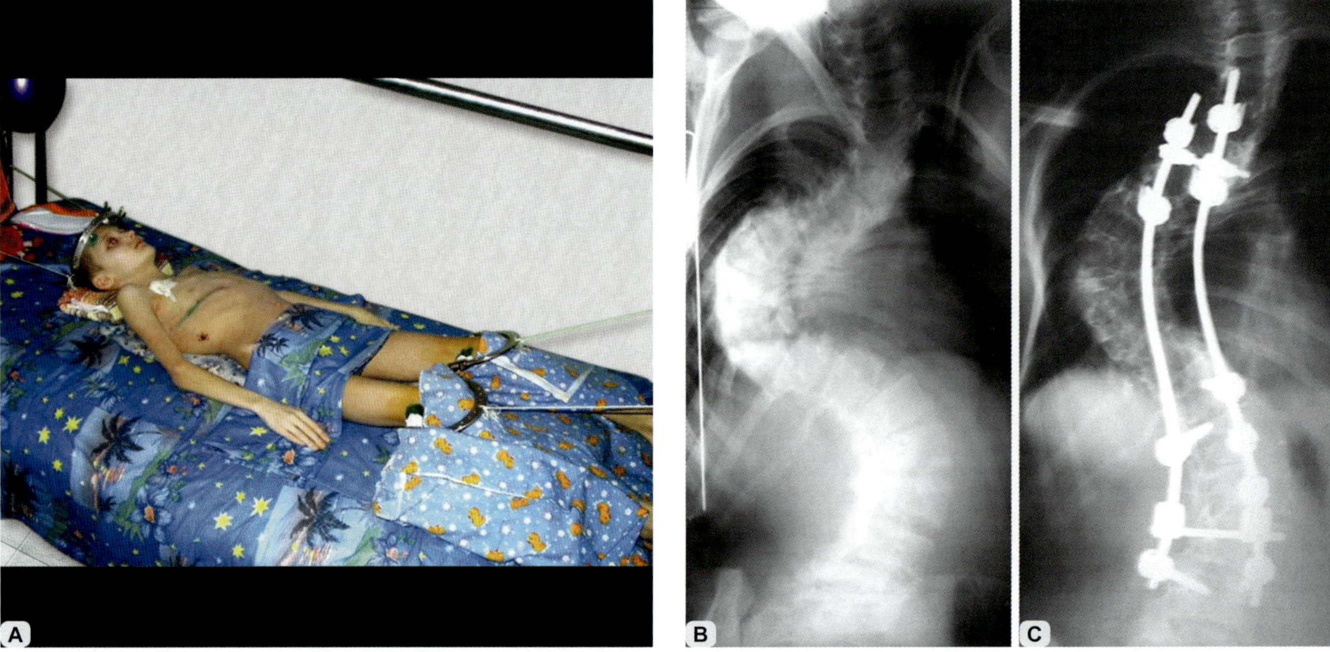

Fig. 20.2 Patient with severe juvenile scoliosis. (A) Halo femoral traction after anterior spinal release; (B) Preoperative AP rentgenogram; (C) Posterior spinal fusion

In patients at the age 8–10 with severe rigid spinal deformities more then 90° anterior and posterior spinal fusion is considerable. This is usually performed in the same day or if patient has contraindications or comorbidities it can be divided into stage surgery with 5–7 days break. Anterior spinal release can be performed endoscopically as well as with the open procedure. It is very important to instrument upper and lower neutral vertebras to avoid curve progression below instrumentation zone – "adding-on phenomenon".[21,22] For better deformity control, it is reasonable to use transpedicular screws with the appropriate size. Pedicular hooks also may be used if pediculum is too small and screw cannot be placed. Because of continued growth in juvenile scoliosis patients it is necessary to achieve solid spinal fusion with autograft, sometimes it could be augmented by allograft.

Growth modulation methods is the alternative for the early spinal instrumentation and fusion. Convex disk stapling for the following growth arrest and deformity self correction is the current trend.[23] But this technique is limited and indicated in mild curves with Cobb angle 25-30°. Precise indications are not well known now and this surgery needs more experience and follow-up.

Another option is anterior convex tethering. In this technique vertebral screws are inserted into bodies and then connected by soft tether. Tightening of the tether creates convex shortening but disck are left intact and limited spinal motion is theoretically preserved. The efficacy of this method needs to be clinically proved in future.

Surgical Management of Adolescent Idiopathic Scoliosis

Adolescent idiopathic scoliosis constitutes the vast majority of the deformity cases. This deformity onset at the age of 10 years old up to adulthood. Approximately prevalence of adolescent idiopathic is 2–3%. Surgical treatment is indicated in skeletal mature patients with Cobb angle greater than 40°, in case of rapid progression and brace intolerance.

For the providing treatment guidelines and better outcomes it was developed many classifications of the adolescent idiopathic scoliosis. King's classification was the most popular since 1983 when it was first published.[24] This classification was popular during Harrington era and only analyzed coronal component of the deformity. Curves were divided into five types. In fact this classification system was the gold standard for the scoliosis surgeons for 20 years, and suffered from bad interobserver reability.[25]

In 2001 Lenke et al. proposed new adolescent idiopathic scoliosis classification. This system provides coronal and sagittal curve analysis, takes into consideration curve flexibility, assesses secondary curves. This classification system is more reliable than that of King and more suitable for the modern polysegmental instrumentation.[26]

The first step in the curve classification is to define its type as presented in Table 20.1 (structural and nonstructural). Structural scoliosis is determined as measured more than 25° on lateral inclination functional radiograph. There are 6 curves patterns (Fig. 20.3). The vertical line extending

Table 20.1 Lenke curve types

Curve type	*Proximal thoracic*	*Main thoracic*	*Thorucolumbar/Lumbar*	*Description*
1	Nonstructural	Structural	Nonstructural	Main thoracic
2	Structural	Structural	Nonstructural	Double thoracic
3	Nonstructural	Structural	Nonstructural	Double major
4	Structural	Structural	Nonstructural	Triple major
5	Nonstructural	Nonstructural	Structural	Thoracolumbar/lumbar
6	Nonstructural	Structural	Structural	Thoracolumbar/lumbar—main thoracic

from the sacrum center upwards on the anteposterior X-ray defined as central vertical sacral line (CVSL) and aimed to assess lumbar spine deviation (A, B, C modifiers). Additionally, sagittal spine modifiers are defined (Fig. 20.3).

Treatment Guidelines

Type I

The most common type of the scoliotic spinal deformities in adolescents. Surgical treatment involves performing selective fusion of the main thoracic curve only. It can be performed with posterior or anterior spinal instrumentation. Posterior implants include screws, hooks or wires. Proximal fusion level is usually T3–T5, distal ends at the last vertebra touched in the part by CSVL (Fig. 20.4). The best candidate for anterior spinal fusion is a patient with Cobb angle 40°–70° and with hypokyphosis (Fig. 20.5). Anterior instrumentation is recommended to extend from the upper end vertebra to the lower end vertebra. In case of rigid thoracic curve anterior open or endoscopic release can be performed.

Type II

This deformity has structural main thoracic and proximal thoracic curves. Elevated left shoulder is the characteristic indicator of this curve type. Both structural curves should be instrumented (Fig. 20.6). The goal is to correct deformity and to get even shoulders. Posterior fusion is recommended in this curve type.

Type III

Thoracic and lumbar curves have similar characteristics and are structural. Proximal curve is nonstructural. If thoracolumbar kyphosis exists then deformity should be managed as double major curve. There is no trunk decompensation because both curves balance each other. The deformity is better corrected by posterior instrumentation (Fig. 20.7). Upper instrumented vertebra is at the T3–T5 levels, lower instrumented vertebra is at L3–L4 levels. Some double major curves can be fused selectively. The prerequisites for this are absence of junctional kyphosis and domination of the thoracic curve.

Type IV

This curve type is rare and has proximal thoracic, main thoracic, and lumbar structural curves. Posterior spinal instrumentation is the treatment of choice. Severe stiff curves require anterior release, but modern screw fixation and osteotomy techniques allow to avoid it in some cases (Fig. 20.8). Proximally fixation ends at T1–T2, distally at L4–L5.

Type V

It is thoracolumbar deformity with the curve apex at T12 and L1 levels. Sometimes it is lumbar if the apex is between L1–L2 disk and L4 body. This curve has C shape. Surgical treatment involves posterior (Fig. 20.9) or anterior thoracolumbar instrumentation (Fig. 20.10). Nonstructural secondary thoracic curve usually resolves one year after the surgery. When the anterior fusion could result in a lumbar hypolordosis due to convex compression it must be avoided by using of interbody cages. If posterior fusion is performed the lower instrumented vertebra is at least one level distal than with anterior techniques.

Type VI

This type combines structural thoracolumbar/lumbar with structural thoracic curve. General recommendation is posterior instrumented spinal fusion from T3–T5 to L3–L4. Anterior approach is considered if residual thoracic deformity will have an acceptable appearance and symmetrical shoulders (Fig. 20.11).

Surgical Methods for Adolescent Idopathic Scoliosis

Posterior spinal instrumentation is the present "gold standard" of the scoliosis surgery. There are many spinal

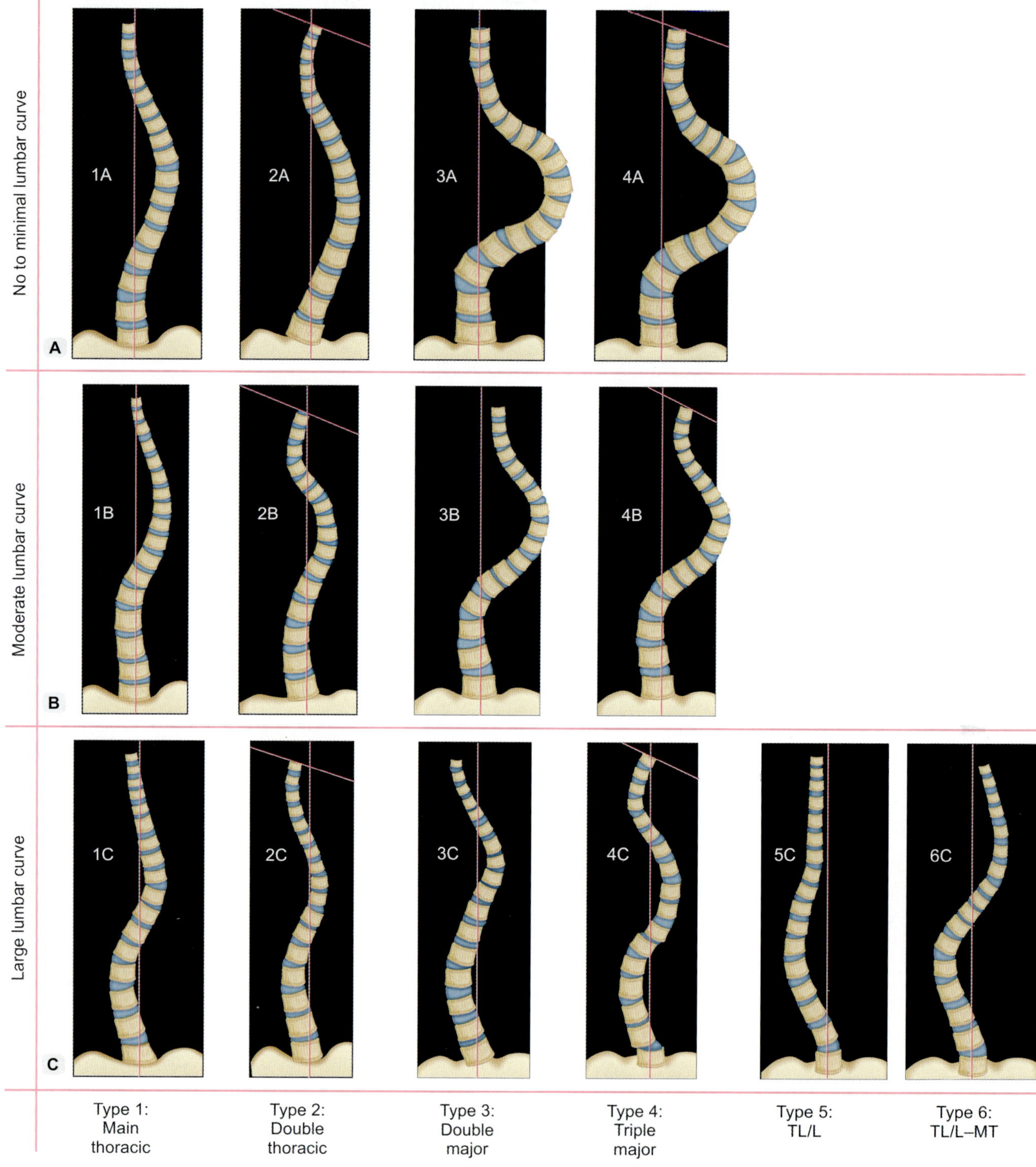

Fig. 20.3 Lenke curve types and lumbar modifiers

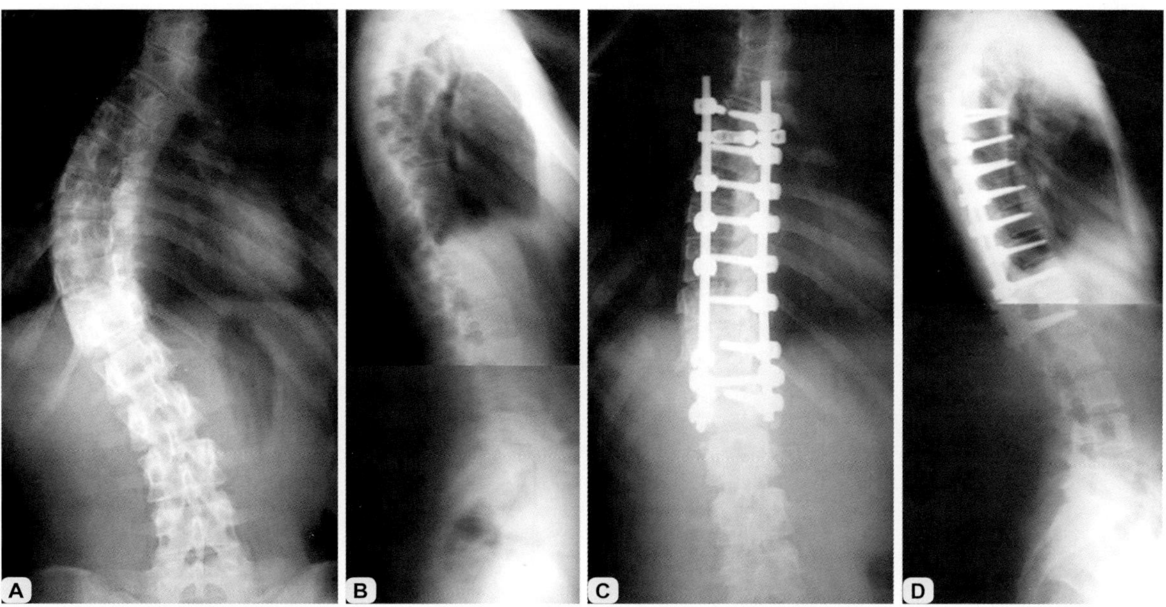

Fig. 20.4 Roentgenograms demonstrate (A and B) Lenke type I thoracic scoliosis; (C and D) Patient was underwent selective spinal fusion T5–L1

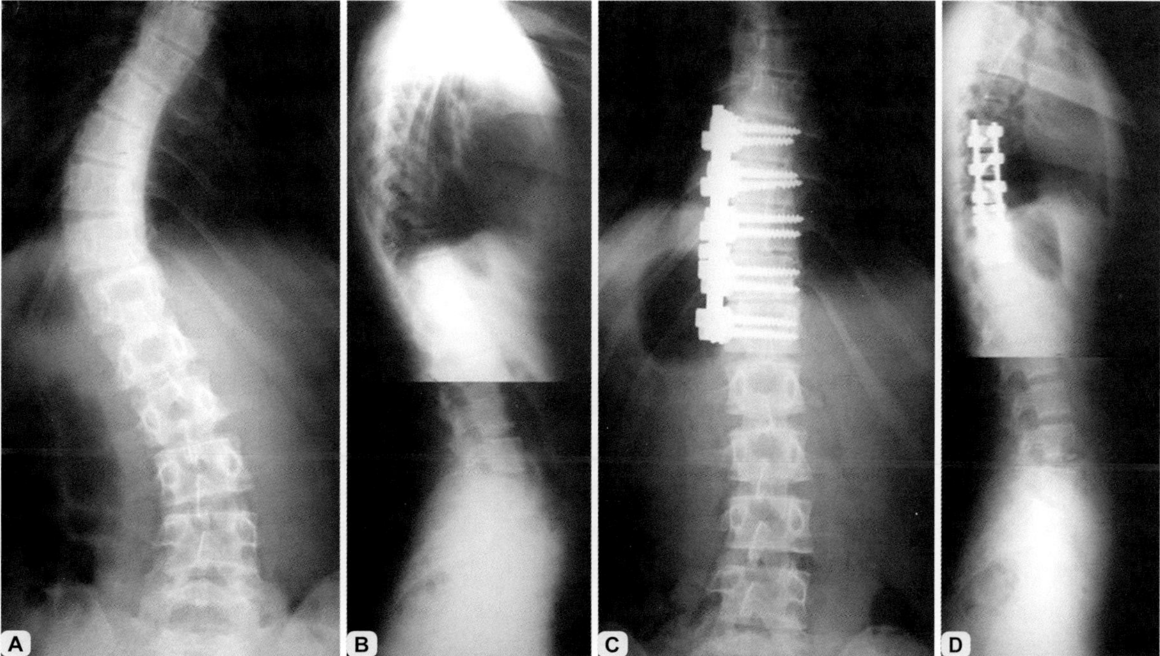

Fig. 20.5 Roentgenograms of the patient with (A and B) Lenke type I scoliotic deformity; (C and D) Anterior short segment bone-on-bone spinal fusion T10–L1 was performed

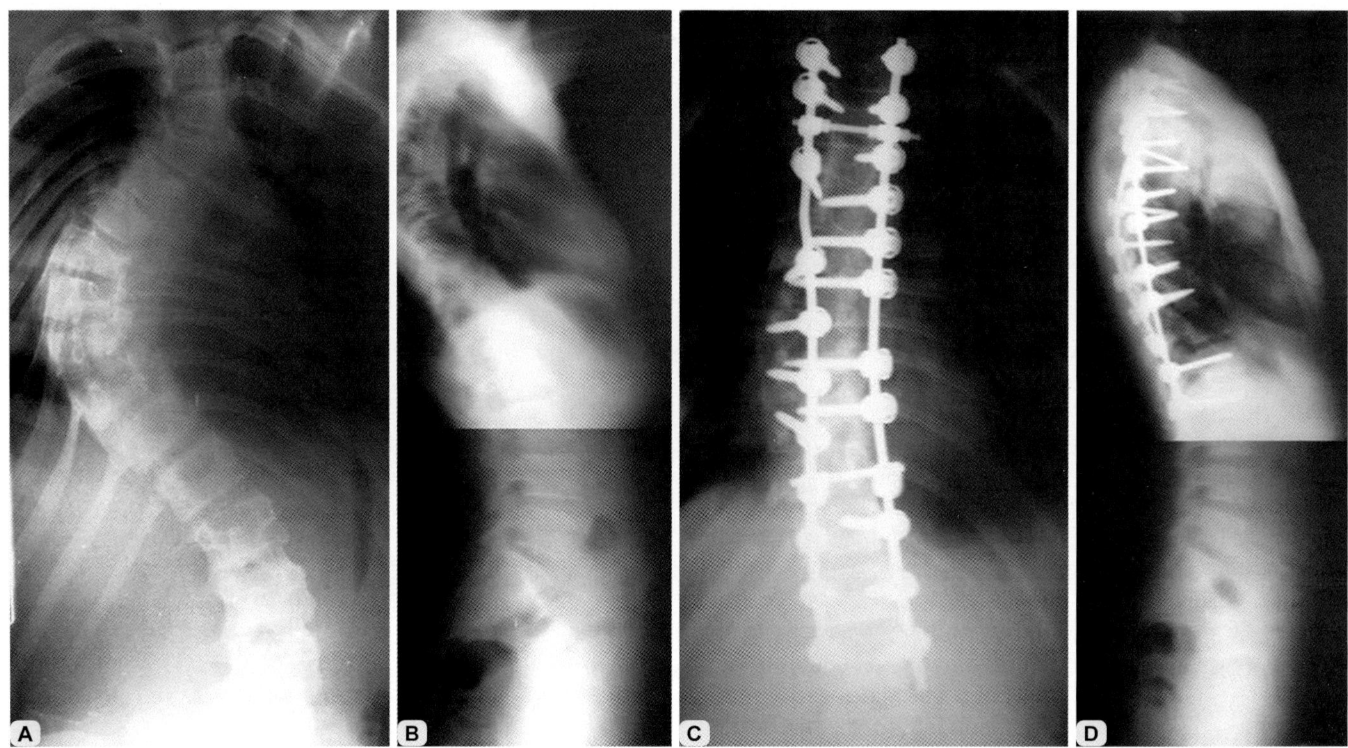

Fig. 20.6 Roentgenograms of the patient with (A and B) double thoracic curve (C and D) Posterior spinal fusion T2–L2 was performed. Even shoulders and coronal compensation were achieved

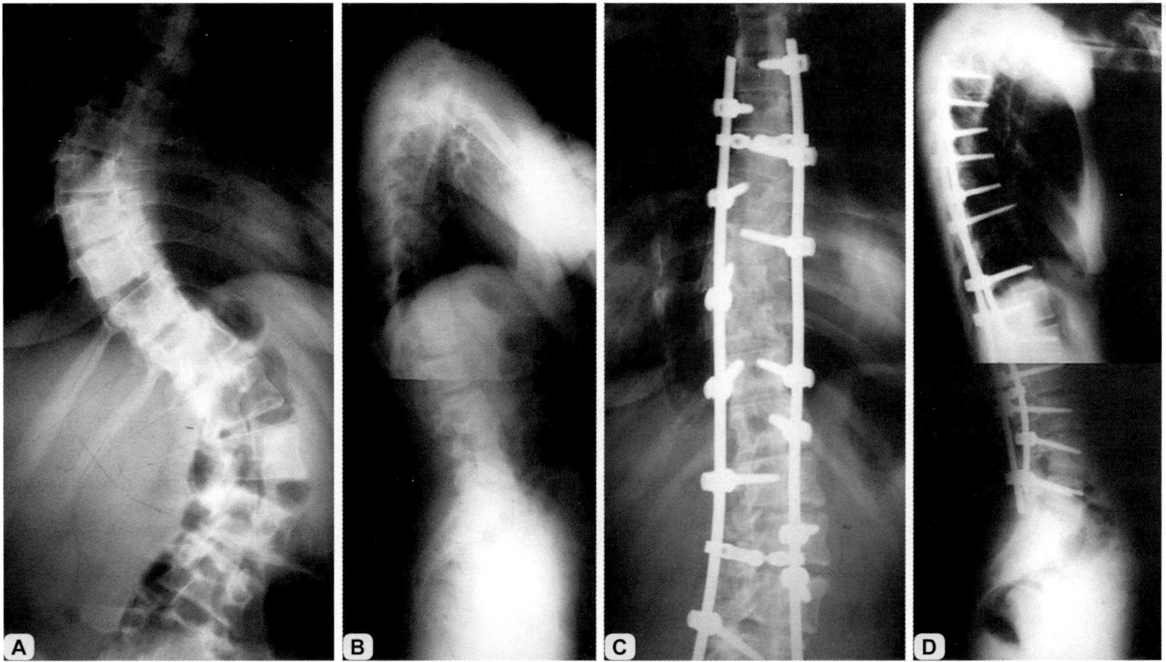

Fig. 20.7 Roentgenograms of the patient with (A and B) Lenke type III curve; (C and D) Instrumented spinal fusion T4–L5 corrected all components of the deformity

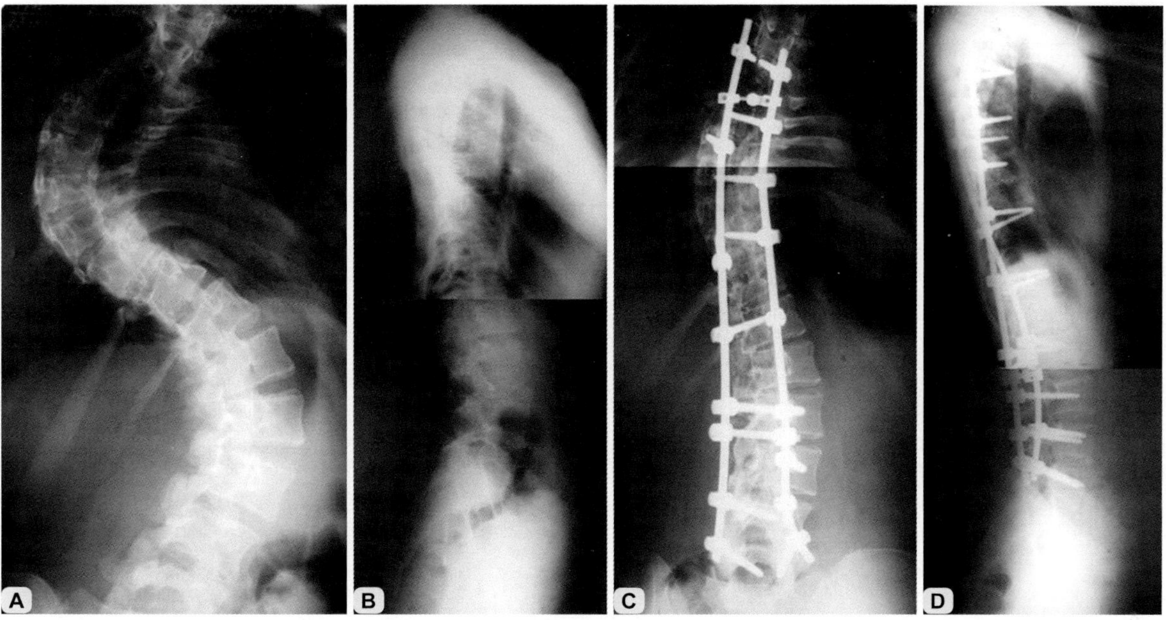

Fig. 20.8 Roentgenograms of the patient with (A and B) Lenke type IV curve; (C and D). Instrumented spinal fusion T4–L5 was performed

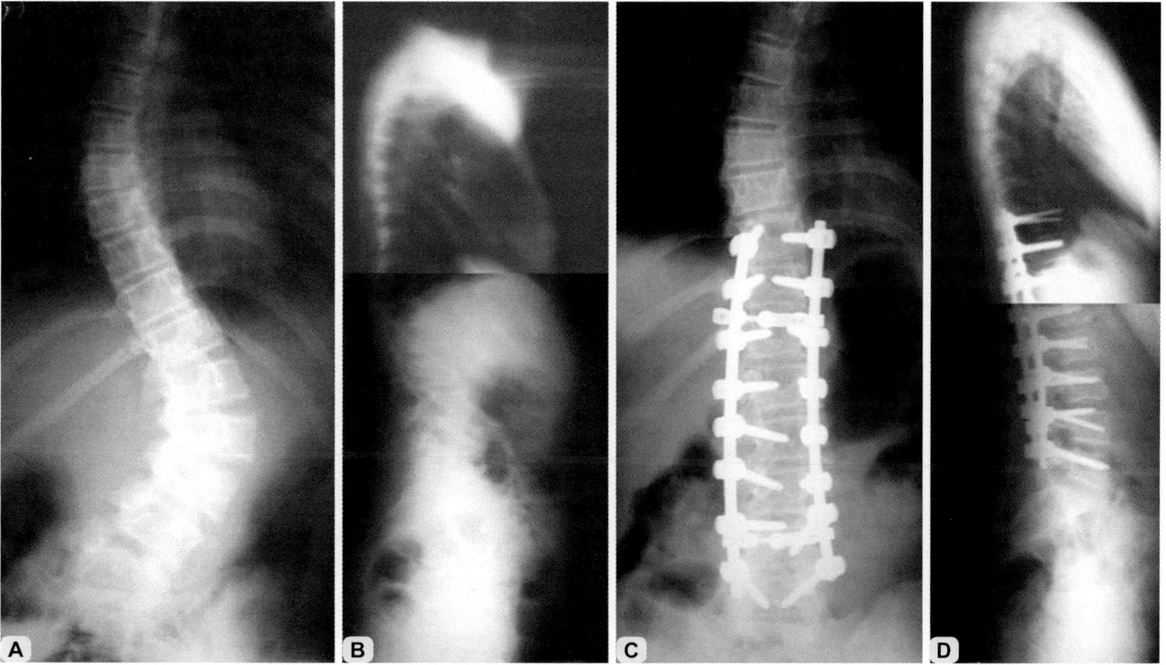

Fig. 20.9 Roentegenograms of the patient with (A and B) Lenke type V curve; (C and D) Because thoracic curve was nonstructural selective spinal fusion T10–L5 was performed

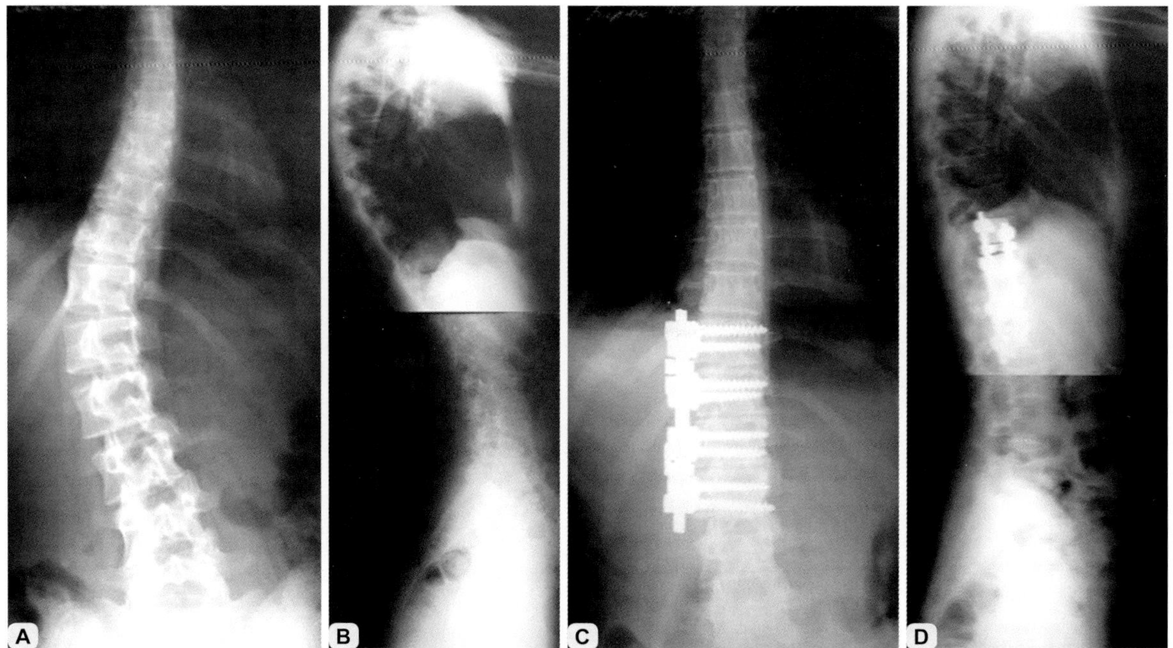

Fig. 20.10 Roentgenograms demonstrate treatment alternative of Lenke type V curve; (A and B) Preoperative roentgenorams show structural thoracolumbar curve; (C and D) Instrumented bone-on-bone spinal fusion T11–L3 was performed

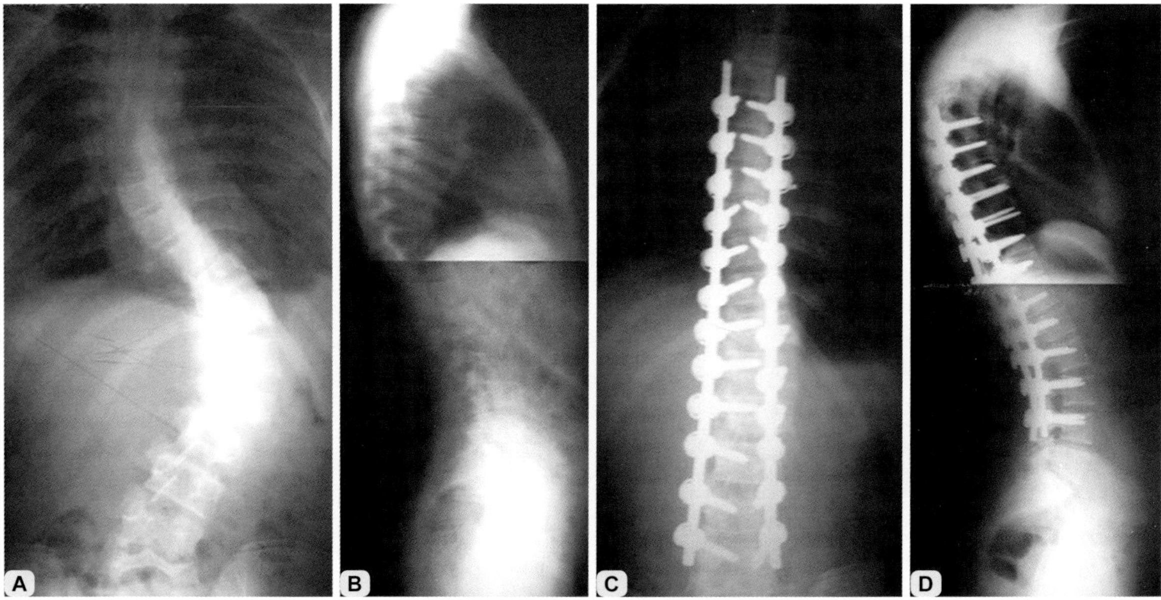

Fig. 20.11 Roentgenograms of the patient with (A and B) Lenke type VI curve; (C and D) Patient underwent instrumented spinal fusion T5–L4

implants utilizing the polysegmental concept of Cotrel and Dubousset proposed in 1980. Current option of spinal anchoring are hooks, wires, and pedicular screws. Screw fixation makes deformity correction very effective, but there is still some controversy in using it, because of small pediculus size especially on the convex size of the deformity. Other concern is flattening of the sagittal spinal profile after the spinal correction with rigid pedicular system and the solid rod. Revision surgery is indicated in some cases. Risk factor for the residual postoperative thoracic hypokyphosis are preoperative hypokyphosis, curves with less main thoracic scoliosis and utilization of 5,5 cm rod.[27] Recent study showed that changes are related to the surgical technique rather than the rod diameter or type.[28]

Modern trend of the posterior spinal fusion is short selective fixation. It is indicated for Lenke type I curve. Short fusion strategy using pedicle screw constructs can produce equivalent correction of the main curve to conventional fusion methods with less surgical time and blood loss.[29] Posterior spinal instrumentation can be combined with convex rib hump resection at the same time. Obtained during the thoracoplasty ribs are used as the autograft.

In case of rigid severe deformity over 80°, curve flexibility less then 50% and if the patient is skeletal immature we perform open anterior release before spinal instrumentation. If anterior release is contraindicated because of the comorbidities posterior spinal ostetomies such as Smith-Peterson, Ponte or pedicular subtractional osteotomy can be used. Vertebral column resection for the severe spinal deformity is highly effective but technically demanding method. This procedure is the last choice when other less aggressive methods are ineffective. Vertebral column resection corrects deformity with spinal cord is the center of the corrective hinge and straightening procedure is at price of spinal cord angulations and rotation.[30]

The study of the complications rate following vertebral column resection in the pediatric group consisted of 84 primary and 63 revision cases was presented. General complication rate was 39%. These complications were 13% neurological and 26% were respiratory. There were no perioperative death or complete neurological deficits. Neurological complications resolved in all patients except one case.[31]

Anterior spinal instrumentation is the treatment alternative for Lenke types I and V deformities. Compared to standard posterior operative methods anterior instrumented fusion offers number of advantages. Anterior construct provides shorter fusion, less blood loss compared to conventional posterior surgeries, low risk of junctional kyphosis, rapid fusion and more effective restoration of the sagittal contour at the cost of diskectomy. It also has reduced postoperative infection rate. Corrective force applied to the spine is compressive with convex side shortening. In comparison with distractional maneuvers spinal cord injuries are minimized. Using of the anterior spinal fixation is limited in deformities with Cobb angle more than 70º, Lenke types 1C and 5C, impaired pulmonary function and previous anterior spinal infection or chest surgeries.

There are many single and double-rod systems for the anterior spinal fusion as well as different approaches. Our personal choice is short segment "bone-on-bone" spinal fusion proposed by R. Gaines. The key for this technique is total diskectomy with removing of posterior longitudinally ligament.[32] Total disk excision allows to limit fixation extend to only those vertebra contained with end vertebras defined on the preoperative anteposterior stretch film. A greater number of noninstrumented vertebra allow to leave spine more mobile with rapid patient's recovery. Recommendation to athletic activity after scoliosis surgery is controversial.[33] However anterior short-segment fusion offers better chance for unrestricted sport life.[32]

In conlusion, the selection of appropriate approach (anterior versus posterior) depends on curve type, surgeon's preferences and training level. The choice of fusion levels is the controversial point remaining disputable question. However, one should remember that fusion should be as short as possible to save spinal function and at the same time enough to provide and maintain deformity correction avoiding junctional problems.

Complications

Possible complications of the scoliosis surgery can be divided into early and late.

Early

- Neurological complications are relatively rare in idiopathic scoliosis patients. Careful preoperative evaluation is very important preventive measure to avoid such outcome. Analysis of the Scoliosis Research Society Morbidity and Mortality Report shows 0.9% of neurological deficits in idiopathic scoliosis. Totally there were 31 cases, 12 patients out of them had incomplete spinal cord injury, 3 had total cord injury and 16 patients had nerve root injury in 6,252 operations. Our experience is 4 total spinal cord injuries in 573 surgeries. Three of them partially resolved during 1 year after the operation and one patient with ischemic myelopathy is in the rehabilitation period 6 month postoperatively.
  Severe spinal deformities, combined anterior and posterior procedures and pronounced kyphosis are the main risk factor of the neurological complications.

To minimize the risk of this problem performing MRI is mandatory in atypical cases (infantile and juvenile curves, left-sided deformity and severe kyphosis). MRI is not recommended in typical scoliosis without any neurological abnormalities in patients.[34] Intraoperative monitoring is the most effective way to define and to avoid spinal cord lesions. Somatosensory and motor potential registration eliminate triggering factor at the early stage making better chances for patient's recovering.[35] It should be emphasized that motor potential depends on anesthetic drugs and every positive signal is recommended to check with Stagnara "wake-up test"

- Infection complications rate is 0.5% and the reoperation rate is about 5-10%. There are studies reported 1.7% infection rate out of 1250 patients with idiopathic scoliosis[36] and 4.7% out of 489 cases.[37] The vast majority of these complications are superfiscial. The risk factors for postoprerative infection are diabetes, rheumatoid arthritis, immunosuppressive conditions and obesity. Risk factors must be optimized before the surgery. It is possible to reduce risk by changing life style: weight loss, associated diseases control, preoperative physical rehabilitation. Prevention of the postoperative infection depends on appropriate antibiotic therapy. Antibiotic should be first generation cephalosporin injected within one hour before incision. Optimal antibiotic dosing is paramount. Postoperative drain in major scoliosis surgery reduces incidence of hematoma and deep wound infection. If infection occurs we use antibiotic medication and irrigation-suction system with antiseptic solutions or specific antimicrobial agents. Wound debridment is indicated if conservative treatment is ineffective. We advocate leaving the construct in a place until fixation of the spine is stable. Blood testing including WBC, ESR and CRP are markers of the treatment efficacy. Recent study shows that prolacitonin is the most specific test for detecting infection[38]
- After anterior approach and rib hump resection pneumothorax or hemothorax are very common complications. Chest tube is required in these cases resulting in quick recovery. A chylothorax is the complication of anterior procedures. It occures rarely and spontaneous reabsorbtion usually occur
- Early implant failure resulting into revision instrumentation mostly associated with hook and wire utilization. Screw instrumentation reduces this complication. Some hypokyphotic patients or who have thoracolumbar junctional kyphosis are at increased risk, especially after posterior spinal instrumentation only.

Late

- Trunk decompensation is the problem of late postoperative period and anticipated in Lenke curve types 2C and 3C.[39] The correction of the spinal deformity with modern polysegmental systems should provide harmonious transition from fused to unfused parts of spine. In case of incorrect choice of the lower instrumented vertebra adjacent to the instrumented spine levels are subjected to increased mechanical stress and this leads to the trunk decompensation. To avoid this complication the lower instrumented vertebra should be touched by CVSL (stable vertebra) or one level upward and it is recommended to take into consideration risk factors such as younger patient's age, larger thoracic curves with apical deviation and using of hybrid constructs[40]
- Loss of the lumbar lordosis is a typical complication of the anterior instrumented spinal fusion in Lenke type 5C curve.[41,42] This situation can be avoided if the correct technique is applied and in defined cases interbody cages should be utilized. Surgeon must be aware to preserve lumbar lordosis in posterior spinal instrumentation
- Correction loss nowadays is not common complication. Its rate was reduced with modern polysegmental spinal instrumentation. Usually this complication occur within two years after the corrective surgery and then spine condition is stabilized. Main reason of the correction loss is pseudoarthrosis which can lead to the rod fracture, screw breakage and displacement. If implant indicated to remove because of delayed infection,[43] prominence or failure, correction loss occurs because of poor posterior fusion[44]
- Transitional zone problems: long-term follow-up demonstrates that spinal fusion with pedicular constructs resulted in well maintained correction without severe major complications. The most important is a good condition of the adjacent segments. The factor which may affect the long-term outcome is the fate of disk below instrumentation zone. Fusion down to L3 or lower can result in a transitional segment disease. Especially this problem could be anticipated in case of the fusion at the L4 and L5 levels. Wedgening of the adjusted disc identified by some surgeons, more often noted when L3 is rotated. Fusion should not be continued beyond the end vertebra in the anterior spinal fusion. In contrast, posterior spinal fusion usually extends lower to the stable vertebra. Some authors suggest this problem can be a causative factor for severe trunk decompensation

especially in patients with lumbar scoliosis. Others think that this question remains uncertain and must be assessed in future.

References

1. Ponseti IV, Friedman B. Prognosis in idiopathic scoliosis. J Bone Joint Surg Am. 1950;32:381-95.
2. Ceballos T, Ferrer-Torrelles M, Castillo F, Fernandez-Parderes E. Prognosis in infantile idiopathic scoliosis. J Bone Joint Surg Am. 1950;62:863-75.
3. Campbell RM Jr, Smith MD. Thoracic insufficiency syndrome and exotic scoliosis. J Bone Joint Surg Am. 2007;89 (Suppl 1): 108-22.
4. Sanders JO, Herring JA, Brown RH Posterior arthrodesis and instrumentation in the immature (Risser-grade-0) spine in idiopathic scoliosis. J Bone Joint Surg.Am. 1995;77:39-45.
5. Betz RR, Kim J, D'Andrea LP, Mulcahey LG, Balsara RK, Clements DH. An innovative technique of vertebral body stapling for the treatment of patients with adolescent idiopathic scoilosis: a feseability, safety and utility study. Spine. 2003; 28:S255-65.
6. Akbarnia BA, Marks DS. Instrumentation with limited arthrodesis for the treatment of progressive early onset scoliosis. Spine: State of the Art Reviews. 2000;14:181-9.
7. Akbarnia BA, Marks DS, Boachie-Adjei O, Thompson AG, Asher MA. Dual growing rod technique for the treatment of progressive early onset scoliosis: a multicener study. Spine. 2005; 30 (17 Suppl.):S46-57.
8. Akbarnia BA, Asher MA, Bagherl R, Boachie-Adjei O, Canale S, Kostial PA, Marks D, McCarthy RE, Mendelow MJ, Poe-Kochert C, Sponseller PD, Thompson GH. Complications of dual rod technique in early onset scoliosis: can we identify risk factors? Annual meeting of Scoliosis Research Society: Monterey, CA;2006.
9. Flynn JM, Tomlison LA, Pawelek J, Thompson GH, McCarthey RE, Akbarnia BA. Growing Rod Graduates: Lessons From 58 Patients Who Have Completed Their Lengthenings. Annual meeting of Scoliosis Research Society; Kyoto, Japan;2010.
10. Winter R. Scoliosis and spinal growth. Orthop Rev. 1997;6:17-20.
11. Lapinksy AS, Richards BS. Preventing the crankshaft phenomenon by combining anterior fusion with posterior instrumentation. Does it work? Spine. 1995;20:1392-8.
12. Burton DC, Asher MA, Lai SM. Scoliosis correction maintenance in skeletally immature patients with idiopathic scoliosis. Is anterior fusion really necessary? Spine (Phila Pa 1976.) 2000;25:61-8.
13. Akbarnia BA, Breakwell LM, Marks DS, et al. Dual growing rod technique followed for three to eleven years until final fusion: the effect of frequency of lengthening. Spine 2008;33:984-90.
14. Luque ER, Cardosa A. Treatment of scoliosis without arthrodesis or external support, preliminary report (Abstract). Orthop Trans. 1977:1:37-8.
15. Rinsky LA, Gamble JG, Bleck EE. Segmental instrumentation without fusion in children with progressive scoliosis. J Pediatr Orthop. 1985;5(6):687-90.
16. McCarthy R, Luhmann S, Lenke L. Greater than two year follow-up Shilla Growth Enhancing System for the Treatment of Scoliosis in Children. Abstracts from:The 2nd International Congress on Early Onset Scoliosis and Growing Spine. Montréal, Québec; 2008.
17. McCarthy R, McCullough F. Growth Guidance Procedure in EOS: Do They Work? Abstracts from: Interanational Meeting on Advansed Spine Techniques. Copenhagen, Denmark; 2011.
18. Mesentsev A., Petrenko D. Growing Polysegmental Construct in the treatment of Juvenile Idiopathic Scoliosis Abstracts from:The 2nd International Congress on Early Onset Scoliosis and Growing Spine, November 7-8, 2008 Montréal, Québec.
19. Botte MJ, Bryne TP, Abrams RA, Grafin S R. Halo skeletal fixation: Techniques of application and prevention complication. Jour. of American Orthopedic Surgeons. 1996;4:44-53.
20. МезенцевА.О., Петренко Д.Є.,Барков О.О Порівняльний аналіз дистракційного ефекту галоапарату та інтраопераційної дистракції при хірургічному лікуванні тяжких сколіотичних деформації хребта. Ортопедия, травматология и протезирование 2008; 4:84-8.
21. Holocomb GW, Mencio GA, Green NE. Video-assisted thoracoscopic diskektomy and fusion. J Ped Surg. 1997; 32:1220-2.
22. Newton PO, Wenger DR, Mubarak SJ, Meyer RS. Anterior release and fusion in pediatric spinal deformity. A comparison of early outcome and cost of thoracoscopy and open thoracotomy approaches. Spine. 1997;22:1398-406.
23. Bertz RR, D'Andrea LP, Mulcuhey MJ, Chafetz R.S. Vertebral body stapling procedure for the treatment of scoliosis in the growing child. Clin Ortop Relat. Res. 2005;434:55-60.
24. King HA, Moe JE, Bradford DS, Winter RB. The selection of fusion levels on thoracic idiopathic scoliosis. J Bone and Joint Surg (Am). 1983;65:1302-13.
25. Lenke LG, Betz RR, Bridwell KH, et al. Intraobserver and interobserver reliability of the classification of thoracic adolescent idiopathic scoliosis. J Bone Joint Surg Am. 1998;80A(8):1097-106.
26. Lenke LG, Betz RR, Harms J, et al. Adolescent idiopathic scoliosis: a new classification to determine extent of spinal arthrodesis. J Bone Joint Surg Am. 2001;83A(8):1169-181.
27. Fletcher N, Hopkins J, McClung A, Brown R, Sucato DJ. Residual thoracic hypokyphosis following posterior spinal fusion in adolescent idiopathic scoliosis: Risk Factors and Clinical Ramifications. Annual Meeting of Scoliosis Research Society; Kyoto, Japan;2010.
28. Ozturk C, Alanay A, karadeniz E, Balioglu MB, Hamzaoglu A. Kyphosis restoration or maintenance with Lenke Type I scoliosis treated by pedicular screw constructs: is it really impossible by using 5.5 mm titanium rods? Abstracts from: International Meeting on Advanced Spine Techniques. Copenhagen, Denmark; 2011.

29. Matsumoto M, Watanabe K, Hosogane N, Okada E, Chiba K, Toyama Y. Short fusion for Lenke Type I thoracic curve using pedicle screw fixation Abstracts from: International Meeting on Advanced Spine Techniques, Copenhagen, Denmark; 2011.
30. Xie J, Wang Y, Zhang Y, Zhao Z. Posterior vertebral column resection for correction of severe rigid spinal deformity. Annual Meeting of Scoliosis Research Society: Kyoto, Japan;2010.
31. Newton PO, Lenke LG, Shufflebarger HL, Sucato DJ, Emans JB, Sponseller PD, Shah SA, Bastrom T. Perioperative complications of pediatric vertebral column resections. Annual Meeting of Scoliosis Research Society: Kyoto, Japan;2010.
32. Brodner W, Yue WM, Moller HB, Gaines RW. Short Segment Bone-on-Bone Instrumentation for Single Curve Idiopathic Scoliosis. Spine 28(205):S224–33.
33. Rubery PT, Bradford DS. Athletic activity after spinal surgery in children and adolescents. Results of survey. Spine. 2002;27:423-7.
34. Winter RB, Lonstein JE, Heithoff KB, Kirkham JA. Magnetic resonance imaging evaluation of the adolescent patient with idiopathic scoliosis before spinal instrumentation and fusion. A prospective, double-blinded study of 140 patients. Spine. 1997; 22:855-8.
35. Pahys JM, Guille JT, D'Andrea LP et al. Neurologic injury in the surgical treatment of idiopathic scoliosis: guidelines for assessment and management. J Am Acad Orthop Surg. 2009;17:426-34.
36. Clark C, Shufllebarger H, Late-developed infection in instrumented idiopathic scoliosis. Spine. 1999; 24:1909-12.
37. Richards B, Emara K. Delayed infections after posterior TSRH instrumentation for idiopathic scoliosis: revisited. Spine. 2001;26:1990-6.
38. Cronk K, Martirosyan N, Theodore. N. Procalcitonin as an early markr for postoperative infection for cases of elective spinal surgery Abstracts from: International Meeting on Advanced Spine Techniques, July 13-16, 2011, Copenhagen, Denmark.
39. Roye DP, Farcy JP, Rickert JP, Godfried D. Results of the spinal instrumentation of adolescent idiopathic scoliosis by King type. Spine. 1992; 17 (Suppl.): 270-3.
40. Hwang SW, Marks MC, Bastrom T, Newton PO, Betz RR, Cahill PJ. Factor associated with loss of coronal deformity correction in patients with AIS. Annual Meeting of Scoliosis Research Society: 2010 Sep. 23; Kyoto, Japan.
41. Lowe TG, Peters JD. Anterior spinal fusion with Zielke instrumentation for idiopathic scoliosis. A frontal and sagittal curve analysis in 36 patients. Spine. 1993;18:423-6.
42. Moskowitz A, Trommanhauser S. Surgical and clinical results of scoliosis surgery using Zielke instrumentation. Spine. 1993; 18:2444-51.
43. Richards BC. Delayed infection followed posterior spinal instrumentation for the treatment of idiopathic scoliosis. J. Bone and Joint Surg (Am). 1995;77:524-9.
44. Padua R, Padua S, Aulisa L, Ceccarelli C, Padua L, Romanini E, Zanoli G, Campi A. Patient outcomes after Harrington instrumentations for idiopathic scoliosis: a 15- to 28-year evaluation. Spine. 2001; 26:1268-73.
45. Dobbs MB, Lenke LG, Bridwell KH. Cureve patterns in infantile and juvenile idiopathic scolisis.

CHAPTER

21

Posterior Correction Techniques in Adolescent Idiopathic Scoliosis

Suken A Shah

Introduction

Idiopathic scoliosis is a three-dimensional deformity: lateral deviation in the coronal plane, thoracic hypokyphosis in the sagittal plane, and rotation in the transverse plane. With pedicle screw fixation and modern corrective techniques, true three-dimensional correction of the spinal deformity can be accomplished. Intuitively, in typical thoracic AIS, this would mean optimal coronal correction, restoration of thoracic kyphosis and realignment of thoracic torsion by lifting the concavity out of the chest and reducing the convex rib deformity without the need for thoracoplasty. There is no single technique for scoliosis correction that will work in every situation. Careful preoperative planning to maximize the usefulness of implants and observation of the correction intraoperatively is mandatory for success. Criteria to be considered are: spinal flexibility, the material properties of the implants being used, the type of vertebral fixation to be employed, and the reduction techniques which are anticipated. With respect to spinal flexibility, an assessment should be made regarding how much correction is possible or necessary. Both coronal and sagittal plane flexibility should be considered. Hypokyphotic or lordotic thoracic deformities are often very difficult to reduce with posterior-only techniques. Is a release required to achieve the necessary correction? If so, what sort of release is needed? Is a simple intraspinous ligament resection with facetectomy sufficient or is some sort of osteotomy required? Flexible spines usually respond to any reduction maneuver. Stiff spines may defy all attempts at reduction until appropriately mobilized with a combination of techniques.

Implant Properties

The material properties of implants are an important consideration during preoperative planning. By varying rod diameter and composition, a surgeon can match the stiffness of the rod to the stiffness of the curve and/or the quality of the bone. Stainless steel (SS) has distinct advantages in deformity correction. The stiffness and strength of SS is a benefit when reducing the spine to the rod as there is increased correction power in conforming the spine to the rod and less potential for rod deformation. For example, for a stiff, lordotic thoracic scoliosis, SS would provide a better correction in both planes than a titanium (Ti) rod which would be expected to bend into the deformity and provide less corrective ability. However, there is such a thing as a rod that is too stiff: if the stiffness of the rod exceeds the strength of the bone-implant interface, implant pullout is possible. The bending characteristics of stainless steel (SS) allows *insitu* contouring for challenging coronal and sagittal plane deformities because it undergoes plastic deformation in a narrower range while the elastic property of Ti does not. Although, SS is stiffer and stronger than Ti; while Ti is more elastic, once the construct is assembled both materials are acceptable, since construct rigidity is also dependent on the number and type of anchors.

Titanium has other cited advantages in the areas of imaging, infection, corrosion and sensitivity.[1,2] Because of decreased artifact creation with Ti, better postoperative computed tomography (CT) and magnetic resonance (MR) imaging has made it more popular than SS, especially in certain situations in which visualization within the canal or evaluation of adjacent segment degeneration is valuable for clinical decision making. Some centers favor the use of Ti for its resistance to infection, since it does not easily allow the formation of bacterial glycocalyx on its surface to harbor organisms that may cause late-onset deep infection; in addition, the surface composition and ion charge are more osteoblast-friendly. Explant corrosion studies cite less corrosion is present in Ti constructs, which may also be a factor in decreasing infection, since host immune responses are tempered.[3] Furthermore, Ti is a better choice in patients who have a known sensitivity to nickel, a component of the SS alloy.

For those surgeons who favor Ti implants, but are frequently disappointed by the lack of strength and stiffness in a deformity application, cobalt chromium (CoCr) rods may offer a satisfactory compromise. CoCr material properties are close to that of SS in the same diameter and are compatible with Ti spinal anchors, so a surgeon seeking to use Ti implants may not need to give up corrective capacity when using CoCr rods. Other materials that may be available in the future are nitinol, a super elastic nickel-titanium alloy that has shape memory properties, and dynamic rods made of PEEK or polyethylene polymers.

The properly contoured and applied rod provides the majority of the deformity correction. There are many reduction maneuvers that can be applied during deformity correction. The most effective reduction maneuvers will be performed while only one rod is in place. The second rod adds stability and resistance to fatigue failure. Occasionally, temporary or working rods may be required to facilitate reduction. These working rods will usually be placed on the side opposite to the correcting or primary rod. Three column osteotomy corrections, large curves with non-harmonious sagittal segments or one long curve with different sagittal contours within it are common indication for temporary or working rods.

To a large degree, the techniques employed to achieve deformity correction depends on the spinal implants used for fixation. Reduction techniques possible with first generation implants using nonsegmental hooks (Harrington) were limited to global *en bloc* distraction of multiple vertebral segments, correcting the coronal plane, often at the sacrifice of the sagittal plane. Second generation implant systems employing "segmental hook" constructs (Cotrel-Dubousset) allowed some flexibility in applying distraction as well as compressive forces across the deformity.[4] Although providing some additional options to achieve reduction of spinal deformity, the hook and wire based systems fell short in several important ways. First, even the "segmental hook" systems did not allow truly segmental (every level) fixation and neither the hook or wire constructs provide rigid fixation, and therefore complete control, over the vertebral segments. Currently available pedicle screw systems overcome both of these failings by allowing truly segmental spinal fixation at every level as well as direct control over each vertebral segment. Now with the ability to directly control each individual segment, the ability to reduce the spinal deformity has more to do with the adequacy of release (i.e. spinal mobilization), the creativity in designing reduction maneuvers that take into account the response of the spine during reduction and the persistence of the surgeon in attempting to achieve complete reduction of the deformity.

The type of vertebral body fixation devices used will also dictate or influence reduction strategies. Monoaxial, uniplanar, polyaxial reduction screws, hooks and wires will lend themselves to specific reduction strategies. The type of implant and its position in the construct should be considered in the preoperative planning stages.

Correction Maneuvers

This text includes a variety of techniques and maneuvers that can be applied individually or in combination to achieve spinal deformity reduction. Where at one time, the technique for reduction of scoliosis was dictated by the implants or by philosophical constraints now multiple techniques can be applied to achieve deformity correction. Not every technique will work equally well in all situations thus the success of scoliosis correction is dependent on the adequacy of spinal release and the skill and experience of the surgeon in applying the techniques.

Compression–Distraction

Distraction on the concave rod decreases scoliosis. In the thoracic spine distraction also increases thoracic kyphosis which is generally desirable, given the frequent loss of normal thoracic kyphosis noted in idiopathic scoliosis deformities. Compression is useful to reduce hyperkyphotic thoracic deformities. Similarly, compression applied to implants along the rod on the convex side of the lumbar deformity both corrects scoliosis and restores or maintains lumbar lordosis. When compression–distraction is used as a primary reduction maneuver, it is important to remember the kyphosing and lordosing effects of these techniques so as not to negatively affect spinal balance in the sagittal plane. However when compression–distraction is used primarily as a technique to fine tune the reduction after both rods are in place and appropriately contoured, the positive and negative consequences of intrasegmental compression and distraction on sagittal profile are probably negligible. This segmental fine tuning is particularly enhanced by using bilateral, segmental, pedicle screws. The possible negative effects of this technique include transmitting assymetric forces to adjacent levels, especially the adjacent uninstrumented levels resulting in junctional malalignment. The use of excessive forces may loosen implants. Fixed-angle or monoaxial screws do not lend themselves to this technique, since they need to either plow through the pedicle or return to their previous orientation (pre-compression or distraction) when the set screws are tightened and the screw head must be perpendicular to the rod for a secure connection. Uniplanar or polyaxial screws are effective in compression–distraction maneuvers. Distraction of the thoracic spine to induce kyphosis in the typical hypokyphotic AIS situation is more effective when adequate releases of the facets and ligamentum flavum are performed, but should be done with caution.

Rod Derotation Maneuver

For a typical lordotic thoracic curve, the classic "derotation" maneuver of Cotrel and Dubousset may be applied.[4] A rod contoured for the coronal plane deformity is placed in the screws on the concave side. The set screws should be engaged within the screw head but not tightened. The rod is then rotated in the correct position. The second rod is then placed. This technique theoretically converts lateral deviation into deviation in the sagittal plane. Given that thoracic curvatures are often hypokyphotic, this maneuver can often both correct coronal plane deformity and restore natural thoracic kyphosis. However, there are some points that should be made regarding this technique. Most important, the derotation really amounts to lateral translation or an *insitu* relocation of the apex when using this "*en bloc*" derotation maneuver. In addition, the desired sagittal contour is rarely concordant with the coronal plane of the scoliotic deformity. Hence, the conversion from coronal plane deformity to kyphosis or lordosis may occur at the wrong location. In addition, the rod must be stiff enough to maintain its contoured shape, the bone is strong enough to withstand screw pullout and the spine is flexible enough to be displaced posteriorly. This technique may not work well with Ti rods which are more flexible than SS and have a tendency to "bend-out" and lose the sagittal contour that was made prior to implantation.

Proponents of the Cotrel-Dubousset procedure believed that rotational correction of the scoliosis would occur with the rod derotation maneuver. This was later disproved with pre- and postoperative computerized tomography (CT) scans of instrumented patients. Labelle et al. used three dimensional digitizers intraoperatively and showed that the Cotrel-Dubousset rod derotation maneuver did exert coronal and sagittal plane correction and relocated the instrumented portion of the spine, but little axial plane rotation had occurred.[5] Hook and wire fixation lack the ability to derotate the spine because force is applied posterior to the instantaneous axis of rotation (IAR) and the moment arm is inadequate to apply sufficient torque. True correction of axial plane vertebral rotation, and consequently, elimination of the convex thoracic or thoracolumbar prominence, is difficult to achieve without anterior diskectomy and chest wall violation with thoracoplasty.

In Situ Contouring

Using appropriate bending tools both coronal and sagittal plane *in situ* contouring can improve spinal alignment. This is a very useful technique to re-establish the coronal contour if the rod bends out during rod rotation. It is much easier to effectively change the coronal than the sagittal plane once all the implants are engaged on the rod. The *in situ* sagittal benders are often very useful in persuading the rod into the implants during difficult rod-to-implant reductions. The sagittal benders are also very helpful in creating lumbar lordosis. Using either technique, great care should be exercised to prevent catastrophic failure of fixation in the vertebral body. This is especially a concern if using hooks for vertebral fixation. *In situ* contouring is not a useful technique with titanium rods because they require too much bend (deformation distance) to reach the plastic range to make to make this technique practical. This technique also does not work well to improve thoracic hypokyphosis.

Coronal and Sagittal Translation

For the correction of thoracic curves, pure translation is very effective. This can be achieved using either sublaminar wires or reduction screws on the concave side of the apical and periapical vertebrae. Reduction screws can be placed in the 4 or 5 apical and periapical levels to facilitate rod placement and deformity correction. The sequence to reduction by translation involves first placing the rod in the distal or proximal implants, which are then closed loosely. Next the rod is sequentially reduced into each adjacent implant, including the reduction implants. The reduction screws are initially left untightened. Rings should be placed on the reduction implants to prevent premature release of the reduction screw flanges. Finally, the rod is introduced into the most cephalad or distal implants which is loosely closed. The rod which has been precontoured into the desired sagittal contour and straight in the coronal plane is rotated into the correct sagittal and coronal orientation. The inner screws on the reduction implants are then slowly and sequentially tightened to achieve reduction of the spine by pulling the spine to the rod. This results in correction of the scoliosis and produces posterior sagittal plane translation, producing kyphosis. The benefits of this technique include that it allows slow reduction of the deformity, taking advantage of viscoelastic creep. It also allows the forces of reduction to be distributed over each segment of the deformity. The screws serve both as the final implants and the tools for reduction, eliminating the need for any additional instrumentation in the operative site. The extended tabs allow rotation of the rod into the final position with little stress applied to the rod. This helps to prevent rod "bend-out". Translation with reduction screws is not as effective with stiff curves or with titanium rods for the reasons mentioned above. Care must be taken to look for screw pull-out. To some degree this is prevented by assessing the flexibility of the curve, the strength of the bone and being satisfied with a reasonable reduction. Maximizing the diameter, length and position of the screw within the vertebral body may also help prevent screw pullout.

"En Bloc" Vertebral Derotation

An alternative reduction technique is regional vertebral derotation. This technique is employed after the Cotrel-Dubousset method of rod derotation when the rod is in its final position. The maneuver involves direct application of force to the entire periapical segment from the convex side. This is achieved by placing devices on the convex pedicle screws that facilitate a derotation moment to be imparted to 3 or 4 of the periapical vertebrae. This produces derotation around the concave rod. Once this is done the set screws are tightened to hold the vertebra in place.

Direct Vertebral Body Derotation

The challenges of three dimensional correction of scoliosis with posterior-only surgery are well addressed with the use of segmental pedicle screw fixation, and, specifically the application of direct vertebral rotation, first described by Lee et al.[6] Pedicle screws extend into the vertebral body, anterior to the IAR and can be manipulated with the use of long derotator instruments attached to the screw heads to achieve true three-dimensional correction of the scoliotic deformity. Segmental fixation with pedicle screws addresses the most rigid, rotated portion of the spine, spreads the corrective force over multiple implants, can pull the concavity out of the chest and will result in little loss of correction over time.

The concept is the same as for regional derotation but instead the maneuver is applied to an individual vertebrae segment. This technique allows segmental derotation incrementally in the same way that repeated compression and distraction maneuvers can be used to incrementally improve coronal alignment. To use this technique, the concave screw must be loose during the derotation. It may also be beneficial to have the vertebra above and below mobile. The sequence can be initiated from either end. Stabilize the distal and proximal end of the construct by tightening the set screws, and then derotate the adjacent level by directly applying a derotation moment to the vertebra through the screw on the contralateral side. Once the desired derotation has been achieved tighten the set screw. Repeat this maneuver at each instrumented level. Additional derotation can be achieved by repeating the process at each level until satisfied.

The goals of vertebral derotation are to achieve true three dimensional correction of the spinal deformity and reverse the torsional asymmetry induced by scoliosis. Intuitively, in typical thoracic AIS, this would mean optimal coronal correction, restoration of thoracic kyphosis and realignment of the thoracic torsion by lifting the concavity out of the chest and reducing the convex rib deformity. The upper and lower instrumented vertebrae would be level and along with the apex, brought into the stable zone as defined by the center sacral vertical line. The rib prominence would be virtually eliminated without thoracoplasty (Fig. 21.1).

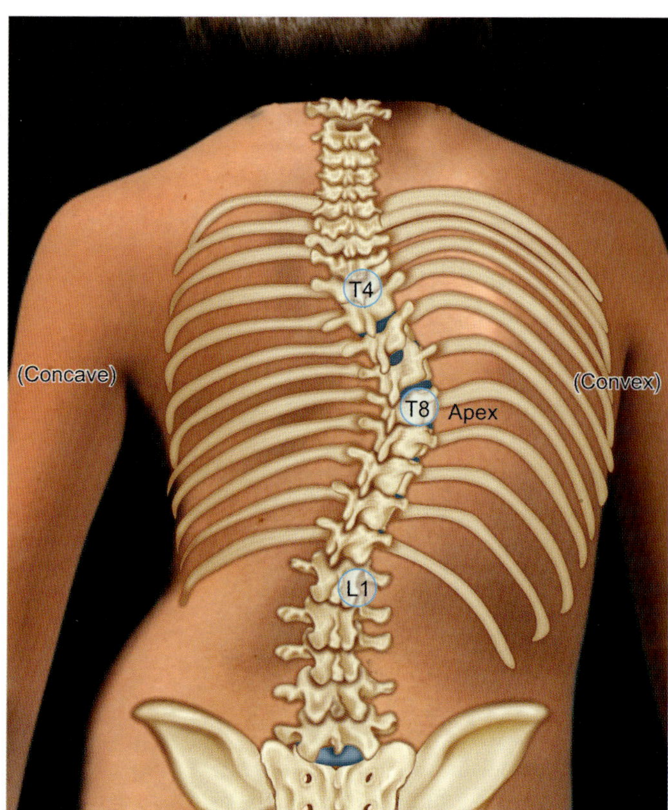

Fig. 21.1 Posterior view of a patient with Lenke type I right thoracic scoliosis showing the typical trunk shift, rib asymmetry, and convex rib prominence

Some technical considerations are important in execution of this technique safely and effectively. Fixed angle pedicle screws offer better axial plane control of the vertebral segment than polyaxial screws [7] and an attempt should be made to employ them in the strategic areas, i.e. the apex of the deformity. Recently, uniplanar screw technology has become available which allows the cephalad/caudad movement of a polyaxial screw, but still remains fixed in the coronal and axial plane for vertebral body derotation maneuvers. Application of force to the screws should be slow, deliberate and controlled, and depends on the bone mineral density and integrity of the bone-screw interface. More force can be applied to the convex screws, as these pedicles are typically larger than the concave pedicles in the apex of the scoliosis[8] and the medial wall of the pedicle is thicker than the lateral wall of the pedicle. [9] When rotated to failure, the convex screws will fracture the medial wall and enter the spinal canal; the concave screws will fracture the lateral pedicle wall, rib/pedicle unit and transverse process and could injure the aorta.[10] Lastly, care must be taken not to transfer torsional forces outside the instrumented segments to compensatory curves or neutrally rotated vertebral levels and create iatrogenic torsion—the neutral end vertebrae must be locked prior to derotation of the apical levels.[11]

Derotation via Differential Rod Contouring

To some degree, differential contouring in the sagittal plane between the convex and concave rod can be used to apply some derotational forces to the apical vertebrae. In a typical right convex hypokyphotic or lordotic thoracic curve, the concave left side of the apical vertebrae needs to be displaced or rotated more posteriorly, while the convex right side of these vertebrae needs to be rotated anteriorly. To produce this derotation moment in the transverse plane, slight hyperkyphosis is contoured into the left rod compared to the hypokyphosis in the right rod.[11] Bilateral segmental pedicle screw fixation can effectively apply these moments to the vertebra. This corrective torque may be helpful in reducing this plane of deformity (Fig. 21.2)

Cantilever Technique

Cantilever techniques find their greatest usefulness in kyphosis. However, in the hyperkyphotic thoracic curve or in the lumbar spine, a cantilever technique can be used to achieve the coronal correction and induce relative or absolute lordosis as needed. In these cases the convex rod may be placed first. Bilateral screws are preferred as vertebral anchors in this circumstance. Rod insertion may be started either proximally or distally. Then using a cantilever maneuver, sequentially reduce the rod into each implant and loosely tighten. This is followed by appropriate compression and distraction to finalize the correction. At this point, if there is no residual coronal deformity, simply retighten the implants and finish. If there is a significant residual coronal or rotational deformity, the inter-vertebral derotation maneuver described above can be performed prior to placement of the second rod. Finally, the second rod is inserted and the set screws tightened.

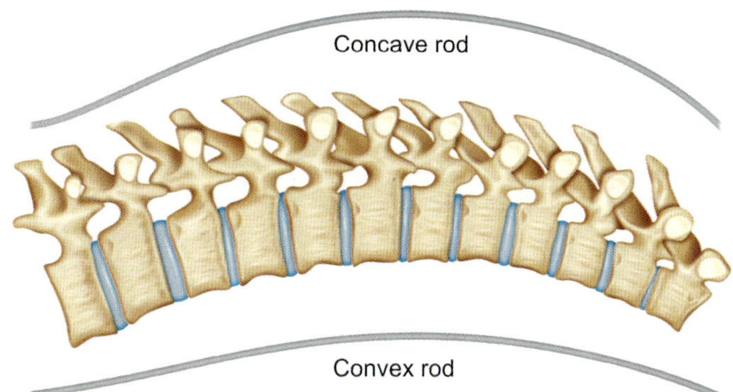

Fig. 21.2 Differential rod contouring: The concave rod will pull the apical vertebrae dorsally out of the chest, and the convex rod is relatively underbent to reduce the convex rib prominence

Traction

Traction has been used extensively in the past, had fallen out of favor as a routine method to achieve correction of deformity as implant technology progressed, but has seen a resurgence in popularity as an option for treatment for rigid, severe curves and early-onset scoliosis. Halo traction can be used preoperatively and is a safe, well-tolerated method of applying gradual, sustained traction to maximize operative correction in patients with severe idiopathic scoliosis and kyphosis. Traction can also be used intraoperatively and between staged procedures. Preinstrumentation traction is facilitated by anterior and posterior releases. The releases can be performed in a staged fashion or together as the initial surgery. This works well for large deformities or in patients who might not be able to tolerate a major anterior posterior reconstruction in one surgical setting. In a multicenter study analyzing the treatment of severe spinal deformities with and without traction, Sponseller et al. found both groups had comparable deformity correction (62% vs. 59%) and complications, but patients in the halo traction group less frequently had a vertebral column resection (Fig. 21.10).[12]

Temporary Working Rods

Working rods are rods that are placed temporarily to facilitate either partial reduction of the entire deformity or a segment of the deformity. The trick to using working rods is to apply them in such a way as to facilitate partial reduction without blocking the ability to reduce the rest of the spine.

The most useful applications of the working rod technique are in the reduction of double curves (Double Major: structural main thoracic and thoracolumbar-lumbar or double thoracic curves: structural upper thoracic and main thoracic curves) and temporary stabilization of spinal osteotomies or resections. If one or both of the curves is very stiff or if the thoracic curves are very lordotic it will be difficult if not impossible to place a single rod the entire length of the deformity and rotate the rod into a corrected position. Attempting to do so will usually result in bending-out of the rod with subsequent ineffective and incomplete reduction. The working rod attempts to overcome this problem by maximizing reduction forces of a rod by applying them to a short segment of the spine which can be more effectively manipulated. Once a segment is realigned then the rest of the deformity can be reduced. For example, placement of a concave lumbar rod in a Double Major deformity as a preliminary step in reduction is especially useful in large highly rotated lumbar curves because the coronal alignment, apical rotation and lordosis can all be addressed independent of the thoracic spine. This part of the reduction often involves a simple derotation maneuver followed by segmental vertebral body derotation and in situ bending if necessary. These maneuvers usually affect significant reduction of the lumbar deformity. With the lumbar spine reduced, the rod bend, insertion sequence, and thoracic reduction maneuvers can then be applied on the thoracic convexity without worrying about the effect that they will have on the lumbar deformity.

A more recently adopted technique involves placement of a rod into the thoracic convexity to achieve partial reduction. This is a useful technique for stiff, lordotic, thoracic curves. The technique must be performed with reductions screws in the concave pedicles and polyaxial screws in the end vertebrae of the thoracic deformity. The rod is contoured into a bit more kyphosis than desired, anticipating that the rod will flatten out some during reduction. The rod is inserted into the screw heads in a scoliotic alignment and rotated into the correct coronal alignment (i.e. straight in the coronal plane and kyphotic in the sagittal plane). The proximal and distal multiaxial screws are locked into place while the reduction screws remain loose. Since the rotation is performed with reduction screws in the apex of the deformity there is only a small amount of stress transferred to the rod and apical reduction screws during the rod rotation maneuver. Once the rod is in the correct sagittal alignment, the reduction feature of the reduction screws is used to slowly translate the spine to the rod. This will affect both translation and derotation. If the curve is not too stiff, complete reduction may be achieved with this maneuver. If the rod begins to bend-out or screw purchase becomes a concern, the reduction on this rod can be temporarily halted. The next step is to bend the contralateral rod into a hypokyphotic sagittal contour and straight in the coronal plane. This rod is inserted into the polyaxial screws on the convexity of the thoracic deformity. Using cantilever forces in both the coronal and sagittal plane, the scoliosis and the convex kyphosis (often due to residual vertebral body rotation) are pushed anteriorly and towards the midline reducing the kyphosis and the scoliosis respectively. This maneuver decreases the forces on the convex working rod. The working rod is now replaced with the permanent concave rod. Once the permanent concave rod is in place the convex screw heads are loosened and final reduction is achieved using the reduction mechanisms on the screws.

Authors' Preferred Technique of Direct Vertebral Rotation in Late-onset Idiopathic Scoliosis

- On the *concave* side: Insert monoaxial or uniplanar screws at every level. Consider using polyaxial reduction screws at the apex of the concavity, particularly for severe curves
- On the *convex* side: Insert monoaxial or uniplanar screws into at least 3-4 convex pedicles at the apex, as well as the proximal and distal foundations
- Confirm placement of screws and check screw length with fluoroscopy or plain X-rays prior to rod insertion.
- Contour the *concave* rod with extra-kyphosis (anticipating that the rod will become flatter during the translation/reduction of the scoliosis) to pull the apical vertebrae dorsally out of the chest, and correct apical lordosis. (Fig. 21.2)
- Contour the *convex* rod with less thoracic kyphosis to push down on the convex side of the vertebral bodies, thus displacing them anteriorly and decreasing the rib prominence. (Fig. 21.2)
- Insert the concave rod into the pedicle screw anchors leaving the set screws loose. (Fig. 21.3)
- The rod can engage the anchors via one or both of the following:
    a. *Translation maneuver*: Insert the rod proximally and distally and tighten the set screws proximally and distally, leaving the rod in the correct sagittal plane. After proximal and distal foundations are connected and locked, apical screws are translated to the rod segmentally by using reduction devices or reduction screws. (Fig. 21.4A)
    b. *Rod rotation Maneuver:* Insert the rod and perform a rod rotation maneuver as in the classic Cotrel-Dubousset Technique (2). In this case, the rod rotates from the midline scoliotic position laterally to the left, approximately 90°. (Fig. 21.4B). During the 90°

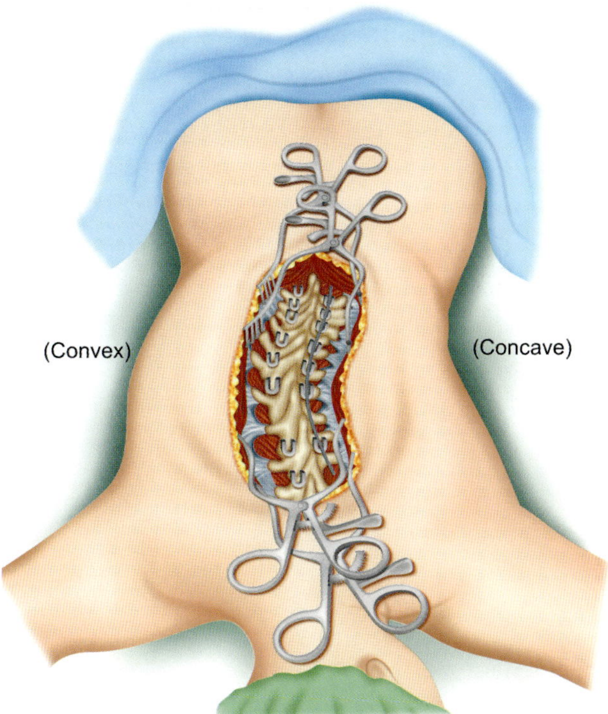

Fig. 21.3 Concave rod inserted with the set screws left loose, prior to translation or derotation

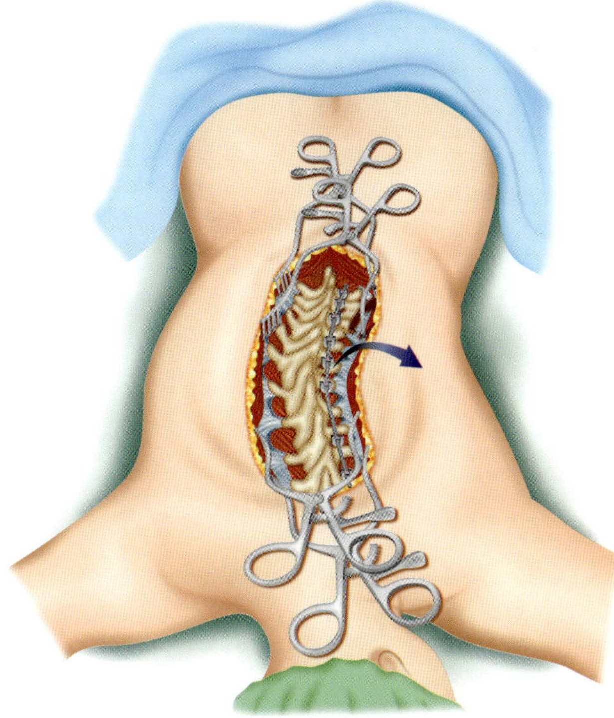

Fig. 21.4B (Alternate method of correction) Rod derotation maneuver with arrow pointing direction of 90° rotation to correct scoliosis in the coronal plane and set rod in the proper sagittal plane

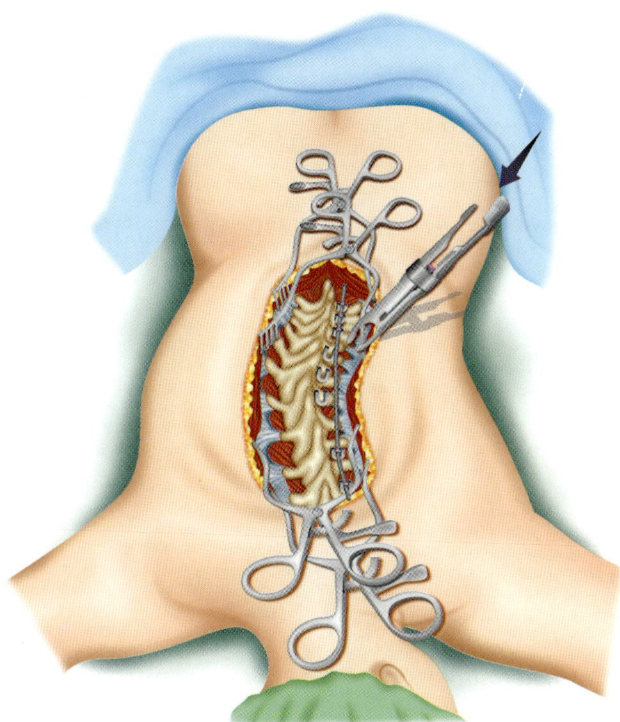

Fig. 21.4A Translational correction of the scoliosis with rod reduction device.

rotation one must have control by pushing down over the convex ribs to avoid aggravating the rib prominence. This accomplishes a translocation of the spine dorsally and medially, but rarely results in true axial plane derotation.

- Finally, proceed with one or both of the Vertebral Body Derotation techniques explained below.

En Bloc Spinal Derotation

- After the concave rod is engaged in all anchors, attach derotation instruments to the apical screw heads on both the concave and convex sides (Fig. 21.5)
- An assistant pushes down on the convex ribs and the convex screws and the concave and convex screws are rotated in the direction that will reduce the rib prominence (counterclockwise in (Figs 21.5 and 21.6). This should be done simultaneously to distribute strain and to limit loading of the bone-screw interface. The rotation of the concave screws will help decrease the torsion and will lift the concavity out of the chest. (Figs 21.5 and 21.6)
- A rehearsal of this maneuver prior to rod insertion can be helpful to gain a sense of how much force is to be applied safely

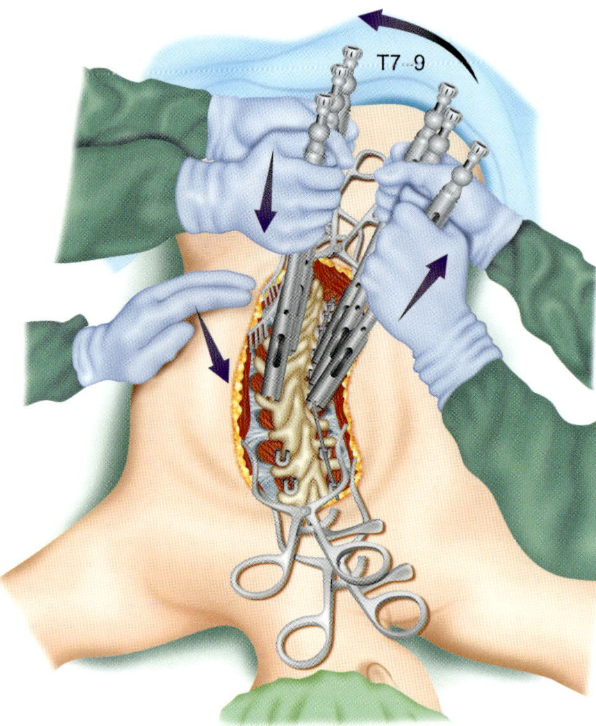

Fig. 21.5 *En bloc* derotation of the thoracic apex with derotators attached to pedicle screws; only the conave rod is implanted at this point, and serves as the axis of rotation

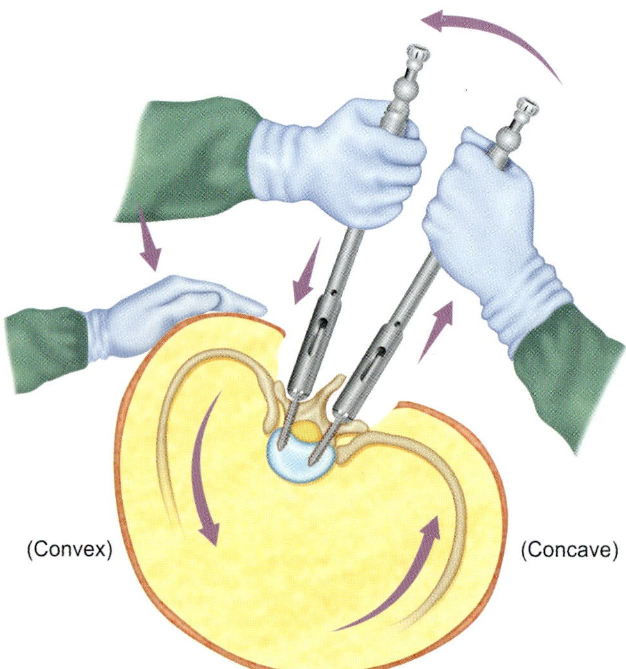

Fig. 21.6 Axial view of the spinal derotation concept: The screws on the concavity are pulled up and over, the screws on the convexity are pushed down and laterally from midline and an assistant pushes down on the convex rib prominence to distribute forces

- Tighten the set screws on the concave rod holding this position and perhaps distracting the screws along the apex to achieve additional coronal correction and better kyphosis restoration (Fig. 21.7A)
- Implant the convex rod and tighten the set screws on the convex side (Fig. 21.7B).

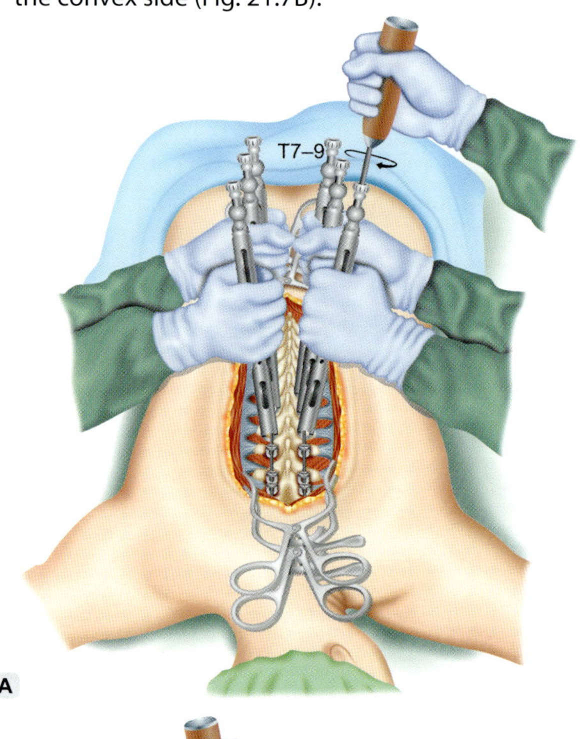

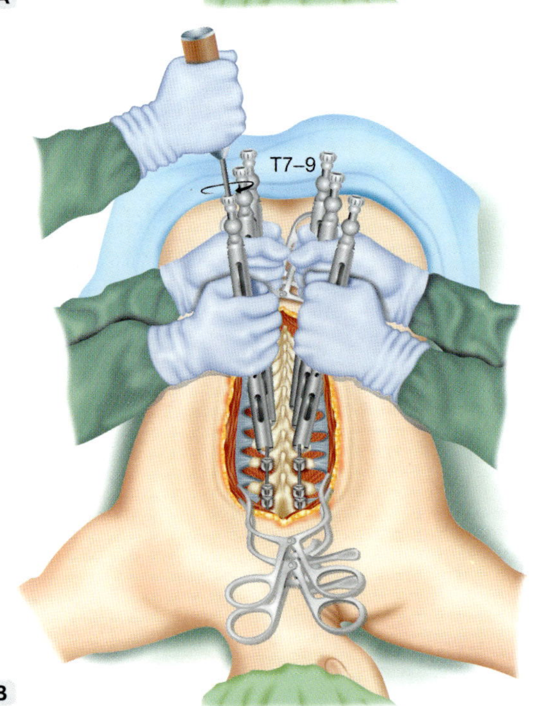

Fig. 21.7 *En bloc* derotation with concave rod implanted and set screws tightened (A), then the convex rod is implanted with rotation held corrected while set screws are tightened (B)

Segmental Spinal Derotation (Individual Vertebral Level)

Segmental vertebral body derotation can be done as the sole derotation maneuver or in addition to the *en bloc* maneuver described above.

- Implant both rods and capture them with set screws. Most set screws should be left loose since lengthening of the spine is expected at each level that will be segmentally derotated. Only the set screws in the distal neutral vertebra should be tightened (e.g. L1 in Fig. 21.8), since derotation will be based on this neutral level and no torsional forces will be transmitted distally.
- Attach two derotators in the distal segment to lock the bottom neutral vertebra. Then attach derotators in the next proximal 1–2 vertebrae. The derotators on the distal vertebra must be held by an assistant to provide counter-rotation force.
- Derotate each proximal vertebral body sequentially to achieve a neutral position in reference to the neutral distal vertebra (Fig. 21.9.). After derotation of each segment, the set screws are tightened. Repeat this process, moving along towards the apex.

Fig. 21.8 Segmental spinal derotation: Starting at the lowest instrumented vertebra in neutral alignment and securing its position with both rods implanted

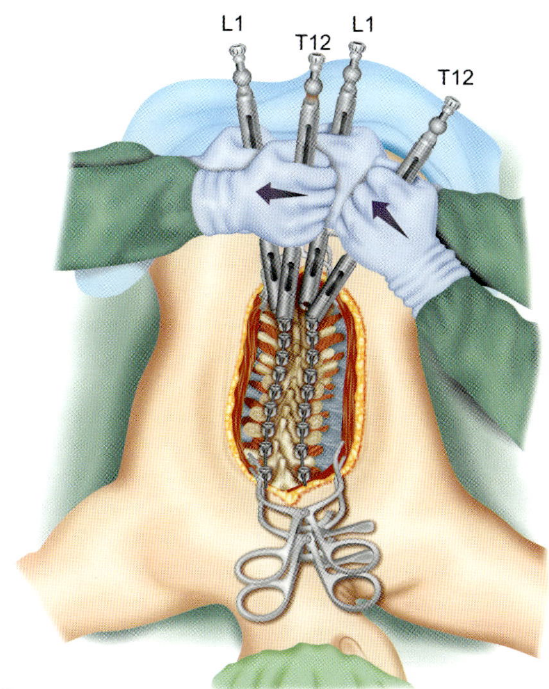

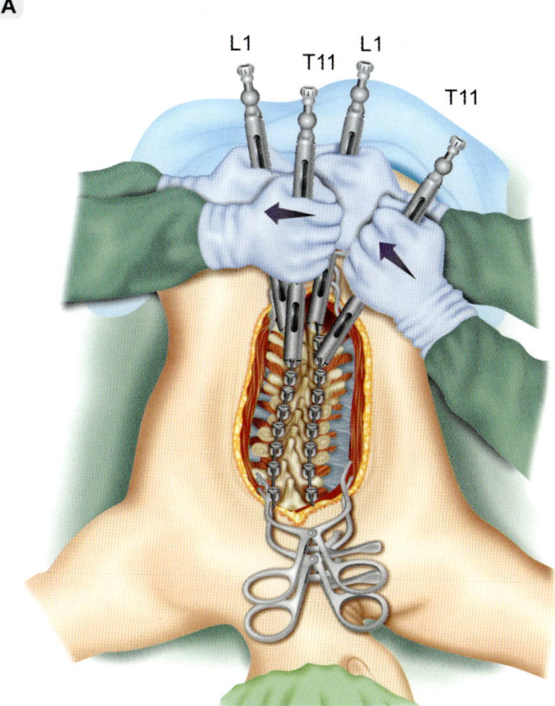

Fig. 21.9 Segmental spinal derotation: With the lowest instrumented vertebra held in counter-torsion, derotators are used sequentially proceeding cephalad, adjusting the axial plane rotation relative to neutral at each segment.

Source: Figures 21.1 to 21.9 by James Millerick, ©2006 DePuy Spine, Inc., used with permission.

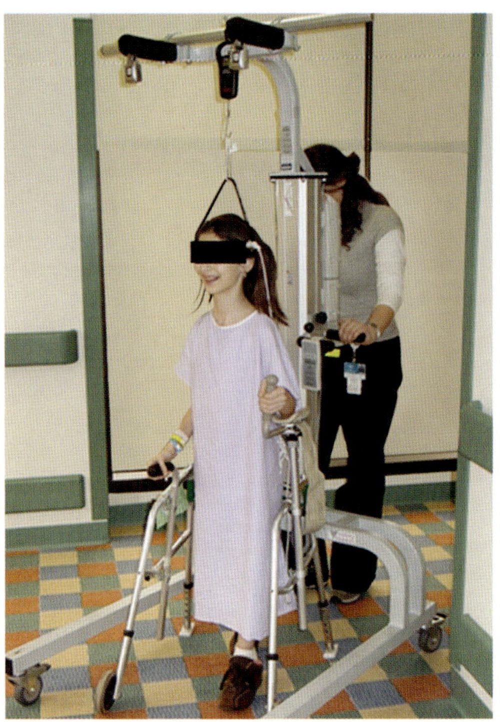

Fig. 21.10 Traction method

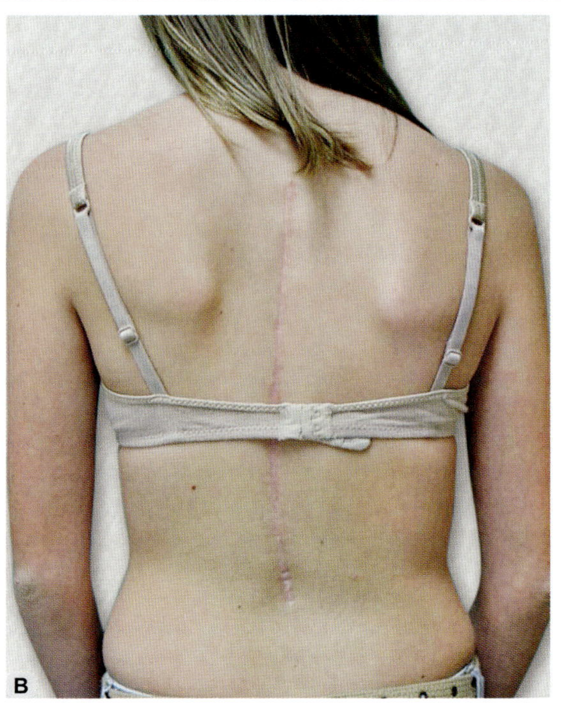

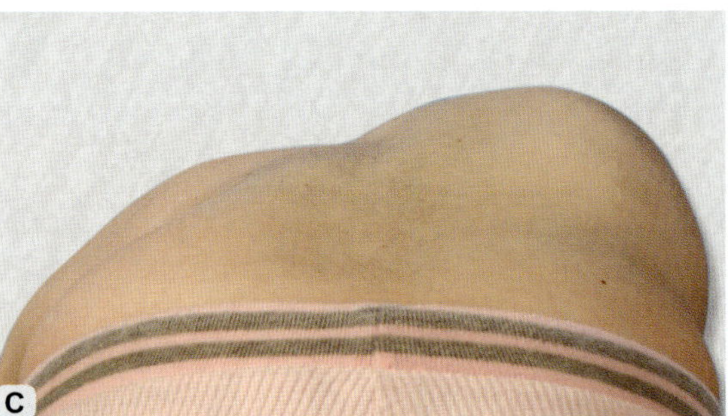

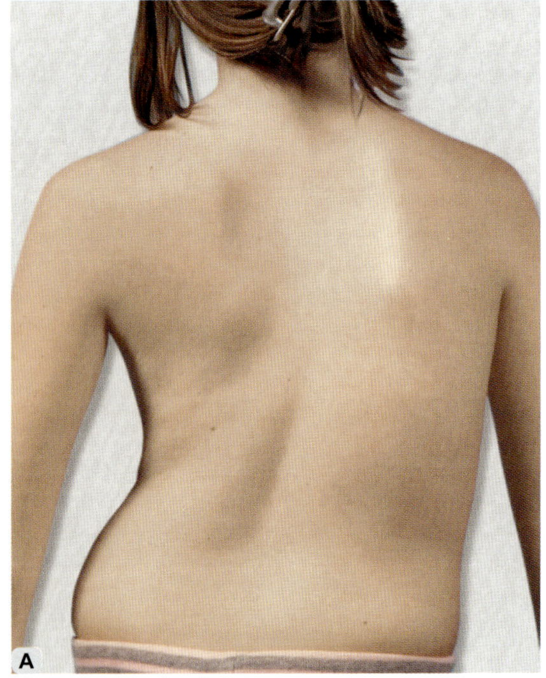

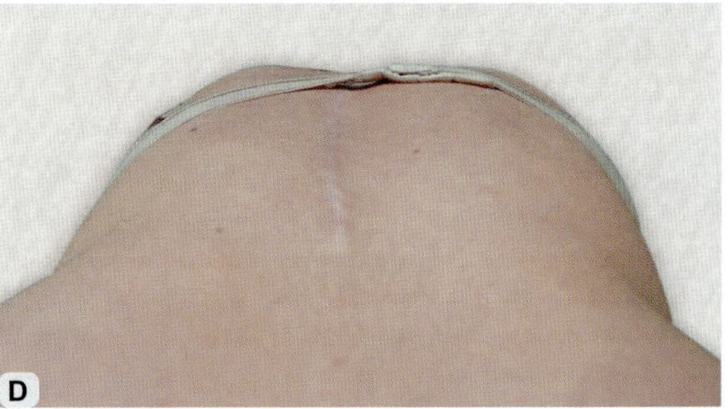

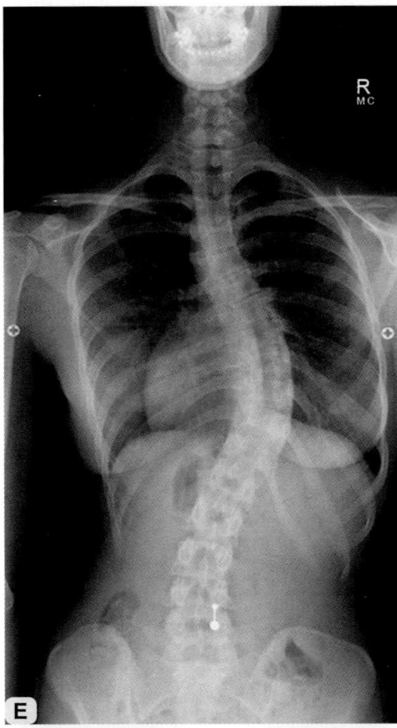

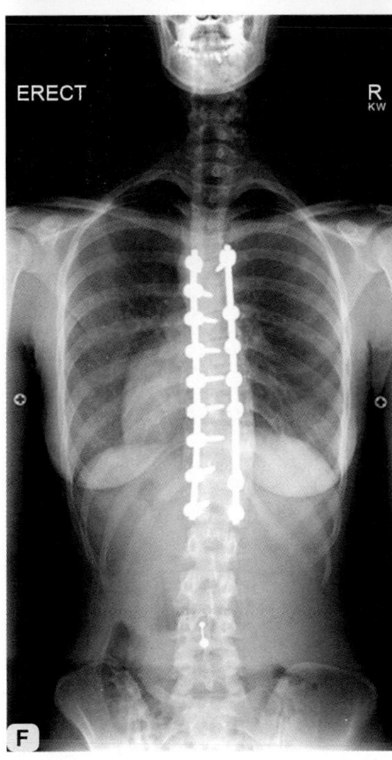

Fig. 21.11 Clinical photos and radiographs: pre- and postoperatively (2-year-follow-up) of a 13-year-old female with adolescent idiopathic scoliosis. Note correction of truncal shift, thoracic torsion, rib asymmetry and rib prominence on forward bend after surgery with segmental pedicle screw fixation and vertebral derotation without thoracoplasty. (A) Preoperative clinical photo; (B) 2-year postoperative clinical photo; (C) Preoperative forward bend photo; (D) 2-year postoperative forward bend photo; (E) Preoperative PA X-ray; (F) 2-year postoperative PA X-ray

- Complete neutral derotation might not be achieved at the apex relative to its torsion to the axial plane. Revisiting the apical levels after a few minutes may allow additional correction due to viscoelastic relaxation of the spine. Care must be taken not to loosen the bone-screw interface while performing the maneuver.
- Repeat the derotation for each segment, until all vertebral levels nearly match the neutrally rotated distal vertebra. During segmental spinal derotation, segmental compression (convexity) and/or distraction (concavity) may be simultaneously applied to effect maximal correction, just before the set screws are finally tightened.

Authors' Preferred Technique of Spinal Deformity Reduction

For typical right convex hypokyphotic late onset scoliosis, the authors use a 5.5 mm stainless steel system and place bilateral segmental pedicle screws, the majority of which are uniplanar screws. In the periapical vertebra, polyaxial reduction screws are placed for larger deformities. On the convex side, uniplanar screws are placed at every level. The concave rod, which is overbent in kyphosis to affect the sagittal plane (technique #7) is placed and a rod derotation is performed to align the rod in the proper sagittal plane (technique #2). Because of the use of periapical reduction screws, this maneuver does not typically result in a significant amount of correction. Coronal translation is achieved as described above using reduction screws (technique #4). If this maneuver results in rod deformation corrective coronal and sagittal *in situ* contouring is performed (technique #3). Next gentle compression and distraction is performed to further decrease the deformity by lengthening the concavity and shortening the convexity (technique #1); this will result in some establishment of thoracic kyphosis as well. *En bloc* vertebral derotation is then performed (technique #5). If additional derotation is necessary direct vertebral body derotation is performed (technique #6) and usually revisited after both rods are implanted and sufficient time for creep and viscoelastic relaxtion has passed. After this maneuver, if any residual apical rotation persists then differential rod contouring is used during placement of the convex rod (technique #7). During this maneuver the concave periapical screws must be loose on the rod to allow derotation of the apical vertebra around the concave rod. The derotation force results from a posterior to anterior cantilever force which is applied as the hypokyphotic convex rod is being seated into the apical screws at the convex apical kyphosis. Once both rods are in place, a final round of compression and distraction is applied to fine tune the segmental correction (technique #1) and to horizontalize the upper and lower instrumented vertebral bodies, when desirable. Once all the instrumentation is in place, the alignment should be checked radiographically. Careful attention should be given to the end instrumented segments to assess how they influence the alignment of the uninstrumented spine, particularly at the junction of instrumented and uninstrumented segments. This will help prevent unacceptable postoperative junctional rotation or tilt (Fig. 21.11).

Summary

There are many techniques to choose from with regard to construct design and deformity correction. Multiple methods can ultimately be chosen and this will depend upon the requirements of the patient's deformity, the preference of the surgeon and the available implants.

References

1. Wang JC, Sandhu HS, Yu WD, Minchew JT, Delamarter RB. MR parameters for imaging titanium spinal instrumentation. J Spinal Disord. 1997;10:27-32.
2. Soultanis KC, Pyroovolou N, Zahos KA, et al. Late postoperative infection following spinal instrumentation: stainless steel versus titanium implants. J Surg Orthop Adv. 2008;17:193-9.
3. Kirkpatrick JS, Venugopalan R, Beck P, Lemons J. Corrosion on spinal implants. J Spinal Disord Tech. 2005;18:247-51.
4. Dubousset J, Cotrel Y. Application technique of Cotrel-Dubousset instrumentation for scoliosis deformities. Clin Orthop Relat Res. 1991:103-10.
5. Labelle H, Dansereau J, Bellefleur C, de Guise J, Rivard CH, Poitras B. Peroperative three-dimensional correction of idiopathic scoliosis with the Cotrel-Dubousset procedure. Spine. 1995;20:1406-9.
6. Lee SM, Suk SI, Chung ER. Direct vertebral rotation: a new technique of three-dimensional deformity correction with segmental pedicle screw fixation in adolescent idiopathic scoliosis. Spine. 2004;29:343-9.
7. Kuklo TR, Potter BK, Polly DW Jr, Lenke LG. Monaxial versus multiaxial thoracic pedicle screws in the correction of adolescent idiopathic scoliosis. Spine. 2005;30:2113-20.
8. Parent S, Labelle H, Skalli W, Latimer B, de Guise J. Morphometric analysis of anatomic scoliotic specimens. Spine. 2002;27:2305-11.
9. Kothe R, O'Holleran JD, Liu W, Panjabi MM. Internal architecture of the thoracic pedicle. An anatomic study. Spine. 1996;21:264-70.
10. King A. Derotation of the thoracic spine using pedicle screws, a comparison of concave to convex screws. Scoliosis Research Society - 39th Annual Meeting. Buenos Aires, Argentina, 2004.
11. Shah SA. Derotation of the spine. Neurosurg Clin N Am. 2007;18:339-45.
12. Sponseller PD, Takenaga RK, Newton PO, et al. The use of traction in the treatment of severe spinal deformity. Spine. 2008;33:2305-09.

CHAPTER

22

Minimally Invasive Surgery of Pediatric Spinal Deformity

Amer F Samdani, Ashish S Ranade

Posterior approaches to the spine are associated with muscle atrophy, denervation, and scarring.[1,2] These can potentially increase postoperative pain and hospital stay, and may lead to chronic long-term pain.[3,4] In order to avoid these problems, minimally invasive surgical approaches to the spine have been utilized to treat various pathologies.In comparing minimally invasive surgery (MIS) versus traditional posterior approaches Several authors have shown similar outcomes, with lesser blood loss and lesser hospital stay.[5-7] In trauma scenario, similar benefits have been documented.[8,9] There is paucity of literature on the utility of MIS in deformity surgery. Anand et al. have presented early results of MIS in 12 patients with degenerative scoliosis.[10] These patients were treated with cicumferential fusion though lateral approach and percutaneous pedicle screw placement.

Rationale

The goals of using MIS techniques to pediatric deformity are decreased blood loss, less muscle disruption, and reduced hospital stay with a faster return to normal activities while obtaining similar clinical results as with open procedures. In adolescent idiopathic socliosis, depending on curve flexibility 70–80% correction of the deformity can be expected with standard posterior approach.[11,12] In comparison to the adult degenerative scoliosis, adolescent spine deformity is more flexible and hence more amenable to MIS techniques. Another obstacle in adult deformity is of achieving solid fusion by using stand alone MIS technique. This is less of concern in pediatric deformity as the spine in pediatric patients may fuse spontaneously.[13] In a randomized study comparing posterior fusion of two groups of patients with AIS using no bone graft and allograft only, only one nonunion was found. This nonunion was in the allograft group.[14]

Indications

We have utilized MIS techniques in 38 patients (Table 22.1). The indications are divided into three groups:

1. At the top of long constructs
2. AIS
3. Pedicle screws placed for growing systems

Table 22.1 Summary of patients studied

Total patients	38
Top of the construct	17
AIS	15
Growing systems	6
Age	10.4 years (range, 6–17 years)
Follow-up	13.5 months (2–35 months)
Preoperative major Cobb angle	58 degrees
Postoperative major Cobb angle	21 degrees
Percent correction	64%

Top of Long Constructs

Proximal junctional kyphosis is known to occur after posterior soinal fusion for AIS or Scheurmann's kyphosis.[15,16] In a study of 410 patients with AIS who underwent posterior spinal fusion, the incidence of proximal junctional kyphosis was 27%.[15] In another study by Loner et al. the incidence of junctional kyphosis was 32% in patients with Scheumann's kyphosis treated with posterior spinal fusion.[16] These studies have shown that the number of levels fused and change in thoracic kyphosis are risk factors for the development of proximal junctional kyphosis. Preservation of proximal soft tissues, ligaments, and facets may decrease the incidence of proximal junctional kyphosis. Thus by using MIS approach for pedicle screw placement may minimize soft disruption. Typically, proximal two levels are instrumented through MIS approach. Figure 22.1 shows an example of patient treated with percutaneous placement of pedicle screws at the top of a long construct.

Adolescent Idiopathic Scoliosis

Stand alone MIS technique can be used for an AIS patient with flexible curve. Typically, these curves bend under 30 degrees, and do not show marked lordosis of the thoracic spine (<10 degrees). We use a single midline incision, followed by percutaneous placement of pedicle screws using commercially available instrumentation. We use polyaxial screws to facilitate subfascial rod passage. After rod passage, coronal correction is achieved with a 90 degree rod derotation manoeuvre. Alternatively, we have used the technique described by Vallespir et al.[17] In this technique two rods are passed through the screw extensions on the convexity of the curve and a forced separation of the rods allows for coronal correction of the curve. After coronal correction, attachments to the screw extensions allow derotation maneuver for axial correction. One should keep sagittal profile in mind as these corrective maneuvers in coronal and axial plane may decrease thoracic kyphosis. Patient positioning with appropriate placement of chest pad is important to optimize thoracic kyphosis. Figure 22.2 demonstrates a patient with AIS treated with posterior only MIS.

Patients with stiffer curves that do not bend less than 30 degrees may be treated with a hybrid/open approach. In the hybrid technique, the proximal and distal fixation is placed percutaneously. The apex of the curve is exposed via open approach and multiple Ponte osteotomies are performed. Then the rod is passed subfascially at the proximal and distal ends, with standard rod reduction achieved across the open segments.

To date, we have treated 15 patients with AIS using a MIS approach. The mean age for these patients is 14.1 years and the mean follow-up is of 8 months. The mean preoperative Cobb angle is 54 degrees. We achieved a mean correction of 67% with the mean postoperative Cobb angle of 18 degrees. The thoracic kyphosis decreased from 31 to 26 degrees. Average surgery time was 470 minutes with the average fluoroscopy time of 192 seconds. Complications include pullout of proximal screws in one patient at 8 months postoperatively. This was treated with revision. Table 22.2 shows summary of results.

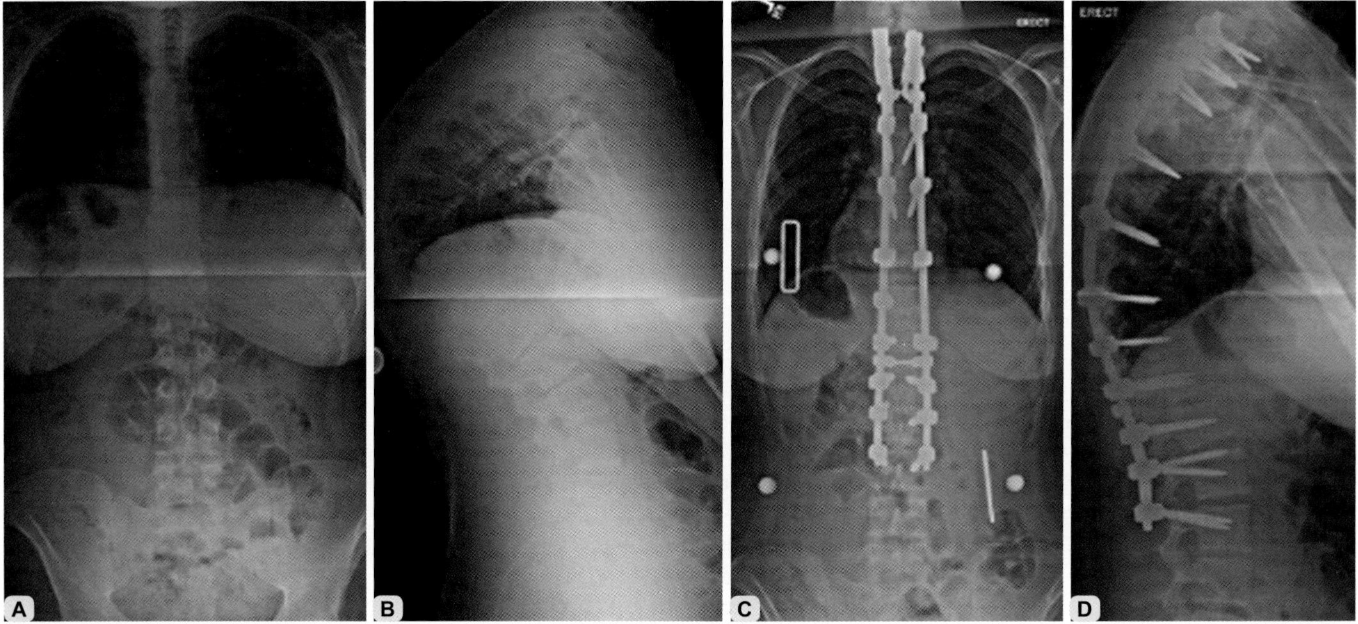

Fig. 22.1 A 15-year-old boy with Scheuermann's kyphosis. Preoperative PA (A) and lateral (B) showed a 96 degree kyphosis with apex at T9. He underwent a T2 – L4 posterior spinal fusion with Ponte osteotomies from T6 to L2 and a pedicle subtraction osteotomy at T9. He underwent MIS placement of pedicle screws at T2–4 bilaterally. Postoperative PA (C) and lateral (D) demonstrated correction of deformity

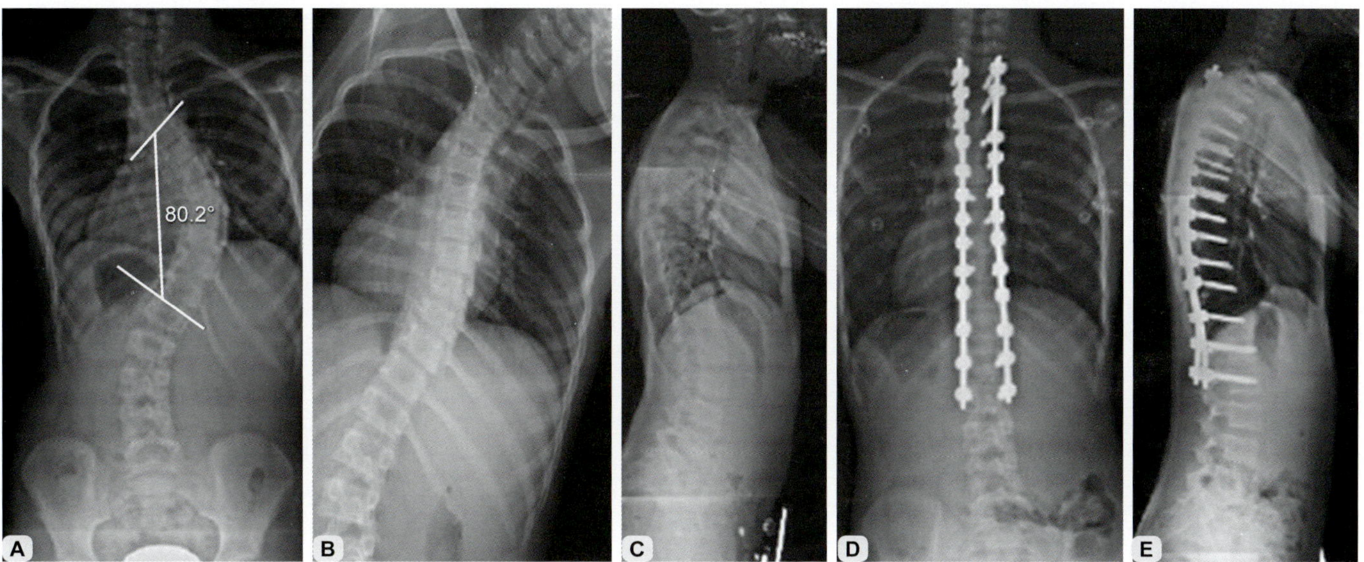

Fig. 22.2 A 12-year-old girl with a right thoracic curve measuring 80 degrees which corrects to 28 degrees on right side bend. Her (A) PA bend film, (B) and (C) lateral are shown. She underwent a T2 to L2 MIS posterior spinal fusion; (D and E) At 18 months postoperatively, good correction was maintained

Table 22.2 AIS patients treated with MIS

Total patients	15
Males	2
Females	13
Age	14.1 years (range, 11–16 years)
Follow-up	8 months (range, 2–35 months)
Major Cobb	
Preoperative	54 degrees (45–82)
Postoperative	18 degrees (9–35)
Percent correction	67%
Thoracic kyphosis	
Preoperative	31 degrees (18–47)
Postoperative	26 degrees (15–34)
Estimated blood loss	254 ml (Range,110–672 mL)
Mean operative time	470 minutes(range, 236–662 minutes)

Growing Systems

Growing systems are used commonly in young children to control spine deformity while allowing for growth.[18] One of the major problems with these growing systems is autofusion of the spine over time.[13] Inadvertent exposure of spinal segments during placement of growing system may be a cause for autofusion. This problem can be minimized by using MIS technique for placement of proximal and distal fixation points.

Fusion Techniques

MIS techniques have concerns about the ability to achieve solid fusion. While using MIS as a standalone treatment for the pediatric deformity, one relies on a facet/lamina fusion. Aggressive decortications with a burr is performed when possible. In addition, curettes were used to decorticate. A mixture of corticocancellous chips with demineralised bone matrix is used and placed prior to pedicle screw placement to ensure appropriate localization. In addition, bone marrow aspirate from the pedicle holes mixed with the bone graft.

The rapid advancement of MIS technology allows for its application for pediatric deformity. The pediatric spine, because of its ability to fuse and inherent flexibility, is ideal for using MIS techniques. Current indications are proximal fixation of a long construct to minimize proximal juntional kyphosis, stand alone treatment of AIS, and percutaneous placement of proximal and distal anchors in growing systems. By utilizing MIS techniques, blood loss is reduced and muscle trauma is minimized; however, operative time and fluoroscopy time are increased especially in the early phases of the learning curve. Clinical results are similar to open procedures for appropriately selected patients. Further studies will refine the indications and clarify the true benefits of using MIS techniques in pediatric deformity.

References

1. Kawaguchi, Y, Matsui, H, Gejo, R, et al. Preventive measures of back muscle injury after posterior lumbar spine surgery in rats. Spine (Phila Pa 1976), 1998; 23, 2282-7; discussion 2288.
2. Kawaguchi, Y, Matsui H, and Tsuji H. Back muscle injury after posterior lumbar spine surgery. A histologic and enzymatic analysis. Spine (Phila Pa 1976). 1996;21:941-4.
3. Sihvonen T, Herno A, Paljarvi L, et al. Local denervation atrophy of paraspinal muscles in postoperative failed back syndrome. Spine (Phila Pa 1976). 1993;18:575-81.
4. Kim DY, Lee SH, Chung SK, et al. Comparison of multifidus muscle atrophy and trunk extension muscle strength: percutaneous versus open pedicle screw fixation. Spine. (Phila Pa 1976). 2005;30:123-9.
5. Dhall SS, Wang MY, and Mummaneni PV. Clinical and radiographic comparison of mini-open transforaminal lumbar interbody fusion with open transforaminal lumbar interbody fusion in 42 patients with long-term follow-up. J Neurosurg Spine. 2008;9:560-5.
6. Park P, Upadhyaya C, Garton, HJ, et al. The impact of minimally invasive spine surgery on perioperative complications in overweight or obese patients. Neurosurgery. 2008;62:693-9; discussion 693-9.
7. Rosen DS, O'Toole JE, Eichholz KM, et al. Minimally invasive lumbar spinal decompression in the elderly: outcomes of 50 patients aged 75 years and older. Neurosurgery. 2004; 60, 503-9; discussion 509-10.
8. Rampersaud YR, Annand N, and Dekutoski MB. Use of minimally invasive surgical techniques in the management of thoracolumbar trauma: current concepts. Spine (Phila Pa 1976). 2006; 31:S96-102; discussion S104.
9. Korovessis P, Hadjipavlou A, and Repantis T. Minimal invasive short posterior instrumentation plus balloon kyphoplasty with calcium phosphate for burst and severe compression lumbar fractures. Spine (Phila Pa 1976). 2008;33:658-67.
10. Anand N, Baron, EM, Thaiyananthan G, et al. Minimally invasive multilevel percutaneous correction and fusion for adult lumbar degenerative scoliosis: a technique and feasibility study. J Spinal Disord Tech. 2008;21:459-67.
11. Lehman RA, Jr, Lenke LG, Keeler KA, et al. Operative treatment of adolescent idiopathic scoliosis with posterior pedicle screw-only constructs: minimum three-year follow-up of one hundred fourteen cases. Spine (Phila Pa 1976). 2008;33:1598-604.
12. Suk SI, Kim JH, Kim, SS, et al. Thoracoplasty in thoracic adolescent idiopathic scoliosis. Spine (Phila Pa 1976). 2008; 33:1061-7.
13. Cahill PJ, Marvil, S, Cuddihy, L, et al. Autofusion in the Immature Spine Treated With Growing Rods. Spine (Phila Pa 1976). 2010.
14. Betz RR, Petrizzo AM, Kerner PJ, et al. Allograft versus no graft with a posterior multisegmented hook system for the treatment of idiopathic scoliosis. Spine (Phila Pa 1976). 2006;31:121-7.
15. Kim YJ, Lenke LG, Bridwell KH, et al. Proximal junctional kyphosis in adolescent idiopathic scoliosis after 3 different types of posterior segmental spinal instrumentation and fusions: incidence and risk factor analysis of 410 cases. Spine (Phila Pa 1976). 2007;32:2731-8.
16. Lonner BS, Newton P, Betz R, et al. Operative management of Scheuermann's kyphosis in 78 patients: radiographic outcomes, complications, and technique. Spine (Phila Pa 1976). 2007;32:2644-52.
17. Vallespir GP, Flores JB, Trigueros, IS, et al. Vertebral coplanar alignment: a standardized technique for three dimensional correction in scoliosis surgery: technical description and preliminary results in Lenke type 1 curves. Spine (Phila Pa 1976). 2008;33:1588-97.
18. Akbarnia BA, Breakwell LM, Marks DS, et al. Dual growing rod technique followed for three to eleven years until final fusion: the effect of frequency of lengthening. Spine (Phila Pa 1976). 2008;33:984-90.

CHAPTER

23

Pedicle Subtraction Osteotomy: Surgical Technique

Munish Gupta

Introduction

Treatment of fixed sagittal imbalance or fixed kyphotic deformities has led to the development of techniques to achieve the necessary correction and restoration of sagittal balance. Techniques, such as Smith-Peterson osteotomy (SPO) as well as pedicle subtraction osteotomy (PSO) have been described and used for over five decades.[1-4] Recently, PSOs have been used to correct sagittal plane as well as coronal plane deformities.[5] The use of PSOs has allowed many surgeons to approach the spine posteriorly alone avoiding anterior release in many cases. The use of PSOs had been used mostly in revision surgeries in the past, but this technique is often used in primary as well as revision deformity corrections.[6] We describe the historical context of the use of posterior wedge resection osteotomies and include a surgical technique as well as pitfalls and pearls for pedicle subtraction osteotomy.

Smith-Peterson et al. first described osteotomies or wedge resection of the posterior elements of the spine in 1945 in patients afflicted with ankylosing spondylitis.[1] From Smith-Peterson's first reports, the technique improved with modifications, such as foraminotomies and ultimately the addition of rigid internal fixation first described by Briggs et al. in 1947.[2] Law et al. published some of the largest series of osteotomies during the 1950s and 1960s with reported lumbar corrections from 20 to 40 degrees.[3,7,8]

The limitation of the Smith-Peterson technique is the lengthening of the anterior column, which may lead to stretching of the cauda equina and possible vascular complications, such as aortic rupture as reported by Weatherley et al.[9] In 1985, Thomasen reported a 3 column posterior wedge osteotomy in eleven patients afflicted with ankylosing spondylitis. He reported in his series that the posterior compression or wedging through the L2 vertebral body did not lengthen the anterior column as in the Smith-Peterson osteotomy; thus, no complications, such as stretching of the cauda equina or vascular complications were noted.[4]

Since Thomasen reported the three-column technique several clinical studies have attempted to document the efficacy of both procedures. In a review of lumbar osteotomies performed in 856 patients with ankylosing spondylitis from 1966 to 1998, Van Royen et al. correctly noted that statistical analysis of the outcomes was not possible based on the lack of standardized outcome data. Therefore, one could not make an evidence based judgment on which technique SPO versus PSO would appropriate for fixed sagittal plane deformity.[10] Recently, Cho et al. assessed the clinical and radiographic outcomes between PSO and SPO in a total of 71 patients. Although there was greater blood loss with the PSO group compared to the SPO. However, no significant difference was noted in the clinical outcome measures. However, when greater than three levels of osteotomies were compared there was a statistically significant difference with correction of sagittal and coronal planes of PSO versus SPO.[6] In reviewing the literature, it becomes apparent that the use of PSO will continue to be an excellent tool for the orthopedic spine surgeon to tackle the difficulty of fixed sagittal plan deformities.

Surgical Indications

Indications for PSOs have widened recently. In the first description, the technique was described for ankylosing spondylitis patients by Thomasen. Nearly a decade later Hehne et al. described the PSO technique in patients suffering from a flatback deformity induced by Harrington distraction instrumentation in the lumbar spine.[5] The PSO technique has been used to treat not only the iatrogenic flatback but also sagittal plane deformities that occur in combination with coronal deformities. The simple example is degenerative scoliosis with significant loss of lumbar lordosis. Using releases, Ponte osteotomies and if needed a PSO can help correct these deformities from a posterior only approach. The author has primarily used PSO in patients who are undergoing revision surgery with fixed sagittal plane deformities (Fig. 23.1). At times, this technique has been employed in revision surgeries of coronal and sagittal plane deformity albeit less frequently.

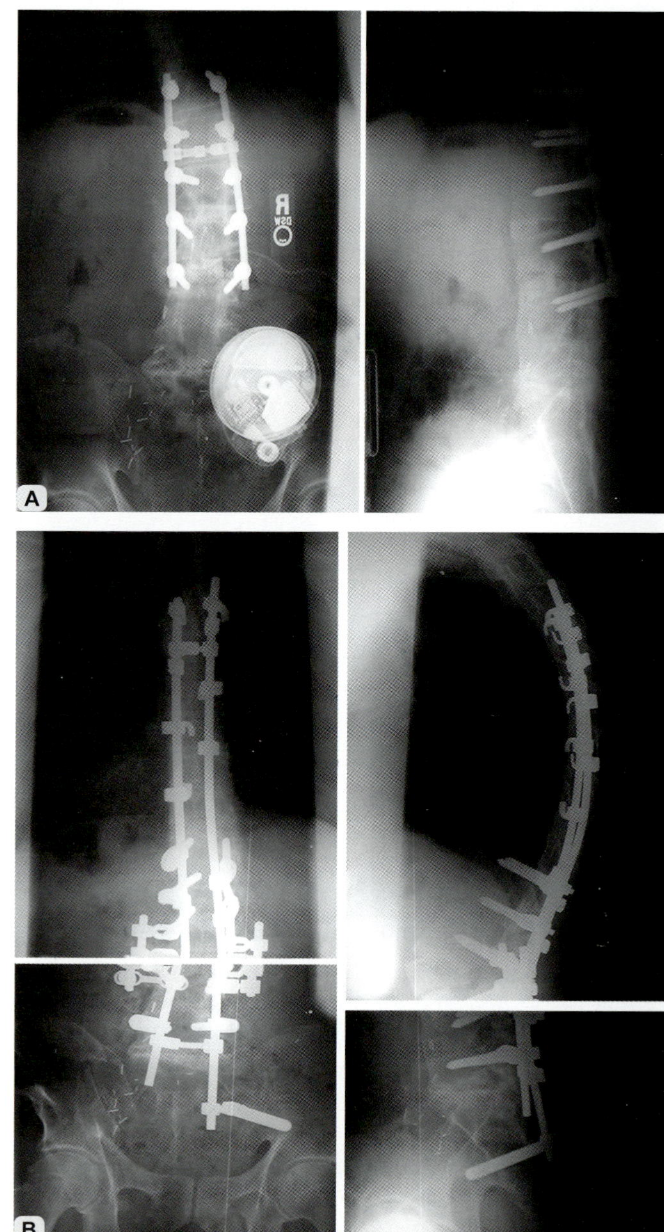

Fig. 23.1 (A) Patient with fixed sagittal plane deformity preoperatively. Patient underwent Anterior L5–S1 fusion with pedicle subtraction osteotomy. Note improvement in sagittal plane in postoperative plain films; (B) Postoperative films status post anterior L5–S1 fusion and PSO

Preoperative Planning

Standard PA lateral radiographs are mandatory. Further radiographs that are helpful are supine AP and lateral radiographs. The supine radiographs help define the flexibility of the sagittal and coronal deformity. The amount of correction necessary can be recalculated if the spine corrects significantly in the supine position. The rigid parts of the spine and the more flexible or compensatory parts of the spine can be identified in this manner. Bending X-rays also are done in a supine position to gain the help of removing gravity while accessing any flexibility of the coronal deformities. In addition, a lateral radiograph while the patient is in supine hyperextension over a bolster is extremely helpful in assessing the flexibility of a kyphotic segment of the spine. The hyperextension radiograph will frequently reveal areas of nonunion in a patient with a previous attempt at arthrodesis such as air in the disk space or angular correction between erect and supine radiographs.

In revision cases, it is essential to define the neural elements and the canal. Arachnoiditis can be found following spinal surgery with clumping of the cauda equina. The presence of arachnoiditis may be a prognostic indicator of subtotal improvement in lower extremity symptoms following decompression and should be discussed with the patient preoperatively. Stenosis, whether central and or foraminal, can be defined properly and addressed during surgery before the PSO. Computed tomography is extremely helpful in outlining the bony land marks and elucidating the extent of the fusion mass, that is, appropriately planning the placement of the spinal instrumentation, such as pedicle screws. CT scan after a myelogram is still a useful tool in cases where the patients that cannot tolerate, e.g claustrophobia, cannot have an MRI due to a pacemaker. The ability to have MRI as well as CT scan preoperatively allows the surgeon to be prepared for the complexity of revision surgery.

Surgical Technique

Perioperative Plan

Preoperative antibiotics such as vancomycin and kefzol are administered 30–60 minutes prior to making skin incision. Use of fibrinolytics, such as tranaxemic acid and amicar have been shown to decrease the operative blood loss in spine surgery.[11,12] A Cochrane review performed by Tzortzopoulou et al. in 2008 showed safety and efficacy of antifibrinolytics in pediatric idiopathic scoliosis patients.[13]

Positioning

The PSO technique requires the patient to be in the prone position with bone prominences well padded with either foam or gel pads and the abdomen to be free during the surgery. The abdomen being free helps increase the venous drainage away from the epidural plexus (Fig. 23.2). The procedure lends itself to increased blood loss due the cancellous bone of the vertebral body as well as violation of the epidural vessels during the procedure.

The bed that reflexes is an extremely useful not only in the initial accommodation or position of the patient with kyphotic deformity, but the method of closing the wedge osteotomy in a very controlled manner by using the bed can be a useful technique. Using temporary rods and the bed that reflexes helps guide the closure safely and effectively.

Technique

After adequate and extensile exposure as shown in (Fig. 23.3) our preference is to begin placement of instrumentation prior to performing PSO. Often we will place temporary rods to control our correction in a gradual manner once the PSO is complete. Once instrumentation is in place, we proceed with laminectomy and removal of the posterior elements (Fig. 23.4). In preoperative planning stages we will decide to correct for coronal plane deformities by adjusting our osteotomy to ensure appropriate cortical contacts for our correction. That is assuming no coronal plane deformity, symmetrical removal of the body can be made. Essentially we are creating a Smith-Peterson osteotomy initially (removal of the posterior element at the desired level). We then turn our attention to removal of the pedicles. During this step it is critical to expose the exiting nerve root just caudad to the pedicle prior to removing them and the transverse process (Fig. 23.5). It is helpful to keep the medial part of the pedicle intact initially to protect the neural elements.

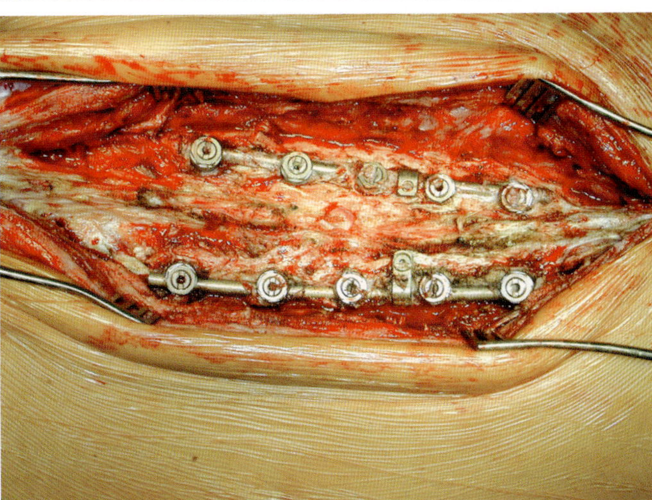

Fig. 23.3 Exposure of the previous hardware and fusion mass

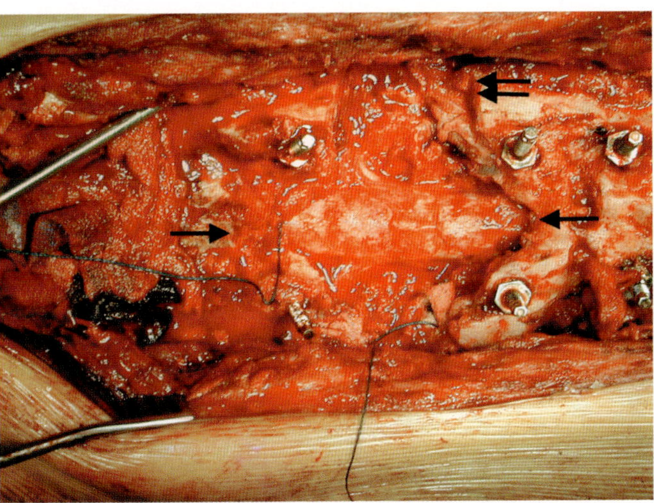

Fig. 23.4 Intraoperative photo showing instrumentation caudal and cephalad to level of the PSO. Single arrow represents midline laminectomies noted above and below level of PSO. Also seen here resection of fusion mass (double arrow)

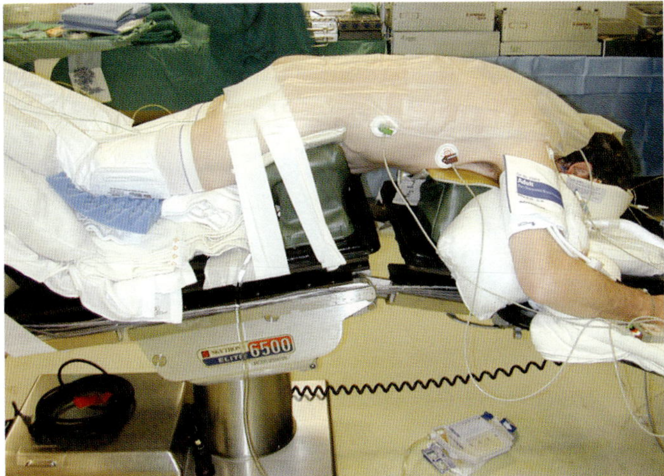

Fig. 23.2 Example of proper positioning of patient on articulating bed. Allows for accommodation of patient's deformity preoperatively. Also note: abdomen allowed to hang free and all pressure points are padded

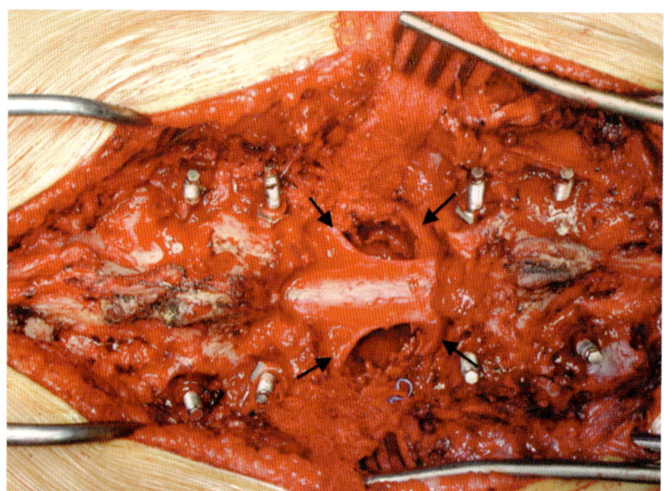

Fig. 23.5 Exiting nerve roots above and below level of PSO are visualized with single arrows

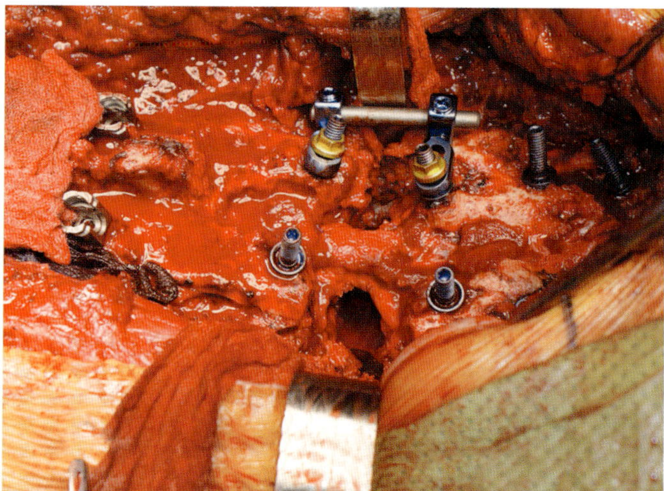

Fig. 23.7 Using temporary rod fixation to aid in the controlled closure of the wedge osteotomy ensuring dura and exiting nerve roots are not in danger

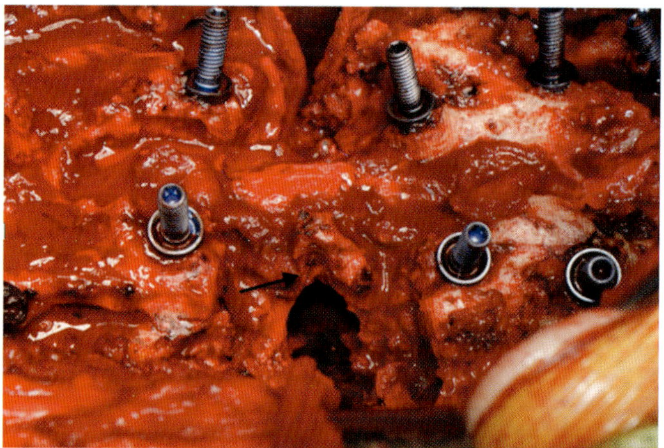

Fig. 23.6 Example of the decancellation of the vertebral body with medial wall of pedicle intact depicted by arrow. The medial wall of the pedicle protects the nerve root during decancellation of the vertebral body

Next we begin decancellation of the vertebral body through our resected or partially resected pedicles (Fig. 23.6). Often we will use a pedicle probe to identify the medial wall of the pedicle and use a Penfield retractor to ensure the thecal sac and the nerve root are not within the field in order to visualize the posterior aspect of the vertebral body. During the decancellation process a combination of curettes and Leksell ronguers are used. Hemostasis is critical at this junction and the use of topical hemostatic agents, such as gelfoam, bone wax, and thrombin soaked cottonoids (particularly if there is bleeding form the epidural vessels). Once adequate exposure of the lateral wall is performed, the lateral vertebral cortex is resected to the level of the anterior cortex (Fig. 23.7). It is at this time where symmetrical resection of the cortex is paramount in order to close the osteotomy with cortical contact.

The next step requires fracturing or resecting the posterior wall of the vertebral body. Often it is necessary to use reversed angled curettes to thin the cortex enough to be able to create a controlled fracture. Great care must be taken to protect the anterior aspect of the dura and the posterior aspect of the vertebral body. Bipolar cautery can be utilized to coagulate the epidural vessels prior to removal of the posterior wall of the vertebral body. Remnants of the posterior cortex are then removed. Note, the fracturing of the posterior cortex does destabilize the vertebral body. Instrumentation and the lateral vertebral walls are intact.

The final step involves closing the osteotomy in a controlled manner. As discussed previously, using a bed that reflexes can certainly assist in this manner. If this is not available hyperextension of the patient's chest and pelvis will also aide in closing the wedge osteotomy or even using pillows or blankets to elevate the thighs. Prior closing the osteotomy, it is important to have loosened the temporary rod to allow smooth motion during the closing of the osteotomy (Fig. 23.8). The surgeon should ensure that there is symmetrical cortical contact when the osteotomy is closed. Once adequate correction is achieved the canal is examined to ensure there is no dorsal impingement of the thecal sac. The longitudinal rods are then placed to lock the osteotomy further (Fig. 23.9). The long instrumented segment achieves additional correction and supports the osteotomy site during the healing process. Finally, the instrumentation is tightened to ensure stability across the PSO.

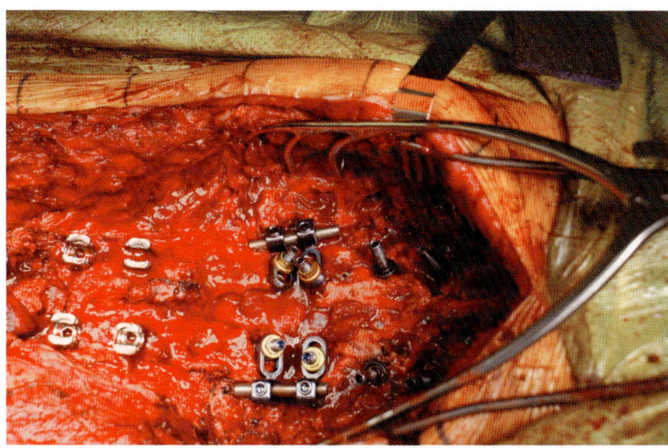

Fig. 23.8 Example of closing the osteotomy using temporary rod fixation

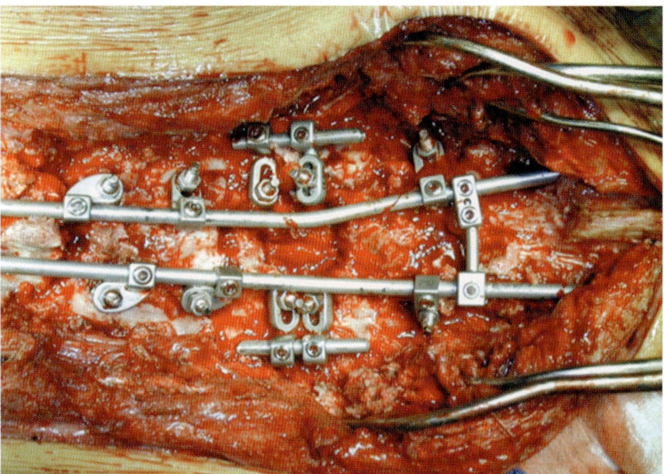

Fig. 23.9 Final construct in place showing longitudinal instrumentation spanning the level of the PSO

References

1. Smith-Petersen MN, Larson CB, Aufranc OE. Osteotomy of the spine for correction of flexion deformity in rheumatoid arthritis. J Bone Joint Surg. 1945;27:1–11.
2. Briggs H, Keats S, Schlesinger PT. Wedge osteotomy of the spine with bilateral, intervertebral foraminotomy: correction of flexion deformity in five cases of ankylosing arthritis of spine. J Bone Joint Surg. 1947;29:1075-82.
3. Law WA. Surgical treatment of the rheumatic diseases. J Bone Joint Surg Br. 1952;34-B:215-25.
4. Thomasen E. Vertebral osteotomy for correction of kyphosis in ankylosing spondylitis. Clin Orthop. 1985;194:142-52.
5. Hehne HJ, Zielke K, Böhm H. Polysegmental lumbar osteotomies and transpedicled fixation for correction of long-curved kyphotic deformities in ankylosing spondylitis. Report on 177 cases. Clin Orthop. 1990;258:49-55.
6. Cho KJ, Bridwell KH, Lenke LG, Berra A, Baldus C. Comparison of Smith-Petersen versus pedicle subtraction osteotomy for the correction of fixed sagittal imbalance. Spine (Phila Pa 1976). 2005; 30(18):2030-7; discussion 2038.
7. Law WA. Osteotomy of the spine. Clin Orthop 1969;66: 70–6.
8. Law WA. Osteotomy of the spine. J Bone Joint Surg Am. 1962;44-A:1199-206.
9. Weatherley C, JaVray D, Terry A. Vascular complications associated with osteotomy in ankylosing spondylitis: a report of two cases. Spine. 1988;13:43-6.
10. Van Royen BJ, De Gast A. Lumbar osteotomy for correction of thoracolumbar kyphotic deformity in ankylosing spondylitis. A structured review of three methods of treatment. Ann Rheum Dis. 1999;58:399-406.
11. Colomina MJ, Bagó J, Fuentes I. Efficacy and safety of prophylactic large dose of tranexamic acid in spine surgery: a prospective, randomized, double-blind, placebo-controlled study. Spine (Phila Pa 1976). 2009; 34(16):1740-1; author reply 141. Spine 2008; 33: 2577-80.
12. Baldus CR, Bridwell KH, Lenke LG, Okubadejo GO. Can we safely reduce blood loss during lumbar pedicle subtraction osteotomy procedures using tranexamic acid or aprotinin? A comparative study with controls. Spine (Phila Pa 1976). 2010; 35(2):235-9.
13. Tzortzopoulou A, Cepeda MS, Schumann R, Carr DB. Antifibrinolytic agents for reducing blood loss in scoliosis surgery in children. Cochrane Database Syst Rev. 2008; (3):CD006883.

CHAPTER

24

Management of Spinal Kyphotic Deformities

HS Chhabra, Ameer S Theruvath

Introduction

Human spine has four physiological curves in the sagittal plane (Fig. 24.1). This includes the cervical and lumbar lordosis as well as the thoracic and sacral kyphosis. The sagittal balance of the spine is maintained by the mutual balancing of these physiologic curves. Kyphotic deformity is a deformity in the sagittal plane, and the thoracic kyphosis is generally considered excessive if it is more than 50 degrees.[1]

Kyphotic deformity, unlike its coronal counterpart or the scoliosis can have more dangerous consequences, in that it has the potential of stretching the spinal cord. This can lead to neurological deficits if the deformity is allowed to progress. From the management standpoint, the surgical strategies to correct a primary kyphosis are relatively straightforward since it is a uniplanar deformity.[2] But it can be fraught with devastating neurological deficits in spite of all precaution.[3] Scoliosis which is a three dimensional deformity involves complicated pathomechanics and treatment principles. However, the chances of intraoperative neurological deficits in a case of scoliosis is quite less compared to kyphosis unless accompanied by a significant sagittal plane deformity.[4]

Scoliosis Research Society defines kyphosis as an abnormally increased posterior convex angulation of the vertebral column.[5] Any degree of kyphosis in the thoracolumbar and lumbar spine is also considered abnormal. Kyphotic deformity ensues if the anterior load bearing capability of the spinal column is jeopardized. Major etiological factors include congenital (e.g. hemi-vertebra), developmental (e.g. Scheuermann's disease), Infective (e.g. Pott's spine), inflammatory (e.g. ankylosing spondylitis), post traumatic/postlaminectomy, degenerative (e.g. degenerative spondylolisthesis) and the senile kyphosis due to multiple osteoporotic compressions.[6]

Etiological classification of kyphosis is as follows:

1. Postural disorders
2. Scheuermann's disease
3. Congenital vertebral anomalies
4. Paralytic disorders
5. Post-traumatic

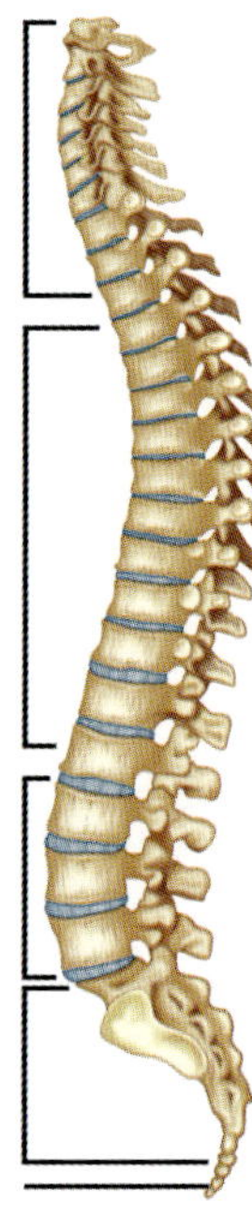

Fig. 24.1 Normal physiological curves of the spine

6. Postlaminectomy
7. Postirradiation
8. Metabolic disorders, e.g. osteoporosis
9. Skeletal dysplasias, e.g. mucopolysaccharadosis
10. Collagen diseases, e.g. Marfans disease
11. Neoplasias benign or malignant
12. Neurofibromatosis.

Pathomechanics

The posterior elements of the spine are designed primarily to resist tension and the anterior elements to resist compression. Disruption of the posterior tension band or the anterior mechanical buttress can result in kyphosis. Once a kyphotic deformity develops the centre of gravity of the body is shifted anteriorly. An increased bending moment is gradually established across the apex of the deformity, which further contributes to increase in the deformity. As the magnitude of kyphosis increase, the susceptibility to further progression increases.[7] The kyphotic deformity may be flexible or rigid. If unattended most flexible kyphotic deformities become fixed over time. Progressive, rigid, large kyphotic deformities of the thoracic spine puts the spinal cord at significant risk of sustaining stretch damage.

Most important factor in the analysis and management of kyphotic deformities is the sagittal plane balance. When a plumb line dropped from the center of the C7 body passes through the posterior aspect of first sacral body the sagittal balance is considered normal (Fig. 24.2). Kyphotic deformity can displace this plumb line anteriorly resulting in positive sagittal balance.

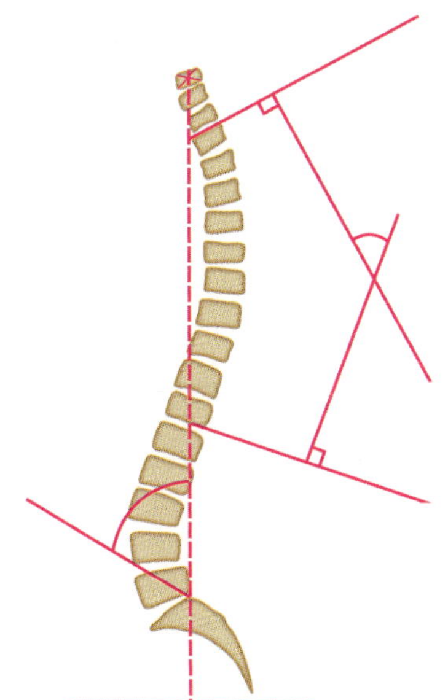

Fig. 24.2 C7 plumb line and the thoracic kyphosis

Management

Kyphotic deformity is surgically correctable by shortening the posterior column or by lengthening the anterior column. Historically, kyphotic deformities were treated by anterior fusion techniques which were mostly instrumented. Later on combined anterior-posterior techniques[8] emerged followed by posterior only procedures. All these techniques have their inherent pros and cons. Anterior procedures involve opening up the normal thoracic cavity and the accompanying morbidities.[9,10] In addition, it is difficult to approach the concavity of an angular deformity if the magnitude of the deformity exceeds 60 degrees. Combined anterior posterior procedures offer excellent decompression, anterior strut placement and deformity correction but is too extensile and may not be tolerated by a frail patient unless done in stages. Posterior only procedures are the current state of the art. Kawahara N et al.,[11] Moon MS et al.,[12,13] and Rajasekaran S et al.[14] have all come out with excellent narrations of technical details of these posterior only techniques. These procedures are now carried out commonly by spine surgeons across the globe with excellent correction of deformity. They are safe even though neurophysiologic monitoring is strongly recommended intraoperatively.

Analyzing the Deformity

Posterior release and resection by osteotomies followed by compression shortening is the mainstay of surgical treatment of kyphosis. This could be achieved through various types of osteotomies like Ponte osteotomy (PO), Smith-Petersen osteotomy (SPO),[15] pedicle subtraction osteotomy (PSO), and vertebral column resection (VCR). The decision making as to which type of resection osteotomy is required demands a thorough analysis of the deformity. The following are the cardinal aspects of decision making.

Type of Imbalance

Sagittal imbalance is classified as type I and type II.[16] In type I imbalance, a portion of the patient's spine is substantially hyperkyphotic, but the patient is able to maintain balance by hyperextending segments above and below. An example is a young adult who has been treated with Harrington rod instrumentation from T4 to L4 but since his /her disks at L4–L5 and L5–S1 are not degenerated as yet are able to maintain balance by hyper extending those 2 segments.

Another example is a post-traumatic kyphosis in which there is a regional kyphosis, but the patient is able to maintain balance by hyperextending segments above and below. Certain congenital kyphosis and many Scheuermann's kyphosis would fall into this category. A type II imbalance is one in which the regional hyperkyphosis is such that the individual cannot balance by hyperextending segments above and below. Examples frequently include patients of ankylosing spondylitis and older patients with a Harrington fusion from T4 to L4 with severe disk degeneration at L4–L5 and L5–S1 such that they are not able to hyperextend the distal segments to maintain balance. Another common situation is that of a middle-aged or older patient who has had surgeries in the distal lumbar spine where the fusion heals in a hypolordotic position and segments above in the upper lumbar spine or distal thoracic spine degenerate and fall into kyphosis. Therein, the patient is not able to stand straight and is pitched forward.

Location

Further characterization of the kyphosis considers whether the kyphosis is based in the thoracic or lumbar spine. The critical point is whether the pathology is in spinal cord or cauda equina territory.

Morphology of the Curve

Another important feature is whether the kyphosis is more of a rounded, long sweeping kyphosis or a short, angular one. A long sweeping kyphosis, such as a Scheuermann's, is more amenable to multiple SPOs, in part because of its multisegmental nature and in part because the pathology is in the thoracic spine/spinal cord territory. A short, angular kyphosis, such as seen with post-traumatic kyphosis, is more amenable to a PSO. Usually, a PSO in the lumbar spine will accomplish approximately 35° of lordosis.[17] In the thoracic spine a PSO will accomplish approximately 25° of lordosis. A SPO will usually accomplish approximately 10° of lordosis. SPOs are rarely performed at one level and are usually performed at 2 or more levels. While it is necessary to have a potentially mobile disk space to achieve correction with an SPO,[18] for a PSO, this is not necessary.

Coexistent Coronal Imbalance

At times, sagittal imbalance will be coupled with coronal imbalance. There are 2 types of coronal imbalance[19] (Fig. 24.3). For the first type (type 1), the shoulder will be high on the side on which the pelvis is low.

In this circumstance, the coronal deformity can be corrected by simply shortening one side of the spine. In the second type of coronal imbalance, the shoulder will be low on the side in which the pelvis is low. The association of the shoulders to the pelvis is such that it cannot be corrected simply by shortening one side of the spine. In this circumstance, a VCR is necessary. In the first type (type 1), an asymmetric PSO will potentially accomplish the correction.

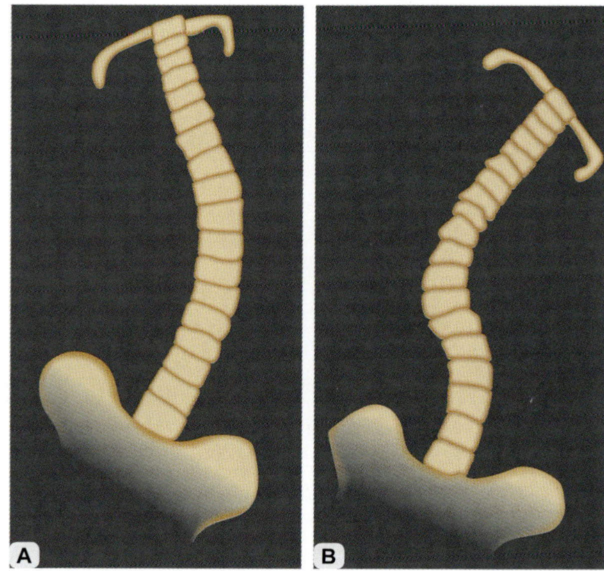

Fig. 24.3 Types of coronal imbalances. (A) type 1; (B) type 2

Spinal Osteotomies

The indication for an osteotomy of the spine is spinal imbalance in the sagittal and/or coronal plane that does not correct on bending radiographs. The options for osteotomy are many. The choice of technique depends on the amount of deformity correction desired and the etiology of the deformity (Fig. 24.4).

Smith-Petersen Osteotomy

Osteotomy of spine was first described by Smith-Petersen[15] in 1945 for ankylosing spondylitis. Smith-Petersen osteotomy (SPO) is a facet based osteotomy performed in a posteriorly fused spine. The same osteotomy if performed in an unfused spine is technically called a Ponte osteotomy. But in majority of the literature these two osteotomies are collectively referred to as the SPO. The structures resected in an SPO include the spinous process of the cephalad vertebra, the facet joints, the margins of the adjoining laminae and the ligamentum flavum bilaterally (Fig. 24.5).

The SPO is often used as an adjunct to facilitate derotation and is more often used in the thoracic spine and at the thoracolumbar junction.[19] The SPO opens the anterior column (disk space), hinges on the middle column (the posterior longitudinal ligament serves as the fulcrum), and closes the posterior column by the amount that is removed posteriorly. The posterior column is thus shortened and the anterior column is lengthened. An open disk space is therefore a prerequisite for closure of the SPO site. Either a collapsed disk or a previous arthrodesis with a completely

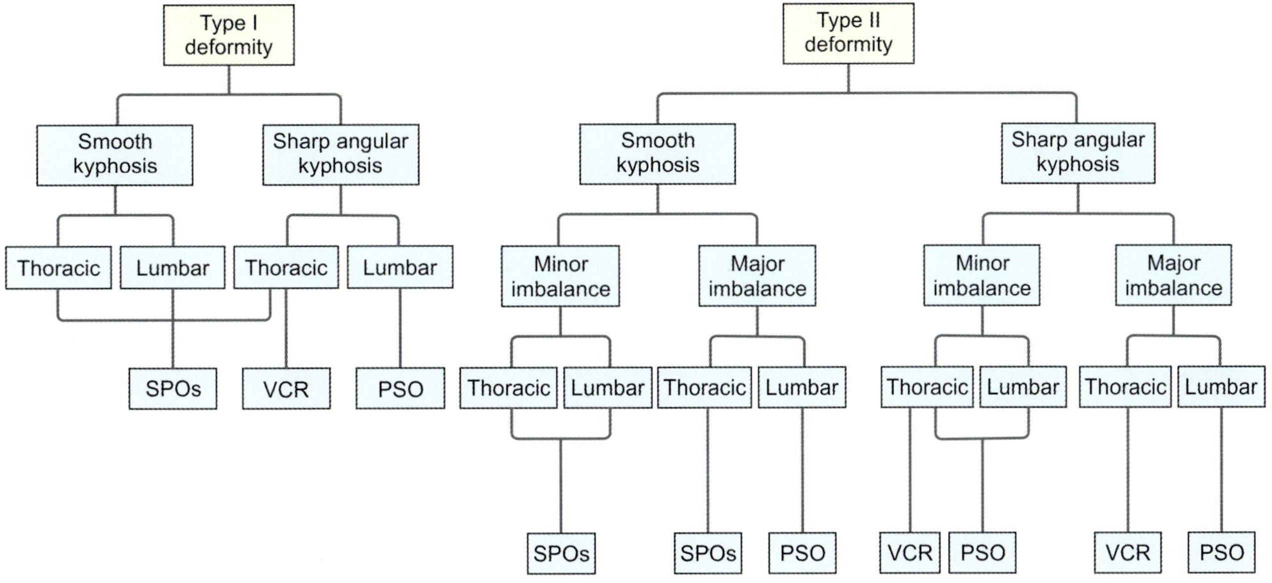

Fig. 24.4 Algorithm for choosing the appropriate osteotomy. POS, pedicle subtraction ostemotomy; SPO, Smith-Petersen osteotomy; VCR, vertebral column resection

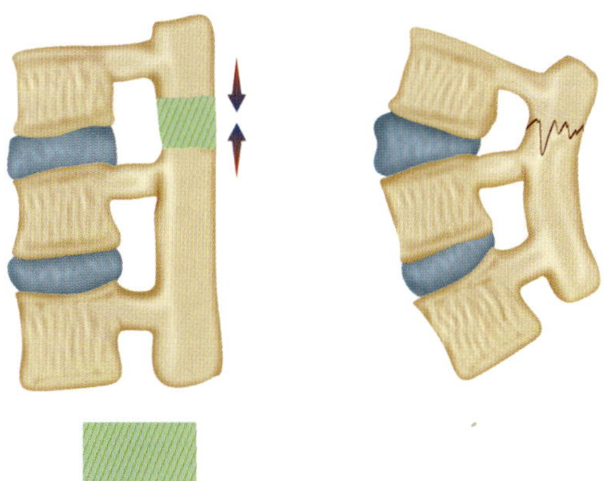

Fig. 24.5 Smith-Petersen osteotomy

immobile disk may limit the amount of correction that can be obtained by a posterior wedge-shaped osteotomy.

Operative Technique

The patient is placed in prone position on an open frame radiolucent operating table. This allows the abdomen to float freely and allows gravity to assist in pulling the lumbar spine into lordosis. The level of osteotomy is dictated by the level of the apex of the deformity. Bilateral facetectomies are then performed throughout the entire length of the intended fusion. Pedicle screw tracts are made but screws are not inserted. These tracts aid in orientation of the osteotomy. The lamina, ligamentum flavum, and superior and inferior articular processes are removed bilaterally. The spinous process of the vertebra just cephalad to the osteotomy site is resected to the base. The osteotomy is then carried laterally to the intervertebral notch using small Kerrison rongeurs. It is important to identify the pedicles above and below the osteotomy site. Care should be taken to inadvertently breach these pedicles as osteotomy proceeds laterally. In addition, the nerve roots sit quite close to the bone that is being resected. The resection is wedge or chevron-shaped, with the tip distally. Width of the osteotomy is typically 8–10 mm. Both limbs of the wedge must be symmetrical, unless concomitant coronal plane correction is also intended. In this case one side of the wedge is widened more than the other side. If the osteotomy is performed at a level with significant rotational deformity, the osteotomy should be opened to a greater degree on the side of the convexity in an effort to decrease the rotational aspect of the deformity. Always undercut the osteotomy to avoid neural compression while closing the osteotomy site—widening the SPO by removing more superior facet may help prevent impingement of the superior nerve root with the compression maneuver. If there is any indication of dural compression during osteotomy closure, the osteotomy should be enlarged centrally. Closure may occur passively as a result of lordosis induced by the surgical frame, or prebent rods can be introduced to the previously placed bone anchors and a combination of cantilever correction and compression should achieve the necessary reduction (Fig. 24.6).

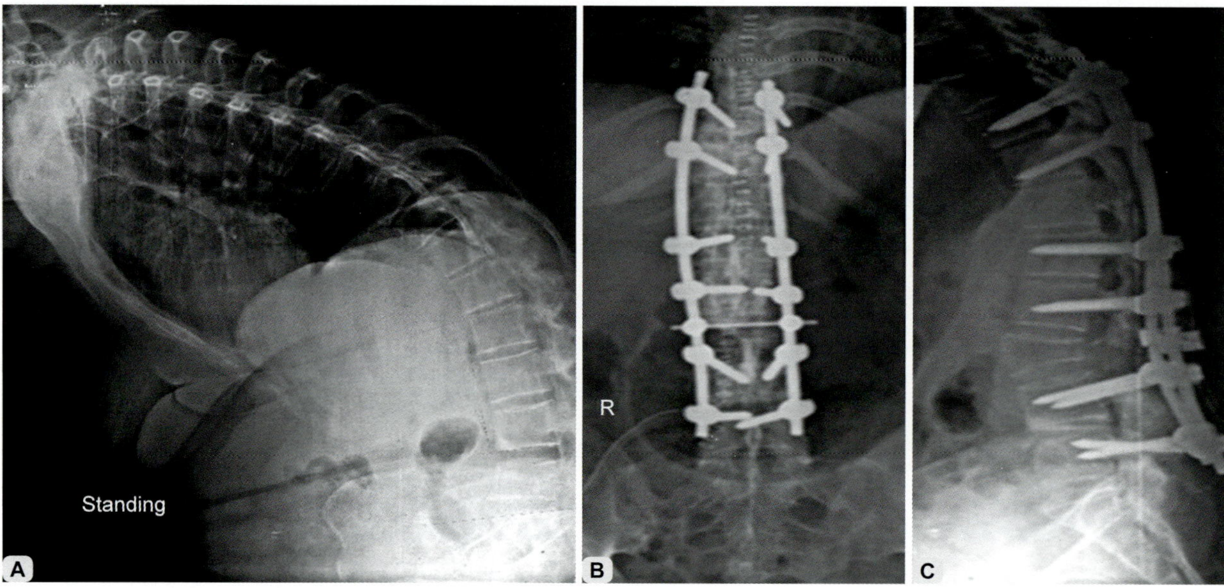

Fig. 24.6 Smith-Petersen osteotomy and instrumented fusion for senile kyphosis with sagittal imbalance

Pedicle Subtraction Osteotomy

Pedicle subtraction osteotomy was first described by Thomasen[20] in 1985. He described it for the management of fixed sagittal plane deformities in patients with ankylosing spondylitis. The PSO is preferably performed at the normal apex of lumbar lordosis, which is either the L2 or L3 vertebra. Owing to the amount of dural retraction and tension created when a PSO osteotomy is closed, it was considered safer to perform the osteotomy distal to the level where cord ends. For stiff global kyphotic deformities, a PSO in the midlumbar spine can be combined with multiple SPOs at the thoracolumbar junction and in the thoracic spine. The technique involves a transpedicular vertebral wedge resection extending from the posterior elements through the pedicles into the anterior cortex of the vertebral body (Fig. 24.7). The PSO has the advantage of obtaining correction through all 3 columns from a posterior approach without lengthening the anterior column, thereby maximizing the correction potential while avoiding stretching of the major vessels.

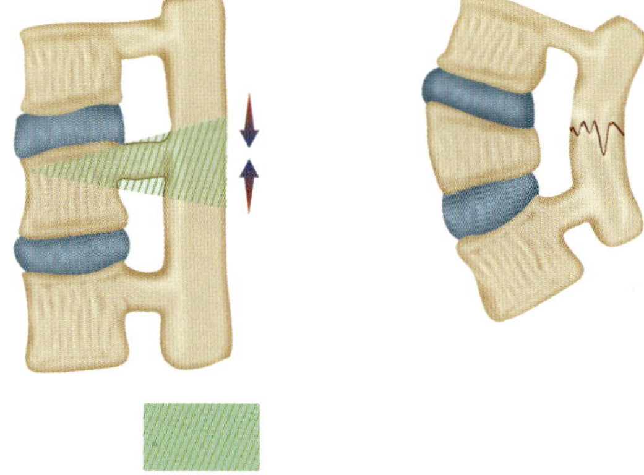

Fig. 24.7 Pedicle subtraction osteotomy

Indications

Positive sagittal imbalance in the lumbar spine is the primary indication for PSO. The typical indication for the PSO procedure is a patient who has a positive sagittal imbalance of greater than 12 cm or a patient who needs approximately 30 degrees of additional lordosis at one level. It is also indicated for patients who have had a circumferential fusion, including multiple vertebrae, which prevents the performance of an SPO as osteoclasis cannot be performed through a fused intervertebral disk.[21] The stability of a PSO is enhanced by bone-on-bone apposition of all 3 spinal columns with proper closure of the posterior column.

Operative Technique

After exposure, the level to be osteotomized is identified. At least 3 screws above and below the osteotomy are necessary to provide appropriate control and stability. The posterior extent of the osteotomy is then outlined on the posterior elements or on an existing fusion mass. Laminectomies and complete bilateral facetectomies are performed at the osteotomy level. Removal of the posterior elements of the spine with a Kerrison rongeur exposes the pedicles, which can then be removed with a rongeur.

Removal of the pedicles allows access to the vertebral body, which is decancellated with a pedicle probe and drill to create a wedge resection. In the absence of a coronal plane deformity, the resection should be made symmetrically on both sides. The pedicles are then isolated and separated from all osseous attachments other than the vertebral body, requiring exposure of the nerve root caudad to the pedicle. Once the pedicles are isolated, the next step is to remove bone from the vertebral body through the pedicles while protecting the dura and nerve roots. Working underneath the posterior vertebral cortex, the surgeon thins the cortex as much as possible with a curette and Woodson elevator. After decancellation and thinning of the posterior wall, the portion of the vertebral body underlying the anterior spinal canal is removed by collapsing this bone into the decancellated cavity with a down-facing curette. The fractured posterior cortex is then removed. Temporary rods should be used to prevent premature uncontrolled closure of the osteotomy. The temporary rods are used unilaterally or bilaterally and may be placed during the decancellation step as the spine becomes more flexible and the osteotomy begins to close. The use of temporary rods is especially important in preventing translation of the spine in patients with long fusion masses above and below the osteotomy. The final step in completing the bony resection of the osteotomy is to remove the lateral vertebral body walls. The lateral vertebral walls are exposed by dissecting the psoas muscle away from the lateral aspect of the vertebral body with a sponge stick or periosteal elevator. This separation is maintained by leaving a sponge or malleable retractor in the potential space until closure of the osteotomy. This separation ensures the psoas muscle will not be entrapped during removal of the lateral vertebral body wall during the osteotomy. Careful attention is needed to ensure that the removal of bone is uniform throughout the vertebral body to ensure symmetric closure of the osteotomy site and appropriate correction of the sagittal deformity. The ventral aspect of the vertebral body acts as a hinge by which the osteotomy site is closed. Disruption of the ventral cortex of the vertebral body will destabilize the spinal column.[22] An extensive posterior decompression of the dura is needed to prevent invagination of the dura with osteotomy closure, which can result in kinking of the neural elements and associated neurological deficit. Bridwell KH[19] suggested the creation of a central enlargement in the lamina cephalad and caudad to the osteotomy such that when the osteotomy site is closed, the thecal sac and nerve roots can be inspected to ensure they are not impinged upon. Closure of the osteotomy can be accomplished by the use of temporary rods to cantilever the spine and also by hyperextending the chest and legs with the operating table or with the manual help of an assistant. When the construct is complete and the osteotomy is closed on both sides, the spinal canal ought to be dissected, first with a nerve hook and then with a Woodson elevator to confirm there is no dorsal compression of the dural sac. The lateral masses should be tightly compressed to promote stability and osteogenesis.

Vertebral Column Resection (VCR)

A VCR[23] entails resection of one or more vertebral segments, including the posterior elements (spinous process and laminae), pedicles, vertebral body, and disks both cephalad and caudad to the resected vertebral body. MacLennan was the first to describe a vertebrectomy procedure via a posterior apical resection with postoperative casting in his 1922 report on the etiology and treatment of severe scoliotic deformities. A posterior-only VCR was described by Suk et al.[23] in 2002, requiring a shorter operative time with less intraoperative instability of the spine.

Indications

The VCR is a powerful technique reserved for the most severe and rigid spinal deformities that cannot be acceptably corrected by less aggressive methods. It is, therefore, indicated for patients with a severe and fixed kyphosis unresponsive to an SPO or PSO or for patients with sagittal deformity in the setting of coronal imbalance that cannot be fully corrected by an asymmetric PSO. Additional indications for a VCR include congenital kyphosis, a hemivertebra, L5 spondyloptosis, and certain spinal tumors.

Operative Technique (Fig. 24.8)

This discussion of the VCR technique will focus mainly on the posterior approach, although a concomitant anterior approach may at times be necessary, especially if there is a preexisting anterior instrumentation/fusion. A wide lateral dissection extending to the transverse processes facilitates vertebral body resection. The resection begins with removal of the posterior elements, including the spinous process, laminae, facets, and transverse processes at the level(s) to be resected. During this step, bilateral total foraminal unroofing exposes the exiting nerve roots. In the thoracic spine, costotransversectomies facilitate removal of the vertebral body.

It is critical to use a temporary rod before destabilization of the spine to prevent dangerous acute translation during this procedure, as the procedure itself temporarily introduces a significant amount of spinal instability. Placement of pedicle screws provides a means of stabilizing the vertebral column during the resection. After insertion of the pedicle screws and removal of the posterior elements,

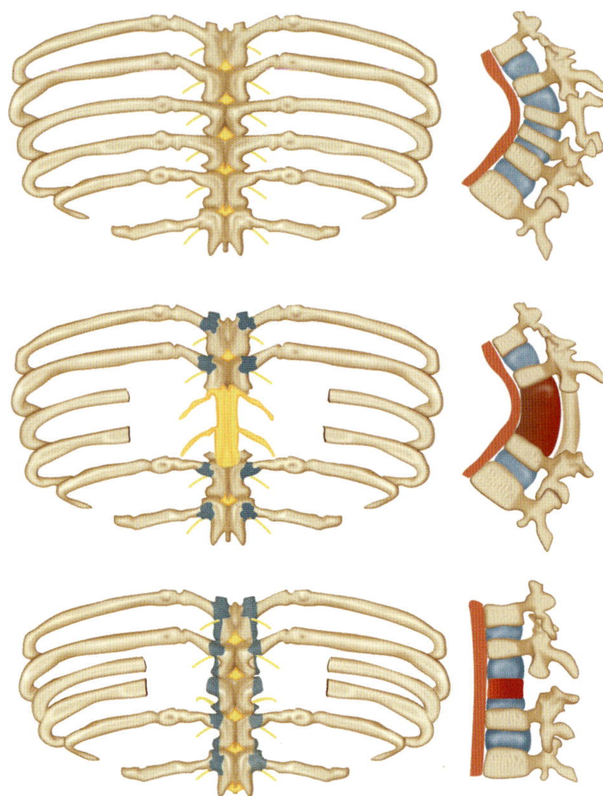

Fig. 24.8 Technique of vertebral column resection

a rod that conforms to the shape of the deformity is placed on one side of the spine. Careful subperiosteal dissection is performed on the side of the spine opposite to the temporary stabilizing rod, following the lateral wall of the vertebral body until the anterior aspect is easily palpable. The pedicle and lateral aspect of the vertebral body are then removed using an osteotome, high-speed drill, and/or rongeurs. Resection of the vertebral body and intervening disks is then accomplished in a step-wise fashion, extending toward the medial side and crossing over to the contra lateral side. A thin shell of medial bone is left behind to protect the dural tube and is removed as one of the last steps in the procedure. Care should be taken to avoid injury to the soft tissues anterior to the vertebral body and to avoid injury to the segmental vessels. A second temporary rod, contoured to fit the shape of the deformity, is secured into position on the side that has now undergone subperiosteal dissection and partial vertebral body removal. The original stabilizing rod is then removed to facilitate complete removal of any residual bone or disc. The last step of the procedure involves the use of a downgoing osteotome to push down on the floor of the spinal canal once the vertebral body has been shelled out. The deformity is initially gradually corrected by repeated compression and shortening of the vertebral column using the temporary rods. After shortening and compressing the resected gap, the temporary rods are exchanged, one by one, with precontoured definitive rods. Additional correction of kyphoscoliosis can be achieved through *in situ* rod bending and segmental compression. Not only during this posterior-only approach, but also during a combined anterior-posterior approach, the spinal cord is particularly vulnerable to injury during the correction and column shortening maneuvers. Appropriate neuromonitoring may provide an early indication of neural compromise and thus may help prevent devastating injury to the spinal cord. The VCR differs significantly from both the SPO and the PSO in that bone-on-bone contact is not achieved with the closure maneuver because of the complete vertebral body removal. Therefore, it becomes important to reconstruct the anterior spinal column using an interbody device after a VCR. In the thoracic spine, it is often adequate to place morselized bone graft anteriorly after a thorough discectomy if the anterior gap is 5 mm or less. If the gap is more than 5 mm a titanium mesh cage filled with bone graft should be used to provide reliable anterior column support without excessive shortening.[24] In the lower thoracic spine and throughout the lumbar and lumbosacral spine, however, intradiscal structural support should be considered most often via allograft bone or an interbody cage that supports the loads applied to the anterior and middle columns through the disc spaces (Figs 24.9 to 24.11).

Halo traction may be used preoperatively or intraoperatively to assist in realignment of the severely scoliotic or kyphotic spine. Preoperative halo traction can be used to maximize preoperative respiratory status in patients with kyphosis greater than 100 degrees or in patients with a concomitant scoliosis deformity greater than 90–100 degrees.[25] It is especially useful in those who will undergo revision and in those who are small or in ill health. When used perioperatively, halo traction can gradually and safely stretch the spinal column and cord while the patient is awake and able to respond to excessive stretching of the neural axis. This strategy may be especially useful in patients who have undergone surgical revision owing to the fact that previous anterior or posterior scar formation from previous laminectomies can put them at increased risk for neurologic complications. When used intraoperatively, the halo device can optimize positioning and thus help achieve optimal deformity correction.

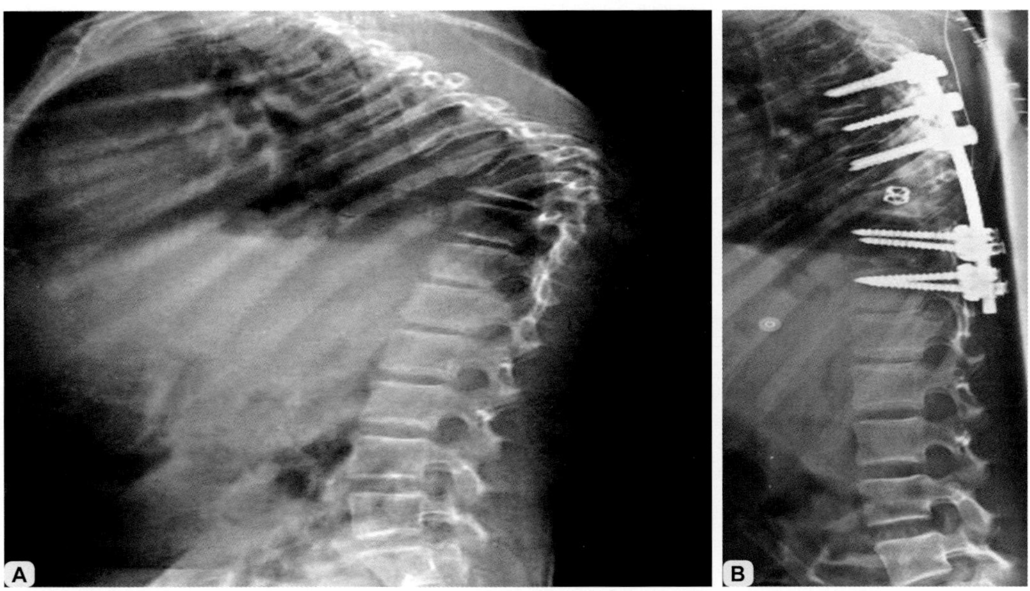

Fig. 24.9 Post-tubercular angular kyphosis corrected (A) by vertebral column resection and 360 degree instrumented fusion (B)

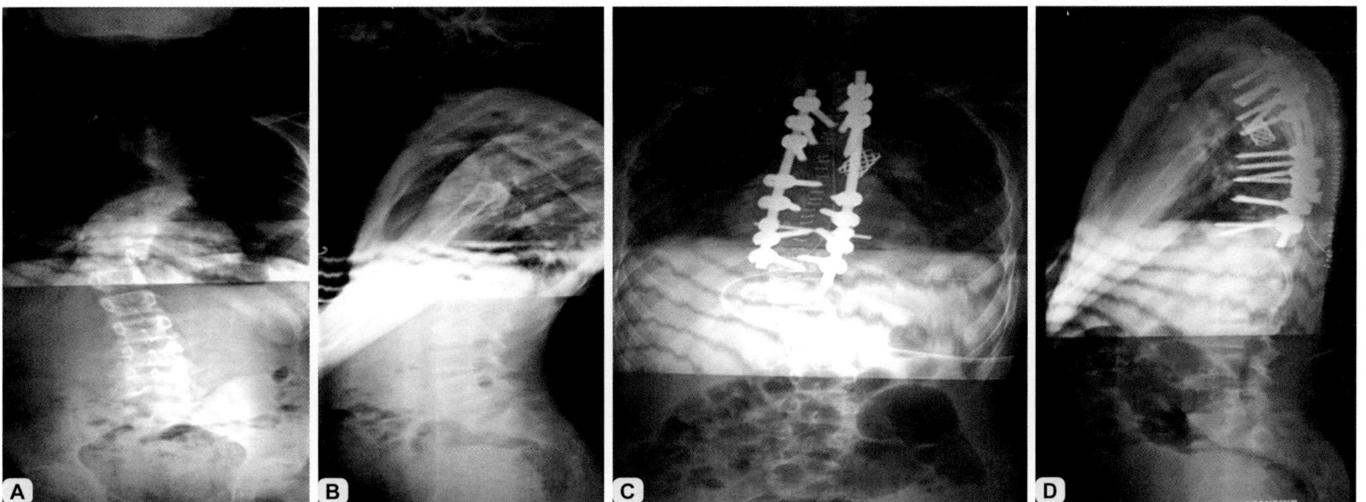

Fig. 24.10 Multiplanar deformity (kyphoscoliosis) treated by VCR

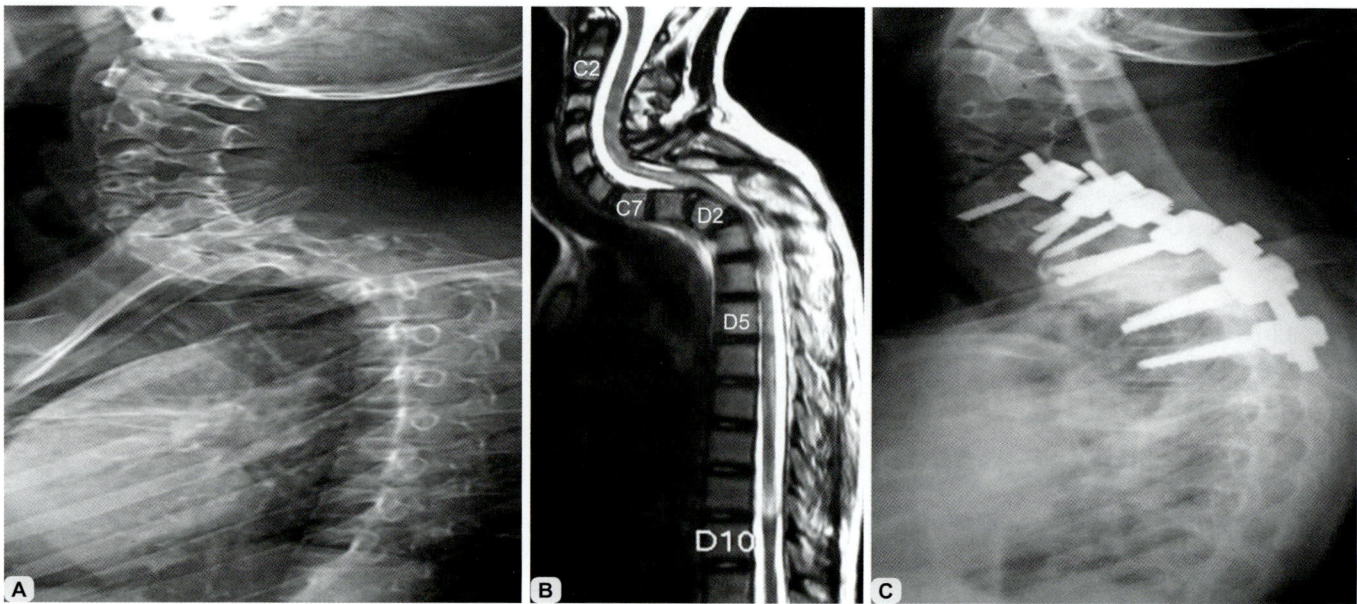

Fig. 24.11 cervicodorsal post-tubercular kyphosis addressed by VCR

References

1. Cobb J. Outline for the study of scoliosis. Insructional course lecture. 1948;5:261-75.
2. Daniel J Sucato. Management of severe spinal deformity scoliosis and kyphosis Spine. 2010; 35(25):2186-92.
3. Bridwell KH, Lenke LG, Baldus C, et al. Major intraoperative neurologic deficits in pediatric and adult spinal deformity patients. Incidence and etiology at one institution. Spine. 1998;23:324-31.
4. Cheh G, Lenke LG, Padberg AM, et al. Loss of spinal cord monitoring signal in children during thoracic kyphosis correction with spinal osteotomy: when does it occur and what should you do? Spine. 2008;33:1093-9.
5. Suken Shah. Scheuermann kyphosis SRS e-text http://etext.srs.org/book/
6. Winter, Hall JE. Kyphosis in childhood and adolescence. Spine. 1978;3:285-308.
7. Panjabi MM,White A. 3rd Johnson RM: Cervical spine mechanics as a function of transaction of components. J Biomech. 1975;327-36.
8. Chen WJ, Wu CC, Jung CH, et al. Combined anterior and posterior surgeries in the treatment of spinal tuberculous spondylitis. Clin Orthop. 2002;398:50-9.
9. Kawahara N, Tomita K, Baba H, et al. Cadaveric vascular anatomy for total en bloc spondylectomy in malignant vertebral tumors. Spine. 1996;21:1401-7.
10. McDonnell MF, Glassman SD, et al. Perioperative complications of anterior procedures on the spine. JBJS. 1996;78-A(6):839-84.
11. Kawahara N, Tomita K, Hisatoshi B, et al. Closing–opening wedge osteotomy to correct angular kyphotic deformity by a single posterior approach. Spine. 2001;26:391-40.
12. Moon MS, Woo YK, Lee KS, et al. Posterior instrumentation and anterior interbody fusion for tuberculous kyphosis of dorsal and lumbar spines. Spine. 1995;20:1910.
13. Moon MS, Lee MK. The changes of the kyphosis of the tuberculous spine in children following ambulant treatment. Korean Orthop Assoc. 1971;6:203-8.
14. Rajasekaran S, Kamath Vijay, Ajoy Prasad Shetty. Single-stage closing–opening wedge osteotomy of spine to correct severe post-tubercular kyphotic deformities of the spine: a 3-yearn follow-up of 17 patients. Eur Spine J. 2010;19:583-92.
15. Smith-Petersen MN, Larson CB, Aufranc OE. Osteotomy of the spine for correction of flexion deformity in rheumatoid arthritis. J Bone Joint Surg Am. 1945;27:1-11.
16. Booth KC, Bridwell KH, Lenke LG, et al. Complications and predictive factors for the successful treatment of flatback deformity (fixed sagittal imbalance). Spine. 1999;24:1712-20.
17. Kalra KP, Dhar SB, Shetty G, Dhariwal Q. Pedicle subtraction osteotomy for rigid post-tuberculous kyphosis. J Bone Joint Surg Br. 2006;88-B:925-7.
18. Macagno AE, O'Brien MF. Thoracic and thoracolumbar kyphosis in adults. Spine (Phila Pa 1976). 2006;31(19 suppl):S161-70.
19. Bridwell KH. Decision making regarding Smith-Petersen vs. pedicle subtraction osteotomy vs. vertebral column resection

for spinal deformity. Spine (Phila Pa 1976). 2006;31(19 suppl):S171-8.

20. Thomasen E. Vertebral osteotomy for correction of kyphosis in ankylosing spondylitis. Clin Orthop Relat Res. 1985;142-52.
21. Hoh DJ, Khoueir P, Wang MY. Management of cervical deformity in ankylosing spondylitis. Neurosurg Focus. 2008;24:E9.
22. Bridwell KH, Lewis SJ, Edwards C, et al. Complications and outcomes of pedicle subtraction osteotomies for fixed sagittal imbalance. Spine. 2003;28:2093-101.
23. Suk SI, Kim JH, Kim WJ, et al. Posterior vertebral column resection for severe spinal deformities. Spine (Phila Pa 1976). 2002;27:2374-82.
24. The textbook of spinal surgery Third edition Keith H Bridwell, Ronald L Dewald Chapter 96. p.1012.
25. Rinella Anthony MD, Lenke Lawrence MD, Perioperative Halo-Gravity Traction in the Treatment of Severe Scoliosis and Kyphosis. Spine. 2005;30(4):475-82.

CHAPTER

25

Lumbar Facet Syndrome

Radchenko Vladimir A, Deduch N, Malyshkina S

Study of the lumbar facet joints has already been a focus of attention in the orthopedic world for many decades. Understanding of the facet syndrome of the lumbar spine involves the notions of structural and fundamental changes in the facet joint.

Background

For many years, the lumbar zygapophyseal joints were the main cause of low back pain.[1, 2]

In 1933, RK Ghormley presented the term, "The lumbar facet syndrome".[3] In this work, he wrote clinical and radiological signs and development of the degenerative process.

The next investigations saw that the role of zygapophyseal joints in clinical and pathomorphological changes of lumbar spinal segment is not simple and play the main role in formation of lateral recess stenosis, foraminal stenosis, radicular pain production.[4-8]

Anatomical Sites and Pathomorphological Study

Facet joints are thought to be integral structural elements of the spine. Along with other components, they provide its supportive, motor, and protective functions. The main peculiarity of the facet joint is their close relationship with the elements of the spinal segment. Together with an intervertebral disk, they compose a so-called tree-joint-complex.[9] Changes in one of the components influence the rest being a morphological basis for reconstructions that result in function disorders of the vertebral column.

Facet joints are formed by articulated processes of the adjacent vertebral bodies and synovial joints, which have all anatomic elements—a fibrous capsule, a synovial membrane, meniscoids (intra-articular synovial folds), ligaments, synovial fluid, and an articular cartilage. Numerous anatomical, clinical, roentgenological, and biological studies prove a significant role in pathology of the facet joints in clinical manifestations of pain and degenerative changes of the intervertebral disks.[10-12]

During this period, the analysis of histologic changes of the facet joints removed in the course of posterior lumbar interbody fusion (PLIF) was carried out.

While studying the joints in 2 patients, we found free intra-articular fragments that noticeably influenced the formation of the clinical picture (Fig. 25.1).

As for the rest patients morphological articular changes corresponded to those in the other joints of the limbs. In unstable segments manifested hyperplastic intra-articular changes that can result in narrowing of the spinal canal were observed.

Structure of the Human Facet Joints at Different Age Periods

The joint surface of the superior articular process is insignificantly concave, and that of the inferior one is convex. In the central part of both facets, the thickness of the articular cartilage is more than in the periphery. On the average, the maximal thickness of the articular cartilage of the inferior process makes up 1.5 – 1.8 mm and the superior one 2.0 – 2.5 mm.

No distinct zone division in location of chondrocytes specific to the articular cartilage of major human joints was found in that of the facet joints though approximately we can identify tree zones (the boundaries are very indistinct). In the Superficial zone, the elongated cells having small but well-manifested processes predominate. However, a bit rounder cells also can be found. The chondrocytes are lying in 2–3 layers locating preferably parallel to the surface. The cells have large hyperchromatic nuclei surrounded with a narrow cytoplasm band.

Single chondrocytes and small isogenic groups (2–4 cells) located irregularly are displayed in a deeper layer.[13] The density of cells in the intermediary zone is the highest. Nucleus–cytoplasm relations in the cells are characterized by a volumetric increase of the cytoplasm where a well developed granular endoplasmic reticulum, Golgi apparatus with multiple secretory bubbles, and large mitochondrias are determined. In the deep zone the giant cells arranged in the isogenic groups (5–7 cells) and oriented by their long axes transverse to the surface appear. The chondrocytes of this zone contain large hyperchromatic nuclei surrounded by a cytoplasm band. In separate individuals (about 30%) in the deep zone, single cells with a part of them being hypertrophic predominate. A calcified cartilage has got thickness within 1/6 of the thickness of all the articular cartilage. A few vascular buds penetrated from subchondral bone into the calcified cartilage.[14]

Changes in the facet joints can be found at young age already but their manifestations cannot be clinically identified. Analysis of structural organization of the articular cartilage of the human vertebral bodies processes at the age of 20–29 indicated violation of cytoarchitectonics connected with absence of cells in the considerable areas of not only in the superficial zone but in the deeper parts as well[15] (Figs 25.2 to 25.4).

Numerous lacunae without chondrocytes are found. The edges of those lacunae are more basophilic than surrounding matrix. In the chondrocytes observed in all

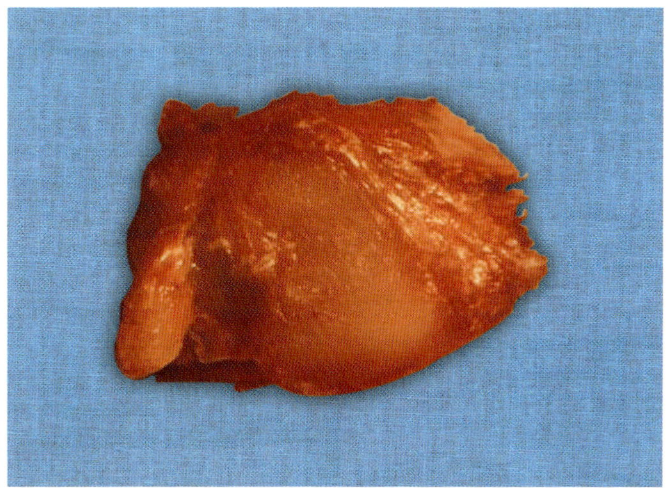

Fig. 25.1 Facet with free intra-articular body

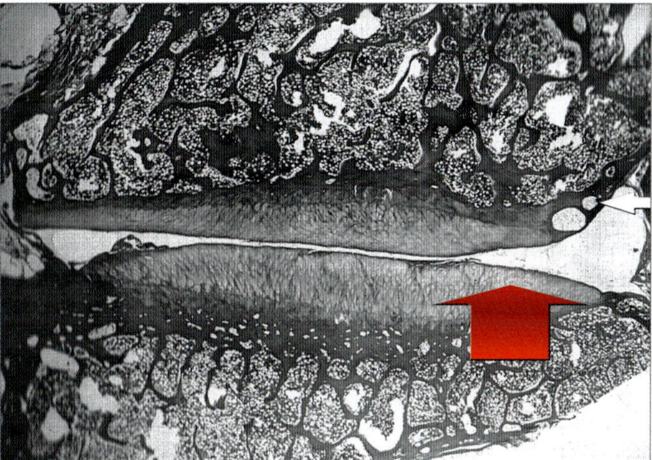

Fig. 25.2 Facet joint of L4–5 vertebral segment in 22-years-old man. Superior articular process L5 (white arrow)—dystrophic changes in articular cartilage. Inferior articular process L4 (red arrow) (H & E × 23)

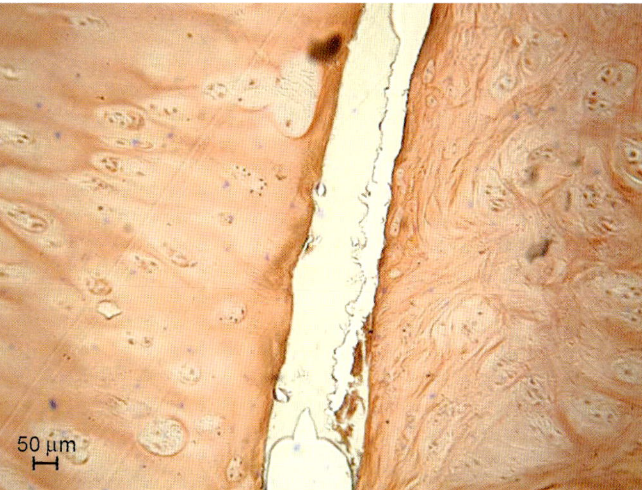

Fig. 25.3 The fragment of Figure 25.1. Lacunae without osteocytes. Pyknosis of chondrocytes (H & E × 100)

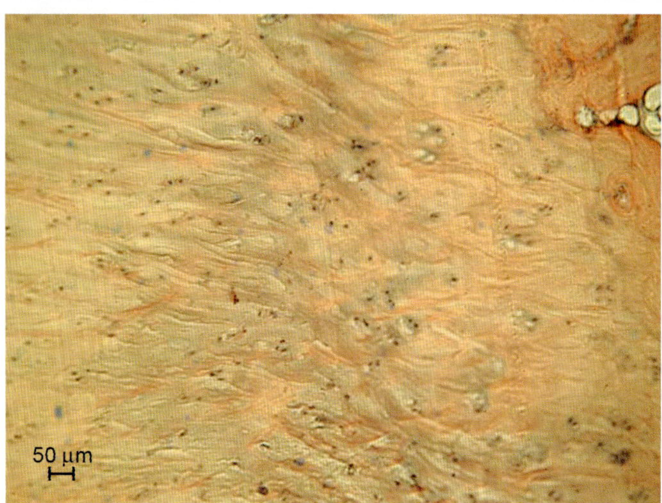

Fig. 25.4 Region of cartilage in facet joint in 22-years-old man, presented in Figure 25.1. Destruction of cartilage surface, appearance of clefts, hypocellularity and pyknosis of chondrocytes (H & E× 100)

zone of the articular cartilage, the nuclei are pyknotic, and cytoplasm is concentrated around the nucleus at one side.

In electron-microscopic study in cytoplasm of some chondrocytes the destruction of the membrane structure, accumulation of glycogen, large lipid drops as well as multiple microfilaments are observed. The nuclei of such cells are wrinkled and polymorphous with condensed chromatin predominated in them. In some lacunae cellular detritus can be seen.

On frequent occasions in the intermediary zone and especially in the deep one large active chondrocytes with their cytoplasm, brightly dyed in toluidine blue can be observed. Also, along with the changed chondrocytes the cells having well-developed and smooth endoplasmic reticulum, Golgi apparatus with a great number of secretory vesicles be seen with the help of electron microscopy that indicates activation of biosynthetical processes in them.

Matrix of the articular cartilage in the areas of destruction is dyed with eosin irregularly, and metachromasia (in reaction with toluidine blue) is not uniform in different parts that indicates change of its sorption properties. Analysis of the magnitude of birefringence of glycosaminoglycans (GAGs) makes it possible to state that in the superficial zone of the facet joints cartilage as well as in the large synovial ones an overall content of GAGs is the lowest. Maximally high magnitudes of GAGs are fixed in the territorial matrix of isogenic chondrocytes groups in deep zone. And the greatest portion of keratan sulfate in the overall content of GAG is determined in the interterritorial matrix.

In the polarized light when using picrosirius red dense and strong bundles of collagen fibers going from the calcified cartilage are observed. They are mainly located vertically but round the cells and change their direction only in the superficial zone where they are thin and loose.

The collagen fibers in the zone are oriented parallel to the articular surface. The magnitude of birefringence of collagen in the zones of articular cartilage is not homogenious. Its maximal value is noticed near the basophilic line. High values of the collagen birefringence are also observed both in the most superficial cartilage parts and deep zone. A significantly lower value of this magnitude is registered in the intermediary zone. These data can be related to a weakly manifested arcade of the collagen fibers in these parts (characteristic to the big joints cartilage).

In the articular cartilage of human vertebral bodies processes of the abovementioned age group more manifested dystrophic and destructive changes in the cells and matrix are fixed. Thus, in some parts of the cartilage surface, there is exfoliation of lamina splendens observed. In such places the cells are practically located on the surface among the loose collagen fibers. In certain samples, foci of matrix fibrillation, granular decay as well as small longitudinal and cross fissures which edges are uneven, brightly basophilically dyed and rather often are without cells or with empty lacunae are observed . Sometimes, the fissures are filled with detritus. Close to the fissures the birefringence of collagen and especially GAGs significantly decreased. A tide mark in the articular cartilages is slightly curved and weakly manifested almost in all the samples of the facet joints. In some cases in the vast territories it is represented by 2 – 4 enlarged lines having a distinctly manifested wavy shape with their peaks penetrating in the deep zone.

When comparing the described structural disorder in the superior and inferior articular processes we have found that for the most part changes in the cells and matrix can be seen in the superior articular process of the lower-lying vertebral body. It mainly relates to decrease of density in the chondrocytes location (especially in the surfaces and intermediate zone), increase in the number of degenerative cells, broadening the matrix fibrillation area and appearing collagen fibers areas, decrease in the birefringence magnitude of GAGs and collagen in some separate parts and growing the areas occupied with microfissures.

In the age groups of 30 – 39 and 40 – 49 years, the character of the observed changes in the cartilage tissue is similar to the above described. On comparing the above disorders in the structural organization of the articular cartilages in the patients' joints of the above age groups we could not state any distinctions, except for the elder age group (40 – 49 years) in which a decrease in the chondrocytes location density, especially in the superficial parts of the cartilage as well as an increase in the number of isogenic groups containing 6 – 9 cells was observed. In some samples of the facet joints, the number of hollow lacunae and chondrocytes with dystrophic changes is growing. Close to those cells, there are some parts of granular matrix decay. In the matrix among the collagen fibrils, the aggregates of dense droplets can be seen electron microscopically. In some lacunae of the dead cells, there were numerous thin collagen fibrils that very often had no distinct regularity. In the deep parts of the calcified articular cartilage hollow lacunae without chondrocytes with basophilic content and occupying significant areas were observed (Fig. 25.5).

In the territorial matrix of the intermediate and deep zones, higher values of birefringence of the keratan sulphates than in the 20 – 29 years age group were found. In 30% of cases in the edge parts of the articular cartilage the areas of chondrocytes hyperplasia were observed. In the articular cartilage in the superior process of underlying vertebral body were marked changes in comparison with than the inferior one. This regularity persists in all age groups.

Thus, in the cartilages of the human facet joints in the 20–29 years age group distinctly manifested changes of structural organization of both cells and matrix components are displayed. Older age (up to 50) insignificantly affects their worsening.

The similarity of structural organization of the facet joints with that of large synovial ones—zonality (though less manifested) in the distribution of cells, GAGs and collagen.[13]

Analysis of developing degenerative changes in the cartilage of facet joints connected with the age shown affinity with changes of articular cartilage of large synovial joints.[16,17]

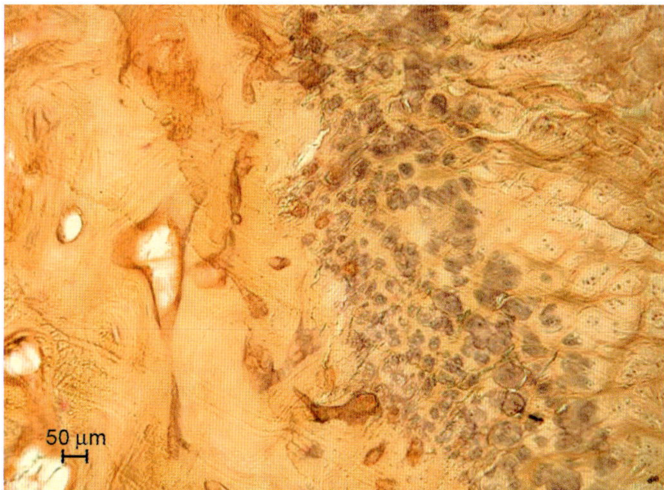

Fig. 25.5 Basophilic lacunae without chondrocytes in the calcified cartilage (H & E × 100)

Comparative research of morphological changes in the cartilage of the knee and hip joint in humans points to absence of those distinctions. The data of our research slow development of degenerative changes in the cartilage of the human facet joints after 30 years are relevant to the numerous data from scientific literature.[17-19] Some author[20,21] stated that their intensity and frequency significantly depends on the age, the others[16,22] noticed a weak rise of degenerative changes from 30 to 60 years.

Thus, a similar character of developing changes due to ageing in the cartilage of the facet and large synovial joints as well as their slow progress after 30 years confirm the existence of general regulations of ageing in the articular cartilage. Certain distinctions of the involutive process in the articular cartilage of that localization consisted in finding earlier (after 20 years) and distinctly manifested degenerative changes in the cartilage of facet joint compared to those in the large synovial joints are also found. The intensity of degenerative changes in the cartilage of facet joints in the earlier age could be connected with the peculiarities of collagen framework, namely the characteristic location of collagen fibers in the intermediate zone (arcades) providing dissipation and softening of pressure forces. Taking into account data of Nachemson[23] concerning the fact that under vertical loading the facet joints take about 20% of its value, and under eccentric loading – even more, one most expect that the cartilage chondrocytes of facet joints undergo increased loading that is a risk factor for developing degenerative changes.

A peculiarity of the facet joints also consists in different intensity of structural changes in the articular facets of a single joint predominating in the cartilage of the superior articular processes of the lower-lying vertebra body.

The facet joints have a capsule similar in structure to the capsule of the other synovial joints. A fibrous part of this capsule consists of dense bundles of collagen fibers interstratified with loose connective tissue and small areas of adipose tissue. Fibroblasts having elongated shape and oval nuclei are located between collagen fibers. A synovial membrane is thin and represented by scarce synoviocytes.

Facet Joint Changes and Low Back Pain

In population, spondyloarthritis is practically found in the equal amount of cases both in men (56.6%) and in women (66.7%). In the age group of 60–69 years, this pathology can be found in 89.2% of individual.

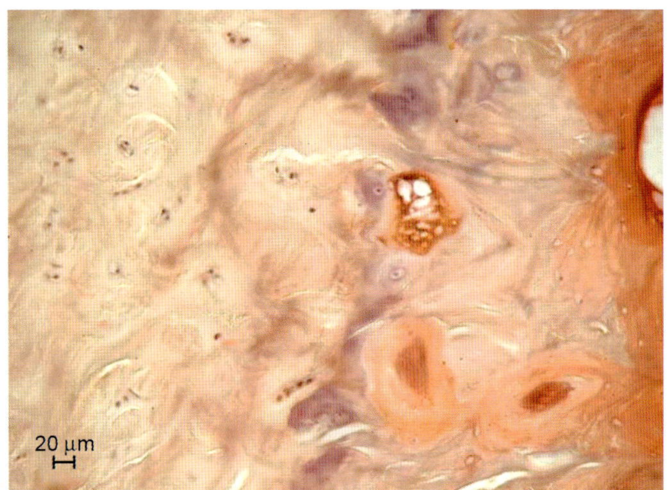

Fig. 25.6 Penetration of blood vessels into the articular cartilage. Pyknosis of chondrocytes. Disorders in matrix organization. Foci of bone formation in the articular cartilage (H & E × 200)

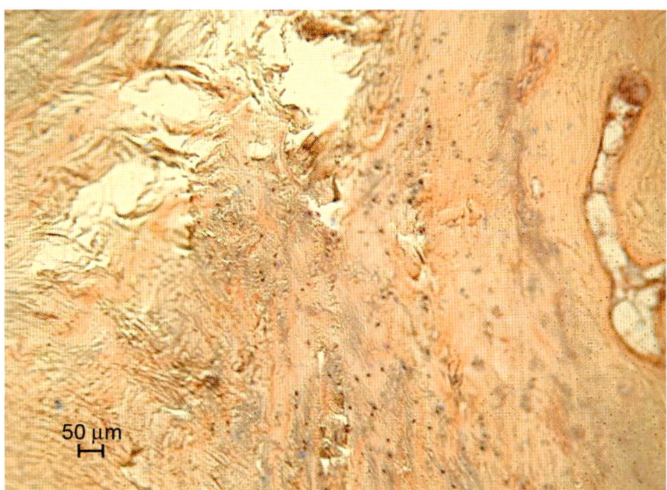

Fig. 25.7 Violation of matrix organization in the articular cartilage. (H & E. × 100)

Most frequently osteoarthritis affects the facet joints in spinal segment L4–L5.[24] Some data show that pain in spondyloarthritis is closely connected with violation of spinal motor segment stability.[25]

With the help of computed tomography, it is shown that the facet joints have a similar complex of pathologic disorders characteristic of the large joints in osteoarthritis: formation of osteophytes, hypertrophy of the articular processes, thinner of articular cartilage, synovial and subchondral cysts, calcification of the articular capsule.[26,27] Blood vessels grow into the articular cartilage, areas of bone tissue form around them (Fig. 25.6) that is evidence to a lack of factor inhibiting the growth of the vessels in this tissue.

Manifested destructive changes can be seen in the matrix of articulare cartilage – foci of ruptures and homogenization collagen fibers, destructive cavities, and fissures (Fig. 25.7).

In the large areas extensive parts having no cells are found. In these parts disorders of the articular cartilage matrix are observed. Scarcely located isogenic groups contain chondrocytes with a basophilic nucleus and a voluminous cytoplasm.

On frequent occasions on the surface of cartilage connective tissue is formed. The tide mark separating the calcified cartilage from the uncalcified one is also involved in the disorders. In some cases, this line is stratified in basophilic lines of different thickness. Sometimes, atypical structures connected with formation of the line in different levels of the articular cartilage are created.

On the vast expanses, the articular cartilage is destructed and found in form of separate segments with inflammatory infiltrates between them.

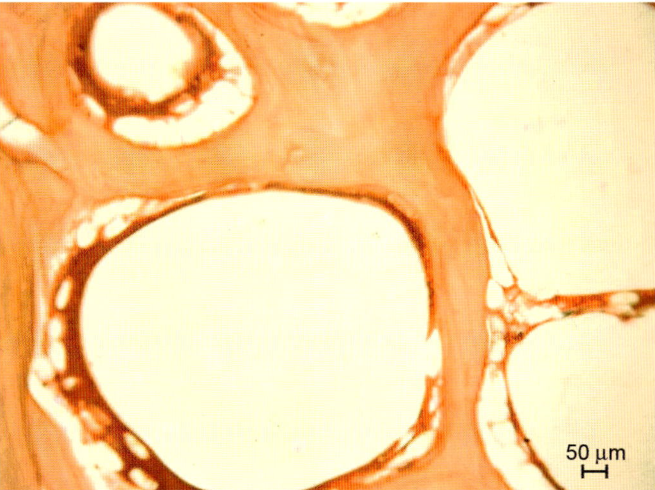

Fig. 25.8 Cyst like cavities in the subchondral bone (H & E × 100)

In the subchondral bone tissue cystlike cavities filled with fluid (Fig. 25.8). The marrow is ruined.

In the synovial membrane and articular capsule inflammatory manifestations can be seen.

At present, it is proved that in osteoarthrosis of the facet joints, synoviocytes and cartilaginous cells discharge a great number of proinflammatory cytokins, prostaglandins, leukotrienes, and metabolites of arachidonic acid supporting inflammatory process in the joint. This substances change metabolism of the matrix macromolecules and chondrocytes.[28,29] Under condition of the inflammatory process in the synovial membrane of the articular capsule biosynthesis of proinflammatory cytokins like TNF-α, IL-1β, IL-6 also rises from the data of Igarashi (2004),[30] the mechanism of pain in the spine does not relate to the impact of mechanic loading on the joints but is based on discharge of great amount of proinflammatory cytokins, which by the way of chemical influence worsen inflammatory process not only in the articular tissues but in the other subsystems of the spine and in the intervertebral disks in particular.

Thus, changes in the facet joints due to aging can be seen in the early age already and have a set of degenerative disorders of matrix and cells with a pain syndrome often being absent. In osteoarthrosis, under condition of manifested inflammatory process, destruction of the articular cartilage takes place on account of biosynthesis of proinflammatory cytokines by cells of the synovial membrane and articular cartilage with a manifested pain syndrome.

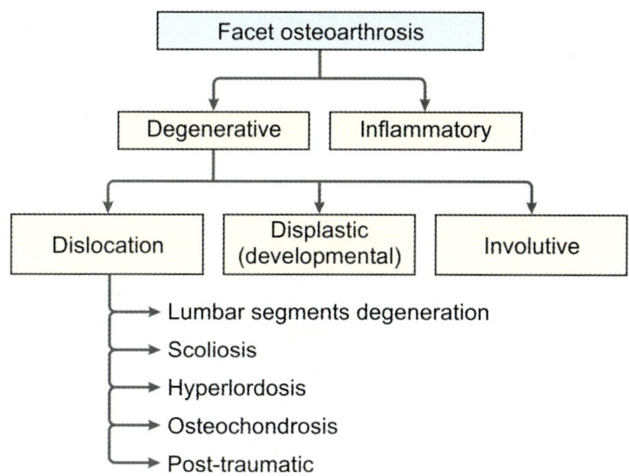

Fig. 25.9 Classification of facet osteoarthrosis

Classification

Facet joint arthrosis classification is usually presented as grade of difficulties of morphological changes and not far from another different joints arthrosis classification.

For example, Weishaupt classification established on the MRI and CT images: Grade 0—normal facet joint space (2–4 mm width); Grade 1—narroving of the facet joint space (<2 mm) and/or small ostophytes and/or mild hypertrophy of the articular process; Grade 2—narrowing of the facet joint space and/or moderate hypertrophy of the articular process and/or mild subarticular bone erosions; Grade 3—narrowing of the facet joint space and/or large osteophytes and/or severe hypertrophy of the articular process and/or severe subarticular bone erosions and/or subchondral cysts.[31]

Clinical classification was presented in Sytenko institute of Orthopaedics and Traumatology (Fig. 25.9).

Clinical symptoms delivery to intra- and extrajoints. Intrajoints realize by changes of cartilage of the facets, synoviits by sebsitivity of medial branch of posterior nervous rami.

Extrajoint clinical symptoms develop as a result of hyperplastic joints process, synovial cysts, lateral recess, and foraminal stenosis (Fig. 25.10). Clinical manifestation are the intermittent radiculo or caudogenic claudication.

The degree of markedness of the facet syndrome in different clinical variants of the lumbar spine degenerative disease was determined.

By functional condition the facet osteoarthrosis is divided into stable and unstable.

Facet Blocks: Diagnosis and Management

Intra-articular facet joints injections are important diagnostic and management procedure.

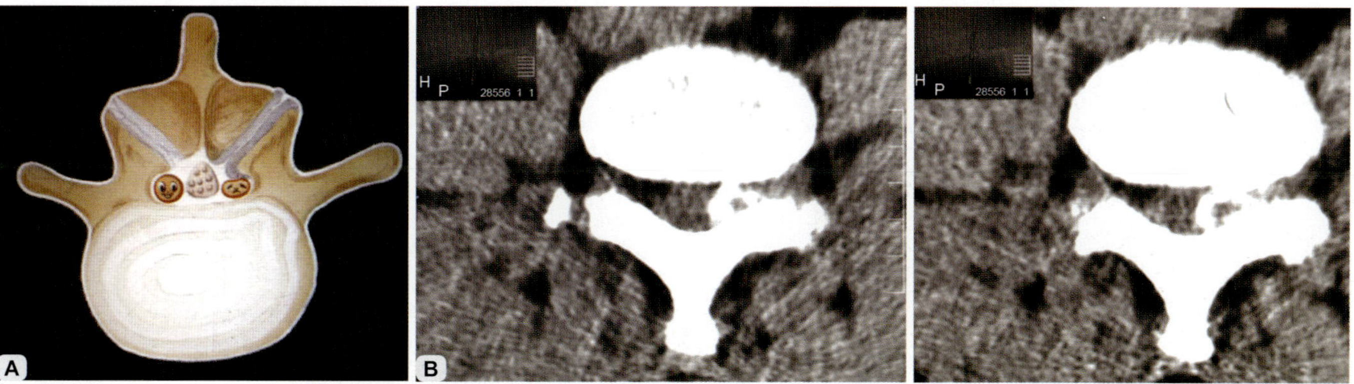

Fig. 25.10 (A) Scheme of facet joint and lateral recess stenosis formation; (B) CT scan of facet synovial cyst hyperplastic calcification

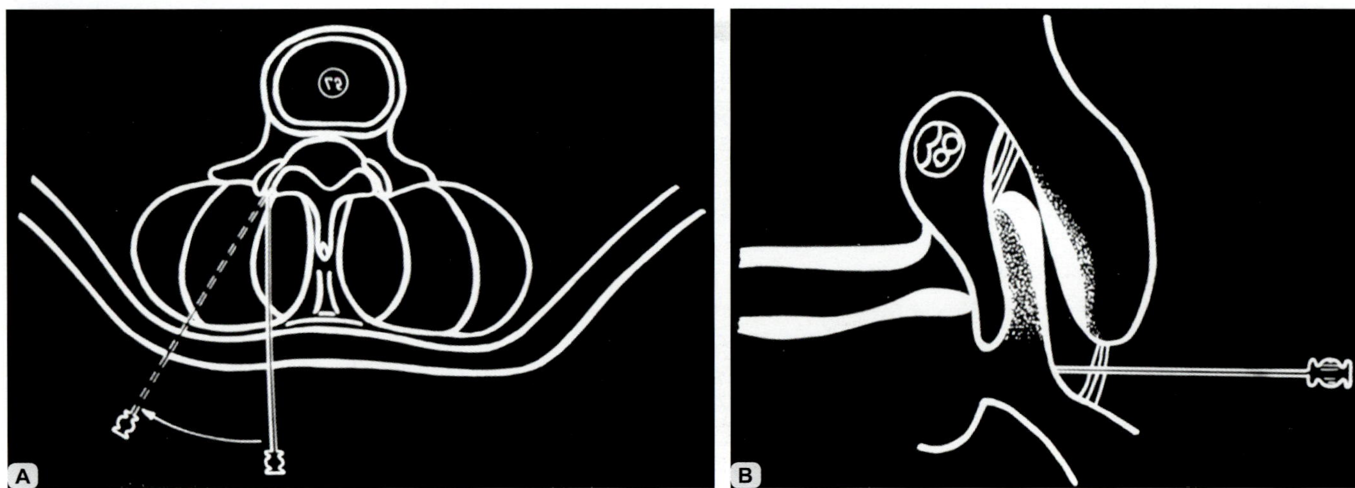

Fig. 25.11 Technique of lumbar facet joint puncture by (A) Mooney and Robertson (1976), (B) Radchenko V (1988)

The first step made of the function of zygapophyseal joint under fluoroscopic or CT scan control.

We used technique of Mooney and Robertson (1976) or Radchenko V (1988)[4, 5] (Fig. 25.11).

After the joint puncture we introduced a water-soluble contrast substance and performed the arthrography. During the introduction of the solution the capacity of the joint is measured. The shape of articular cavity on arthrograms was different. It depended on the extent of degenerative changes and instability growth in the spine.

As a rule in instability the joint capacity increases by our data, in two cases up to 2.5 mL, and that is fully reflected on arthrograms – i.e. enlarging of the contrast shadow square in the recesses of the joint (Fig. 25.12).

In two patients a diverticulum of the upper recess of the facet joint is revealed (Fig. 25.13). This fact greatly influences the clinical symptoms caused by the degeneration of the spine.

In 6 observations, we noticed ruptures of the joint capsule which occurred more frequently in the area of the upper turn. On the arthrograms it is seen that the contrast substance spreads extrajointly, with little reservations intrajointly (Fig. 24.14). We did not find any capsule rupture on the anterior surface of the joint, i.e. precisely on the segment which directly related to the spinal canal.

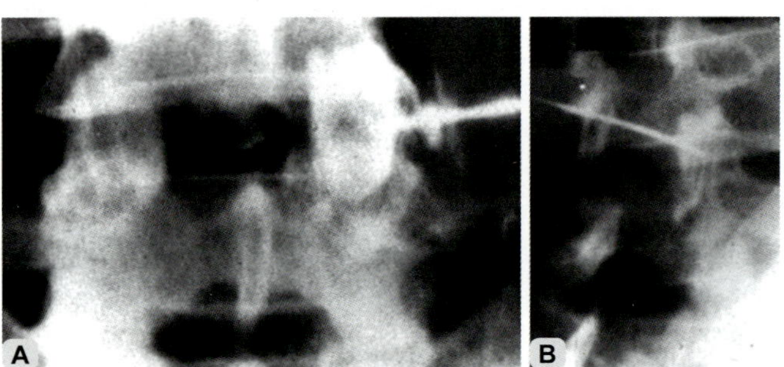

Fig. 24.12 Arthrogram showing enlargement of contract shadow square in the recesses of the joint

Understanding of structural and functional changes in the spinal segments greatly influences the choice of correct methods of treatment of pain syndromes caused by osteoarthrosis of the facet joints.

Along with medicamentous anti-inflammatory treatment, physiotherapy and other traditional means the blocade of the facet joints with corticosteroids is an important additional method for the treatment. When utilizing the blocades of the facet joints we arranged 2 groups of patients (Fig. 25.15):

Group I – the blocades performed under radiologic control with a primary arthrography, i.e. confirmed intra-articular introduction of a needle.

Group II – so-called – para-articular blocades, i.e. without a primary arthrography.

The results of the intra-articular blocades in the first group were good 65%, satisfactory 33%, and unsatisfactory 2%. In the second group, they were good in 58%, satisfactory 35%, and unsatisfactory 7%.

The study demonstrated more effective intra-articular introduction of medical preparations compared to the para-articular one.

Facet Denervation

The next efficient means to fight with pain syndromes of the facet joints is their denervation proposed by Rees in 1971.[32] It became particularly spread after the article by

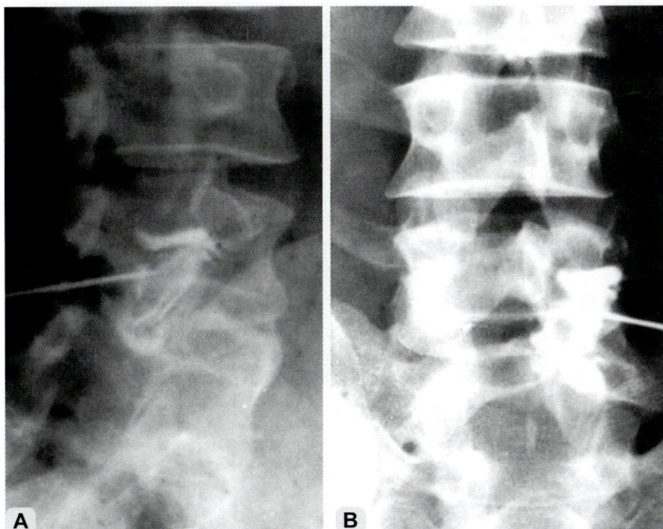

Fig. 25.13 Diverticulum of the lumbar facet joint L4–5. (A) X-ray in oblique projection; (B) X-ray in A/P projection

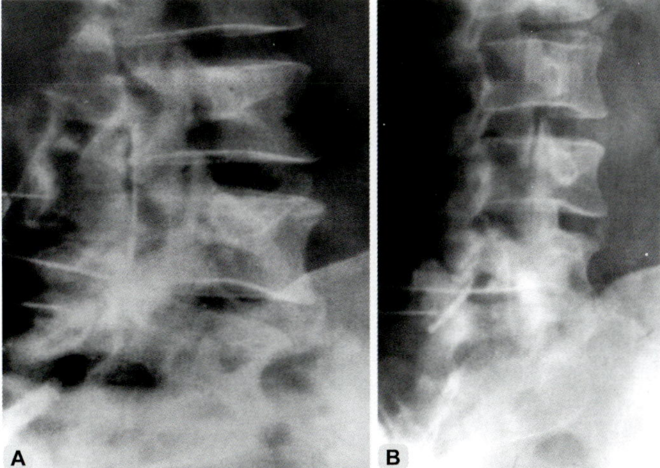

Fig. 25.14 X-ray in (A) oblique and (B) A/P projection. Extra-jointly contrast shadow

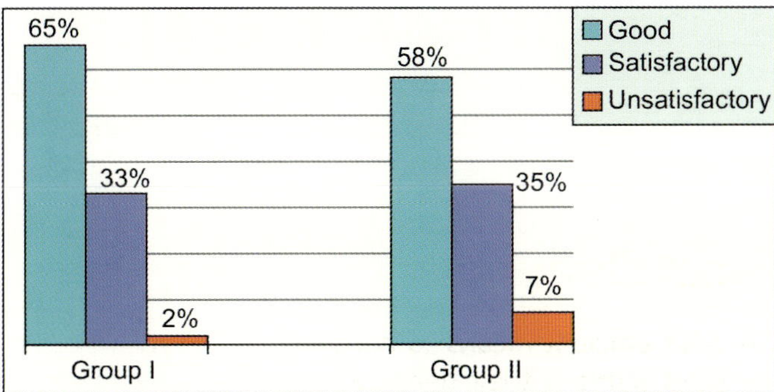

Fig. 25.15 Results of facet intra- and extra-articular blocks

Shealy W published—the journal "*Clinical Orthopaedics and Related Research*" in 1976.[33] He proposed to perform destruction of the posterior ramus of the medial branch by way of radiofrequency destruction. Since that time the denervation is performed by way of laser or cryodestruction and other means.

We performed the denervation of the facet joints in the lumbar spine by way of electrocoagulation and cryodestruction (Fig. 25.16).

The results of the facet denervation were satisfactory in the first group 72% and in the second group 76% (Fig. 25.17).

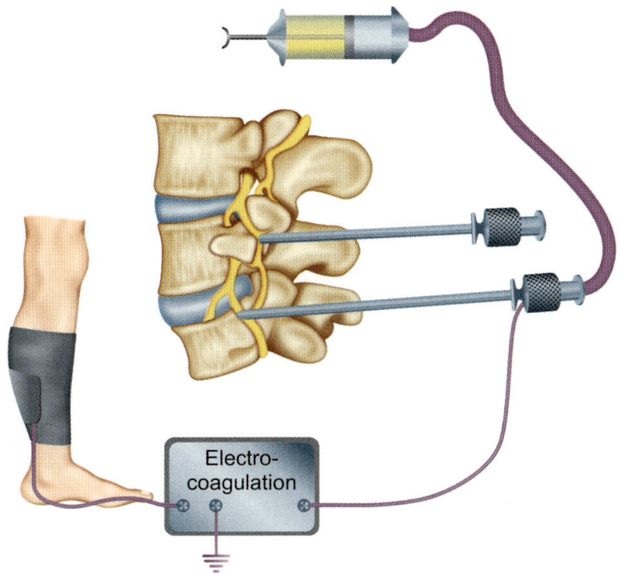

Fig. 25.16 Scheme of lumbar joints denervation by electrocoagulation

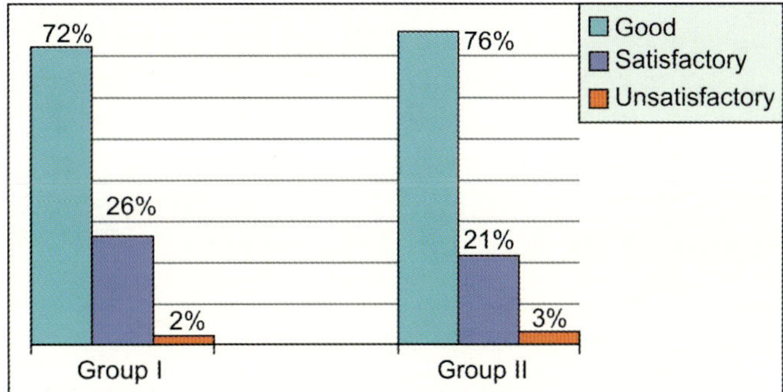

Fig. 25.17 The results of lumbar facet joint denervation by electrocoagulation and cryodestruction

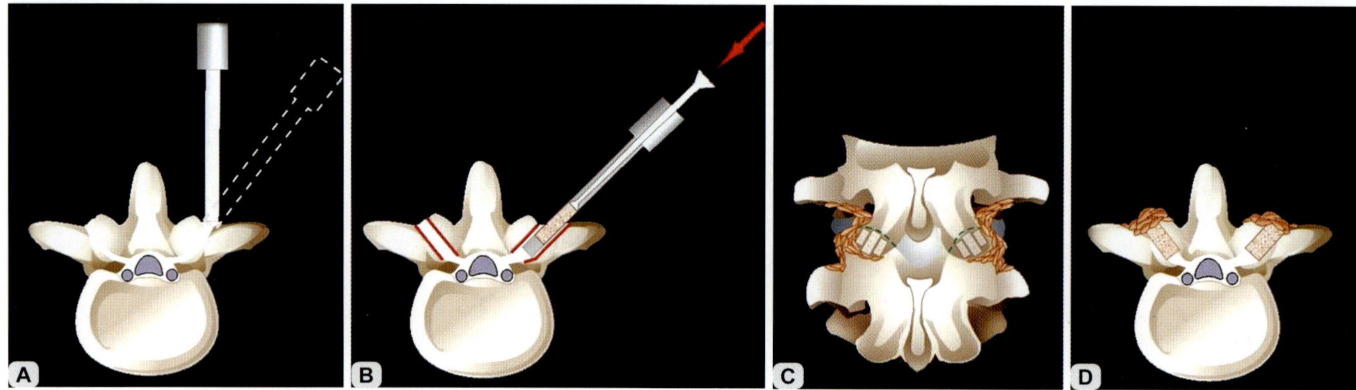

Fig. 25.18 Scheme of technique of percutaneous lumbar facets spine fusion

Percutaneous Facet Joint Fusion

The most radical methods of management of spondyloarthrosis are stabilization of the lumbar vertebral segments and arthrodesis of the facet joints in particular.

The potentiality of facet joint arthrodesis of the lumbar spine has been attracting surgeon's attention for along time. For this purpose King (1948) used bone transplants from tibia and osteous processus,[34] Boucher (1959)[35] applied method of the transarticular fixation by means of screws and bone autoplasty taken out from the ilium and interposed them between vertebral arches.[35]

Necessity of the percutaneous arthrodesis of the facet joints emerges not frequently. However, such a type of surgical intervention must be seriously regarded and applied by spinal surgeons.

The first experience a new technique of percutaneous arthrodesis of the lumbar zygapophyseal joint was presented by Radchenko in Zurich symposium (1998)[36-38] and publicated in *the Journal of Minimally Invasive Spinal Technique* (2004).[39]

The first experience in USA presented by J Chiu in the Rome Spine Congress (2006).[40]

Indications to the operation were the facet syndrome (17 cases) the conservative treatment of which stayed unsuccessful as were as degenerative lumbar spine instability (3 cases).

Control and assessment of the results were performed 3,6, and 12 months later after the operation.

Technique of Percutaneous Ceramic Fusion of the Lumbar Facet Joints

The patient is placed in a prone position with a slight flexion in the hips under radiologic control.

On the first stage of the operation the puncture of the joints is performed by means of a long needle. For the puncture of the joint use Mooney and Robertson (1976) thechniques.[3]

After the joint puncture, we introduced a water-soluble contrast substance and performed arthrography.

After assessment of additional data, received by means of arthrography, in turn, on both sides, the performing of arthrodesis of the facet joints is started (Fig. 25.18).

The working tube for percutaneous arthrodesis has an internal diameter of 5.5 mm.

After stabbing the skin and fascia by scalpel, a cannular set with an obturator is introduced up to the joint on the level of the middle portion of the articular fissure and bent under the angle coinciding with the joint processes plane.

The obturator is extracted, and instead of it a milling cutter is introduced. The cutters used are of different shape-conical, round, cylindrical. In order to form the canal the drills are also applied. In the course of drilling and cutting operations the cartilaginous layers are cut up to the bone tissue.

The formation of the canal is finished by means of cylindrical cutter.

After extraction of the cutter an implant of biologically, inactive material of cylindrical form is hammered. For this purpose we use a medium porous ceramics of cylindrical form (dimension of pores – from 50 to 300 μ.

Then the canal in the inferior part of the joint is performed and bone allotransplant is introduced into it.

In the superior part bone matrix is introduced.

After the completing of this stage through the tubus by means of cutters decortications of the posterior surface of the facet with a transition to the transverse processes of the adjacent vertebrae is performed.

Along with the operation at the same time denervation of the facets using advanced technique by Shealy (1976), through the electric coagulatition of a medical branch of the posterior ramus of the spinal nerve according to innervation was performed.[33]

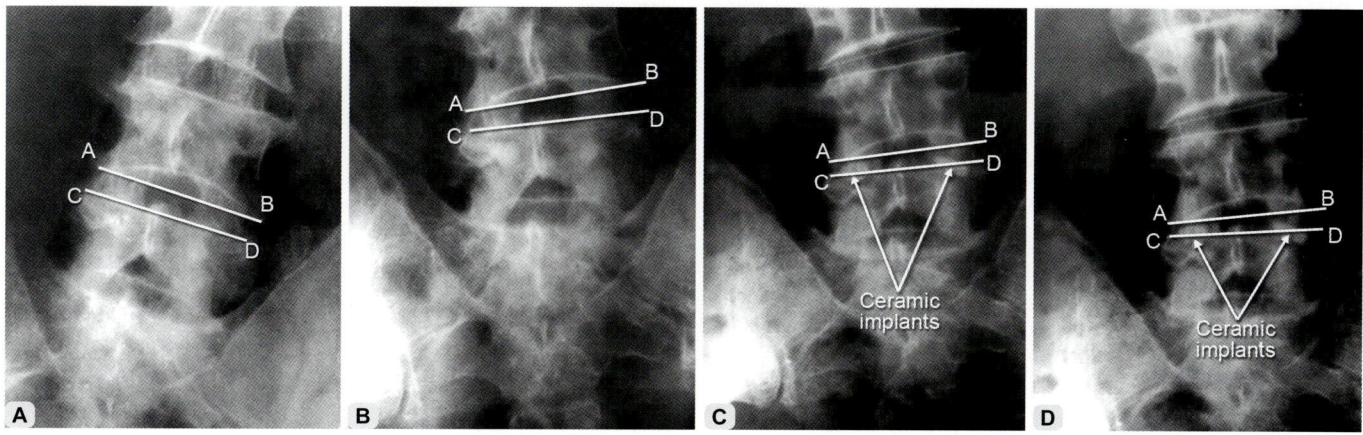

Fig. 25.19 X-ray showing clinical examples

In two patients cryodestruction was made.

After removing of the cannular set, we introduced electrodes for electrostimulation of regeneration using direct current.

Control and assessment of the results were performed 3,6 and 12 months later after the operation.

Clinical Examples

During the postoperative period the intensity of pain syndrome decreased immediately and gradually disappered maximum a week later after the operation.

In two patients, the pain syndrome still remained relatively severe, that demanded to introduce anti-inflammatory corticosteroids to stop the pain.

The tension of paravertebral muscles after intervention gradually was decreasing for 3 weeks; however, in a vertical position, it was renewed. During the wear of a corset rigidity and constraint in the lumbar spine which disappeared max. 5–6 months later was observed.

Moving exercizes for the lumbar spine including hydrokinesiotherapy and others were allowed 9–12 months later after the operation.

In 3 patients an increase in the movements amplitude was accompanied by pains of low intensity which were eliminated of nonsteroid anti-inflammatory substances.

Step by step, the range of movements increased and the patients renewed their working activity. Two of them are busy with physical job now.

In three cases the validity of the osteoceramic bloc was doubtful.

X-rays of clinical example are introduced in Figure 24.19.

References

1. Goldwaith JE. The lumbosacral articulation an explanation of many cases of "lumbago", "sciatica" and "paraplegia". Boston Med Surg J. 1911;164: 365-72.
2. Putti V. New conceptions in the pathogenesis of sciatic pain. Lancet. 1927; 2:53-60.
3. Ghormley RK. Low back pain with special reference to the articular, facets, with presentation of an operative procedure. JAMA. 1933;101:1773-7.
4. Mooney V, Robertson J. The Facet Syndrome. Clin Orthop Relat Res. 1976;115:149-56.
5. Radchenko V. Z-arthrosis. Kharkov.1988. p.192.
6. Prodan A, Paschuk A, Radchenko V, et al. The lumbar facet arthrosis. Kharkov. 1992.
7. Prodan A, Radchenko V, Malyshkina S. Facet joints changes and artrography. Orthop., Traumat., 1990; No. 8: p.21-6.
8. Sak L. The lumbar facet syndrome. Magnitogorsk, 2001.p.100.
9. Yong-Hing K, Kirkaldy-Wills H. The pathophysiology of degenerative disease of the lumbar spine. Orthoped. Clin North Amre. 1983;14(3):491-504.
10. Kenesi C, Lusur E. Orientation of the articular processes at I. L and S. Possible role in pathology of the intervertebral disc. Anat Din. 1985; 7(1):43-7.
11. Singer K, Gules L, Day R. Intra-anicuiar synovial folds cf thoracolumbar junction zygapophyseal joints. Anat Rec. 1990; 226: 147-52.
12. Taylor J. Lumbar zygapophyseal incongruity as a sign of motion segment instability. J Anat 1989; 165:299-303.
13. Dedukh NV, Malyshkina SV, Kern M, Pankov YeYa. Age changes of the intercellular substance hyaline and collagen-fibrous cartilaginous human tissue. Archive anat. 1988;94(4):35-9.
14. Dedukh NV, Malyshkina SV, Radchenko VA. Morphology of the articular cartilage of facet joints and intervertebral discs in the humans at young age. Tavrichesky Medico-Biological Bulletin. 2006; 9(3):45-9.

15. Radchenko VA. Dedukh NV, Malyshkina SV. Histological changes in facet joint and disc degeneration. The practice of minimal invasive spinal technique. New York: AAMISS Press; 2005. p.75-81.
16. Hough AG, Webber R.J. Aging phenomena and osteoarthritis: cause or coincidence. Ann Din Labor Sci 1986; 16(6):502-10.
17. Vignon E, Ariot M, Vignon G. The ceil density of human femoral head cartilage. Clin Orthop. 1975;121:303–08.
18. Armstrong CG, Gardner DL. Thickness and distribution of numan femoral head articular cartilage. Ann Rheum Dis. 1977; 36(5):407-12.
19. Lequesve M. Senescence et arthrose. La fin d'un litige de frontiers'7 Nouv. Presse med. (Paris). 1973; 2:619-20.
20. Pemcone E, Poaimoski M. Failure of proteoglycans to form aggregates in morphologically normal aged human cartilage Arch Rheum. 1977; 20(7):1372-80.
21. Venn M. Chemical composition of human femoral head cartilage. Ann Rheum Dis. 1979; 33(1):57-62.
22. Stockwetl R. The interrelationship of ceil density and cartilage thickness in mammalian articular cartilage. J Anat. 1971;109: 411-12.
23. Nachemson A. Recent advances in the treatment of low back pain. Int.Orthop. SICOT. 1985; 9:1-10.
24. L Kalichman, L Li, DH Kim et al. Facet joint osteoarthritis and low back pain in the community-based population. Spine. 2008; 33(23):2560-5.
25. Fujiwara A, Lim TH, An HS. The effect of disc degeneration and facet joint osteoarthritis on the segmental flexibility of the lumbar spine et al. Spine. 2000; 25(23): p.3036-44.
26. Carrera GF, Haughton VM, Syversten A et al. Computed tomography of the facet joints. Radiology. 1980;134:p.145-148.
27. Resnick R, Niwayama G. Degenerative disease of the spine. Diagnosis of bone and joint disorders, 3rd ed. – Philadelphia, PA: WB Saunders, 1995; c.1372-462.
28. Willburger R.E. Prostaglandin release from lumbar disc and facet joint tissue. Spine. 1994;19:2068-70.
29. Iwanaga T, Shikichi M, Kitamura H. Morphology and functional roles of synoviocytes in the joint. Arch Histol Cytol. 2000;63:17-31.
30. Igarashi A, Kikuchi S, Konno S, Olmarker K Inflammatory cytokines released from the facet joint tissue in degenerative lumbar spinal disorders. Spine. 2004;29(19):2091-5.
31. Weishaupt D, Zanetti M, Boos N. et al. Skeletal radiology. 1999;28:215-9.
32. Rees WS. Multiple bilateral subcutaneous phizolysis of segmental newes in the treatment of the intervertebral disc syndrome. Ann Yen. Pract. 16:126-7
33. Shealy C.N. Facet, denervation in the management of back and sciatic pain. Clin Orthop. 1976;115-64.
34. King D. Internal fixation for lumbosacral fusion. J Bone J Surg. 1948;30(A):560-8.
35. Boucher H.H. A method of spine fussion. J Bone J Surg. 19598; 41(B):258-64.
36. Radchenko V. Lumbar pertcutaneous arthrodesis of zygoapophyseal joints. 16th Course for Percutaneous Endoscopic Spinal Surgery and Complementary Techniques.- Symposium with international guest faculty and work- shop/ technical exhibichion. Zollikerberg: Zurich; 1998; p.26
37. Radchenko V. Percutaneous fusion of the lumbar facet joints. The practice of minimally invasive spine technique – Wyndham Hall Press in Lima, Ohio; 2005; p.537-9.
38. Yeung AT, Savitz MN, Chiu JC. Endoscopic removal of 3 incidental synovial cysts of the lumbar facet. J Minim Invasive Spinal Tech. 2003;3:42-5.
39. Radchenko V. Percutaneous fusion of the lumbar facet joints Minim Invasive Spinal Tech. 2004;4:51-2.
40. Chiu JC. Evolving endoscopic spine surgery. Rome spine 2008, Electronic presentation, Rome, Italy; 2008.

CHAPTER

26

Degenerative Lumbar Scoliosis: Controversial Issues and a New Challenge

Myung-Sang Moon, Sung-Soo Kim, Bong-Jin Lee, Jeong-Lim Moon, Seog In Moon

As the current population ages, clinicians are confronting more complex degenerative spinal conditions with increased frequency. One such condtion is the degenerative lumbar scoliosis (DLS) which is usually seen in the elderly patients with unilaterally wedged degenerative disk and advanced facet degeneration.

Scoliotic spines are seen frequently and are known to be caused by the various etiologies: congenital, disease-related (neuromuscular diseases, fibrous dysplasia, spondylolysis), idiopathic, degenerative, and postlaminectomy origins (Fig. 26.1). Among the various types of scoliosis the most common one is the DLS, which is more symptomatic than the others.

However, it is true that up to now most physicians have interested more in the idiopathic scoliosis in the adolescent than DLS, though the management of idiopathic scoliosis is rather cosmetic than the symptomatic purpose.

DLS is not a new entity,[1-18,21-27,29-43] and in the past, this condition was known as a senescent lumbar deformity, i.e. those elderly people with the deformity was named as a hunch-backed grand-mom or -pa, and the deformity was regarded as a natural process of senescence in the lumbar spine. When those patients had stenotic symptoms and signs, they were treated under the diagnosis of lumbar stenosis,[19,20] multisegmental spondylosis and/or unstable back without paying attention to the crooked back. It was true that the deformed back in the elderly was lowly regarded as a disease entity regardless of size of the curve, and that surgeons in the past paid more attention to the patient's pain complaints, and not to the crooked (deformed) back.[28,31-37]

In the elderly people, two different types of bone qualities are observed: some have osteoporosis without spondylosis, while others have relatively good bone quality with spondylosis. The elderly with osteoporosis suffers more frequently from back pain secondary to bony vertebral column collapse, while the elderly with good bone quality suffers more from the limb pain and/or back pain due to spondylosis associating stenotic symptoms. The elderly people with symptomatic back suffer from one of these two conditions.[1-13]

DLS has also been referred as "collapsing scoliosis" and "senescent lumbar scoliosis". The DLS patient has additionally lumbar kyphosis instead of lordosis with antelisthesis and/or rotatory lateral olisthesis at another segment.

DLS is a *de novo* deformity of the spine occurring after the fourth or fifth decade of life in adults with no history of scoliosis in the growing age. As its name implies, DLS preferentially affects the lumbar spine particularly the lower segments, although occasionally the upper lumbar spines are also involved (Fig. 26.1). In general DLS is a progressive deformity, and the curve may increase in size between 2° and 6° per year. Disk degeneration leading to segmental instability in the coronal plane may result in degenerative scoliosis with or without olisthesis.[11,15]

Robin et al. reported that a scoliotic angle of 10° or greater was noted in 30% of 554 symptomatic patients, and that 10% had new curvatures during the 7- to 14-year follow-up period. They listed the 3 risk factors: genetic background, gender, and disk degeneration.[42] Others listed the following factors, such as degree of apical rotation, the Cobb angle,

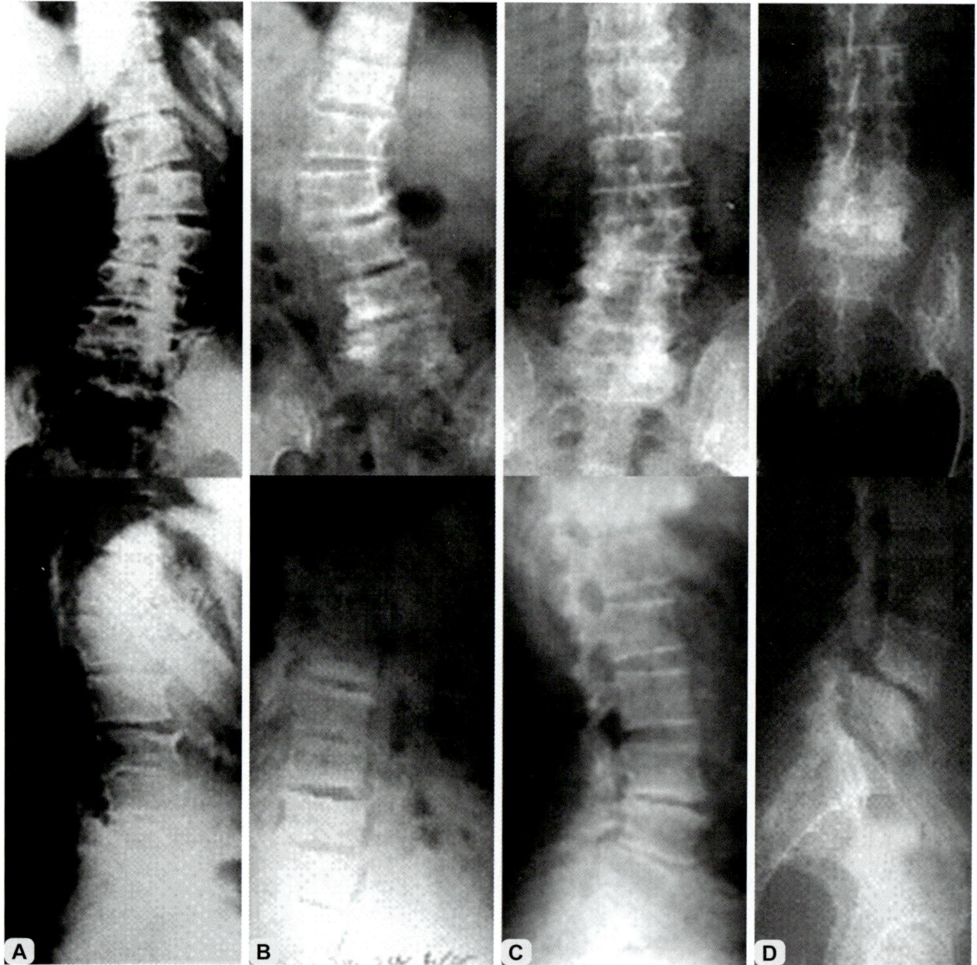

Fig. 26.1 Radiographs of four types out of 7 scoliosis of the different origins. (A) Adolescent idiopathic lumbar scoliosis (rotatory slip of L3); (B) *de novo* degenerative lumbar scoliosis (rotatory slip of L3); (C) Postlaminectomy degenerative scoliosis (angular tilt of L3–4); (D) Degenerative scoliosis secondary to spondylolysis (angular and rotatory tilt and anterior slip of L4)

the relation of L5 to the intercrestal line, while Pritchett and Bartel suggested that DLS may start with instability at the L3–L4 and L4–L5 disks.[40]

DLS is a condition causing mainly stenotic symptoms. Therefore, it is thought that DLS should be included in the category of the degenerative spinal diseases causing stenosis. It seems better to be treated under the diagnosis of spinal stenosis in the clinical sense.

Subject Gender and Age Incidences

Some reported that the gender incidence of DLS was equal,[16] while the other reported that the incidence in females is twice more than the males.[7] In the current authors' series the incidence was also higher in females.

The reported overall incidences of DLS according to Vanderpool et al.[44] Fujita and Yamakawa,[15] and Perennou et al.[39] were 6% (patients over 50 years), 8.3%, and 7.5% (671 low back patients), respectively.

The age-related incidence of the DLS were 0.3% in the patients under age of 40 years, 2.8% in 5th decade, 5.1% in 6th decade, 8.1% in 7th decade, 18.0% in 8th decade, 15.0% over 80 years of age.[13] The mean Cobb's angle was 14.9° (10°~56°).

Pathogenesis

Although its cause was not completely understood, it seems to result from the asymmetric degeneration of the disks which might associate the unilateral erector spine weakness. However, recently according to Shim et al. DLS may be predisposed by genetic factors that control the quality or quantity of protein expression, and was considered that the expression of DLS is supported by various typical copy number variations (CNV-s)-associated structural variants of the genome.[45]

Clinical Findings, Pathomorphology, and Pathophysiology

Jackson et al. graded the severity of the degenerative changes of the scoliotic lumbar spine into four grades (Table 26.1).[22]

Table 26.1 Grades of degenerative changes in the lumbar curve (modified from Jackson's criteria)

Grade 1	Only mild disk narrowing with evidence of degenerative changes
Grade 2	Moderate disk degeneration, end-plate sclerosis, osteophyte-associated slipping
Grade 3	Severe disk degeneration, sclerosis, osteophytic lipping, slipping and vertebral body wedging
Grade 4	Marked disk degeneration, sclerosis, osteophytic lipping, slipping and vertebral body wedging

The relationships of the clinical findings, pathomorphology and pathophysiology in DLS are shown in Figure 26.2. In DLS the etiology, clinical symptoms and signs, and the deformities are very closely related (Fig. 26.2). [14,39] When the deformity progresses the symptoms and signs become worse, and the unsightly trunk shift is frequently seen.

According to Moon et al., there was no direct relationship between age and degree of curvature, whereas there was a linear relationship between the severity of degenerative changes and increase in curvatures.[32-34,37] The primary pathology in degenerative scoliosis is lateral listhesis, coupled with lateral wedging of the vertebral body and angulation secondary to asymmetric degeneration of the facet joints. Degenerative spondylolisthesis may often be associated with degenerative scoliosis.[41]

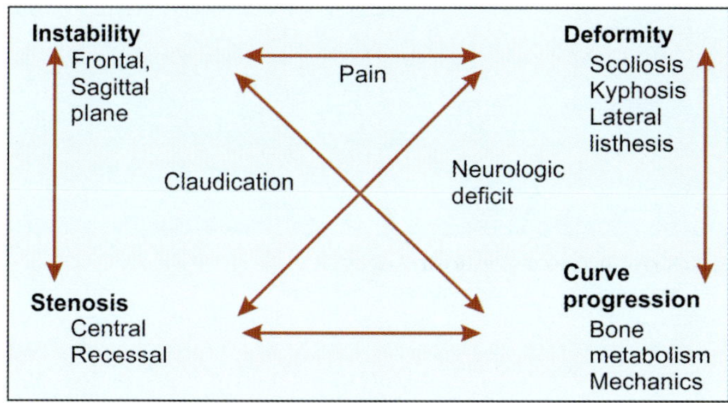

Fig. 26.2 Complexity of the relationship between clinical symptoms and signs and pathomorphology and pathophysiology of lumbar scoliosis

Table 26.2 Characteristic features of polysegmental degenerative lumbar scoliosis and adult idiopathic lumbar scoliosis with secondary age-relateed spondylosis.

Disease entity / *Features*	*De novo DLS*	*Idiopathic adult scoliosis*
Curve • Size	Small (mild)	Larger (severe)
• Secondary curve	Rather minimal and flexible	Rather larger and rigid
• Associated deformity	Kyphosis	Lordosis
• Rigidity	less (flexible)	Rather rigid
• Rotatory slip	Frequent	Rare
Anterior vertebral column and canal length	Equal	Anterior column is longer than canal
Curve correction	Easier	Difficult

DLS differs from adult idiopathic scoliosis with secondary degenerative changes (Table 26.2), because there is minimal structural vertebral deformity, advanced degenerative changes, and a lower lumbar curve. Therefore, the advanced multisegmental DLS has kyphoscoliotic deformity, while the adult idiopathic scoliosis with advanced spondylosis has lordoscoliotic deformity.[15-17,32-35]

Clinical Type Classification

The *de novo* DLS were classified into three types by Toyama (Table 26.3),[46] and two types by Moon et al. due to the numbers of the involved disks making the curve:[33-37]

1. oligosegmental type (1~2 motion segment involvement) and
2. polysegmental type (3 or more motion segments are involved in making the curve).

Table 26.3 Toyama et al's classification of degenerative lumbar scoliosis (1990)

Type		*Accessory changes*
I	Laterally wedged L4–5 disk Severe degenerative change in the facet joint of concave side of L4–5	Mild scoliosis in the upper level with small Cobb angle and right rotation. * Bony lipping on the concave side of L1–2, and L2–3
II	Scoliosis due to multilevel disc degeneration of mid-lumbar region. Deformity and rotation are more remarkable than type I	
III	Other type (combined I and II)	

Curve features and the incidence of the curve types are presented in Table 26.4.

In the oligosegmental type there are three subtypes; mono- and bisegmental origin in the 3 different levels; upper, middle, and lower type. Polysegmental DLS is also classified by its curve shape; C-curve and double reciprocating types. In both curves, some have the apex of the curve in the right, and other have the apex in the left.

Clinically, the upper type of oligosegmental DLS took the better clinical course than the lower types. In the polysegmental type, C-curve DLS took the more benign clinical course than the double reciprocating type. Stenotic symptoms were more frequently found in the double reciprocating type and the lower type of oligosegmental DLS.

Up to now the polysegmental type has been known to represent the classical degenerative lumbar scoliosis. Most of the symptomatic early oligosegmental DLS was not accepted as DLS, and was treated under the diagnosis of the degenerative lumbar stenosis. The current authors strongly propose that oligo- and polysegmental DLS should be managed equally under the same therapeutic protocol, though those two are different entities from the start as far as the curve length on basis of numbers of the participating degenerative disks is concerned.[31-34]

The radiograms of the two polysegmental (Figs 26.3 and 26.4) and the one oligosegmental DLS (Fig. 26.5) are shown.

Polysegmental DLS has two subtypes: single C curve and double reciprocating curves. However, there have been controversies whether the oligosegmental DLS is the early

Table 26.4 Curve features

Curve pattern	*Author's series No. of patients (%) (n = 141)*
Shape of curve	
C-shape	75 (53.2)
S-shape	66 (46.8)
Direction of curve	
Right side	73 (51.8)
Left side	68 (48.2)
Apex of curve	
L2	22 (15.6)
L3	91 (64.5)
L4	26 (18.4)
Number of segments involved	
5	4 (2.8)
4	23 (16.3)
3	37 (26.3)
2	77 (54.6)
Mean: 2.8 segments	
Range: 2–5 segments	
Degree of curve	
11–20°	98 (69.5)
21–30°	37 (26.2)
31–40°	6 (4.3)
Mean: 16.4°	
Range: 10-32°	
C-shape: single curve	
S-shape: double reciprocating	

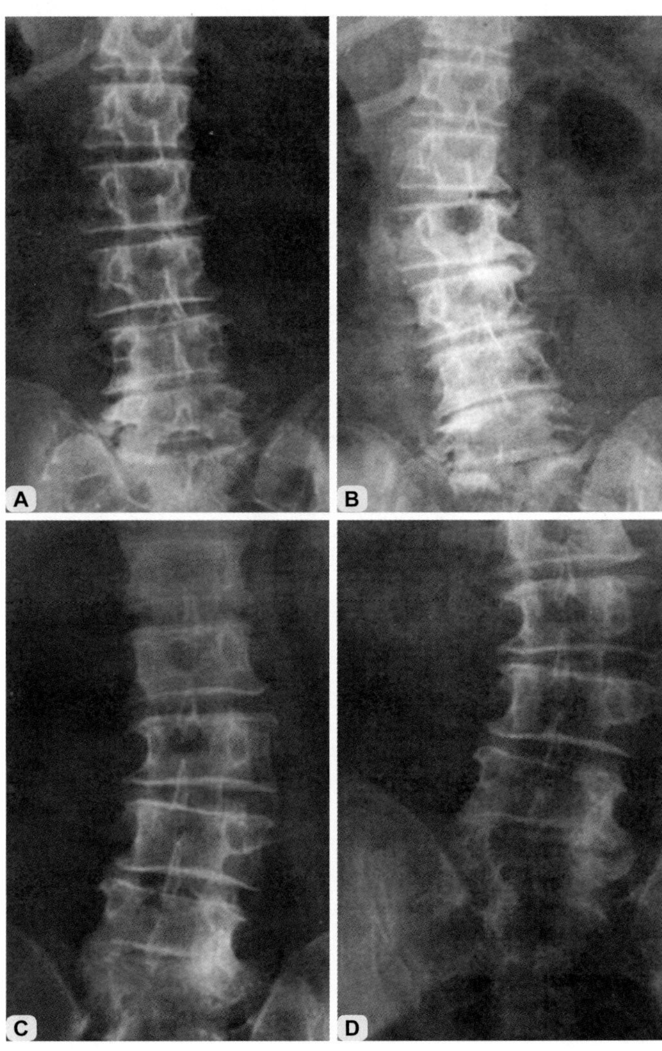

Fig. 26.3 Two examples of conservatively treated polysegmental DLS. (A) Radiograph of a 61-year-old male with mild single C-curve left lumbar scoliosis with L4 rotatory left listhesis; (B) Radiograph of same patient at 77-years of age show moderate curve progression with more advanced degenerative changes; (C) Radiograph of a 54-year-old female with mild single right C-curve polysegmental de novo degenerative lumbar scoliosis; (D) Radiogram of the same patient at 66 years of age shows curve progression and slightly advanced degenerative changes

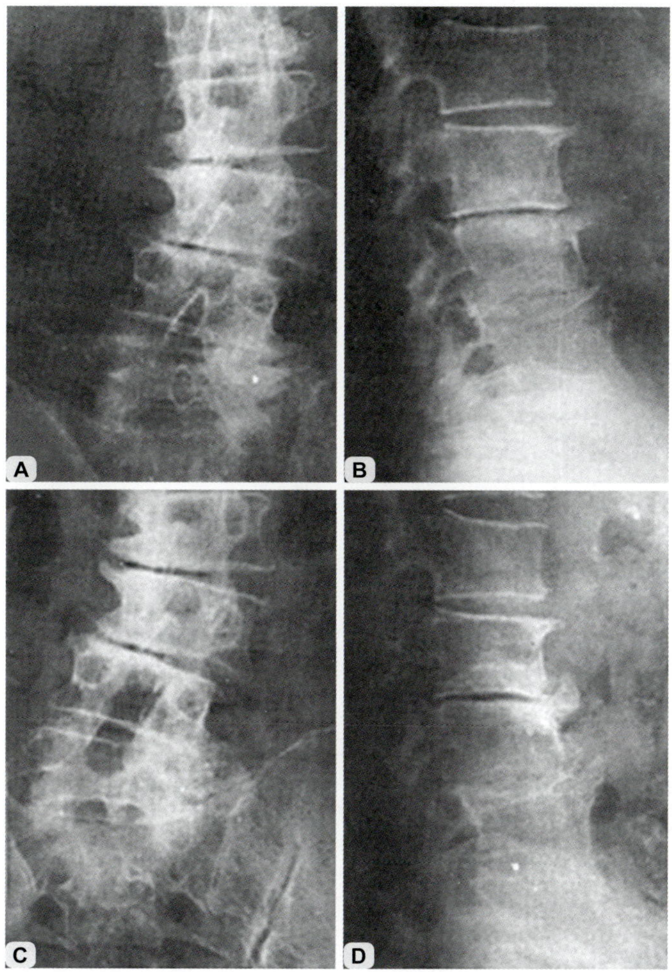

Fig. 26.4 A case example of decompression surgery alone. (A and B) X-rays of a 63-year-old female patient who underwent laminectomy at L4–L5; (C and D) There was no curve progression except mild retrolisthesis for postoperative 5-year. Big stabilizing anterior buttress bony spur is seen at upper margin of L3 and L4

manifestation of the polysegmental DLS, or independent entity.[34-37]

Polysegmental C-curve and upper monosegment DLS precipitated infequently clinical symptoms, while the short double reciprocating polysegmental DLS and lower oligosegmental DLS precipitated more frequently the clinical symptoms.[37] However, as far as coronal decompensation is concerned, truncal shift is more frequently seen in case of the polysegmental C-curve DLS than the double reciprocating type.

Oligosegmental Type

The coronal hemivertebra develops the scoliotic tilt, and congenital kyphosis due to sagittal hemivertebra (anterior vertebral body defect) develops less frequently the clinical problems such as unsightly kyphosis. Thus, it is considered that the coronal plane deformity in the lumbar spine will be not only functional problem but also the aesthetic problems.[31-34] Unilateral advanced disk degeneration in coronal plane of the lumbar spine gradually leads the upper segment of spine to tilt laterally, and then complicates gradually the vertebral body rotation of the upper segments of spines.

The current authors' view is that the upper and middle segment types are rather benign clinically in nature in comparison with the lower segment type. (Fig. 26.6).

Toyama classified the polysegmental DLS into 3 types (Table 26.3). But he did not recognize the oligosegmental type as an independant entity. Type I has less vertebral rotation, while type II has more severe rotation. Rotatory lateral slip can associate in type I and II. Type III is the other type.[46]

Fujita and Yamakawa classified the polysegmental DLS into single and double curve patterns. They found the single curve pattern in 66 patients and the double curve pattern in 43 patients, and the greatest degenerative wedge deformity of the disk space was found at L3–4 in single C curve (48.0%) and L4–5 in double curve (83.7%).[13]

As regards the progression of the curve, it is known that the large curve increases more than the smaller one, and the curve in the lower type of oliogosegmental DLS progresses more in comparison with that of the upper type.

In polysegmental type the curve normally ranges from T12 or L1 to L3 or L4. There is often a short compensatory curve from L3 or L4 to S1 in the double reciprocating type. The lower end vertebra (L3 or L4 vertebra) is markedly tilted and a more lateral slip as well as pedicular download is observed.

Risk Factors for Curve Progression

Eight risk factors suggesting rapid curve progression are listed : (i) ladies, (ii) 7° of curve difference in standing and supine AP radiograms in early stage of the disease, (iii) tilt angle of L4 body over 15°, (iv) vertebral body rotation of grade II or III, (5) Cobb angles of L4 body over 30°, (vi) the segmental instability, (vii) severe off-balance (truncal shift), and (viii) narrower AP diameter of L4 body.[36,37]

Segmental instability in the curve is indicated by presence of Knuttson's vacuum sign, facet joint fluid sign, degenerative spondylolisthesis, and/or lateral listhesis of more than 3 mm.

Clinical Symptoms and Signs

Clinical presentation of DLS varies greatly. Truncal shift is more frequently seen in the advanced polysegmental C-curve DLS than the double reciprocating type. The scoliotic deformity is often associated with axial rotations,

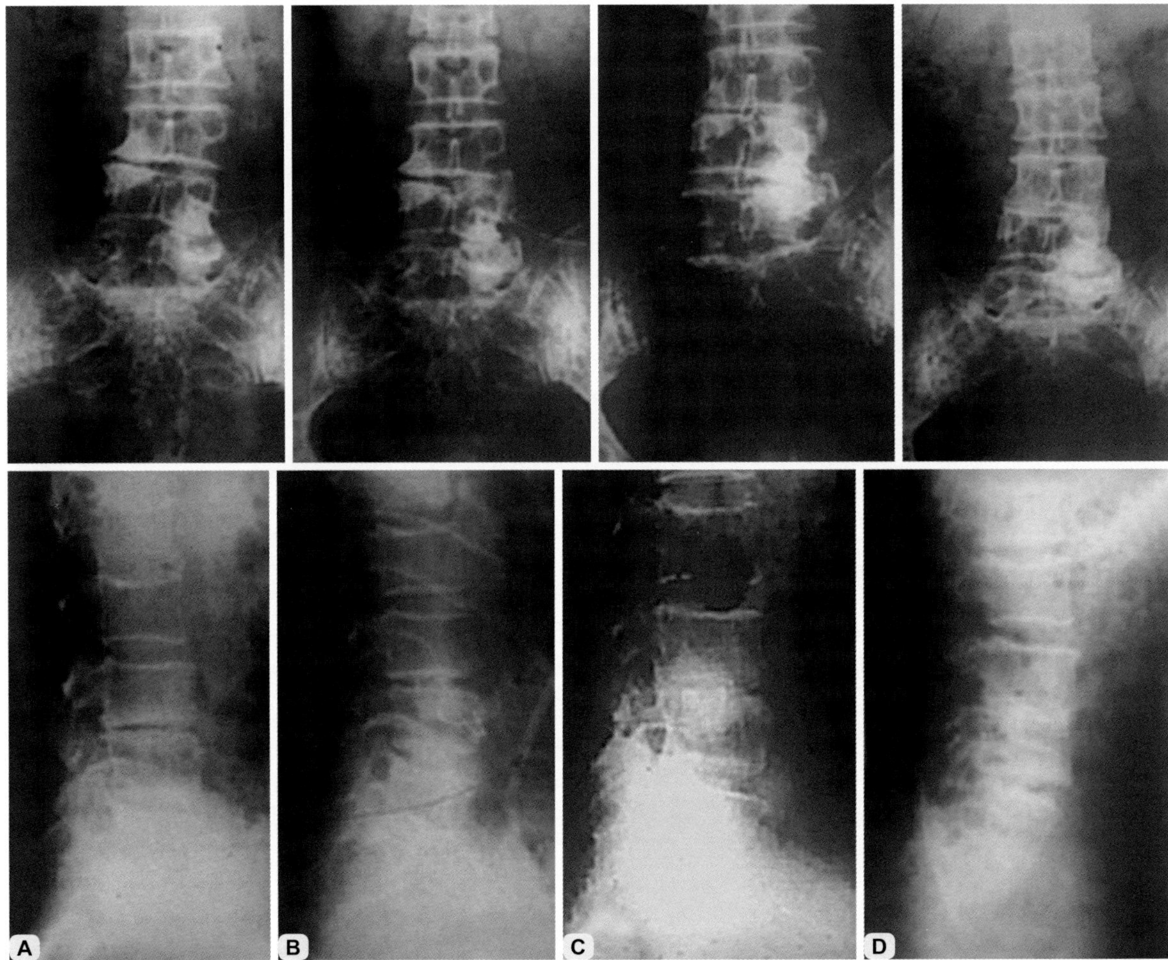

Fig. 26.5 (A) Anteroposterior and lateral radiograms of a 44-year-old lady with worsening incapacitating low back pain and mild sciatica over a year show the advanced degenerative changes at L3–4 and L4–5, and mild scoliosis having reciprocating double curve with an apex at L3–4 disk; (B) Radiograms after anterior interbody fusion between L3–4 and L4–5, showing well-placed bone grafts and well aligned lumbar spine in coronal plane; (C) Radiograms, taken at postoperative 6 months showing the fused L3–5 in normal coronal alignment; (D) Radiograms, taken at postoperative 5 years and 4 months, showing the solid fusion between L3–5 without any evidence of adjacent joint problem

loss of lordosis, antelisthesis, lateral listhesis, and spinal stenosis. Back pain develops even at an early stage of the disease though the spinal deformity is not evident ostensibly, and the stenotic symptoms develop gradually as the deformity progresses.[25] Typical initial presenting complaint in most patients is the radicular pain in the lower extremity. The patient may report concomitant back and buttock pain as well (Table 26.5). That is, majority have progressive symptoms of spinal stenosis, including (i) worsening of buttock pain, (ii) increased paresthesias, and (iii) limb weakness with standing or walking, cauda equina syndrome, intermittent claudication, and (iv) physical sign such as truncal shift.[18,29,30,32-34]

Stenotic symptoms can be elicited by the degenerated disk(s) of the normal and malaligned spines. In the scoliotic spines sagittal and/or coronal malalignments are seen. In

Table 26.5 Clinical symptoms

Clinical features	*No. of patients (%)*	*Total*
Low back pain		141 (100)
Low back pain only	16 (11.3)	
Associated neuropathy	125 (88.7)	
Radiating pain		110 (78.0)
Convex side	62 (56.3)	
Concave side	16 (14.5)	
Both sides	32 (29.1)	
Claudication		68 (48.2)
Motor and/or sensory		67 (47.5)
Low compensatory curve	47 (70.1)	
At the apex	20 (29.9)	
Laseque test positive		13 (0.2)

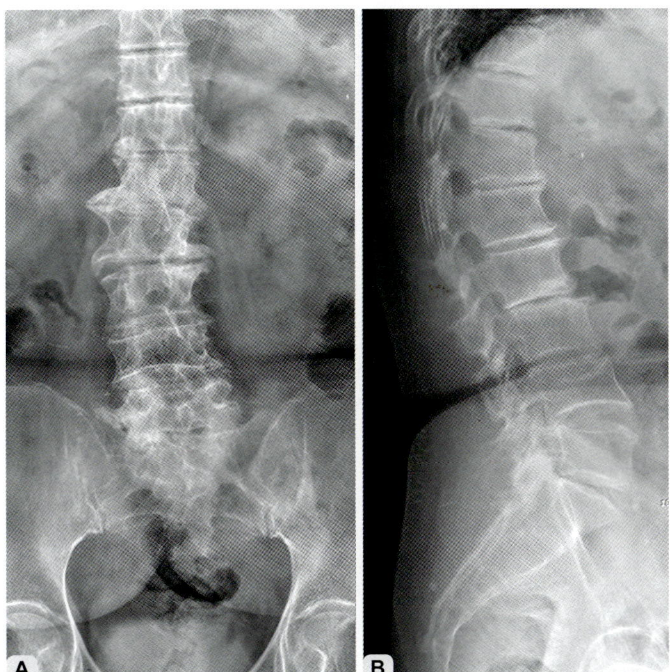

Fig. 26.6 An example of an upper type polysegmental DLS showing the C-curve. Apex is located L1–2 and L2–3. She complained only low back pain. This type of DLS is a benign form

those patients with malaligned spines, their activities are affected mainly by pain and not by the deformity. Curve features are also presented in Table 26.4.

Site of Compression and Symptomatic Nerve Roots

According to Liu et al. the compression factors of L3 or L4 roots and those of L5 and S1 were different which still remained to be clarified.[31] In degenerative lumbar spinal stenosis with normal alignment, L5 and S1 nerve roots were most likely affected by lateral recess or central canal stenosis at the L4–5 level. However, they found in DLS that the loading line crossed through the lateral recess zone of the convex side at L4–5 or L5–S1, and the foraminal or extraforaminal zone of the concave side at the L2–3 or L3–4. Therefore, at the lateral recess of the convex side at L4–5 or L5–S1 segments, by the concentrated mechanical stress more degenerative changes apparently was seen. In contrast, L3 or L4 nerve root entrapment which was caused by pedicular kinking, facet joint subluxation and foraminal or extraforaminal disk herniation occurred at the foraminal or extraforaminal zone on the concave side of the curve.[6,31]

Diagnosis

Differential diagnosis of de novo DLS with scoliosis of the other origins is essential, such as adult idiopathic scoliosis complicating secondary degenerative spondylosis, adult scoliosis associated with congenital scoliosis, and scoliosis of spondylolysis origin, etc.

Diagnostic studies, such as conventional radiographs, CT scans, and MRI scan must be performed and interpretted within the context of the clinical presentation.

The key points in making diagnosis of DLS are listed: *de novo* polysegmental DLS has the scoliokyphotic deformity with less rigidity, and it more frequently associates the anterior and/or lateral rotatory slip.

Treatment

There are two academic schools for treatment of DLS; Robin regarded the DLS as natural senescent process and was against treatment,[40] while Kostuik recommended the active treatment.[22,24,41-44,46,47,49,50]

Asymptomatic scoliosis in the elderly seldom becomes a clinical problem as far as deformity is concerned. Moreover, it appears that back pain is not a significant problem in those people.

Treatment is tailored to the specific symptomatology in each patient. Primary aim of the treatment of the adolescent idiopathic scoliosis is the prevention of the progress of the curve and/or correction of the deformity for cosmesis, but is not so in the DLS. Once the diagnosis of DLS is established, an individualized treatment plan should be formulated.

Treatment aims primarily at alleviation of clinical symptoms by any means, and does not primarily aim at the deformity correction and fusion. Treatment consists of medical and surgical means.

The treatment depends on many factors, and may include physical therapy, epidural or nerve root injections, a laminectomy and/or a spinal fusion procedure with or without deformity correction.[34] Bracing is occasionally recommended for a short period of time, but does not play a significant role in the treatment. Most patients probably do not require surgical treatment as back pain usually responds to conservative treatment.

When the pain is the primary reason for which the adult with scoliosis seeks treatment, it is important not to overlook this aspect in evaluating the patient and making decision on the role and extent of surgical intervention. When consideration is given not only to the structural problem but also to a comprehensive evaluation of pain, more feasible results will be obtained by surgery of the DLS in the elderly.

The surgical complication rate is high for an aged group in which the health and quality of life may already be compromised. Optimal surgical goals have yet to be established in this population.

It is believed that the primary goal of surgery should be the decompression of the neural elements and secondly the establishment of a stable, pain-free spine. However, the treatment of this complex condition remains controversial, and raised several questions: (i) purely for pain relief, (ii) restoration of truncal balance, (iii) improvement of spinal function, and (iv) cosmesis.[37]

Functional improvement through pain relief must be the primary aim of surgery. Correction of the deformity is a secondary consideration which may contribute in relieving pain.

The surgeon is left with his or her own inherent biases and very little solid evidence to support the selection of one type of decompression versus another. Options range from simple laminectomy to complete deformity correction and arthrodesis.

It is stressed that instrument-aided correction and stabilization of the scoliotic deformity should be carried out on the sound preoperative assessment, but that the procedure should not be adopted as the primary choice of treatment.

The rational approach in the surgical management of the symptomatic moderate and severe DLS is the decompression of the stenotic segment and instrument-aided deformity correction and stabilization and fusion. Correction of the scoliotic spine may open the stenosed foramen. This may be achieved with a single operation, either anteriorly or posteriorly, or a combined circumferential approach. The past consensus was that circumferential spinal fusion with posterior decompression and instrumentation provided the best results in achieving fusion, relief of pain, and improved function.[31-37] (Fig. 26.7 and Table 26.6).

Conservative Treatment

Generally, it is given to all the symptomatic early cases.[32-34,36] Elderly patients with DLS do not become uniformly disabled with age, and disability can not solely be predicted by radiographic findings. These informations should be considered when the conservative treatment is contemplated. There were reports that the nonoperative treatment did not improve the patient's quality of life, while operative treatment did significantly improve the QOL in the DLS patients.[28,44,49,50]

Two conservatively treated patients who were followed over 10 years are presented: the curves progressed, but were well balanced without causing stenotic symptoms (Fig. 26.3A and B, case 1; Fig. 26.3C and D, case 2).

Table 26.6 Treatment option in DLS

Type of Treatment (Measures)			*Advantages*	*Disadvantages*	*Remarks (Comments)*
Nonoperative			Least morbid and least costly	Patient may not respond, curve may progress	Initially treated
Operative	**Stabilization alone (fusion)** **Anterior / Posterior ± instrument**		• Good for back pain relief • Provide stability • Correct deformity	Increased surgical morbidity will not relieve limb pain	Parafusion segment (adjacent) disease
	Decompression	**Laminotomy**	Preserved stability, Obviate need for fusion	High neural injury Benefits for fusion Skill required	Excellent alternative No need for fusion Highly selective decompression 96% improved leg pain 80% improved back pain
		Laminectomy	Better decompression (Wider)	Further destabilized spine 82% good at 5 years 57% good at 10 years	May require fusion
		+ fusion:	Single stage procedure	Surgical time, cost, morbidity	Good choice for DLS
		• **PLF**			
		• **PLIF**	Increase fusion rate and correction (Single stage procedure)	Technically demanding. Additional morbidity	Rarely primary procedure
	Osteotomy	**± Decompression + Instrumented correction + fusion**	Correction of malaligned stiff spine	High surgical morbidity	Performed for unbalanced severe deformed spine

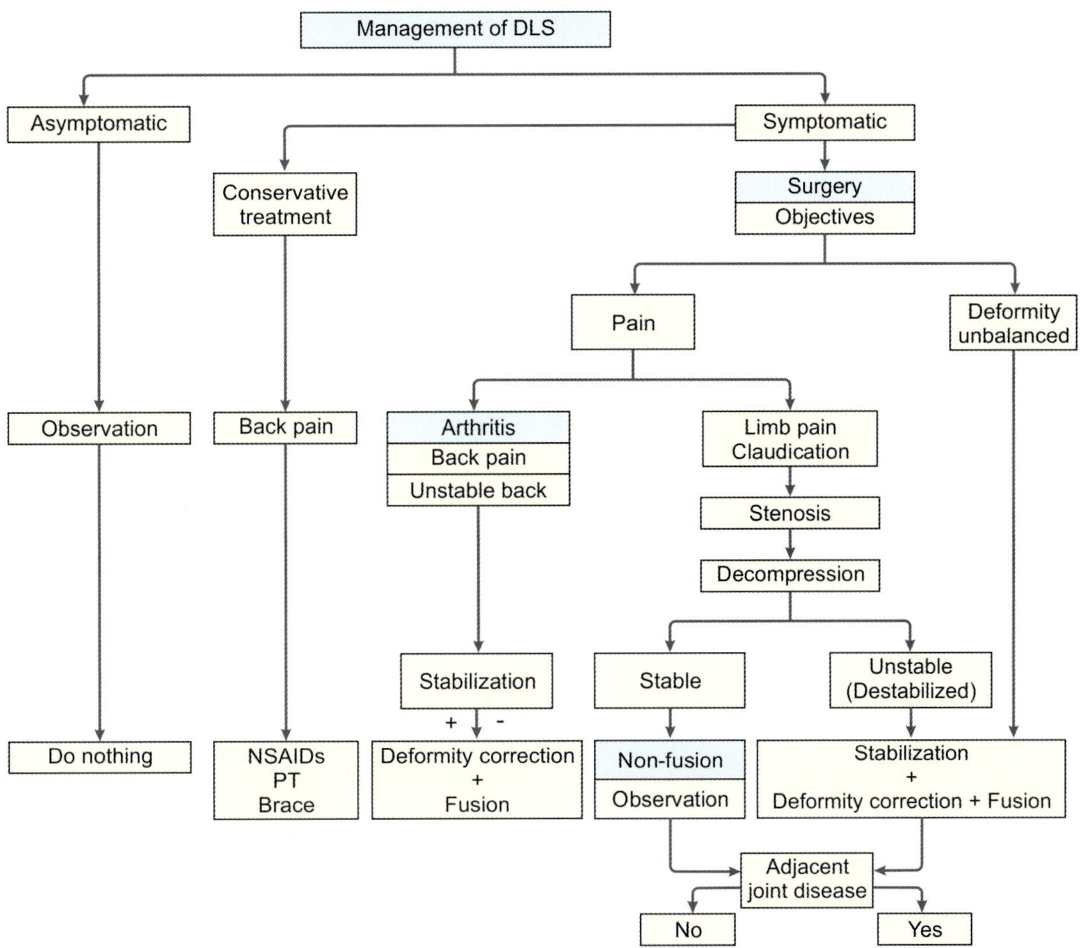

Fig. 26.7 Flowchart showing management of degenerative lumbar scoliosis. Management must be focused primarily on the pain relief and not on the deformity correction

Surgical Management

We are not allowed to state the generalized principle that surgical intervention has no role in the treatment of the adult with scoliosis. Operative treatment for patient with adolescent idiopathic scoliosis was driven by increased coronal plane deformity. Conversely, pain and disability mandated treatment for DLS patients, independent of radiographic measure. The operative treatment is a challenge to achieve the greatest benefit with least amount of intervention.

The extension dynamic stenosis often mimic the degenerative kyphosis with sciatic tilt or DLS. The surgeon should always know that dynamic extension stenosis in itself causes patients to lean forward, and that interspinous decompression block relieve the symptoms. Therefore, it should be differentiated from those two conditions.[36]

The surgical rules for treating adolescent idiopathic scoliosis do not offer gratifying result in the treatment of degenerative scoliosis. The objective of surgery for the symptomatic DLS is primarily the pain relief procedure such as fusion alone, decompression alone or decompression and fusion for root symptoms. Deformity correction is the secondary one.

"Scoliotic deformity" is not a significant factor in the causation of pain, and the pain may not be lessened by curve correction and spinal fusion. However, when the conservative treatment fails, surgery for pain relief through decompression, curve correction and/or fusion should be opted. The goal of surgery should be the effective decompression of the neural elements along with establishment of a pain-free stable and normally aligned spine by instrumentation.[36,37] Treatment of structural problem alone is not likely to offer relief.

For the patients with minimum scoliosis and stenotic symptoms, decompression alone relieve the symptoms. Great care must be taken to preserve the pars interraticularis and the facet joints as much as possible.[36] In the elderly patients a weakened pars can later induce fracture and results in progressive deformity. Thus, maintenance of the stability of the decompressed segment(s) have been the issue. However, when there is huge anterior butress osteophytes, the posterior surgical destabilization does not affect the segmental stability. Any sign suggesting the presence of instability usually necessitates a surgical stabilization. Patients with curves over 30° should be a candidate for instrumented fusion of the entire curve together with restoration of the spinal alignment after decompression surgery.

Decompression Surgery

It is important to differentiate DLS from the other degenerative spinal disorders presenting the similar clinical pictures, because the prognosis and treatment considerations are different.[37] Unlike most of the patients with similar spinal disorders, patients' pain is not reliably relieved by reversing their lumbar scoliosis.

According to Liu et al. it is important to bear in mind that L3 or L4 root were more strongly compressed by foraminal or extraforaminal stenosis at the concave side of the curve, whereas L5 or S1 nerve roots were affected more by lateral recess stenosis at the convex side of the curve.[37] Therefore, central and lateral recess stenosis are relatively easy to diagnose by MRI or myelography. However, it may be difficult to determine foraminal or extraforaminal stenosis from the neuroradiological point of view.

When the conservative treatment fails to relieve the patient's stenotic pain complaints over 6 months, those patients with stable curves are firstly subjected to decompression surgery. Surgical intervention of this disabling radiculopathy is becoming more necessary. Before decompression surgery, it is necessary to determine the symptomatic nerve roots and their compressive factors. Preoperative accurate assessment of the stenotic segments and zones are essential for the successful decompression (Fig. 26.2).

Surgical decompression alone is indicated for those cases with (i) large anterior bony buttress spur indicating hyperstable segment, (ii) no rotatory lateral subluxation, and (iii) single root decompression with possible preservation of facet joint.

Highly selective decompression is most desirable if possible which does not destabilize the decompressed segment and does not require the stabilization procedure.

There are conflicting reports about the need for stabilization after decompression for DLS (Fig. 26.4). Because many of these patients have already begun the natural spinal restabilization process with bridging osteophytes and hypertrophy of the lateral masses. Therefore, the decompressed segment seems unlikely destabilized after laminectomy and foraminotomy. For this reason, it should be prudent in dealing with a decompressive procedure which must be followed by close follow-up for the possible curve progression.

Although stenosis can be relieved by laminectomy alone, resulting instability may compromise a successful outcome, especially in large curves which are more likely to progress. Correction of the deformity may facilitate the relief of foraminal stenosis and thereby relieve pain.

Fusion

The potential benefit to be obtained by spinal fusion must be measured against the operative risks. Fusion alone for the disabling back pain is one of the surgical options, though it is rarely indicated.

Anterior lumbar interbody fusion (ALIF): ALIF for oligo-segmental DLS is an effective stabilization procedure which also accomplish the deformity correction and indirect decompression through reduction of collapsed disc space and sagittal and/or coronal vertebral slips, and also do not damage the nerves (Fig. 26.5).

Posterior Instrumentation

Deformity correction and fusion after decompression are the another surgical option for the painful limb and back, and/or unbalanced back.

Reposition of the slip and restabilization of the decompressed segment(s) close to the normal functional alignment is the final goal. Also achieving a sound fusion is important for a successful outcomes.

However, it is reminded that age, comorbidities and sagittal balance did not influence the treatment modality for DLS.

In summary surgical options range from simple laminectomy to complete deformity correction and arthrodesis for prevention of the recurrent stenotic symptoms, though it sacrifices the segmental mobility.

Mistake should be avoided in surgery: It is important to begin and end the fusion at neutral and stable vertebrae. "Neutral" means that the pedicles are neutrally rotated, and "stable" means that the vertebrae are within the stable zone. The worse thing the surgeon can do is to end the fusion next to a rotatory subluxation. At times, it may be a reasonable alternative to end a fusion somewhat out of the stable zone if the adjoining segments have very large osteophytes and are relatively stiff and immobile. Big mistake is to stop an instrumentation and fusion at the apex of a sagittal curve. Stopping instrumentation and fusion at apex of thoracic kyphosis will almost certainly lead to fall-off over the top and sagittal unbalancing.

The effort should be made to improve the lumbar lordosis during instrumentation. The usual apex of thoracic kyphosis is between T5 and T9, and the usual apex of lumbar lordosis is at L3–4 with L3 pointing in a 3 o'clock direction. The weight-bearing line should fall behind the L3–4 segment. Normal sagittal vertical axis of the spine should be restored and maintained.[37]

In the posterior instrumentation surgery, there are as yet several critical issues: (i) is restoration of normal sagittal and coronal alignment and truncal balance and its maintenance essential? (ii) is limited fusion of the decompressed segment acceptable, and (iii) is fusion of the entire curve including the degenerated disks out of the curve in fusion or to extend up to T10 mandatory.

A common mistake is to end a fusion next to a level that has rotatory subluxation. This will almost invariably lead to worsening of the subluxation and a poor surgical result. However, there was extreme opposing view that the instrumented correction of stiff degenerative scoliotic spine should not be done.[36,37,47]

Instrument-aided posterior stabilization is indicated only for the cases with:

1. Preoperative instability with rapid curve progression,
2. Post-surgical instability,
3. Unbalanced fatiguing trunk.

For instrumented fusion, it is advisable to use pedicle screw fixation, and to put together a surgical construct in which the top and bottom of the fused vertebrae are neutral, horizontal, and centered on the stable zone over the sacrum in coronal plane together with normalized sagittal alignment, and to make the fused spine pain-free and stable (Figs 26.8 to 26.17).

Corrective and Balancing Spine Surgery

Before surgery the 4 raised questions would be preferable to be revisited. To achieve the normal functional alignment, the corrective and balancing surgeries in sagittal and coronal planes should be done.

Before instrumented deformity correction in the elderly, following factors should be considered:

1. Can the deformity correction improve the activity of daily life (ADL)?
2. How much the patients will be benefitted from surgery? and lastly
3. What are the disadvantages of this procedure?

Will the instrument-related stiff back and junctional problem be unavoidable (?), and will the well-balanced stiff back be beneficial or detrimental for the ADL, including the oriental floor life.

Spinal decompensation in the coronal plane is more often seen in the advanced DLS.[36,37] In instrumentation surgery, to improve spinal function and to minimize the junctional problem, restoration of the spinal balance in coronal plane is most important together with the horizontal positioning of the tilted end-plates of the fused upper and lower vertebral bodies and restoration of normal sagittal curve. Restoration of sagittal alignment should be preceded before restoration of coronal alignment. Restoration of single vertical column axis in coronal plane is essential to treat the trunk shift and prevent and/or minimize the incidence of the late junctional problems.

Surgeon must know that sagittal balance will be lost when correction of the coronal curve is performed by rod distraction technique instead of rod derotation technique. That is, scoliotic curve correction should be carried out by rod rotation in the concavity of the lumbar curve.

It is reported that pedicle instrumentation must be used to obtain correction and stabilization of coronal deformity in order to prevent future spinal nerve root compression from increasing deformity, which is usually caused by pedicle migration. However, this statement does not apply in prevention of the transitional syndrome.

Anterior Spinal Column and Canal Length Ratio

In the idiopathic scoliosis anterior column is longer than the canal, while in DLS both lengths are equal. In the past the Harrington (H) distraction rods were used in the treatment of idiopathic scoliosis. In that occasion by over-distraction of the spinal column for coronal deformity correction cord was stretched together with the flattening of the sagittal curve, and resulted in palsy and shift of normal vertical sagittal axis of spine. However, when anterior column shortening by total anterior disectomies and/or spondylectomy equalized the anterior column and canal length. Consequently, H distraction-rod could be safely used for deformity correction without inducing the spinal flattening and cord stretch.[37]

Curve Correction Technique

Both scoliotic and kyphotic deformities could be corrected by rod derotation of the contoured rods, while pedicle-screw-plate system has been used for scoliotic curve correction by some.[30] In the DLS cases with stenotic symptoms, complete decompression is essential to avoid the root damages during instrumented curve correction, particularly in cases having rotatory slip. After the curve correction, the residual vertebral body rotation can be additionally corrected by using the segmental screw rotation technique.[9,10]

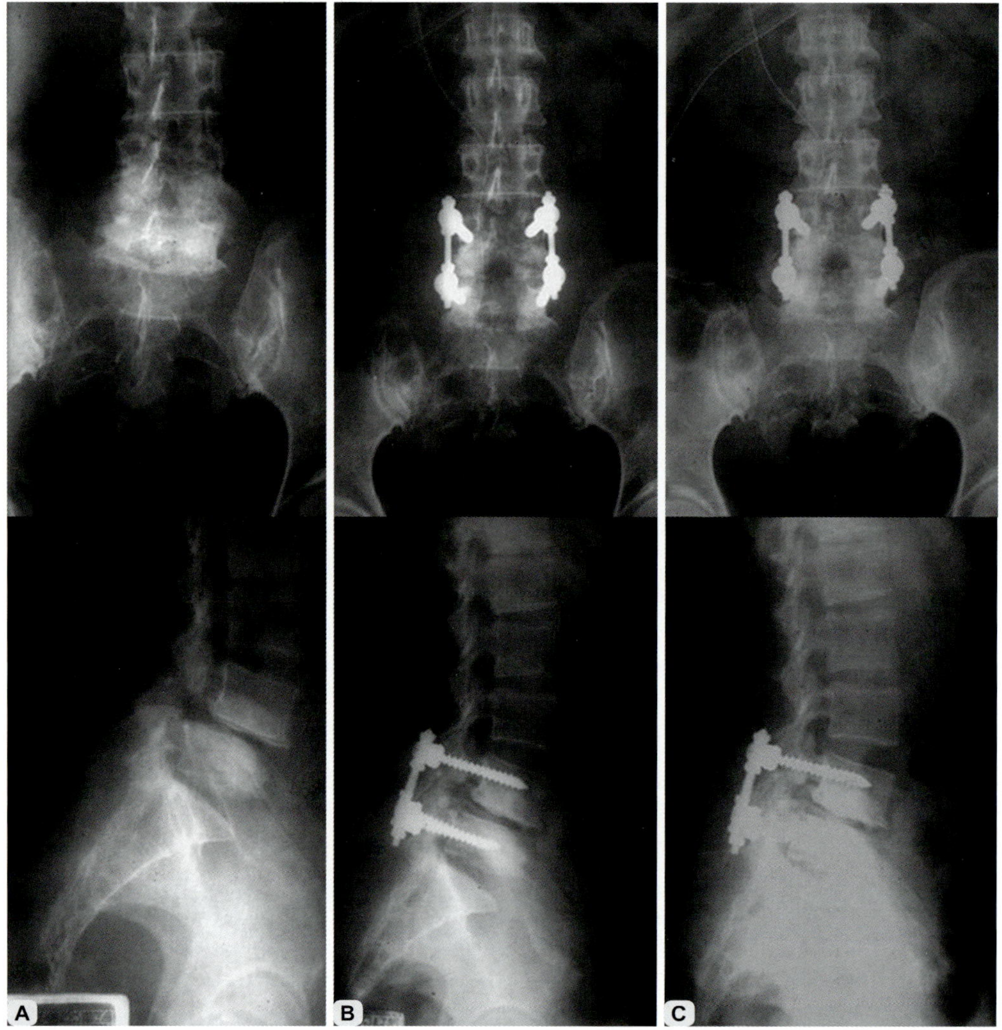

Fig. 26.8 Symptomatic oligosegmental scoliosis secondary to grade 1 isthmic spondylolisthesis with severe L4–5 disk degeneration in a 55-year-old lady. She had persisting back pain associating the stenotic symptoms. After decompression, posterior instrument-aided curve correction, stabilization and PLF of L4–5 were carried out. The postoperative 3 years and 3 months follow-up roentgenograms show the good PLF masses and maintenance of the normal lumbar alignment. No evidence of the adjacent segment disease at L3–4 and L5–S1 is seen

Postoperative Complications and Long-term Outcomes

In general the elderly patients with DLS are more likely to have perioperative complications, and also the late adjacent segment diseases after instrumented spinal fusion which will subsequently convert the early good outcome into poor. Therefore, early and late postoperative complications should be minimized or nullified.

Current Issues Related to Management

There are as yet a lot of controversial issues related with the management of DLS which should be solved in the coming years.[37-39,45]

Presently raised and unanswered questions are:

1. What is the clinical significance of DLS?
2. What are the predictors of deformity progression?
3. What are the treatment options for DLS?
4. Is deformity correction necessary, and if so is the goal the complete or partial correction and stabilization?
5. What would be the most appropriate surgical intervention for each patient?

Preoperative patient selection and decision-making, and clinical factors related with the DLS were more complicated than those in the young idiopathic scoliosis patients.

There is considerable controversy regarding surgical indication; role for decompression alone, and decompression and fusion with or without instrument-aided deformity correction.

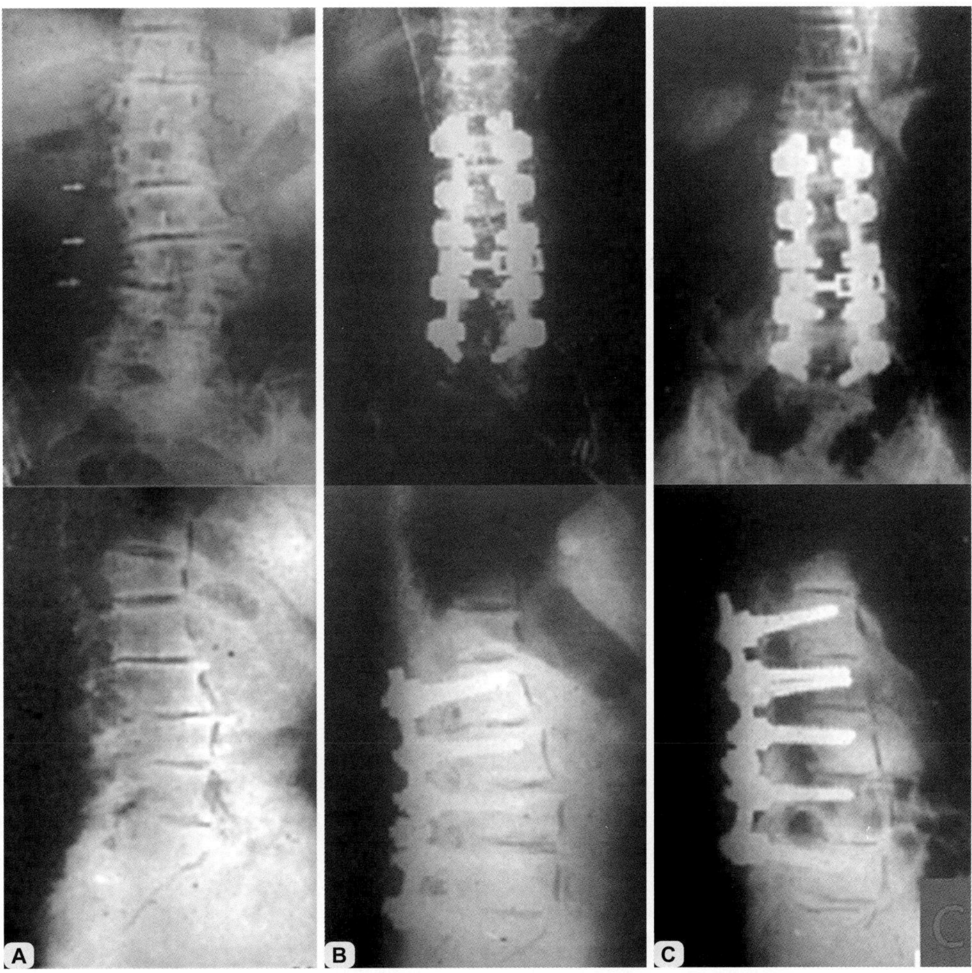

Fig. 26.9 An example of successful instrumented curve correction and stabilization for polysegmental C-type DLS. (A) A 64 year-old lady presented clinically severe stenotic symptoms; (B) After decompression of L3–4, instrumented curve correction and stabilization between L1–L5 and posterolateral fusion was performed; (C) Radiograms taken at postoperative 6 years show no adjacent joint disease at T12–L1 and L5–S1

The long-term efficacy of surgery for the symptomatic DLS is currently unproven (Pritchett, 1993),[41] but Grubb et al. stated that the long-term efficacy of surgery seemed to be dependent on the gradual deterioration of symptoms in cases of decompression alone by the curve progression and recurrence of the stenotic symptom.[18] In cases of the instrumented surgery junctional problem was the key factor which deteriorated the immediate postoperative symptomatic recovery (Grubb et al. 1994). By postoperative 4 years, 50% of the patients reported increasing pain, and had documented additional spinal pathology not present at the initial assessment, and 36% had undergone reoperation.[18]

The facts which was pointed out by the other previous authors that sagittal curve correction and restoration of body balance were the most important factors that influenced the incidence of low-back pain and junctional problem. The persistence of a flat back after surgery clearly correlated with continuous lumbar pain. It was pointed out that restoration of normal lumbar lordosis and vertical sagittal axis was important.[6]

The current issues related with the instrument-aided fusion in management of DLS are:

1. How much physiological lumbar lordosis should be provided to ease the daily living.
2. To fuse or not to fuse the destabilized segment after decompression.
3. To minimize the fusion segments to maintain the pain-free and stable spinal mobility.
4. How to minimize the fusion syndrome (add-on syndrome), and finally
5. How to obtain long lasting successful outcome.

Surgeons should pay attention (i) not to destabilize the decompressed segments by doing the highly selective decompression surgery which is most important to maintain pain-free spinal stability, (ii) to avoid the instrumented

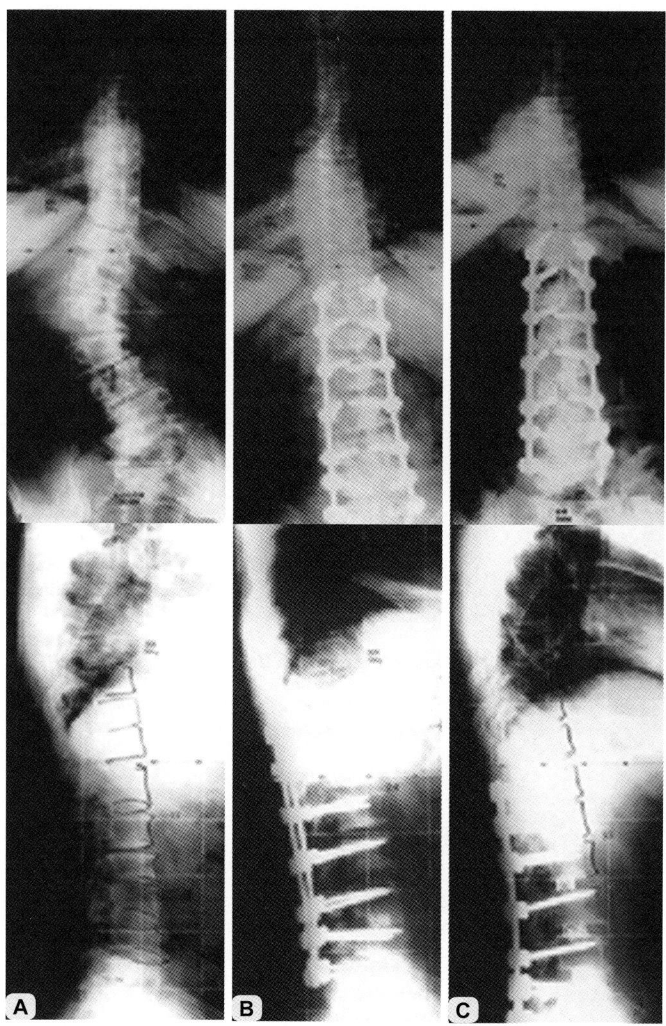

Fig. 26.10 An example of instrument-aided curve correction, stabilization, and posterolateral fusion after L4–5 decompression. (A) Initial radiograms show the double reciprocating polysegmental degenerative scoliosis. Main primary lesion was severely degenerated and unilaterally wedged L4–5 disk; (B) Immediate postoperative radiograms show corrected coronal curve, instrumented stabilization and PLIF (T12–L5). However, residual flat back deformity was seen. Normal sagittal vertical axis of the spine could not be restored; (C) Follow-up radiograms taken at 3½ years show no add-on symptoms in spite of upper screw failure

fusion, and (iii) postfusion syndrome which is suggested through case illustrations.

For the successful surgery and minimization of the surgery-related immediate and late untoward complications, accurate assessment of the stenotic segment(s) and selection of the best surgical procedure are most important. That is, (i) accurate assessment of the root compression sites, (ii) careful and meticulous surgery, and (iii) adequate decompression before instrumented curve correction and fusion should be carried out. In the cases with rotatory slip there is high neural complication during decompression and slip reduction procedures.

It is important to bear in mind that L3 or L4 roots are more strongly compressed by foraminal or extraforaminal stenosis at the concave side of the curve, whereas L5 or S1 nerve roots are affected more by lateral recess stenosis at the convex side of the curve of the large polysegmental DLS (Epstein, Liu).[14,36]

It was reported that the results of a highly selective decompression compared favorably with those of a traditional laminectomy. By selective decompression back and leg pain relief was obtained together with maintenance of segmental stability and reduction of long-term deterioration. Based on

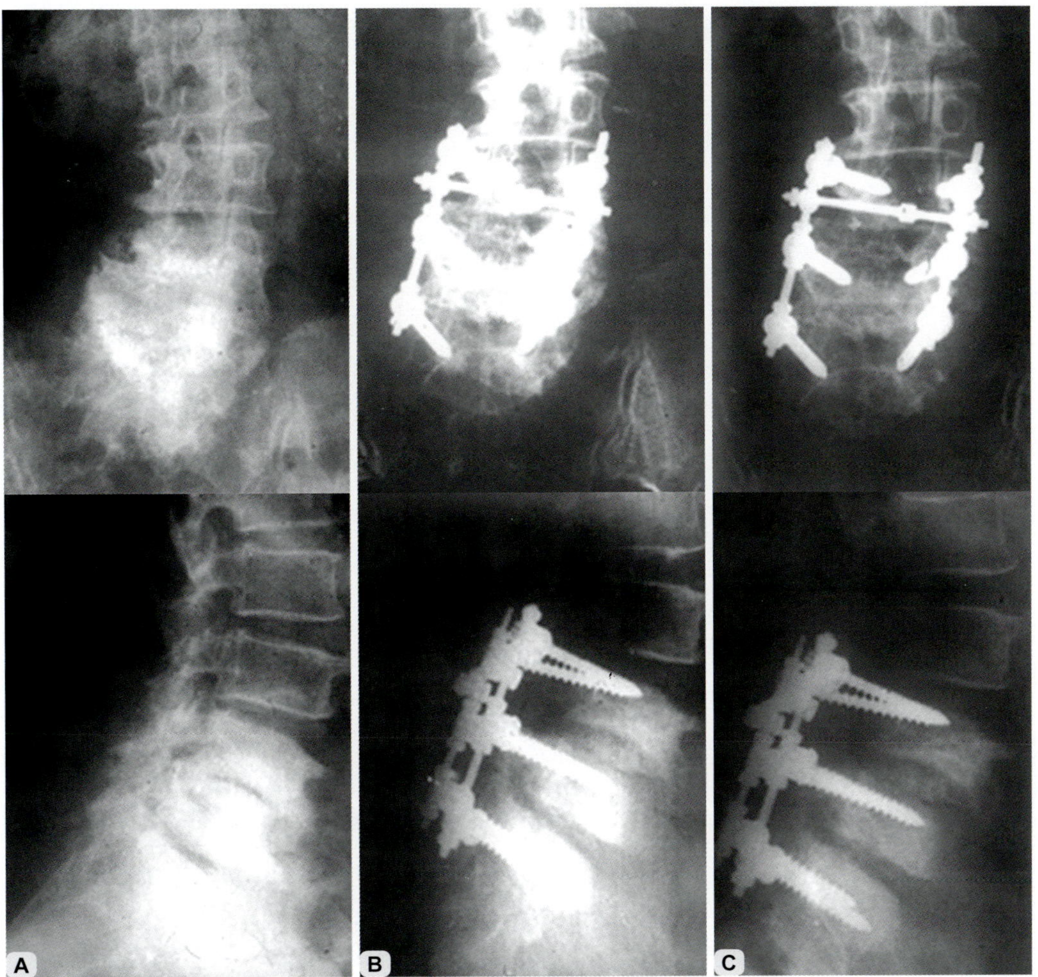

Fig. 26.11 (A) Radiograms of a 57-year-old lady with oligosegmental degenerative lumbar scoliosis who presented the severe sciatica and weakness of legs due to bilateral L5 and S1 radiculopathy. Severe bony sclerosis of L4 and L5 and anterolisthesis of L_4 is shown. Posterior decompression, posterior interbody fusion and posterior pedicular fixation between L4–S1 was performed; (B) Postoperative radiograms show the iatrogenic lamina defect, bone graft between L4–5 and L5–S1 disc spaces and posterior fixation instrument (MOSS system). However, the scoliotic curve was not corrected; (C) Radiograms taken at postoperative 4 years show the progressing scoliotic curve at L3–4 disk level

those results the highly selective decompression surgery is strongly recommended if possible.[19,30,41-44,49]

Once in the past, noninstrumented posterior fusion was practiced for stabilization after decompression surgery primarily to relieve back pain.[41,42] Anterior interbody fusion was also once popularly practiced for the same. Now non-instrumented fusion became the obsolete practice.

With the extended life spans and greater patient's expectations, and the advances in spinal instrumentation and technology, surgical treatment of DLS has become increasingly popular though it has a lot of controversies. However, the issues related to the high surgical complication rates of the long segment instrumentations raised the questions whether the corrective and stabilizing instrumentation surgery was the beneficial procedure. The overriding evidences also indicated that fusion failure resulted in a poor outcome in most instances.

Instrument-aided Deformity Correction and add-on Syndrome

Postoperative long-lasting good outcome after the instrument-aided deformity correction and stabilization surgery related closely with the untoward incidence of the add-on syndrome. The incidence is known to be highest in the cases of *de novo* degenerative lumbar scoliosis.[36,37] Therefore, it is thought that it is a timely and appropriate to deal with the add-on syndrome at this section.

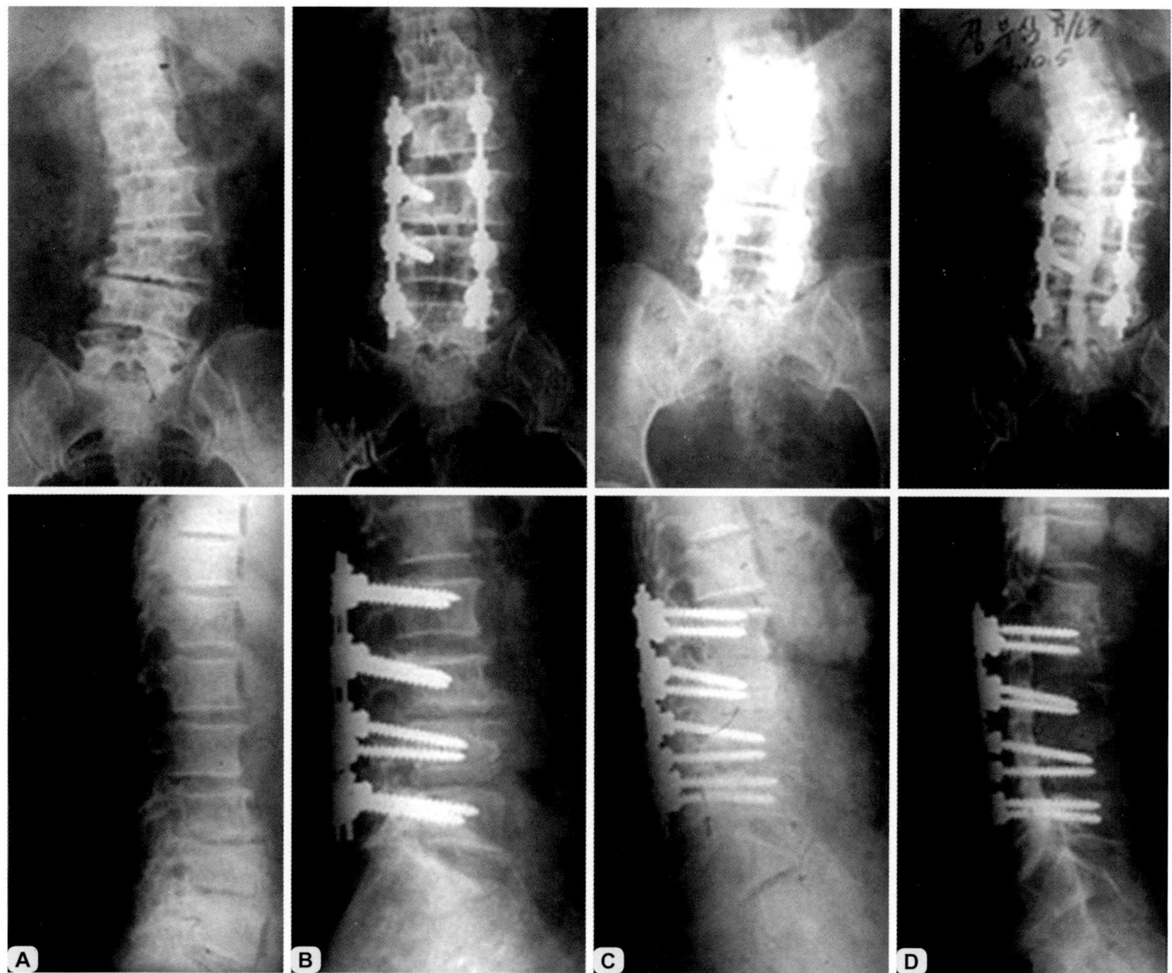

Fig. 26.12 (A) Preoperative radiograms of a 54-year-old lady with polysegmental large C-curve scoliosis presenting stenotic symptoms. No olisthesis is seen; (B) Immediate postoperative radiograms show good correction of the scoliotic curve, stabilization instrument (MOSS system) and posterolateral fusion after limited decompression (L3–5). Some residual kyphoscoliotic deformity and flattened lumbar curve are seen; (C and D) Radiograms taken at postoperative ((C) 1 year and (D) 3 years) show gradual left lateral tilt of L1 over L2

Junctional syndrome is a representation of the failure of the parafusion segments and bone against the transferred load and motion from the fused segments, because the parafusion segments and bones were overloaded and could not adapt to the change in load and motion secondary to the instrumented fusion.

Various factors influencing the fate of the adjacent motion segments are listed: (i) extent of fusion segment(s), (ii) degree of curve correction, (iii) positioning of parafusion disk in coronal plane, (iv) restoration of anatomical single vertical axis in coronal plane to treat trunk shift, (v) degree of degeneration of parafusion segment disks, and (vi) method of fusion: PLF < PLIF = ALIF < instrumented fusion.[20-25]

Instrumentation is necessary at correction and stabilization surgery.[9,10] The goals of instrumentation surgery are to provide stability, to correct deformity, and to promote fusion. However, it should be the last procedure to be carried out. There is a definite indication for such conditions: (i) very unstable segment with rapid curve progression, (ii) previous laminectomy, and (iii) severely off-balanced trunk making the patient walking difficult.[11-13]

As regards the effect of posterior instrumented fusion on the parafusion segment, Shirado stated that monosegment posterior pedicle screw instrumentation produced stress at the adjacent level that was more than twice the amount of stress produced with PLIF alone. It could be imagined from his statement that instrumentation could be the cause of parafusion segment failure.

Iizuka and Yamada reported that the combined decompression, deformity correction and PLIF procedure only limited to the neurologically affected levels may be one of the surgical procedures to challenge DLS.[22] The opposite

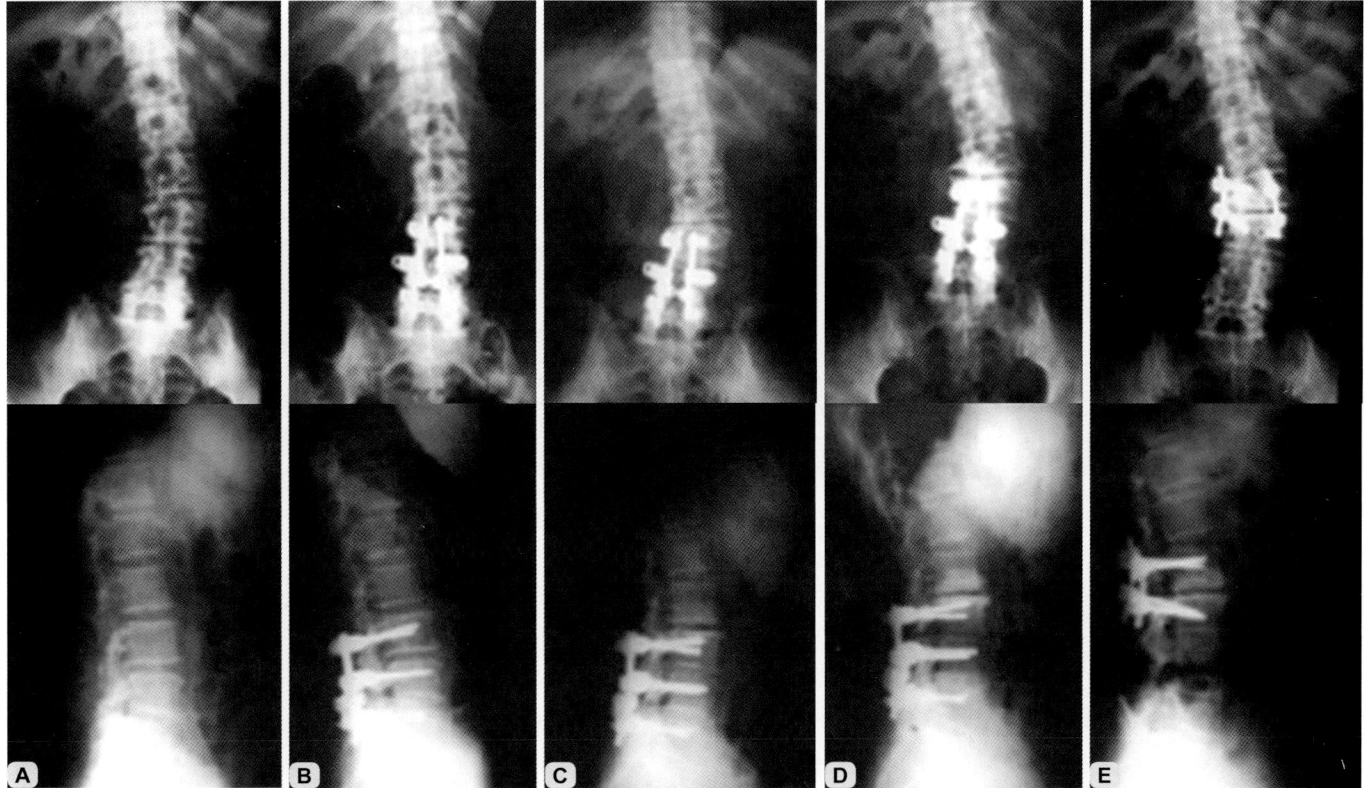

Fig. 26.13 An example of limited stabilization of decompressed segments. (A) Initial radiograms show polysegmental single C curve type of DLS without olisthesis in a 54-year-old lady with back pain and intermittent claudication; (B) Immediate postoperative radiograms show surgical lamina defect of L4, instrumented stabilization of L3–L5 and posterolateral fusion. Entire curve correction was not attempted; (C and D) Radiograms taken at postoperative 1½ and 4 years show progressive left lateral tilt of L2 over L3. Mild truncal shift to right is seen; (E) After removal of initial instrument, L2–3 floating instrumented stabilization was performed again by the initial surgeon

opinion was that instrumented one or two segment in-situ floating fusion of the curve, localized only to the decompressed segments developed rapidly the lateral angular tilt at the upper segment in all. However, in patients with complete curve correction the junctional problem complicated infrequently during period of observation. Therefore, it is reminded that floating and/or limited segmental fusion is not the recommendable procedure.[41-43]

In the instrument-aided deformity correction surgery the importance of horizontal positioning of both parafusion segment disks and restoration of single vertebral column axis in coronal plane including the parafusion segments together with restoration of normal sagittal curve should be kept in mind.

Nine risk factors giving ill-effect on the adjacent segments after instrumented fusion are listed:

1. Advanced age (>60)
2. Female gender
3. Post-menopausal status
4. Osteopenia/osteoporosis
5. Preop adjacent segment instability (disk degeneration): "floating" fusions (not anchored to thoracic or sacral spine).

*6. Long fusion segment (length):[15] { 2 segments: 78%; 3 or more segments: 100% }

7. Loss of coronal and/or sagittal balance
8. Obliquely aligned disks of parafusion segments in coronal plane.
9. Two vertical axis of spinal column in coronal plane.

To minimize the adjacent segment disease in fusion surgery, coronal and sagittal anatomic realignment of the deformed lumbar spine is essential. However, the need to extend the fusion in surgery of the nonscoliotic degenerative spine to include the mild or moderately degenerated adjacent disk is controversial.

The spectrum of recovery was significantly wider, and recovery from surgery particularly in multisegmental DLS usually took longer than that of oligosegmental DLS and the similar conditions in the young.

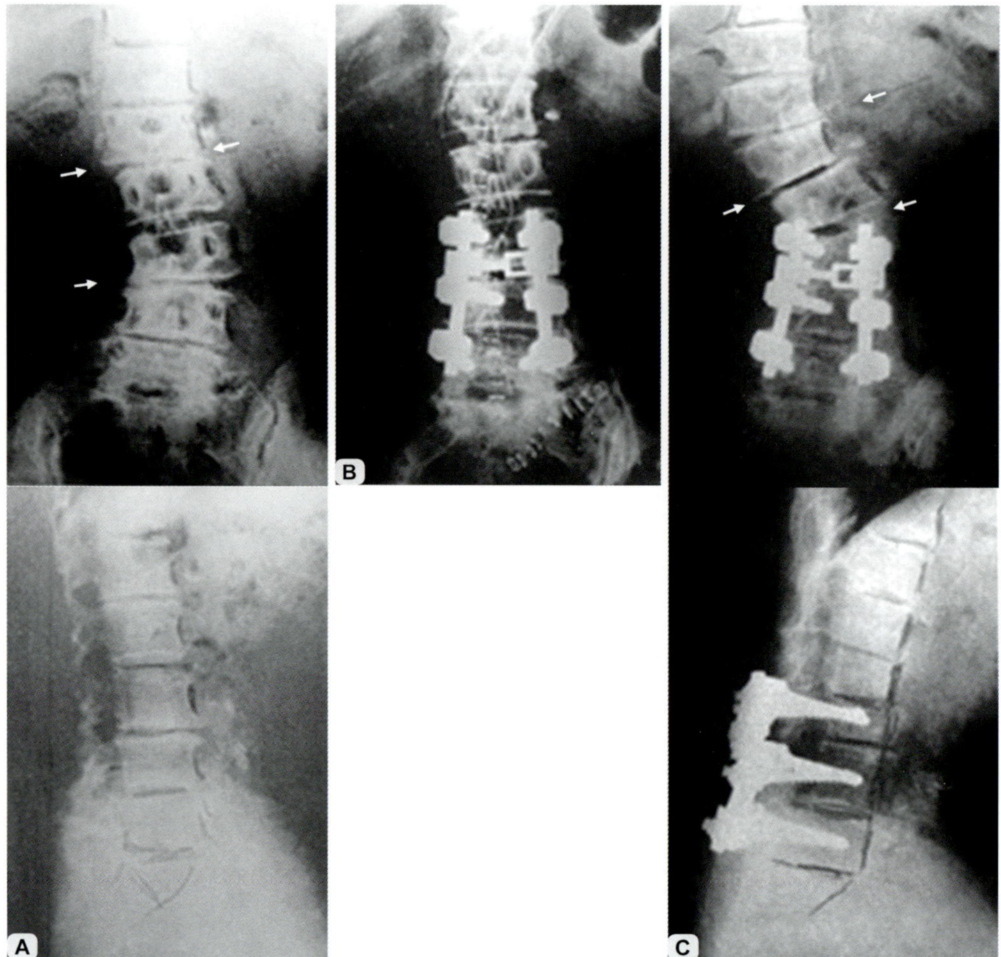

Fig. 26.14 An example of failed limited instrumentation and (A) 56-year-old lady with polysegmental DLS presented initially severe stenotic symptoms in the lower limbs. Two level decompression and limited instrumentation localized only to L3–L5 and posterolateral fusion were performed. Normal lumbar lordosis was not restored by surgery; (B) Postoperatively she did well for 3 years, and then developed again the worsening back pain; (C) Radiograms taken at postoperative 6 years show the acutely tilted L2 over L3

Postfusion Average Time Interval to Adjacent Segment Failure Due to Fusion Type

According to Schlegel et al. the junctional problem developed 13 years after the noninstrumented posterior spinal fusion,[50] while according to Etebar and Cahill the junctional problem developed 26.8 months after posterior instrumented fusion and the shortest interval was postop 3 months.[15]

Nine measures should be considered to minimize or to avoid the junctional syndrome (the add-on syndrome) at parafusion segment:

1. Type of fusion: anterior vs posterior
2. Less rigidity of the fixation
3. Complete curve correction and restoration of normal sagittal and coronal alignment.
4. Reduction of numbers of fusion segment when the sagittal and coronal balances are restored.
5. Horizontal position of the disks of the parafusion segments in coronal plane.
6. Avoidance of *insitu* floating fusion in malaligned spine.
7. Preservation of posterior ligamento-osseous complex at the parafusion segment.
8. Parafusion segments with disk degeneration should be included in fusion.

However, some argue the need to extend the fusion segment to the mild or moderately degenerated adjacent discs outside the scoliotic curve.

In summary, most of the DLS patients are elderly ones. Therefore, surgical treatment should be safe and effective, and also the long-lasting successful outcomes should be maintained.[28] Highly selective minimal decompression

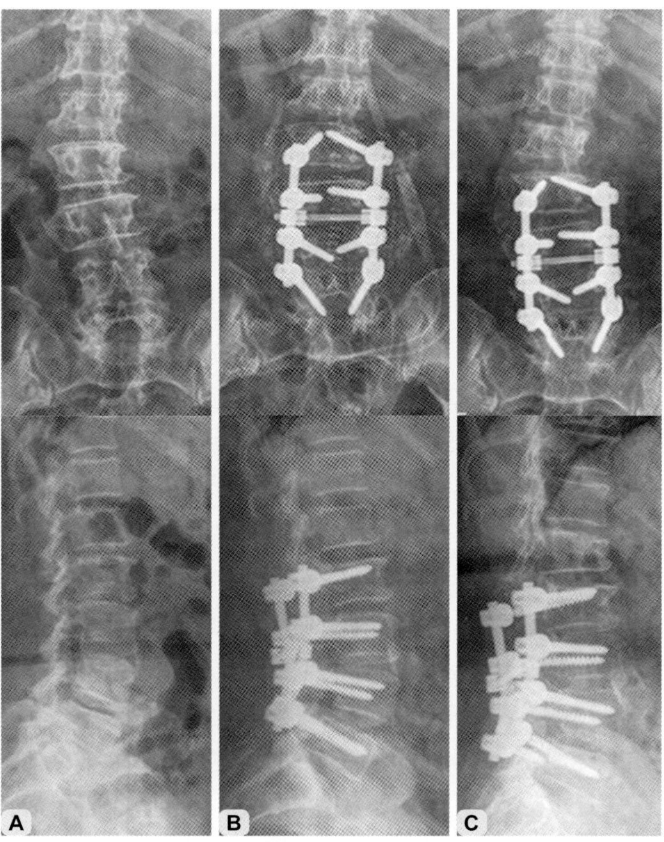

Fig. 26.15 (A) A 68-year-old female has polysegmental reciprocating DLS (L1–L5) with a scoliotic curve (15°) and disk wedge (2.7°) at L1–2; (B) After the posterior decompression and instrument-aided curve correction (L2–L5) and posterolateral fusion, Cobb angle and disk wedging became 11° and 3.2°; (C) One year postoperatively Cobb angle and disk wedging became 16° and 4.1°, and also L1 compression (Denis type B) fracture and screw breakage and screw loosening were complicated. Main cause of failed instrumentation is the limited instrumentation and incomplete curve correction

surgery to avoid segmental destabilization was a desirable procedure as first step. Despite an increased immediate postoperative success rate, complications remained significant in the instrumented cases. Incidence of junctional syndrome was higher, especially in the cases of multilevel instrumented fusion and partial correction, and also floating fusion in the polysegmental DLS, which could be listed as the most important risk factors inducing transitional syndrome. Sagittal and coronal plane balance remains critical for avoiding potentially disabling iatrogenic deformities at the parafusion segments in the future. Complication rate was higher in our early instrumentation series than the late ones, because in the past early era of DLS surgery multisegment instrumentation without rigid surgical indication were performed.

In situ floating fusion of polysegmental DLS is not recommended. Regardless of the clinical types, entire curve should be fused after complete restoration of normal alignment.

Up to now the importance of the instrument-aided deformity correction and stabilization for the symptomatic DLS spine had been overstressed, though long-extended multisegment instrument-aided stabilization and fusion procedures were reported to be accompanied by substantial postoperative early complications including the high rates of adjacent bone and/or joint diseases. Therefore, the best surgical procedure should be judiciously selected on the basis of the surgical strategy.

The current authors do not agree with the statement that in DLS patients without substantial problems related with the coronal or sagittal plane balance, stabilization and fusion of the scoliotic spine must be confined only to the decompressed area.

There are as yet insufficient evidences to conclude that (i) the decompression alone can suffice in alleviation of root pain, (ii) that one stage or staged fusion is essential to stabilize, (iii) that what is the desirable degrees of curve correction (allowable residual scoliosis), and (iv) that the

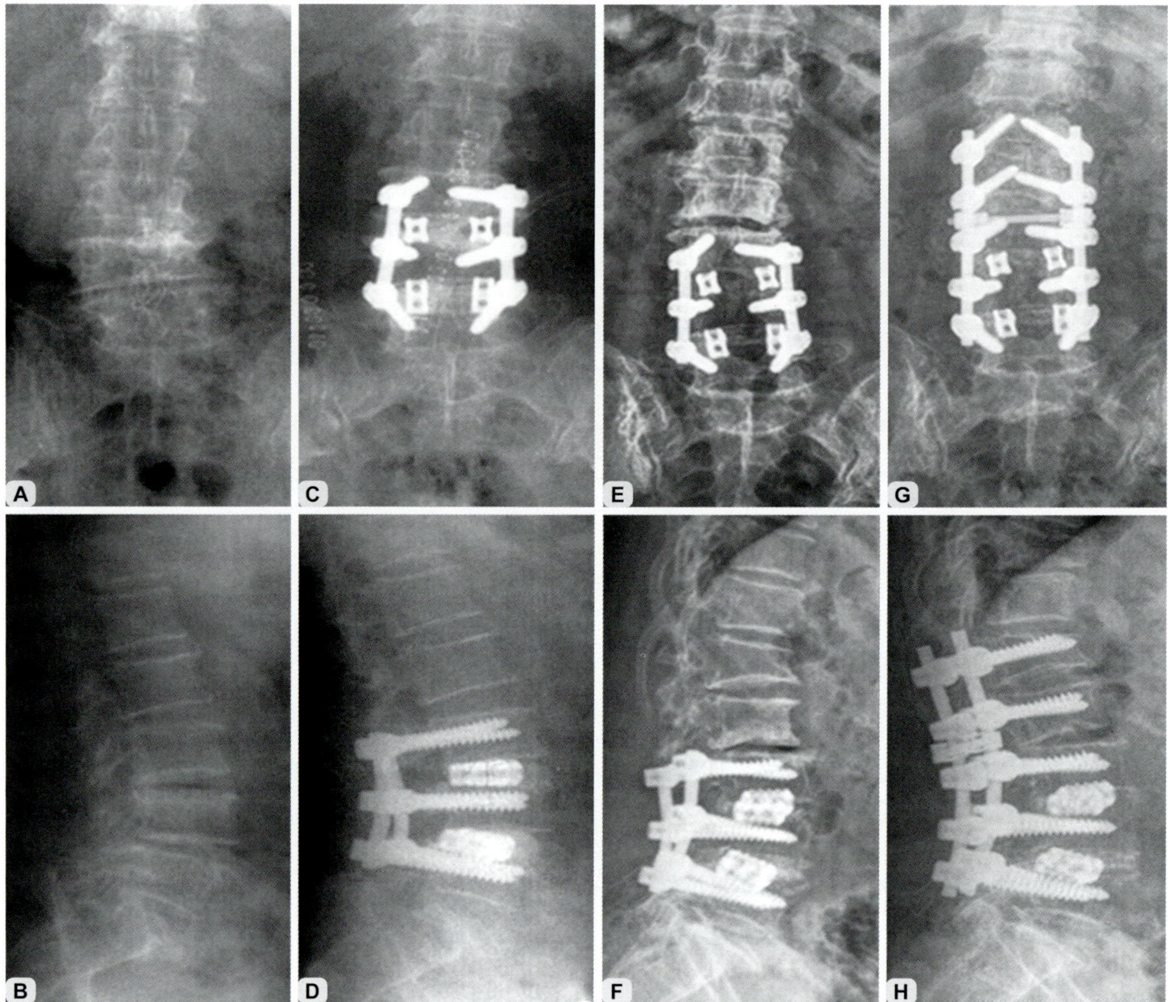

Fig. 26.16 A 69-year-old lady with polysegmental degenerative scoliosis (L1–L5). (A and B) 15° of scoliotic curve and 1.2° of disk wedge (L2–3) associated with L4 spondylolisthesis; (C and D) After posterior decompression and instrument-aided deformity correction (L3–L5) and posterior interbody fusion, Cobb and disk wedge angles became 7° and 1.8°; (E and F) At postoperative 3 years, advanced disk degeneration and Knuttson's sign (L2–L3) at upper adjacent segment and compression fracture of L1 was complicated. Cobb angle, disk wedge angle became 14° and 2.7°; (G and H) Extended stabilization surgery was performed up to L1

most desirable extent of fusion from S1 or L5 up to T6 ~ T10, in cases of polysegmental DLS.

Conclusion

1. Decompression is the essential primary surgery for the patients presenting neurologic symptoms.
2. Instrument-aided curve correction and stabilization for the patients presenting only the arthritic back pain should not be done as the primary procedure, and should be reserved only for the destabilized cases.
3. ALIF procedure for the oligosegmental DLS provided the gratifying results with least complication, though delayed postoperative mobilization was listed as one of the demerits.
4. While the short-term results of the instrumented stabilization and fusion after decompression in our series were gratifying, the long-term outcomes were variable with progressive deterioration in the results because of the junctional syndrome.
5. Mid-term results of decompression, instrumented stabilization and fusion after complete sagittal and coronal curve correction were most gratifying with less parafusion segment syndrome.
6. To avoid or minimize the adjacent segment diseases, the following measures should be taken:
   i. Preservation of the posterior ligamento-osseous complex at the parafusion segment.
   ii. Avoidance of partial floating fusion in malaligned spine.

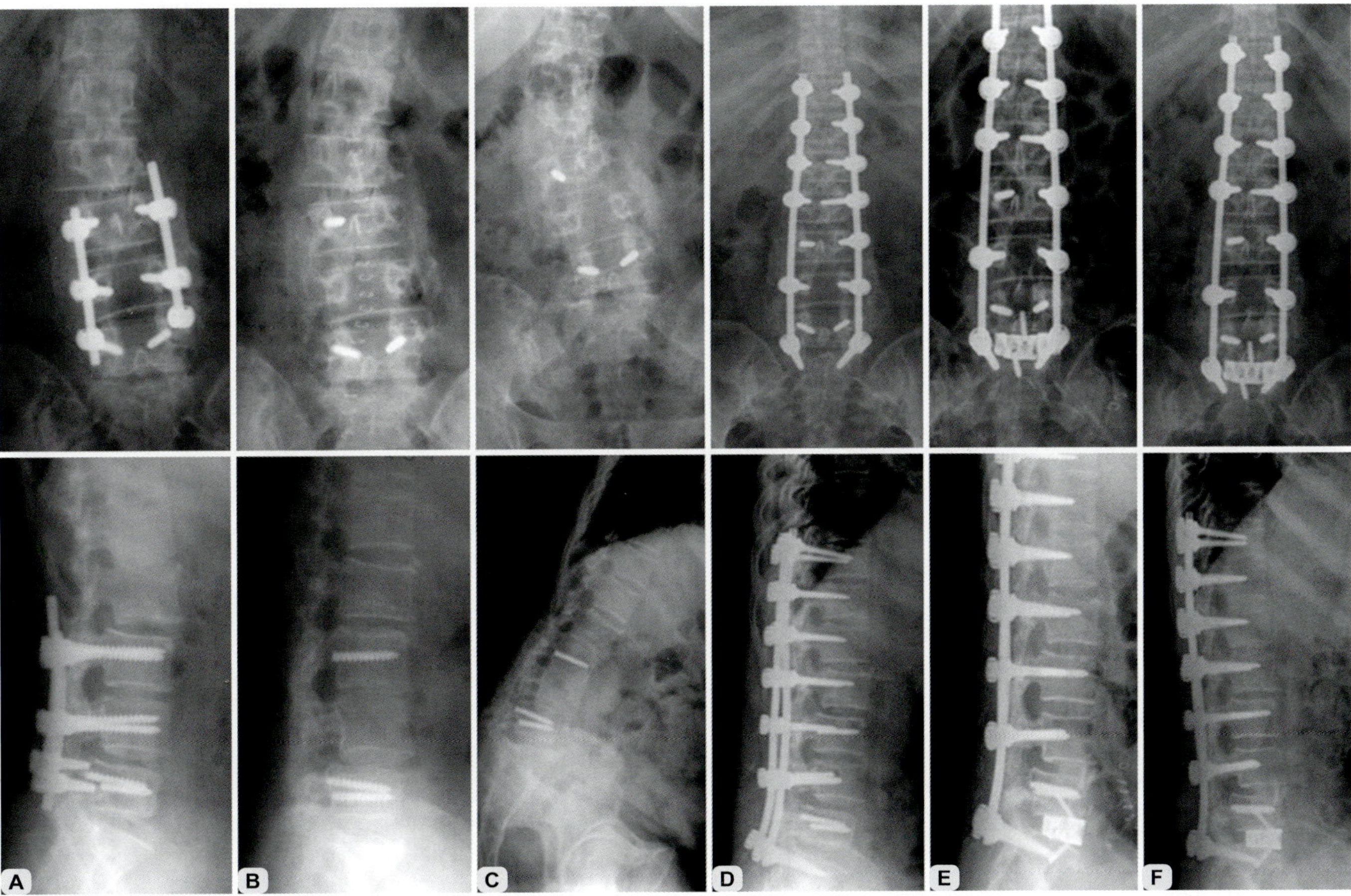

Fig. 26.17 An example of fixation failure in a 56-year-old DLS patient. Screw failure is seen in L3 and L5 bodies. The spine was re-implanted from T11–S1, and anterior Hartshill horseshoe cage between L5–S1. However, lumbar spine became flattened in spite of good restoration of coronal alignment. Finally, S1 screw gradually became loose

iii. In case of multilevel fusion, normal alignment should be restored, and undercorrection of the malaligned spine at time of fusion should not be allowed.

iv. Inclusion of the adjacent degenerated disk in fusion.

With the increased pre- and postoperative vigilance, continued refinement in technology and surgical techniques, the rate of success may increase and the rate of complications may drop.

Finally, the treating surgeons should sharpen their indications and operate only where effectiveness and efficacy have been demonstrated.

The surgeons should not operate only with too much zeal for the new and contempt for what is old. Otherwise, they will encounter the failure if they operate the patients with only zeal and without certain judgment.

References

1. Aebi M. Correction of degenerative scoliosis of the lumbar spine: a preliminary report. Clin arthop. 1988;232:80-6.
2. Akbarnia BA, Ogilvie JW, Hammerberg KW. Debate: Degenerative scoliosis; To operate or not to operate. Spine. 2006; 31:S5195-S5201.
3. Baron EM, Berven SH, Bridwell KH, Dewald CJ, Hu SS, et al. Adult spinal deformity focus issue. Summary statement. Spine. 2066;31(19):S202.
4. Benner B, Ehni G: Degenerative lumbar scoliosis. Spine. 1979; 4:548-52.
5. Bess S, Boachie-Adjei, Burton E, et al. Pain and disability determine treatment modality for older patients with adult scoliosis, while deformity guides treatment for younger patients. Spine. 2009;34(20):2186-90.

6. Bradford DS. Adult scoliosis: current concepts of treatment. Clinical Orthop. 1988;229:71-87.
7. Bridwell KH, Glassman S, Horton W, et al. Does treatment (nonoperative and operative) improve the two-year quality of life in patients with adult symptomatic lumbar scoliosis. Spine. 2009;34(20):2171-8.
8. Cho KJ, Suk SI, Park SR, Kim JH, Kim SS, Choi WK, et al. Complications in posterior fusion and instrumentation for degenerative lumbar scoliosis Spine. 2007;32:2232-7.
9. Cho KJ, Suk SI, Park SR, et al. Short fusion versus long fusion for degenerative lumbar scoliosis. Eur Spine. 2008; 17: 650-76.
10. Daffner SD, Vaccaro A. Adult degenerative lumbar scoliosis. Am J Orthop. 2003;2:77-82.
11. Daubs MD, Lenke LG, Cheh G, Stobbs G, Bridwell KH. Adult spinal deformity surgery: complications and outcomes in patients over age 60. Spine. 2007;32(20):2238-44.
12. Epstein JA, Epstein BS, Jones MD. Symptomatic lumbar scoliosis with degenerative changes in the elderly. Spine. 1979;4:542-7.
13. Etebar S, Cahill DW. Eisk factors for adjacent-segment failure following lumbar fixation with rigid instrumentation for degeneratie instability. J Neurosurg. 1999;90:163-9.
14. Freadman BA, Horton WC, Rhee JM, Edwards CC, Kuklo TR. Reliablity analysis for manual radiographic measures of rotator subluxation or lateral listhesis in adult scoliosis. Spine. 2009;34(6):603-8.
15. Fujita Y, Yamakawa T. Personal communication, 2009.
16. Grubb SA, Lipscomb HJ, Suh PB. Result of surgical treatment of adult onset scoliosis. Spine. 1994;19:1619-27.
17. Gupta MC. Degenerative scoliosis positions for surgical management. Orthop Clin N Am. 2003;34:269-79.
18. Ha KY, Moon MS, Park SY. Effect of instrumented stabilization and fusion of degenerative lumbar scoliosis on infused adjacent segment. J Korea Spine Surg. 1995;2:270-5.
19. Ha, KY, Moon MS. Effect of instrumental stabilization and fusion of degenerative lumbar scoliosis on unfused adjacent segments, J. Jpn Orthop Assoc. 1996;70(2)(3):S66.
20. Harms J. Jeszenszky D. Die operative Behandlung der degenerativen Lumbarskoliose: ed. Matzen KA. Chronischer Kreuzschmerz alter Menschen. W. Zuckschwerdt Verlag. Muenchen. Bern. Wien: New York; 1966.
21. Iizuka T, Yamada S. Challenging degenerative lumbar scoliosis with segmental corrective fusion surgery. J Musculoskeletal Res. 2006;10:141-50.
22. Jackson RP, Simmons EH, Stripinis D. Incidence and severity of back pain in adult idiopathic scoliosis. Spine. 1983;8:749-56.
23. Kim YJ, Bridwell KH, Lenke LG, et al. Pseudarthrosis in primary fusions for adult idiopathic scoliosis: incidence risk factors and outcome analysis. Spine. 2005;30:468-74.
24. Kim YT, Lee CS, Lee MH, Shin SJ. Operative treatment of degenerative scoliosis. J Korea Spine Surg. 2001;8:491-6.
25. Korovessis R, Piperos G, Sidiropoulous P, Diamas A. Adult idiopathic lumbar scoliosis. A formula for prediction of progression and review of the literature. Spine. 1993;19: 1926-32.
26. Kostuik JP, Hall BB. Spinal fusions to the sacrum in adults with scoliosis, Spine. 1983;8:489-500.
27. Kusaka G, Kuno S, Inoue T, Shoda M, Sano H. Surgical strategy for degenerative lumbar scoliosis: clinical outcome of posterior lumbar interbody fusion with pedicle screw fixation. J Spinal Surg. 2010;1:178-82.
28. Laohacharoensombat W, Wajanavisit W, Chaiyakit P. Preliminary results on the surgical treatment of disabling degenerative scoliosis. J Musculoskeletal Res. 1997;3:285-303.
29. Lee SM, Suk SI, Chung ER. Direct vertebral rotation: a new technique of three-dimensional deformity correction with segmental pedicle screw fixation in adolescent idiopathic scoliosis. Spine. 2004;343-9.
30. Lin JF, Moon MS: The lateral retroperitoneal approach to the fifth lumbar disc. J Spinal Surg. 2009;1:12-7.
31. Liu H, Ishihara H, Kanamori M, Kawaguchi Y, Ohmori K, Kimura T. Characteristics of nerve root compression caused by degenerative lumbar stenosis with scoliosis. Spine J 2003;3:524-9.
32. McPhee IB, Swanson CE. The surgical management of degenerative lumbar scoliosis: posterior instrumentation olare verus two stage surgery. Bulletin H for Joint Dis. 1998; 57: 16-22.
33. Moon MS, Lee KS, Lim CI, Kim YB, Lee HS. A clinical study of degenerative lumbar scoliosis. J Korea Orthop Assoc. 1992;27:946-55.
34. Moon MS, Lee KS, Lim EI, Kim YB, Lee HS. A clinical study of degenerative lumbar scoliosis. Lumbar fusion and stabilization. eds. Yonenobu K. Ono K. Takemitsu Y. Springer-Verlag: Tokyo, Berlin; 1993. pp. 98-112.
35. Moon MS, Ha KY, Moon YW. Results of surgical treatment of painful degenerative lumbar scoliosis. J Jpn. Orthop Assoc. 1996;70(2)(3) S65.
36. Moon MS, Lee BJ, Kim SS, Lin JF. Evolution of management of spinal deformities: controversial issues and current concept review. J Spinal Surg. 2010;2(1):295-305.
37. Moon MS, Kim SS, Lee BJ, Lin JF. Degenerative lumbar scoliosis – an update – controversial issues and a new challenge. J Spinal Surg. 2011;2(3):439-50.
38. Oskovian RJ, Shaffrey CI. Degenerative lumbar scoliosis. Neurosurg Clin N Am. 2006;17:299-315.
39. Perennou D, Marcelli CH, Risson CH, Simon L. Adult lumbar scoliosis—epidemiological aspeets in a low back pain population. Spine. 1994;19:123-8.
40. Ploumis A, Transfeldt EE, Gilbert TJ, Mehbed AA, Dykes DC, Perra J. Degenerative lumbar scoliosis. Radiographic correlation of lateral olisthesis with neural canal dimension. Spine. 2006;31:2353-58.
41. Pritchett JW, Bartel DT. Degenerative symptomatic lumbar scoliosis. Spine. 1993;18:700-3.
42. Robin GC, Sparn Y, Stlinberg R, Makin M, Menczel J. Scoliosis in the elderly: A follow-up study. Spine. 1982;7:355-9.
43. Schlegel JD, Smith JA, Schleusener RL. Lumbar motion segment pathology adjacent to thoracolumbar, lumbar and lumbosacral fusion. Spine. 1996;21:970-81.

44. Vanderpool DW, Jmanes JI, Wynne-Davies R. Scoliosis in the elderly. J Bone Joint Surg. 1969;51A:446-55.
45. Shim JH, Ha KY, Cheung Y-J, Chung S-H. Genetic predisposition of degenerative lumbar scoliosis due to the copy number variation. Spine. (Phila Pa 1976)2011;36:1-11.
46. Toyama Y. Surgical treatment of degenerative lumbar scoliosis. In Yonenobu K, Ono K, Takemitsu Y (Eds). Lumbar fusion and stabilization. Springer-Verlag: Tokyo, Berlin; 1993. pp. 113-25.
47. Shufflebarger H, Suk SI, Mardjetko S. Debate: determining the upper instrumented vertebra in the management of adult degenerative scoliosis: stopping at T10 versus L1. Spine. 2006;31:S185-94.
48. Simmons EH, Jackson RP. The management of nerve root entrapment syndromes associated with the collapsing scoliosis of idiopathic lumbar and thoracolumbar curves. Spine. 1979;4:533-41.
49. Simmons ED: Surgical treatment of patients with scoliosis. Clin Orthop. 2001;384:45-53.
50. Zurbriggen C. markwalder TM, Wyss S. Long-term results in patients treated with posterior instrumentation and fusion for degenerative scoliosis of the lumbar spine. Acta Neurochirurgica. (Wien). 1999;141:21-6.

CHAPTER

27

Degenerative Lumbar Kyphosis: Pathogenesis and Global Standard for Management

Myung-Sang Moon, Sung-Soo Kim, Bong-Jin Lee, Min Geun Yoon, Jeong-Lim Moon

Introduction

In the aged spine, two sagittal deformities are frequently seen: increased thoracic kyphosis and decreased lumbar lordosis.[1-12] The loss of lumbar lordosis based on its severity was first named as flat back or degenerative lumbar kyphosis (DLK) by Takemitsu et al.[13,14] As yet there is no report on DLK among the Europeans in English literatures. Patients with advanced DLK have walking difficulty due to the forward trunk stooping. DLK is not only a cosmetic but also a functional one (Fig. 27.1). *De novo* lumbar kyphosis in the elderly drew the physician's attention in Japan and Korea since mid-1980s.[15-19] The physicians in the aged community now have expressed their regret for the past graceless neglect of their duty in the management of the spinal deformity of the elderly.

DLK is a rare spinal deformity seen in the females in 5th and 6th decades of life which results in truncal imbalance in standing in its late stage, and needs the balancing management while the dynamic stabilizers of the lumbar spine, pelvis, and hips still do their role.[1-19] This deformity is mostly seen in the oriental women who do their works in long-standing sitting positions, including squatted farm works. In most clinical cases there is a trend that the increased or decreased thoracic kyphosis accompanies the decreased or increased lumbar lordosis in the presence of the mobile segments, and consequently both curves are balanced. However, there is exceptionally a lumbar spinal deformity in the elderly women which cannot be balanced.

To make diagnosis of DLK, standing lateral view of entire spine should be taken (Fig. 27.1).[2-4,6,20-25] X-rays localized to lumbosacral spine should not be prescribed, because it cannot provide the information related with sagittal vertical axis of spine. In DLK patients dorsal spine gradually becomes lordotic and the lumbar spine becomes kyphotic, and infrequently the cervical spine becomes kyphotic. For this reason standing lateral view of whole spine should be taken. To describe the spinopelvic morphology, up to now different parameters have been used on basis of the standing lateral radiograms.[26-29]

Characteristic Features (Figs 27.2 to 27.5)

When in standing the trunk is raised from the fully flexed position, the movement is initiated by the hip extensor which becomes activated before the lumbar extensor (Fig. 27.5).[15-17] When the pelvis tilts anteriorly in the balanced spine, the lumbar lordosis is increased. This is counter-balanced by the contraction of the extensor muscles of the hip. When these gluteal muscles contract they tend to tilt the pelvis posteriorly. In this movement, these muscles can be actively aided by the abdominalis. So both the hip extensor and abdominalis muscles create a force couple to tilt the pelvis backward (the force couple of abdominalis and hip extensors), and thereby flatten the lumbar spine (Fig. 27.5).

It should be known that the spinal imbalance in DLK is confined not only to the spine but also to pelvis, hips and knees. Failure after the corrective and stabilizing surgery for DLK relates closely with the inefficient dynamic stabilizers of the pelvis, hips, and knees.

Symptomatic deformity, such as dynamic lumbar extension stenosis (dynamic flat back) should be ruled out as the first step from the structural one.[21-25]

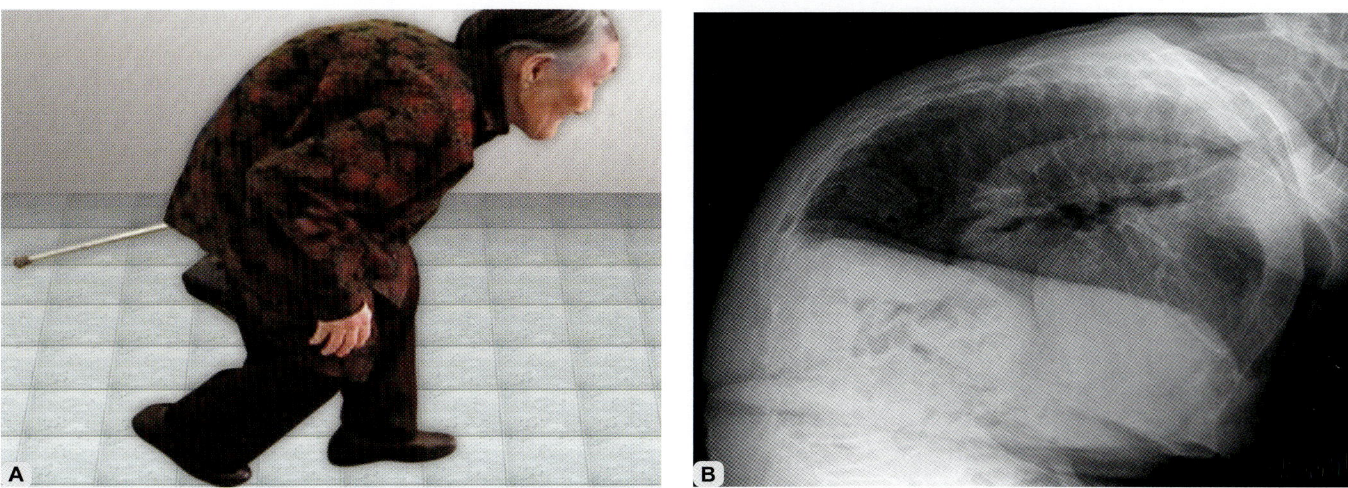

Fig. 27.1 An example of senile dorsolumbar kyphosis (dorsal round back due to osteoporosis. This is not the classical case of DLK due to lumbar disk degeneration. (A) Clinical appearance; (B) Lateral radiogram

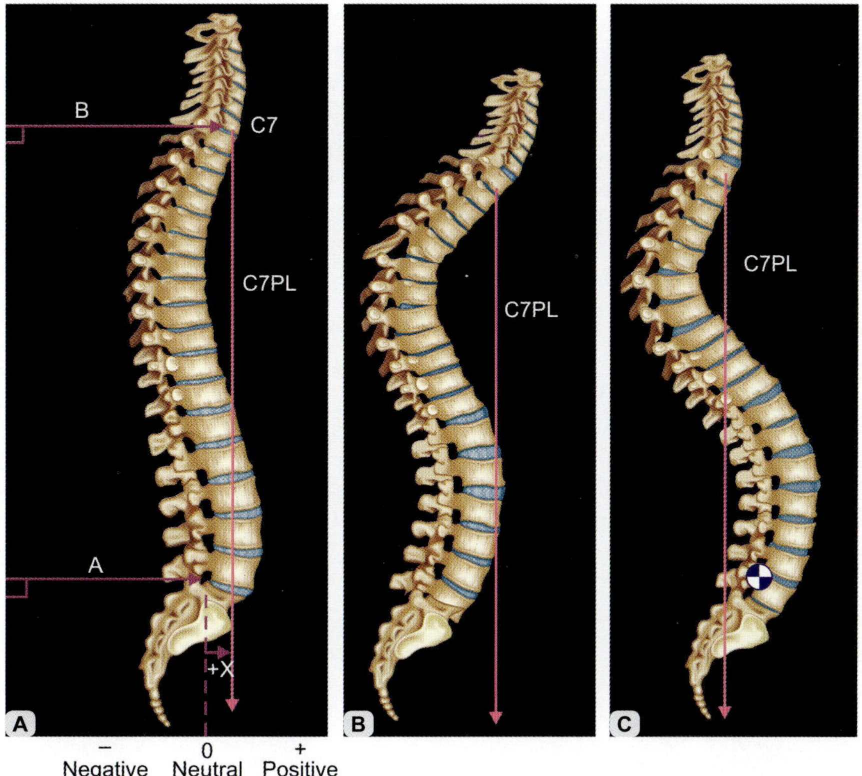

Fig. 27.2 (A) Neutral sagittal balance, B = A: negative balance: B < A; positive balance, B > A; +X = positive distance; (B) Positive sagittal balance; (C) Negative sagittal balance. SVA passes far front of S1 posterosuperior corner it is defined positive sagittal balance, while SVA passes far behind the corner it was defined negative sagittal balance

Deformity severity ranges clinically from mild to severe. Patient's complaints are low back pain, easy fatigability, and gradual stooping with walking difficulty which relates closely with erector spinae muscle weakness. Also pelvic extensor contributes greatly in accentuation of severity of DLK. Also segmental forward flexion instability of the lower lumbar segments is an adjunctive contributing factor for the development of DLK.[26-31]

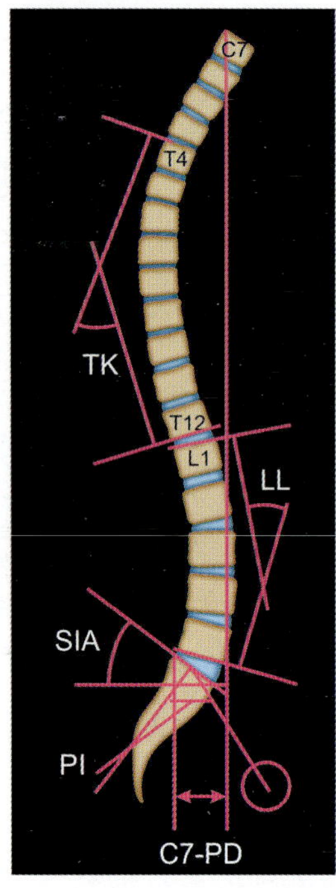

Fig. 27.3 Radiographic measurement of the sagittal spinal and pelvic parameters. TK, thoracic kyphosis; LL, lumbar lordosis; SIA, sacral inclination angle; C7-PD, C7 plumbline distance; PI, pelvic incidence

According to Lee et al. initial chief complaint is the truncal stooping in standing, though it is not seen in sitting.[15-17] The truncal stooping becomes worse on walking. In the early stage of disease, the patient tries to walk reclining the upper trunk backward by protruding the anterior chest forward and placing both shoulders widely spread and backward. The patient tries to shift the vertical loading line more posteriorly by flexing the hips and knees.[15,16]

In Takemitsu et al. types 1 and 2 DLK, patients have the flexed hip and knee deformities, though hip joints show ostensibly extension deformity. The reason is that the patients' trunks lean over backward to disguise the flexed hips to be seen extended. This is very important in management of DLK. Secondly, they cannot lift the weight placed in front with arms. Thirdly, during kitchen work they support the anteriorly inclined trunk by placing the elbow to the kitchen table. Lastly, they complain difficulty in walking upstairs or hill. All those listed above are the cardinal complaints of DLK. Except those listed above, DLK patients complain the nonspecific symptoms, such as low back pain and sciatica.

Patients with extension dynamic stenosis walk in stooped position to relieve pain. Therefore, afore-mentioned dynamic spinal stenosis and symptomatic early *de novo*

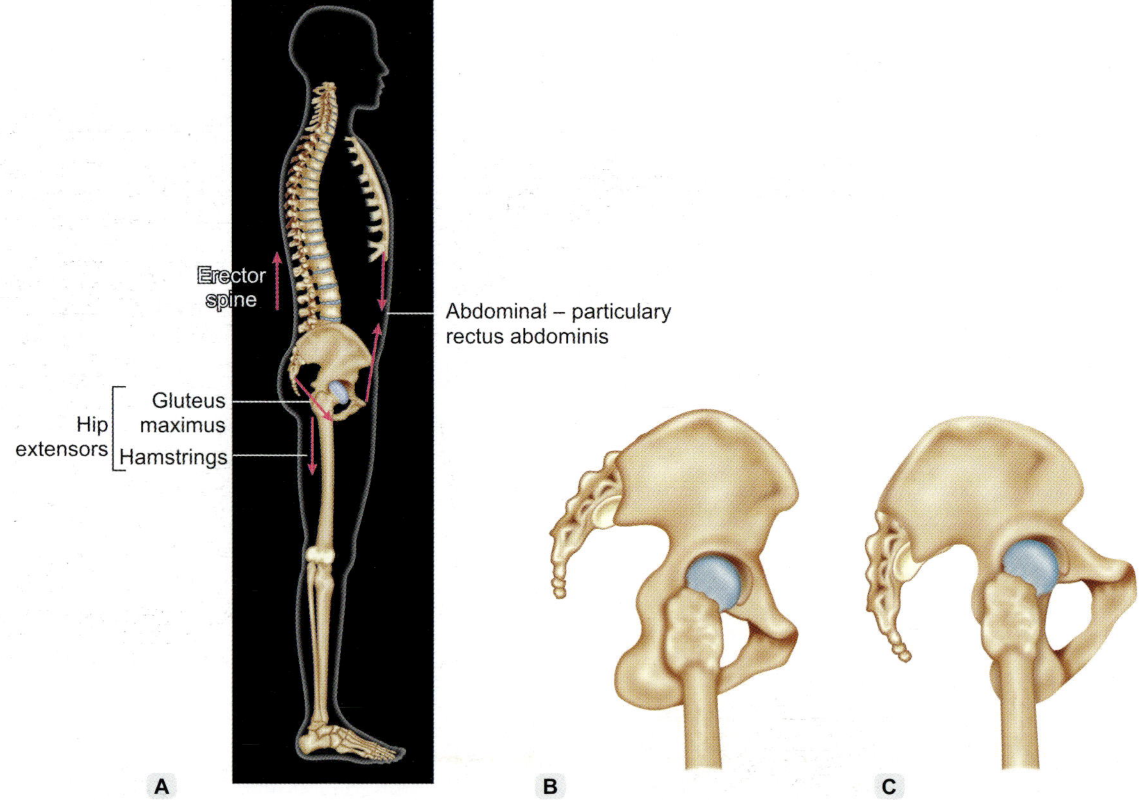

Fig. 27.4 The force couple of the abdominals and hip extensors rotate the pelvis backwards around the axis through the two hip joints from position (B) to position (C). There is also an accompanying flattening of the lumbar spine which is not shown in the diagram

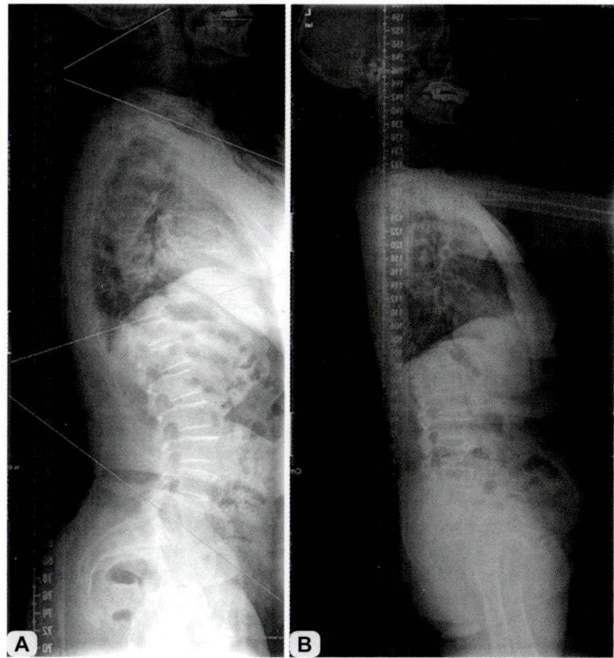

Fig. 27.5 (A) Sagittal radiograph of the spine and pelvis; (B) An example of Takemitsu's type 2 and Lee's group 1 DLK

degenerative lumbar kyphosis should be carefully assessed and to be differentiated each other.

In healthy spine, anterior pelvic tilt directly develops the compensatory lumbar lordosis at the mobile segments, and also indirectly gives influence on the femoral head coverage by the acetabulum. Posterior pelvic tilt decreases the femoral head coverage by the acetabulum which leads to the coxarthrosis. It was demonstrated that when sacral inclination angle changes from 35° to 10° femoral coverage by acetabulum (DLK hip) was decreased by 21%.[31] Takemitsu et al.'s study disclosed that the DLK hip is loaded 5 times more than the normal subject in standing. Also it was confirmed that pelvic inclination index (PII) approximately correlates with pelvic angle of Jackson, and that in stooped posture the hip muscles showed hyperactivity during walking comparing to the normal condition.[20,30,31]

Classification by Deformity, Severity and Evolution

DLK was classified into 4 types by Takemitsu et al., based on its disease evolutionary stage (severity) (Figs 27.6 and 27.7).[13,14,20]

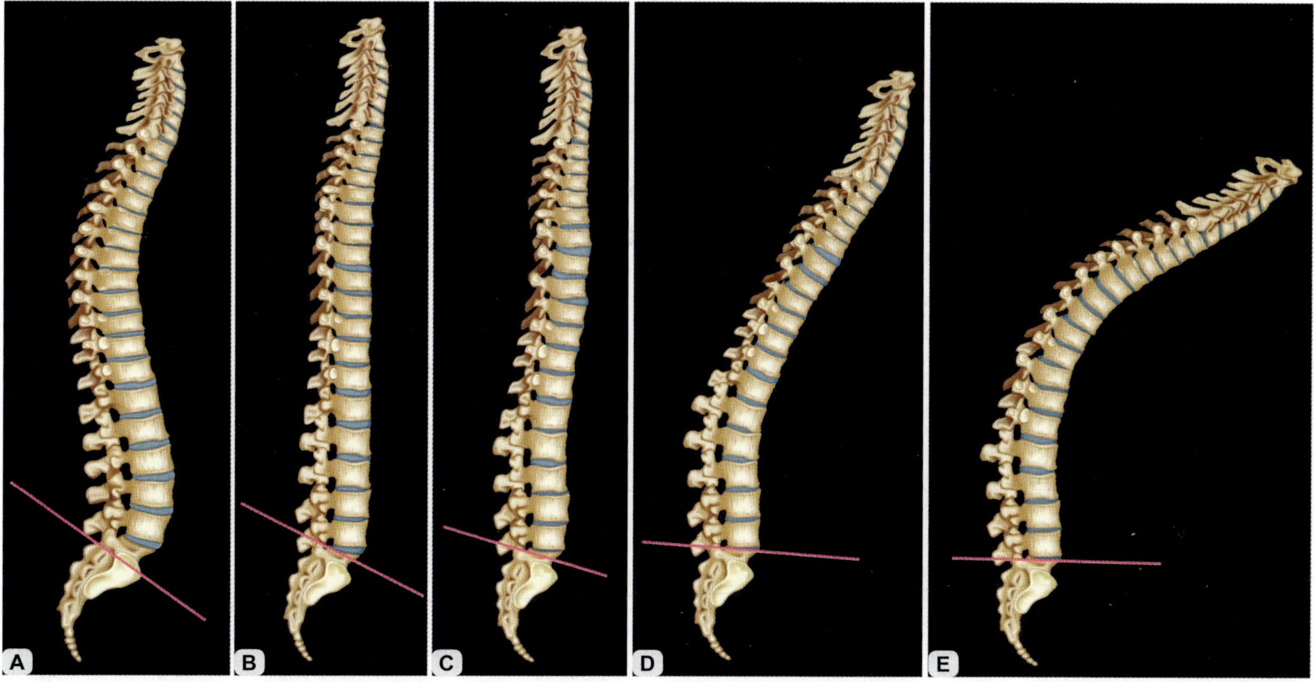

Fig. 27.6 Takemitsu's classification of four types of degenerative lumbar kyphosis due to the disease progress. Gradual posterior tilt of the normal sacrum is illustrated, based on its progress. In type 4 DLK, sacrum is positioned rather vertically (horizontally positioned sacral dome). However, group I of Figure 27.8 shows the posteriorly tilted pelvis, while group II of Figure 27.8 shows the anteriorly tilted pelvis. When the positive imbalance redevelops, the pelvis is rotated posteriorly; thereby, sagittal balance can be restored when gluteal muscle are intact. (A) Normal standard; (B) Type 1: Straight back; (C) Type 2: Mild kyphosis; (D) Type 3: Moderate kyphosis; (E) Extended and back

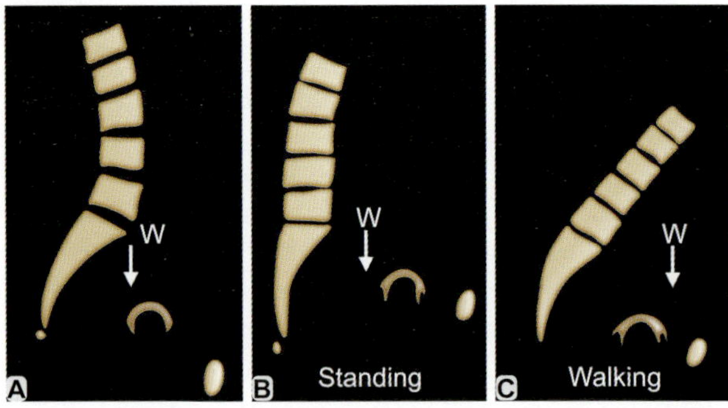

Fig. 27.7 Standing sagittal view of lumbar spine in normal and DLK persons: Biomechanical correlation between lumbar spine, hip joint, and center of gravity line are illustrated. In this figure illustration, Takemitsu et al. showed the vertically aligned sacrum on standing and anterior tilted sacrum on walking. However, their illustration of DLK classification shows the gradual posterior sacral tilt (horizontal sacral dome) when the DLK progress. For this, there is no plausible explanation. The current authors' view on it is that such sacral position change is the result of gluteal and hamstring muscle activity and passive tightening of the muscle and its fascia and stabilizing ligaments. (A) Standard; (B and C) Lumbar degenerative kyphosis: (B) Standstill posterior pelvic tilt and (C) Dynamic anterior pelvic tilt

- Type 1: Straight back
- Type 2: Mild lumbar kyphosis
- Type 3: Moderate lumbar kyphosis
- Type 4: Extended round back.

However, they did not provide the numerical data of the spinopelvic parameters related with the sagittal balance; plumb line shift distance and overhang distance of S_1.

The spinal column in DLK becomes more positive in balance in its progress. Patients with type 1 and 2 DLK can stand and walk unaided, while patients with type 3 and 4 can hardly stand upright unaided and depends more on cane or puts their hands above the knee-caps on walking to prevent the knee buckling. Some patients try to support their low backs posteriorly with their clenched hands.

Two Groups of DLK by Lee et al.

The advanced DLK (types 3 and 4) were grouped into two by Lee et al., based on the conditions of the erector spinae and gluteus muscles.[15-17]

Group I (DLK with weakness of erector spinae only).

Group II (DLK with weakness of erector spinae and gluteus muscles).

In case of weakened erector spinae muscle alone, stooping could be compensated by gluteal muscle activity which induced the posterior pelvic tilt. Most of the DLK patients (80%) belonged to this group. The patients' spine (Group II) with weakened erector spinae and the associated excessive anterior pelvic tilt due to weakened gluteal muscles, was nominated by Lee et al as "sagittal spinal and pelvic decompensation state (SSDD)" (20%). For the latter case, instrument-aided correction and stabilization surgery is contraindicated, because the persistent stooping lasts even after corrective surgery.[15-17]

It is difficult clinically to differentiate the two groups, particularly at its early stage of the disease. Also it is uncertain whether the group I DLK progress to group II DLK or two groups are different from the start of the disease. Most reliable differential diagnosis is the standing sagittal radiograms of lumbosacral spine, taken on flexion, neutral and extension of the spine. Assessment of pelvic tilt on upright standing is crucial in differentiation of the two groups; erector spinae atrophy type or combined erector spinae and gluteal muscle atrophy type. Also stage of disease and compensated and decompensated groups can be searched by assessment.[15-17]

Clinical Types Due to Involved Disk Level (Apex of the Curvature)

There are two types: in the upper type the apex locates above L3, while that of the lower type locates below L3. According to Lee et al., among the 98 DLK patients 79 had lower type and 19 had upper type. The lower type DLK was reported to have clinically poorer prognosis than that of the upper type DLK.[15-17]

Classification by Curve Flexibility

Lumbar kyphosis is a flat back deformity which is seen in ankylosing spondylitis, vertebral fracture, and various iatrogenically and naturally induced deformities. Most of those flat back deformities are rather stiff. However, DLK in some patients is rather flexible, while in others rather rigid. It is due to evolutionary stage of disease. Based on these informations the surgery must be carried out under different indication.

To test the flexibility of the involved segments, fulcrum bending test is essential.[19] The correctable deformity by fulcrum bending test is the flexible type, and non-correctable deformity is the rigid type. For diagnosis standing and recumbent AP and lateral roentgenograms of whole spine are essential.

Classification by Segmental Stability

There are two forms: stable (hypomobile) and unstable (hypermobile). Segmental instability is detected by lying, standing and stress radiograms. This classification together with flexibility classification is helpful in preoperative assessment of limitation of the instrument-aided correction surgery.

Differential Diagnosis

Diagnosis can be made by clinical symptoms and signs including typical external body appearance in walking. Clinical symptoms and signs are (i) pain, (ii) functional impairment, and (iii) spinal deformity.

Chief complaint of a patient with disk herniation is the pain, and that of the idiopathic scoliosis is the deformity.[8] The cord injured patient's chief complaint is the functional impairment, and those of cervical spondylotic myelopathy are pain and the functional impairment. In those patients listed above their chief complaints are one or two, while DLK patients present 3 typical findings: (i) pain, (ii) functional impairment, and (iii) deformity (Figs 27.1, 27.7, 27.9, 27.10, 27.11 to 27.15).

Pitfalls in Diagnosis

Common low back pain disorders in patients of 6th to 7th decades are spondylosis with or without stenosis and disc herniation. Therefore, the treating surgeons easily miss the diagnosis of early DLK. Because the patients with extension dynamic stenosis walk on stooped position to relieve the pain. Secondly DLK should be differentiated from the senile kyphosis secondary to osteoporotic vertebral compression fractures mostly of the lower dorsal and dorsolumbar spines. DLK is seen in age group between 40 and 60 years in whom the advanced disk change with some associated bony abnormality is seen.

The sacropelvic angle of Jackson is the static standstill radiographic findings,[8] and is not the dynamic one such as the radiogram on walking. That is, the increased or decreased pelvic tilt during walking is dynamic, while Jackson's sacropelvic angle is the unchangeable static one. Parkinson's disease also should be differentiated, because corrective DLK surgery in this condition fails. In the management of the senile kyphosis, corrective lumbar surgery was often erroneously done without good preoperative assessment. Utmost attention should be paid not to make misdiagnosis of DLK.

Treatment

Up to now no standardized regimen was proposed except Takemitsu et al. and Lee et al.[13-17]

Conservative Management

Patients with early DLK are subjected to this treatment which is also indicated when the surgical management is impossible or contraindicated. The conservative treatment should aim both at the back pain alleviation and prevention of progression of stooping. However, the therapeutic effects were not promising, because it was not proven as yet (Flowchart 27.1).

Low Back Pain

general pain management protocol is applicable. NSAIDs and muscle relaxants are prescribed.

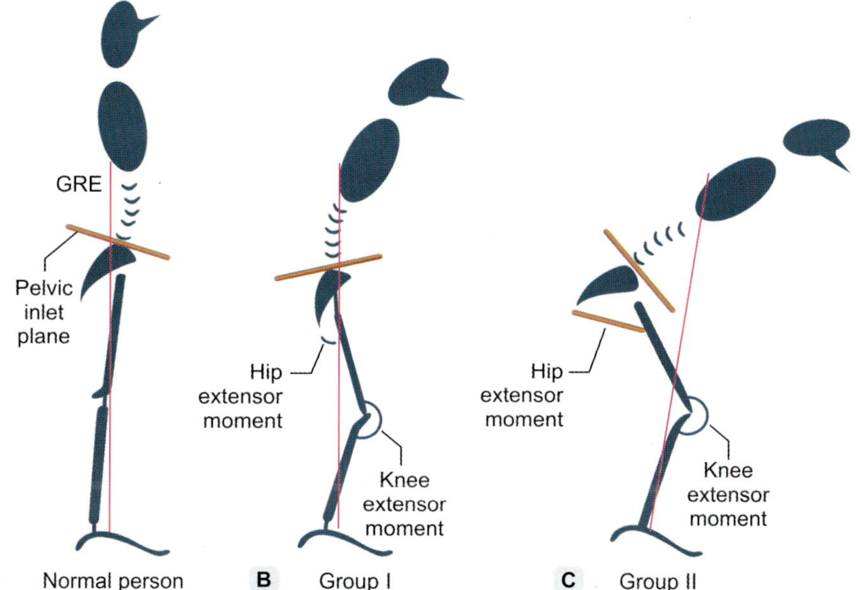

Fig. 27.8 Ground reaction force (GRF) on kinetic gait analysis. GRF passed just anterior and close to the hip joint in group I, whereas it was displaced far anterior to the hip joint with increased hip extensor moment in group II. These figures also show two types of degenerative flat back according to pelvic tilt on gait analysis: posterior pelvic tilt in group I and marked anterior pelvic tilt in group II. This different result is due to dynamic difference in gluteal and hip extensor muscle activity, evident only during walking. Those phenomenon can be seen in some cases of type III–IV DLK. Therefore, in defining the pelvic balance, the concept of dynamic and static imbalance should be brought in interpretation of spinopelvic alignment

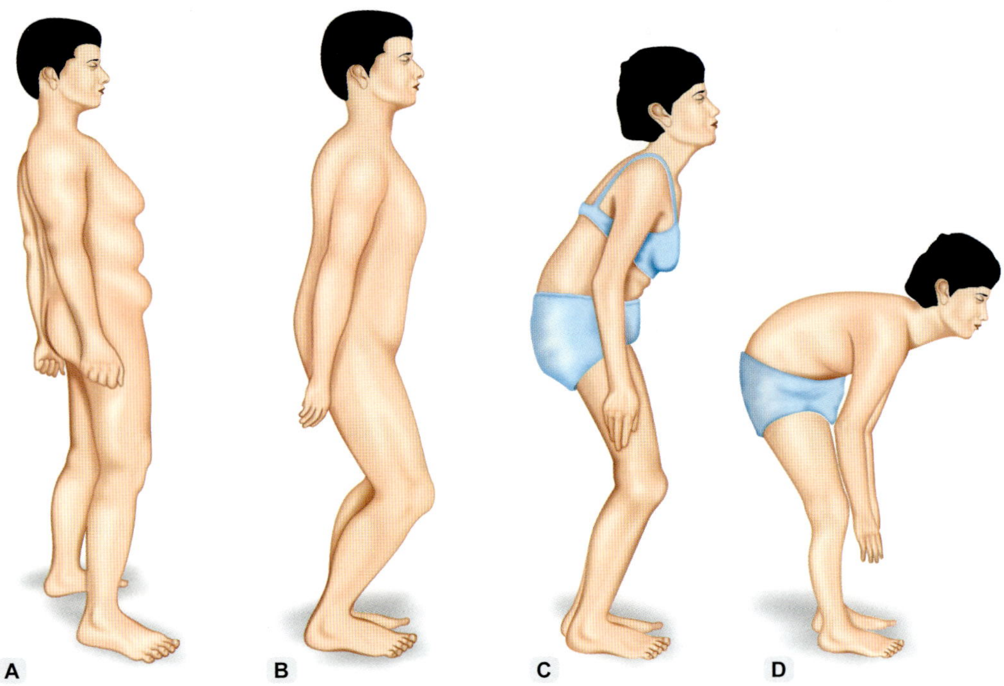

Fig. 27.9 Two lateral postures to stand upright in (A and B) Type 2 DLK; (C) Type 3 DLK; (D) Type 4 DLK

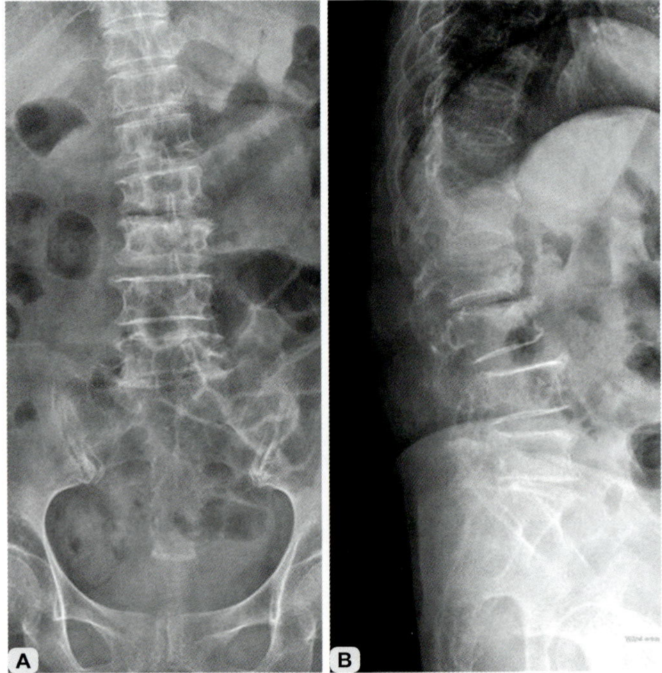

Fig. 27.10 An example of the Takemitsu stage 2 upper type DLK (L2–L3) with L3 wedging. Knuttson sign is seen at narrowed L2–3 disk

Muscle Strengthening Exercise

Powers of the back and pelvic extensor muscles should be carefully assessed before exercise. Strengthening exercise for back extensor muscle is primarily indicated, because the primary cause of DLK is the weakness of the back extensor muscles. However, its efficacy is doubtful when there is the established fatty fibrotic atrophies of erector spinae muscles. Also pelvic extensor muscle strengthening exercise should be combined. Muscle strengthening exercise can retard the progress of the deformity, but cannot cure the condition if there are definitely the established back and pelvic extensor muscle atrophies, and advanced disk degeneration. However, success of the correction and stabilization surgery depends more on the plevic extensor muscle strength than the erector spinae muscles. Therefore, preoperatively muscle strengthening should be prescribed and assessed, and also should be maintained even after corrective surgery.

Surgical Management

Surgery aims at the instrument-aided correction of the kyphotic spine in normal alignment and maintenance of the corrected spine but cannot restore the normal lumbar function.[19-27]

Preoperatively to fulfill the objective of the surgery the physical and psychological conditions should be considered. The informed consent also should be obtained. The treating surgeon let the patient and his or her family members understand the surgical objective, and the final result. Also he or she, the family members should know the

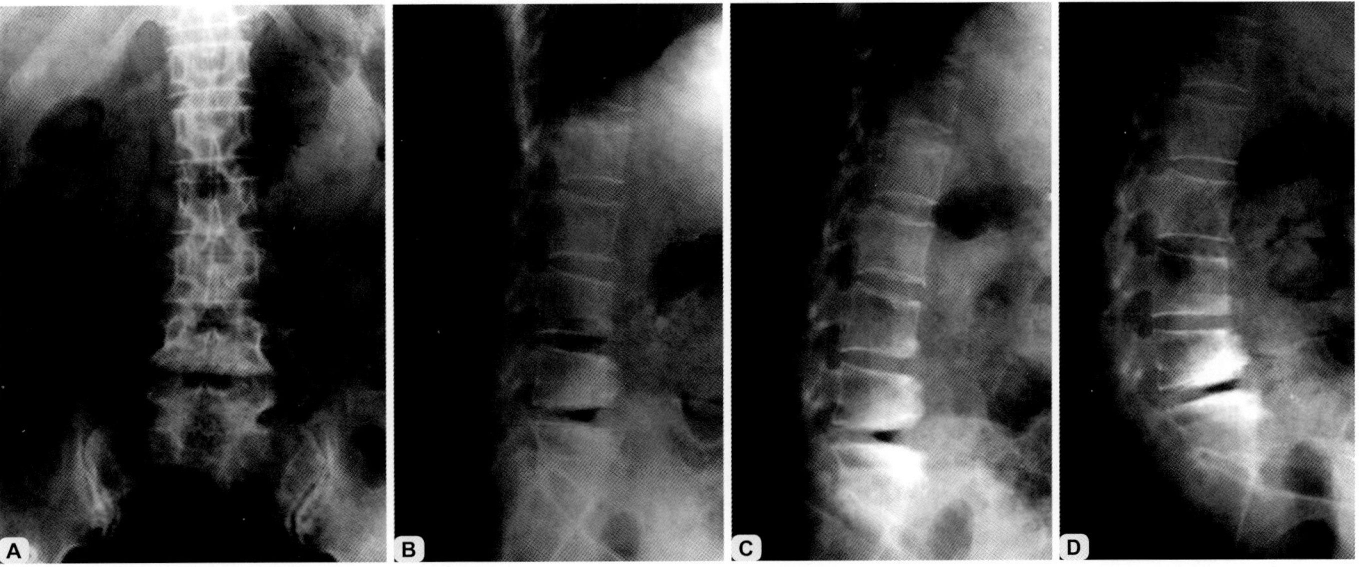

Fig. 27.11 Stage 1 lower type DLK in a 69-year-old lady. Mirror sign in L4 and L5 and Knuttson's sign at L4–5 disk are seen

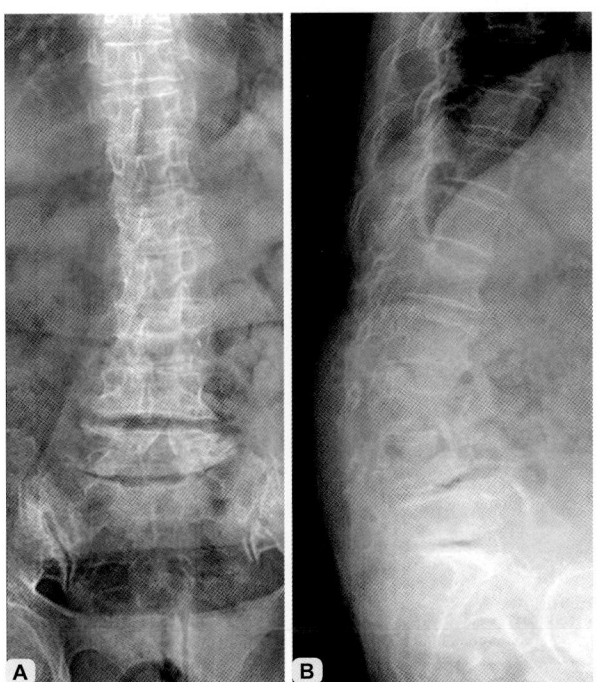

Fig. 27.12 Lower type DLK in late stage 2 in a 75-year-old lady (Koh, S-D). Knuttson's sign is seen at L4–5 and L5–S1 disks

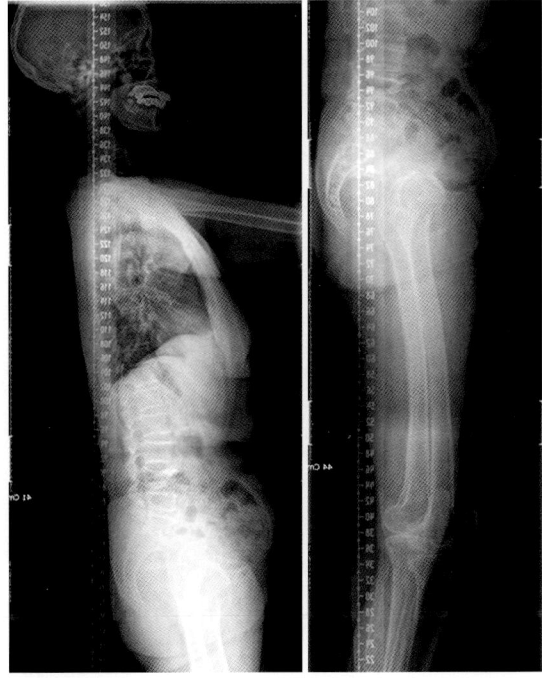

Fig. 27.13A This is a whole spine AP and lateral view in a 65-year-old lady with lower type 2 group 1 DLK. Flattened whole spine sagittally with posterior tilted pelvis

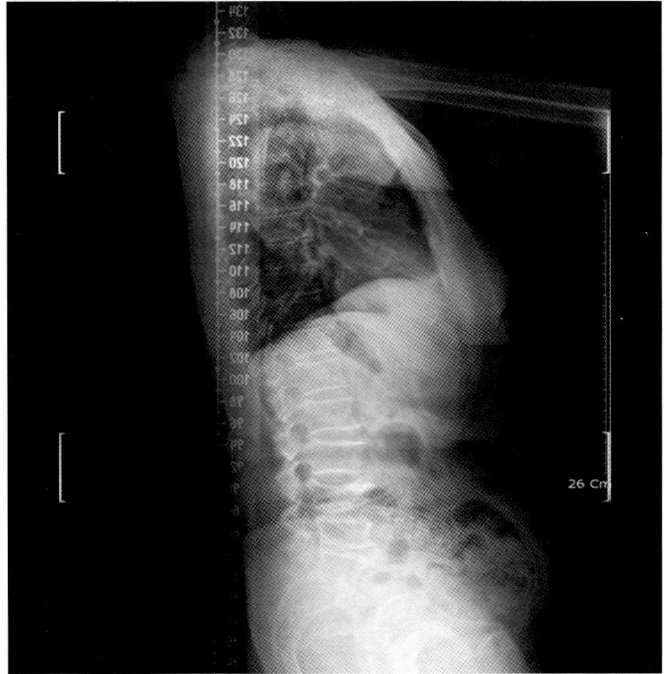

Fig. 27.13B Sagittal spinal view from C5 to sacrum hip. Collapsed L4 vertebral body is shown with vertically situated sacrum (posterior pelvic tilt).

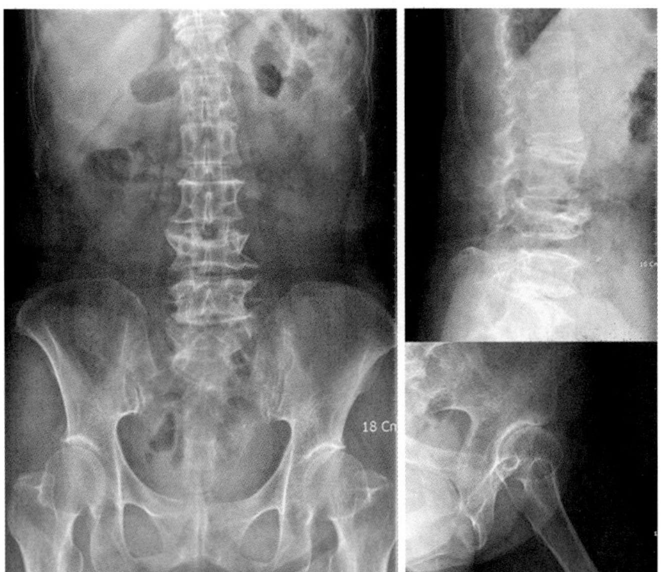

Fig. 27.13C Lumbar spine (AP and lateral views) and an arthritic hip are shown together with uncover anterior part of the femoral head. Posterior pelvic tilt uncovers the femoral head by acetabulum, though posterior pelvic tilt stabilize the lumbosacral joint in standing when the gluteal muscles are intact while it gives ill-effect on hips.

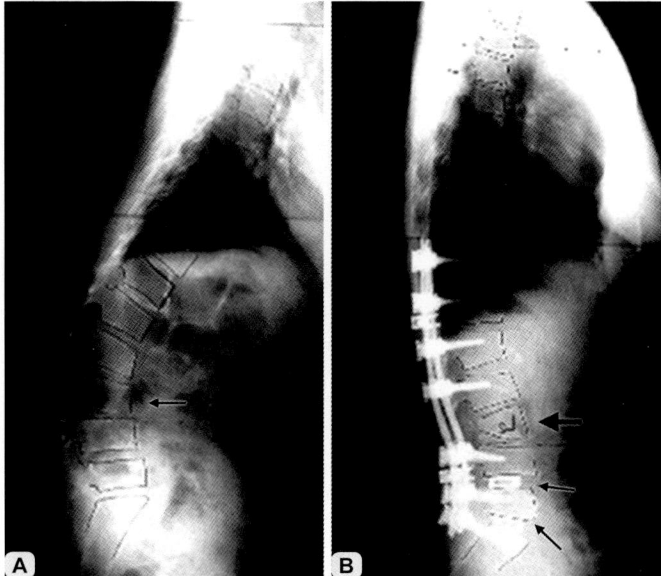

Fig. 27.14 An example of (A) Takemitsu's type 3 upper type degenerative lumbar kyphosis, which was corrected and stabilized with (B) the posterior rods and pedicle screws and anterior cages at L4–5 and L5–S1 (T11–S1)

patients' comorbidity. Because patient should tolerate the surgical stresses, and should have the good bone quality for instrumentation. Otherwise, the instrumentation will fail because of bone and/or instrument failure. For successful surgery instruments should maintain the corrected alignment without failure until fusion.[27-29]

The primary objective of the surgery for the balanced and unbalanced deformed spines are different: The surgery for the severely deformed balanced spine aims primarily at the deformity correction for aesthetic reason, while surgery for the unbalanced (decompensated, maladjusted) spine must be the balancing one. Therefore, it should be known that the skeletal deformity correction alone cannot restore the trunk balance if there is no extraskeletal dynamic stabilizers. Lee et al. recommended the preoperative muscle strength study of erector spinae, gluteal, and hip extensors.[15-17]

Some surgeons recommend the corrective surgery for all the lumbar kyphosis and thoracic lordosis. Because their view on the lumbar deformity is that DLK is the byproduct of skeletal deformity unrelated with stabilizers' weakness, though the de novo DLK is truly the secondary deformity due to erector spinae muscle atrophy like the deformity in the neuromuscular diseases, and the adaptive change of the vertebral body deformity due to the advanced disk changes. Therefore, surgery, aiming only at the skeletal deformity correction without considering the erector spinae and gluteal muscles' condition will result in therapeutic failure. The corrective surgery is not simple, and frequently develops complications.

In summary, it should be known that the lumbar spine can be normally aligned and stabilized by instrumentation surgery, but results in stiff back. Therefore, preoperatively

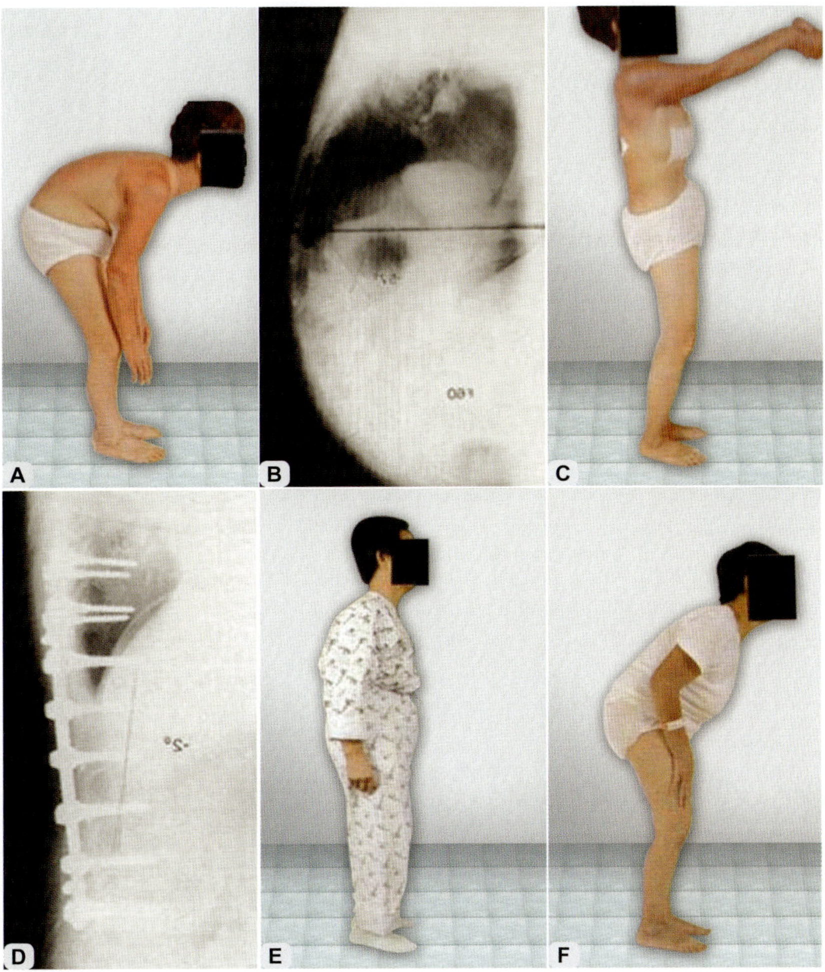

Fig. 27.15 Persistent stooping after corrective and stabilization surgery in the absence of gluteal and hip extensor muscles. (A) Initial body appearance in sagittal plane; (B) Initial sagittal radiogram; (C) Supported standing lateral view; (D) Instrumented flattened spine from T11 to S1; (E) Upright stand-still posture; (F) Restooped posture on walking. Also insufficient lordotization (flat back) seems to be the one of persistent stooping. Lumbar lordosis should be restored over 35° to shift the load more posteriorly

the advantages and disadvantages should be intensively studied for the successful outcome and patients' benefit, and those informations should be known to the patients and their supporters.

Surgical Objectives and Indication

The primary surgical objective of DLK is to restore the normal sagittal alignment of the kyphotic spine through the instrument-aided deformity correction and stabilization. That of surgical management of the other pain-provoking aged spines, such as DLS is to control the pain, and deformity correction is the secondary one.

Instrument-aided deformity correction and stabilization surgery should not be done solely on basis of the image findings alone without considering the clinical findings. Surgery is not indicated for the asymptomatic early DLK patients without difficulty in ADL, very old patients, and Parkinson's disease and other osteopathy patients.

The DLK patient's chief complaints are low back pain and stooping. Patient with dynamic extension stenosis shows the stooping posture to relieve pain. Therefore, based on the misinterpreted data, decompression surgery for early DLK patient was often carried out under the diagnosis of spinal stenosis in the past[27](Fig. 24.16).

Preoperative Patient's Condition and Surgical Indication

The elderly patient with DLK should have the good physical conditions tolerable for surgery. However, only for the following three conditions surgery is indicated; (i) severe

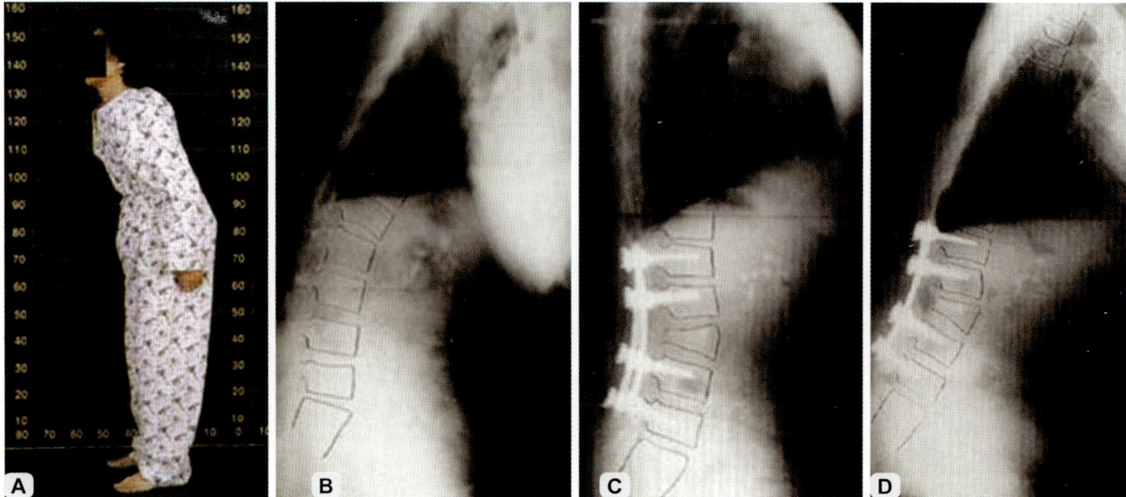

Fig. 27.16 (A) Persistent stooping after corrective surgery because of hip flexion due to gluteal and hip extensor muscle atrophy; (B to D) Posterior pelvic tilt is seen

difficulty in ADL because of stooping, (ii) better bone quality, and (iii) physically active patient wishing to continue her professional life for many more years. However, surgery is contraindicated for very old patient with poor general condition and severe osteoporosis.

Postoperatively far anteriorly displaced C7 plumb line (positive balance) should be shifted to normal range of sagittal vertebral axis.

Surgically realigned curve could not restore the normal balance in some patients. In some of the DLK patients (15–20%) surgery was wrongly indicated, because stooping persisted postoperatively in spite of good correction. Those patients were found to have weakness of the erector spinae, gluteus maximus and hamstring muscles (persistent stooping). In those patients, surgery was judged "failure".

Lee et al. reported that in flat back deformity active posterior pelvic tilt by pelvic extensor muscle was considered to be the most important compensatory mechanism to overcome stooping from sagittal imbalance which was manifested as a vertical sacrum on standing radiogram.[16,17]

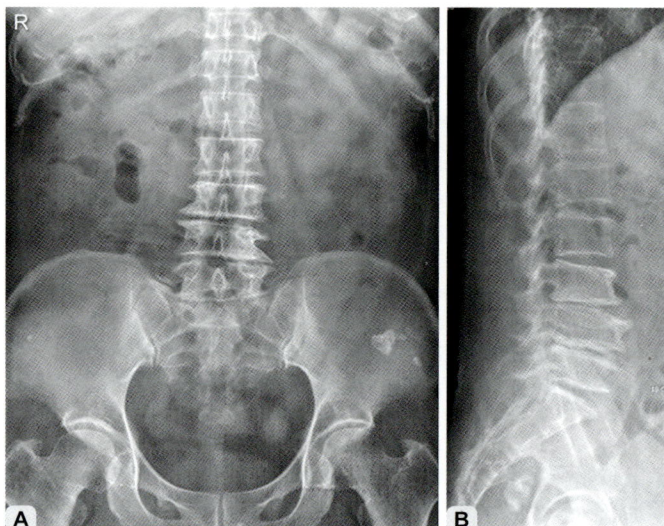

Fig. 27.17 An example of Takemitsu's type 1 and Lee's group I DLK. Whole spine in sagittal plane is flat with normal pelvic tilt

Surgical Methods

Instrument-aided posterior correction

this procedure is indicated for the flexible curve. Surgery is best done by rod derotation technique, utilizing the contoured rod and pedicle screws. To make the lumbar spine lordotic, patients should be placed on operating table in prone with 20°–30° of hip flexion and 60°–70° knee flexion, and thus brings the pelvis in anterior rotation. Subsequently the extent of instrumentation should be decided. In general spinal segments from lower thoracic (T10) or upper lumbar spine (L1) to L5 or S1 and/or ilium are included in instrumented stabilization. Stooping force (load and motion transfer) after surgery concentrates at upper or lower adjacent segments and/or both, but mostly at L4–5 or L5–S1 (Fig. 27.17).[15-18,25,28]

Anterior and posterior correction procedures

The rigidity of the kyphotic deformity should be assessed preoperatively by bending test. The rigid segments should be released by anterior and posterior approaches before instrumented deformity correction. All the contracted soft tissue around disks should be released or resected together with disk excision which is followed by distraction of the involved disk space. To correct the deformity and to maintain the corrected alignment, anterior interbody fusion cage and/or strut bone graft are inserted into the excised disk spaces, and then posterior instrument-aided sagittal curve correction and stabilization should be followed. This combined surgery gives the physical burden a lot to the patient. Therefore, preoperatively comorbidity should be carefully examined to minimize the intra- and postoperative surgical complications. This procedure is nowadays less frequently used because of the graveness of the surgery.[15-18]

Posterior instrument-aided correction with posterior lumbar interbody fusion

this procedure replaced the combined anterior and posterior correction procedure. After expansive laminectomy, disk excision and anterior release through posterior route is done before posterior interbody fusion and instrumented stabilization. This procedure is less effective in kyphosis correction than the combined anterior and posterior correction procedure. However, it is more effective in patient with highly flexible and hypermobile spine.

Decancellation or posterior wedge resection osteotomy

decancellation procedure is known as transpedicular decancellation osteotomy, pedicle subtraction osteotomy, and egg-shell procedure.[24-28] After expansive laminectomy, the cancellous bone of the vertebral body is curetted out through pedicle route which is followed by the instrument-aided axial compression to induce the posterior wedge-shaped vertebral body collapse. Two and three vertebral bodies are decancellated for full correction. One bone decancellation provide around 30°–40° of correction. Also posterior wedge resection osteotomy does the same role. Lehmer et al. (1994) recommended not to correct over 35° by single level osteotomy.[21] Otherwise, dural buckling can occur which may require dural plasty (Fig. 27.9).

Selection of type of Surgery

DLK spectrum is variable due to stage and severity of the disease, and rigidity of the deformed segments. Therefore, surgery should be individualized on the basis of (i) site of involvement, (ii) severity of kyphosis (stage of disease), (iii) flexibility of the affected segment, and (iv) segmental instability.[15-16]

Severity of kyphosis

Disease severity initially was classified into 4 stages by Takemitsu et al. However, neither Takemitsu et al and Lee et al did present the numerical data related with the balanced and unbalanced spine, utilizing the distance between C7 plumb line and S1 upper surface, though presently severity of stooping in standing can be assessed and expressed by numerical grading system; anterior or posterior shift of C7 plumb line from S1 dome.

Site of involvement

Segments forming kyphosis is important. There are two types: upper and lower lumbar types; 20% are upper type, and rests are lower type DLK.

Flexibility of kyphotic segments

When the kyphosis is corrected by fulcrum test it is flexible curve, and when the kyphosis is not corrected by the test it is the rigid curve. Most of the upper types are the flexible type. In lower kyphosis types there are again two types: flexible and rigid.

Instability of affected segments

Instability is seen at one or two segments in a half of the DLK patients, and is thought to be one of the causes of DLK. By radiograms taken in standing and lying positions, and flexion-extension sagittal radiograms instability can be assessed. However, the current authors' view is that surgical management is same in both flexible and unstable types. Unstable type has ligamentous (basic) stabilizer insufficiency. Therefore, more deformity correction can be obtained easily, but more rigid stabilization is required.

DLK Classification Based on Segmental Stability and Indicated Surgery

Lee et al classified DLK by the degrees of mobility of the involved segments into four types: (i) upper flexible type, (ii) lower flexible type, (iii) lower unstable type, and (iv) lower rigid type (Table 27.1). The flexible type has normal or subnormal ROM, while the unstable type has abnormally widened ROM.[15-18]

1. *Flexible upper DLK:* Most of the upper types are flexible. If rigidity is found in the upper type it may not be the DLK. Most of the flexible type can be corrected by posterior instrumentation. Decancellation osteotomy is infrequently indicated for more correction of the kyphosis.
2. *Flexible lower DLK:* Deformity can be corrected by posterior instrumentation. For enough correction infrequently decancellation osteotomy is combined, because infrequently there is a limitation of correction by posterior instrumentation alone without anterior release.
3. *Unstable lower DLK:* Main focus of pathology is located at the unstable segment. Therefore, the disk of the affected segment should be resected and fused with strut bone graft or cage. Posterior instrument-aided correction and PLIF is the most desirable procedure.

Table 27.1 Surgical approaches for four types of DLK due to segmental stability (Lee et al.)

Clinical type by segmental stability	*Indicated Surgical approach*	*Remarks*
Flexible upper type (normo- or hypomobile)	Decancellation osteotomy Posterior instrumented correction	Floating fusion is not Preferred.
Flexible lower type (normo- or hypomobile	Decancellation osteotomy Posterior instrumented correction	More rigid fixation is needed. Long operation time needed.
Unstable lower (hypermobile) type	Anterior and posterior release Posterior instrumented correction + PLIF	Instrument-aided correction is possible. More rigid fixation should be obtained.
Rigid lower type (nonmobile)	Decancellation osteotomy	Anterior release, posterior osteotomy and rigid posterior instrumentation is need.

Flowchart 27.1 Moon et al's modified Lee et al.'s therapeutic algorithm in degenerative flat back

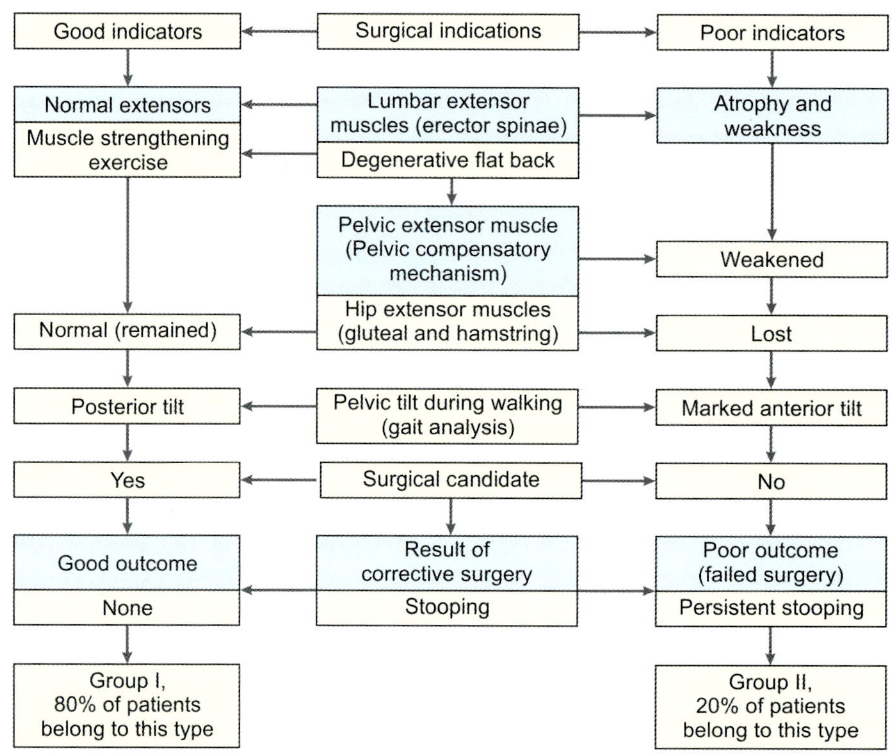

4. *Rigid lower DLK:* In most cases of this type of DLK, combined anterior and posterior release and decancellation is indicated, because posterior instrument-aided correction is inadequate for sufficient correction.

The current authors simply classified DLK based on the segmental mobility of the affected segments into two for therapeutic purpose; mobile (flexible) and nonmobile (rigid) types. This classification seems more practical in the surgical management. More deformity can be corrected easily in the flexible and unstable DLK, while less correction will be obtained without anterior release and/or posterior closed wedge osteotomy in the rigid type of DLK.

Postoperative Management

DLK patients have atrophies of erector spinae and pelvic extensor muscles.[13-17] Therefore, to prevent the postoperative restooping, patients should be taught preoperatively how to do the muscle strengthening exercises after surgery. In the kyphotic lumbar spine of other origin erector spinae and pelvic extensor muscles are normal. Strengthening of the gluteal and hamstring muscles participating the pelvic extension (posterior pelvic tilt) is very important in upright standing. Corrective surgery cannot be successful in patients with weak gluteal muscles. Also quadriceps strengthening exercise and one leg standing exercise should be carried, because DLK patients have had flexed knees in standing over years.

In summary strengthening exercise program of all extensor muscles of the low back, pelvis and lower limb should be formulated and established.

Postoperative Outcome Assessment

Improvement can be assessed clinically and radiologically.

1. Clinical improvements are assessed on basis of improvement in walking ability and improvement of ADL (elimination of difficulty in ADL), degree of back pain relief, truncal appearance, and finally, the patients' overall satisfaction.
2. Radiological improvements are assessed by restored sagittal alignment, including lumbar lordosis, and pre- and postoperative C7 plumb line shift to S1 within normal range.

Postoperative Complications

It is reminded that DLK is the product of degenerated disks and degenerated dikc-associated segmental flexion instability due to the lumbar dynamic stabilizer weakness, and is not the primary product of the skeletal diseases. Therefore, lumbar kyphosis and thoracic hypokyphosis of the other origin should not be subjected to corrective surgery under the same surgical treatment protocol of DLK. There are two types of complications; general and specific.

General Complication

Wrong patient selection should not be done. Patients with senile osteopathic kyphosis and/or senile spinal deformity associating Parkinson's disease are not candidates for surgery. Poor bone quality can be listed as a cause of fixation failures after instrumented deformity correction and stabilization. Therefore, treatment of osteoporosis should be preceded before the planned instrumented deformity correction. The treatment of osteoporosis only with teriparatide can elevate BMD over 1.0 in a short period of time, though it takes time and is expensive. Lastly, insufficient correction (incomplete restoration of lumbar lordosis) less than 35° of lumbar lordosis can be listed as a cause of failure of surgery which is led to restooping.

Specific Complications

Problems can arise in the adjacent segments and bone after the instrumented stabilization, and also in fixated bone (screw toggling or screw failure).

1. *Shift of stooping force to the unfused adjacent part (joint and bone) of the spine:* In patients with kyphosis secondary to ankylosing spondylitis and iatrogenic flat back, corrective surgery can solve the clinical problem. However, in DLK surgery preoperatively, deformity type and dynamic extensor muscles of lumbar spine, pelvis and hips should be scrutinized. If there is erector spinae and gluteal extensor muscle weakness or atrophy, the deformity correction surgery can fail soon postoperatively because of the early shift of the stooping force which induces gradually the adjacent joint disease - rather earlier junctional kyphosis. Once in the past Lee et al explained this force shift was seen only in DLK.[15,16] But this stooping forces act on the upper adjacent joint even in the normally aligned fused spine with normal erector spinae and gluteal extensor muscles.
2. *Concentration of stooping force within the "fused part" of the spine":* These are the examples of fixation and/or fusion failure (screw toggling or screw failure) of the posteriorly instrumented spine, and vertebral fracture within the instrumented segments. Anterior column fusion with bone graft or cage can minimize this complication.

Persistent Stooping

Stooping seen in senile round back, ankylosing spondylitis, and tuberculous kyphosis is static, while stooping in DLK is dynamic. In the former, spinal deformity does not change on walking, while that of DLK changes on walking and is time-dependent.

Compensation Mechanism

When sagittal truncal balance is lost on standing, patient clinically presents forward stooping posture or forward truncal shift. For this decompensated spine, the body itself mobilizes its compensation mechanism. In case of early DLK, activation of this compensation mechanism is seen: To correct and/or compensate the stooping posture, patient walks with upper trunk posteriorly swayed (the chest anteriorly protruded and widely opened and extended both shoulders) and flexed hips and knees. In the DLK most effective compensation mechanism is the "posterior pelvic tilt". However, in a patient associating pelvic extensor muscle weakness the pelvis cannot tilt posteriorly to stabilize lumbosacral segment. On this occasion, the passive stabilizers are mobilized to tilt the pelvis posteriorly in type 4 DLK.

Erector Spinae and Gluteal Muscles

"Lumbar pelvic rhythm" was already explained; In forward bending between 0° and 45° flexion occurs mainly in lumbar spine, while flexion between 45° and 90° occurs mainly in pelvis. To prevent sudden flexion, eccentric contraction (isotonic muscle contraction with lengthening) of erector spinae (lumbar extensor) does the role, and regulates smooth and slow flexion, and eccentric contraction of gluteal muscle does the role in pelvic tilt.

In raising the stooped trunk to upright position from 90° to 45° gluteal muscle does the main role, and subsequently the erector spinae muscle takes over the role (Fig. 27.17).

In summary DLK develops primarily due to disk degeneration secondary to the weakened erector spinae muscles, and secondly stooping by weak gluteal muscles. Most effective compensating mechanism for the stooped trunk is the posterior pelvic tilt. For the effective posterior pelvic tilt, gluteal muscles must be normal. Thus, when gluteal muscle becomes atrophic and loses its muscle power, the compensatory mechanism will be lost. When posterior pelvic tilt occurs, lumbosacral angle decreases (vertical sacrum).

Loss of Pelvic Compensatory Mechanism

The existence of the pelvic compensatory mechanism (intact pelvic extensor muscles) is expressed by sacral angle that is associated with lumbar lordosis.

When the pelvic compensatory mechanism is lost in DLK due to the inefficient gluteal muscle power, anterior pelvic tilt develops together with stooping at the trans-coxal axis. However, the patient can stand still alone with the stooped posture by passively tilting the pelvis posteriorly with the passive tightening of the passive stabilizers (ligaments and muscle fascia) and flexed hips and knees, though she or he cannot stand upright unsupported. This is the main cause of postoperative persistent stooping.[16,17]

Conclusion

It is important to know how the spinal column maintain its balanced stability harmoniously and effortlessly in the upright posture. The key components are primarily the static stabilizers, such as bone and disk column and ligaments, and secondly the dynamic stabilizers (muscles). When either stabilizing component fails, the subsequently spinal column instability and deformity will ensue. To prevent and treat the age- and/or specific work- or disease-related spinal deformity, those stabilizers listed above should be assessed carefully whether those are diseased or not. DLK is known to be caused by the age- or work-related chronic extensor muscle atrophy of the low back and pelvis and subsequent disc degeneration, while pure laterally wedged disc degeneration without extensor muscle atrophy is the primary cause of DLS in which no lumbar extensor muscle atrophy though unilaterally wakened erector spinae can be a factor.

It should be known that for successful corrective surgery of DLK preoperative gluteal and erector spinae muscles particularly the gluteal and hamstring muscles must be good in power.

Acknowledgments

We would like to acknowledge Mr. Seog In Moon for his good assistance in material collection and analysis, and secretary works, and finally to acknowledge Prof. Y Takemitsu's comments and help in obtaining the referencing papers.

References

1. Berthonnaud E, Dimnet J, Roussouly P, Labelle H. Analysis of the sagittal balance of the spine and pelvis using shape and orientation parameters. J Spinal Disord Tech. 2005;18:40-7.
2. Roussouly P, Gollagly S, Berthonnaud E, Dimnet J. Classification of the normal variation in the sagittal alignment of the human lumbar spine and pelvis in the standing position. Spine. 2005;30:346-52.
3. Jackson RP, McManus AC. Radiographic analysis of sagittal plane alignment and balance in standing volunteers and patient's with low back pain matched for age, sex, and size: A prospective controlled clinical study. Spine. 1994;19:1611-18.
4. Bernhardt M, Bridwell KH. Segmental analysis of the sagittal plane alignment of the normal thoracic and lumbar spines and thoracolumbar junction. Spine. 1989;14:717-21.
5. Bonlay C, Tardieu C, Hecquet J, et al. Sagittal alignment of spine and pelvis regulated by pelvic incidence: standard values and prediction of lordosis. Eur Spine. J 2006;15:15-422.
6. Schwab F, Lafage V, Boyce R, Skalli W, Farcy JP. Gravity line analysis in adult volunteers: Age-related correlation with spinal parameters, pelvic parameters, and foot position. Spine. 2006;31:E959-E967.
7. Vedantam R, Lenke LG, Keenley JA, Bridwell KH. Comparison of standing sagittal alignment in asymptomatic adolescent and adults. Spine. 1998;23:211-5.
8. Jackson RP: Spinal balance, lumbopelvic alignments around the hip axis, and positioning for surgery. Spine State Art Rev. 1997;11:33-8.
9. Basmajian JV. Muscles alive. 4th edn. Baltimore Williams and Wilkins Co. 1978.
10. Farcy JP, Schwab FJ. Management of flat back and related kyphotic decompensation syndromes. Spine. 1997;22:2453-57.
11. Joseph J. Man's posture: Electrographic studies. Springfield: Charles C Thomas; 1960.
12. Globler LS, Moe JH, Winter RB, Bradford DS, Loustein JE. Loss of lumbar lordosis following surgical correction of thoracolumbar deformities. Orthop Trans. 1978;2:239.

13. Takemitsu Y, Harada Y, Iwahara T. Low back pain and aging change of spine in Japanese farmers aged more than 40 years. J Jpn Orthop Assoc. 1984;58:551-2.
14. Takemitsu Y, arada Y, Iwahara T, et al. Lumbar degenerative kyphosis: clinical, radiological and epidemiological studies. Spine. 1988;306:64-72.
15. Lee CS, Kim YT, Kim E. Clinical study of lumbar degenerative kyphosis (in Korean). J Korea Spine Society. 1997;4:27-35.
16. Lee CS (Ed). Degenerative lumbar kyphosis. Seoul: Gunja, Publishing Co; 2000.
17. Lee CS, Lee CK, Kim YT, Hong YM, Yoo JH. Dynamic imbalance of the spine in degenerative flat back. Spine. 2001;26:2029-35.
18. Moon MS, Lee BJ, Kim SS, Lin JF. Evolution of management of spinal deformities: controversial issues and current concept review. J Spinal Surg. 2010;2(1):295-305.
19. Luk K, Lu D, Cheng KM, Wong YW. A prospective comparison of the coronal deformity correction in thoracic scoliosis using four different instrumentations and the fulcrum bending radiograph. Spine. 2004;29:560-3.
20. Takemitsu Y, Atsuta Y, Kamo Y, et al. Operative treatment of lumbar degenerative kyphosis. Proc. 5th Int. Conf. Lumbar fusion an stabilization. Tokyo: Springer-Verlag; 1993. pp.150-9.
21. Lehmer SM, Keppler L, Biscup RS, Enken P, Miller SD, Steffee AD. Posterior transvertebral osteotomy for adult thoracolumbar kyphosis. Spine. 1994;19:2060-7.
22. Nakai O, Yamaura I, Kurosa Y, et al. Posterior stabilization for lumbar degenerative kyphosis: In situ fusion in maximum extension on Hall's frame. Proc. 5th Int. Conf. Lumbar fusion and stabilization. Tokyo: Springer-Verlag; 1993. pp. 135-49.
23. Bridwell KH, Lewis SJ, Lenke IG, Blanke K. Pedicle substraction osteotomy for the treatment of fixed sagittal imbalance. J Bone Joint Surg Am. 2003;85:454-63.
24. Bradford DS, Tribus CB. Vertebral column resection for the treatment of rigid coronal decompensation. Spine. 1997;22:1590-9.
25. Jang JS, Lee SH, Min JH, Han KM. Lumbar degenerative kyphosis (in Korean) J Korea Spine Society. 1997;4:27-35.
26. Jang JS, Lee SH, Min JH, Han KM. Lumbar degenerative kyphosis – radiologic analysis and classifications. Spine. 2007;32(24):2694-99.
27. Cho KJ, Lenke LG, Bridwell KH, Kamiya M, Sides B. Selection of optimal distal fusion level in posterior instrumentation and fusion for thoracic hyperkyphosis. The sagittal stable vertebral concept. Spine. 2009;34:765-70.
28. Cheng KW, Cheng CW, Chen HC, Chang KL, Chen TC: Closing-opening wedge osteotomy for the treatment of sagittal balance. Spine. 2008;33:1470-7.
29. Joseph SA Jr, Moreno AP, Brandoff J, Casden AC, Kuflik P, Newwirth MG. Sagittal plane deformity in the adult patient. J Am Acad Orthop Surg. 2009;17:378-88.
30. Iwahara T, Takemitsu Y, Watakabe M, Goto E, et al. Roentrenologic and biomechanical study of lumbar degenerative kyphosis with special reference to effect of sacral inclination and hip joint (in Japanese). Rinsho Seikei Geka (Clin Orthop). 1988;23(7):811-9.
31. Goto E. Biomechanical effects of lumbar degenerative kyphosis on the hip joint–Study of electromyography of the muscles around hip joint in patients with lumbar kyphosis (in Japanese) J Joint Surg. 2004;23(4):56-61.

CHAPTER

28

Sagittal Spinal Alignment and its Clinical Implication

Myung-Sang Moon, Sung-Soo Kim, Bong-Jin Lee, Min Geun Yoon, Jeong-Lim Moon

Introduction

The vertebral column is an aggregate of articulated, superimposed segments, each of which is a functional unit. Standing is not a static position—a person does not stand completely still even if trying to do so. The upright position is maintained by the alternating action of antagonistic muscle groups which prevents overbalancing. This results in a continuous slight sway of the body, keeping the total body center of gravity over the area covered by the feet —"the base". The upright standing posture is inherently unstable because the body's center of gravity situated high above a relatively small base. Thus, the body as it moves constantly challenging and neutralizing the force of gravity. In standing the body segments may be considered as being like a movable segmented up-side-down curvilinear cone block stacked and linked one on top of the other (Fig. 28.1). Ideally the line from the center of gravity of each of these segments should be centered over its supporting base—the segment below—for balance to be maintained with minimal muscular activity. That is, its function is to support a man in upright position, mechanically balanced to conform to the stress of gravity, permitting locomotion, and assisting in purposeful movement.[1-20]

Body proportions alter during the life cycle, and in addition, there are changes in the curve of the spine. In the neonate, the whole spine is flexed, forming a long "C" curve convex posteriorly from the sacrum to occiput. When the child begins to gain head control a counter-curve evolves in the cervical spine. Later as the child begins to sit and stand a second curve evolves in the lumbar region. Once the standing position is achieved and during adult life the four curves are present. In normal standing state, those 4 sagittal curvatures are well-aligned and-balanced with least energy-consumption, though there is an individual variations in a certain range.[23] When compared with the neonate, spinal flexibility is now greatly reduced. These structural changes of the spine and their accompanying effects on neighboring soft tissues, account in part, for the characteristic appearance of the posture typical of different age groups. Spinal column has tridimensional alignment in coronal, sagittal and axial planes, and has 2 different sagittal curvatures at four different levels; cervical and lumbar spine have lordotic curves, while in the dorsal and sacral segments have kyphotic alignment in normal adults (Figs 28.1 to 28.5).

In the aged, the shape of the spine tends to reverse back to the long "C" shaped curve. However, in many elderly people the cervical curve may increase as they try to keep their eyes directed parallel to the floor, so that they can look ahead.[20,22]

In normal spine with normal mobile segments, a coupled motion between kyphotic and lordotic segments can be observed. The spine, pelvis, hips and knees are all involved in maintaining sagittal balance.[12] The pelvis cannot be separated from the torso in the analysis of trunk muscle activity, as it is an integral part of the whole spinal system. Muscles of the lower torso, pelvis and upper leg work in concert for control of pelvic posture. Gluteus maximus activity about the pelvis has been observed in the beginning of lifts, presumably to provide a stable pelvis against which the erector spinae can act to produce extension of the trunk. It is important to understand the normal and abnormal spinal and pelvic alignment. In this

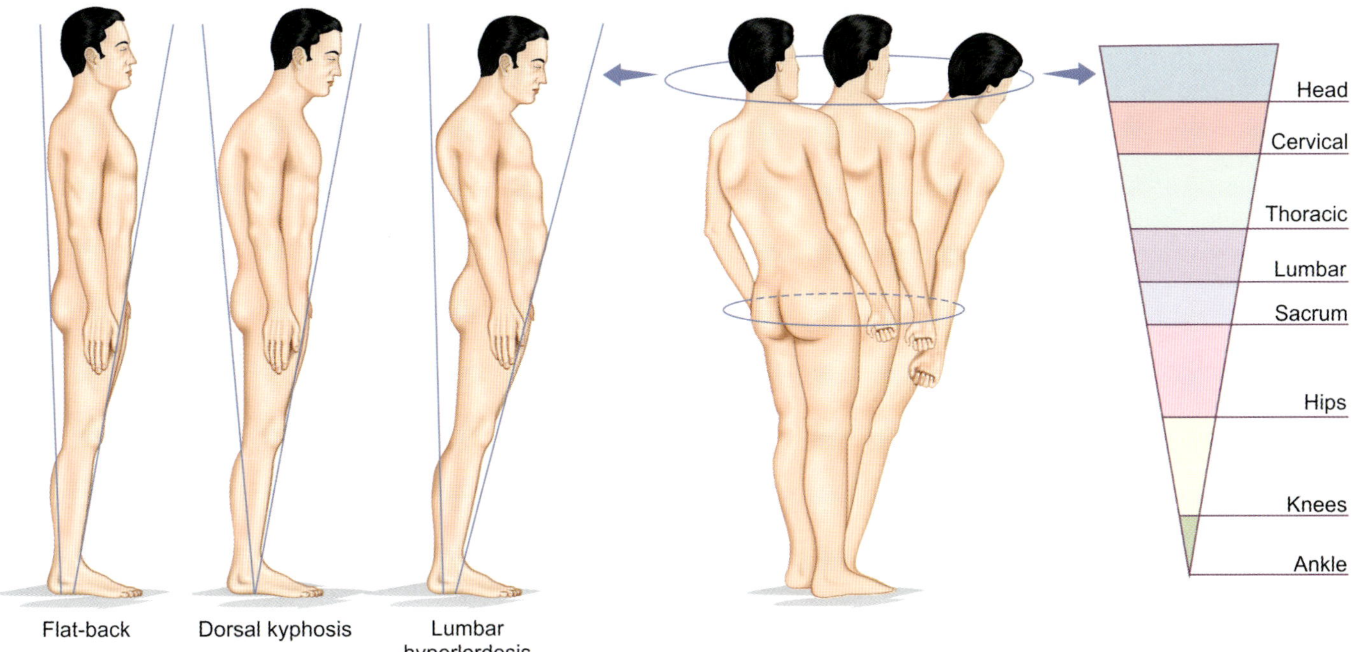

Fig. 28.1 In a narrow range of cone base, the upper trunk sways all around in which the body can remain balanced without external support and with minimal effort (least energy consumption) when all the segments are mobile with normal spinal guy musculatures. Standing is not a static (rest) position—a person does not stand completely still even if trying to do so. The upright standing posture is inherently unstable because of the body's center of gravity is situated high above a relatively small base. Thus, the body as it moves is constantly challenging and neutralizing the force of gravity. Consequently, body segments may be considered like a segmental up-side-down curvilinear cone block stacked and linked one on top of the other.

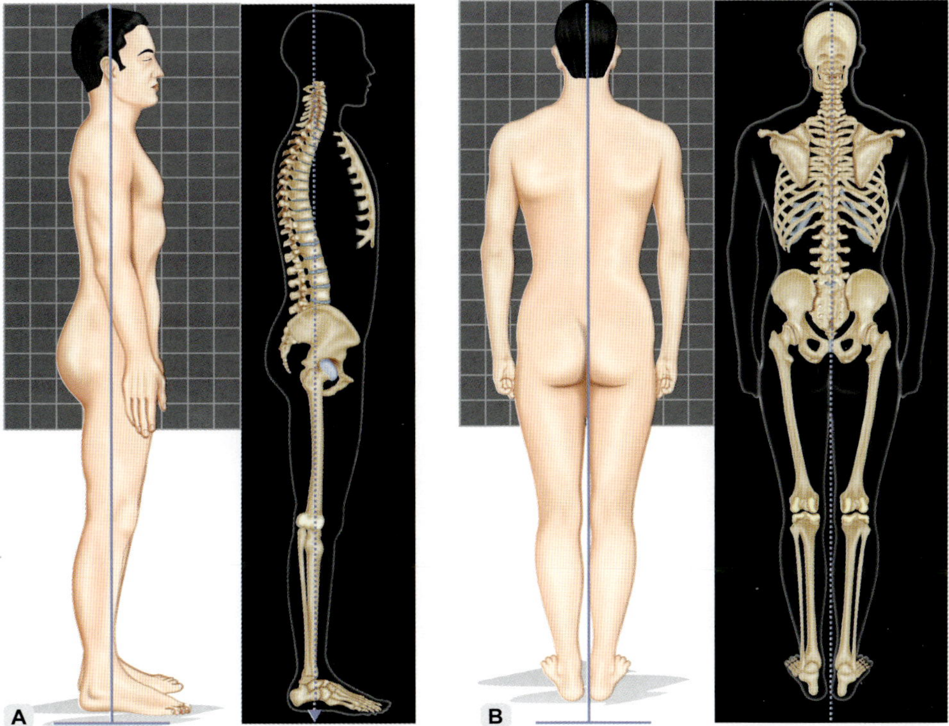

Fig. 28.2 Line of gravity in an ideal normal erect posture passes through the mastoid process, just in front of the shoulder joint, through the hip joint or just behind it, just in front of the center of knee joint, and approximately 5 cm in front of the ankle joint. (A) Lateral view (sagittal); (B) Posterior view (coronal)

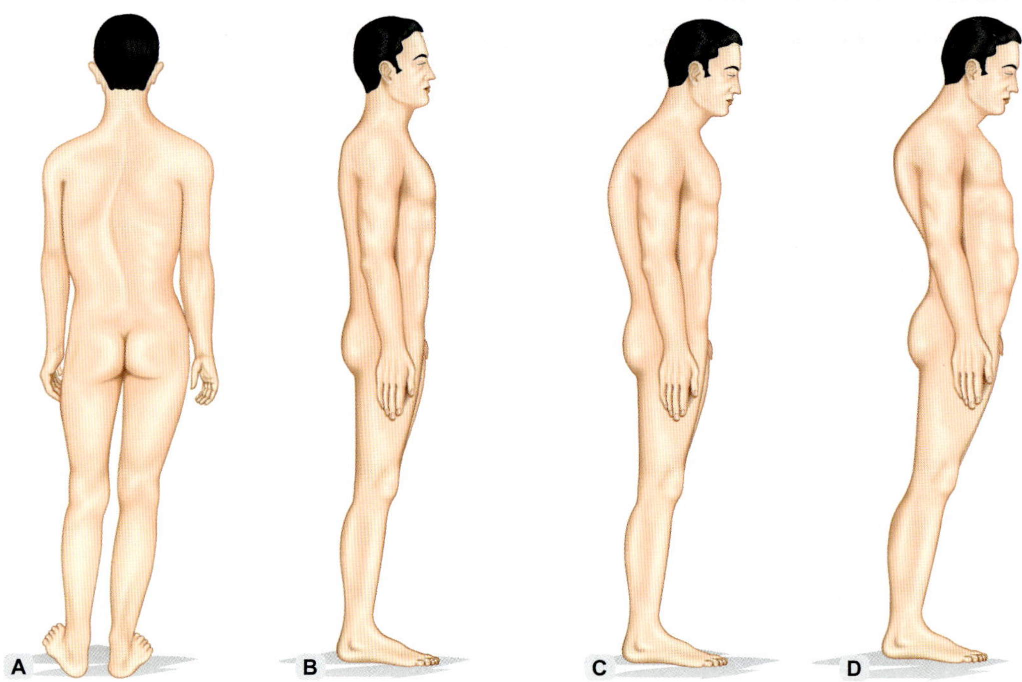

Fig. 28.3 Common body posture abnormalities (A) Scoliosis; (B) Flat-back; (C) Dorsal kyphosis; (D) Lumbar hyperlordosis

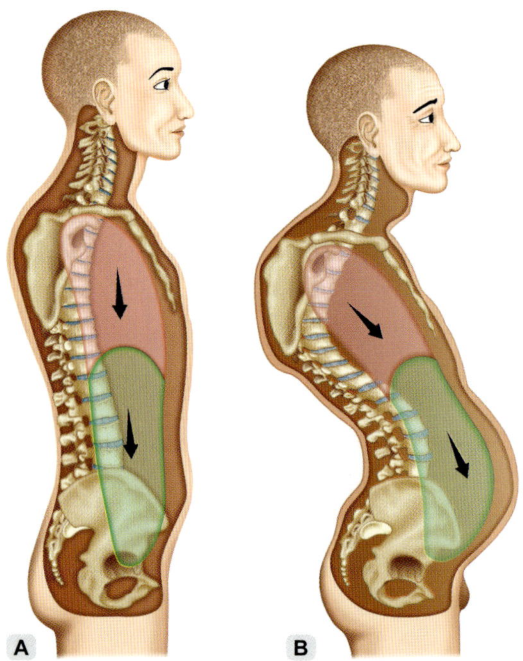

Fig. 28.4 (A) Normal distribution of the body weight on physiologic weight-bearing structures; (B) and its disturbance causing a continuous strain on some muscles and ligaments in compensatory hyperlordosis of lumbar spine secondary to dorsal kyphosis

review, the authors confined to use the term "balanced trunk in upright standing" to indicate the unsupported neutral and comfortable upright standing position.

Significance of Sagittal Alignment

Legaye et al. previous barycentrimetrical study demonstrated that the axis of gravity of the upper body segment is located behind the lumbar vertebrae and the femoral heads, thus, ensuring economical energy expenditure and stability.[17,18] Upright standing position for economical balance is most desirable.

Since muscle tone, strength and neurological mechanism affect the standing posture in an individual, it is thought that it is necessary to consider these factors of foremost importance to understand the control of the standing posture and the gravity line position.[4] Also, it should be known that the sagittal morphology of the pelvis, hips and knees determines the amount of lumbar lordosis needed for each individual. The pelvis should be balanced on the femora in an arbitrary neutral position neither too far forward nor too far back.

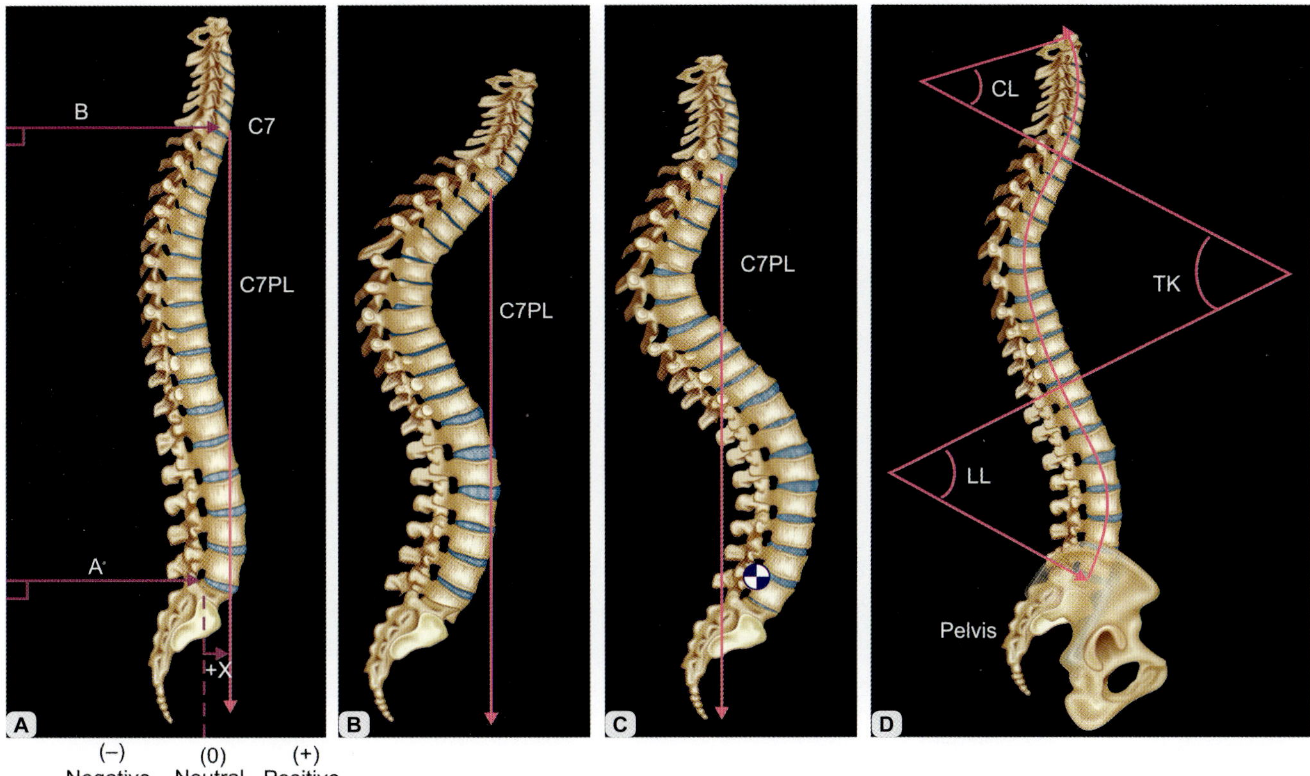

Fig. 28.5 (A) Neutral sagittal balance: B = A, negative balance, B < A, positive balance B > A, + X = positive distance; (B) Positive sagittal balance; (C) Negative sagittal balance; (D) A method showing measurement points of cervical, dorsal, lumbar and sacral curves is illustrated. SVA passes far front of S1 posterosuperior corner it is defined positive sagittal balance, while SVA passes far behind the corner it was defined negative sagittal balance

In studying the sagittal spinal alignment abnormalities, such as flat back, dorsal hyperkyphosis, and degenerative lumbar kyphosis (DLK), it is important to understand what are normal and abnormal with respect to thoracic kyphosis and lumbar lordosis as well as to the body's sagittal vertical axis (SVA) and C7 plumb line (Figs 28.5 to28.7).[6,12]

To express the harmony of the sagittal shape of the spinal column and of the spinopelvic morphology, many descriptive terms are used: static, neutral, stable and unstable equilibrium; economical balance, unfavorable sagittal balance, positive and negative balance; balanced and unbalanced (imbalance) spine; compensated and decompensated spine; economical standing position for economical balance, and unbalanced and maladjusted pelvis. Those terms have resulted in substantial confusion in taxonomy. The terms balanced and unbalanced pelvis is concerned in the cases of high grade isthmic spondylolisthesis, it has not yet achieved universal acceptance, because the patient can stand upright unsupportedly in any pattern of the slip.

Greater variation in SVA can be tolerated if compensatory mechanisms at the mobile segments are present to maintain standing balance. Lordosis in the lumbar spine should be 30° or more than the amount of kyphosis in the thoracic spine.[20]

Energy dissipation during trunk flexion is known to be about 4-folds greater than the trunk extension on the average.[20] During trunk flexion, lumbar kyphosis showed the most energy dissipation.[1,18-20]

Interpretation of Standing

Interpretation of upright human standing, based on the barycentric concept (cone of economy), upper trunk is similar to the straight block cone base, and foot is the tip of the sharp cone.[21] Therefore, sharp cone tip standing like thin tall pole is very unstable, and falls easily when there is no external support. In such cone tip standing, standing balance should be obtained only by the external supporter, such as guy ropes or wires, anchored to the cone base and ground. In human standing, internal extraskeletal support for the crooked curvilinear segmented cony body build is provided basically by static (ligaments), and dynamic (muscles) guy stabilizers.

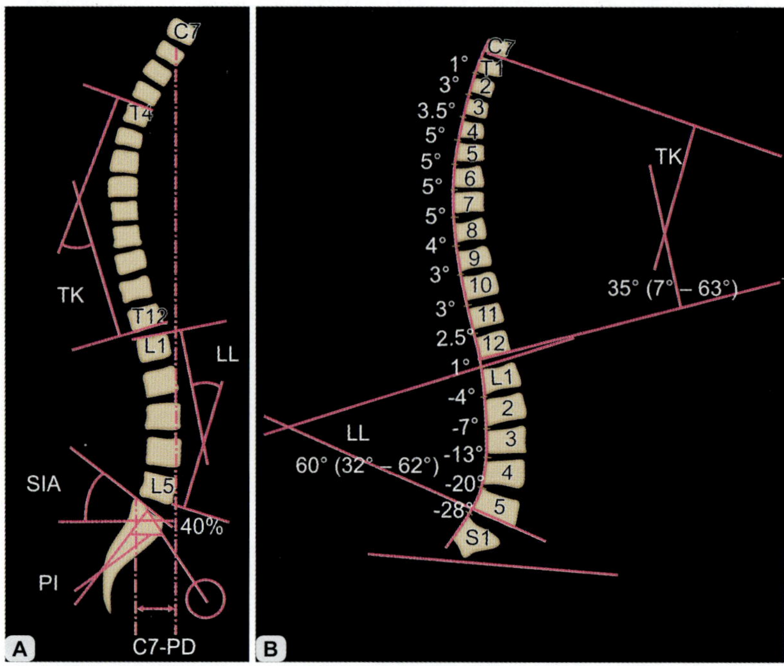

Fig. 28.6 (A) Radiographic measurement of the sagittal spinal and pelvic parameters. TK, thoracic kyphosis; LL, lumbar lordosis; SIA, sacral inclination angle; C7-PD, C7 plumbline distance; PI, pelvic incidence. Lumbar lordotic curve must exceed the thoracic kyphosis over 30–35 to maintain the most economical standing; (B) A measurement of dorsal and lumbar sagittal curves: Percentile contribution of each lumbar segment in formation of lumbar sagittal curve: L1–2: 5%, L2–3: 10%, L3–4: 20 %, L4–5: 30%, L5–S1: 40%. TK: thoracic kyphosis, LL: lumbar lordosis

Thoracic kyphosis: normal: 10° – 40° Hyperlordotic: >70°

Lumbar lordosis: Normal: 40° – 60° Kyphotic: <5° (some defined <10°)

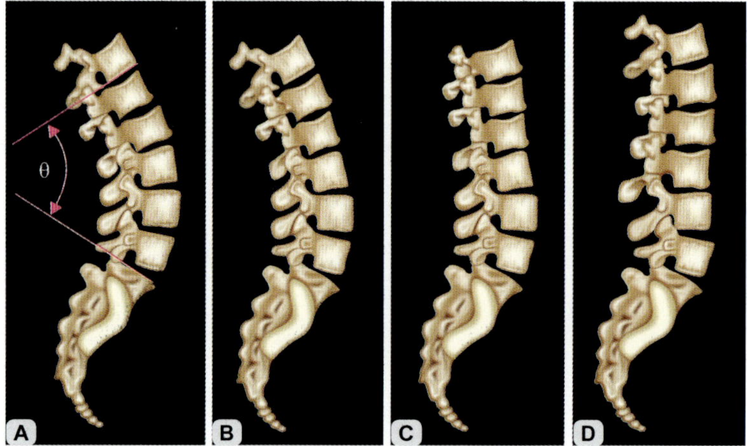

Fig. 28.7 Lumbosacral joint model with respect to lordosis. Lumbar lordotic angle is defined by the angle between the upper plane of L1 lumbar vertebrae and the upper S1 sacral vertebrae. Excessive lordosis (EL) is over 75°, normal lordosis (NL) is 40°, hypolordosis (HL) is in the 20°, and lumbar kyphosis (LK) is 5.° (A) Excessive lordosis (75°); (B) Normal lordosis (40°); (C) Hypolordosis (20°); (D) Lumbar kyphosis (5°)

In a healthy spine, the stability and balance is not only consciously or unconsciously controlled by the dynamic stabilizer's activity, but also in the absence of those active stabilizers' activity the passive stabilizers (ligament and joint capsule) and postural change take passively over those muscles' role in maintaining and/or restoring the spinopelvic balance and stability. Therefore, in assessing the lumbar and lumbosacral alignment primarily the conditions of those muscles, such as erector spinae, gluteus, hamstring and abdominalis muscles should be evaluated. Erector spinae muscles (largest group of intrinsic back muscle) which lie posterolaterally to the vertebral column and attach to sacrum, iliac crest and spinous processes with broad thick tendon are the primary extensors of the vertebral column and head. Acting bilaterally, they straighten the back, returning it the upright position from a flexed position, and pull the head posteriorly. They also participate in controlling vertebral column flexion by contracting and relaxing in a coordinated fashion. Erector spinae muscles participate in the lordotization and stabilization of lumbar and lumbosacral spine posteriorly, and the gluteal muscle secondarily participate in the pelvic tilt posteriorly and the hamstring and abdominalis muscles participate in hip extension and stabilization. When the excessive posterior pelvic tilt destabilizes the hip by reducing the femoral head coverage by the acetabulum, it finally causes the hip–spine syndrome.

The spine in an upright manner bears axial load to support the body. When the upper trunk of the upright human body alone sways around in all directions, it makes a upside-down cone motion without fall within a certain range, while the truncal motion exceeds the allowable range the lower parts of cone can hardly neutralize the imposed motion-associated load to stabilize the moving upper trunk.

Postural abnormalities change the weight-bearing axis of the spine. It is reminded that the C7 plumb line and the center-of-gravity line are not identical. However, in clinical situation C7 plumb line is used for the convenience to replace the center-of-gravity line. The C7 plumb line should pass within a few millimeters of the posterior-superior corner of S1. Vedantam et al. showed that the mean SVA moved forward with age, from –5.6 cm in adolescent to –3.2 cm in middle-aged and elderly persons.[11-23]

When spine develops a deformities, such as kyphosis, lordosis, and scoliosis at a certain level, the proximal and distal mobile segments of the spine should develop a compensatory curve to maintain the spinal balance. However, if those proximal and distal segments cannot make a compensatory curve, the spine fails to maintain the balance. As a consequence, excessive truncal shift in sagittal or coronal planes develops. It should be known that the stiff segments cannot form the compensatory curve, and the spine becomes unbalanced.[17]

The individual active muscular activity necessary to keep the center of gravity controlled in standing might be the key to understand the different clinical presentation of patients with the same sagittal malalignment. Different parameters have been used to describe the spinopelvic morphology on basis of the standing lateral radiograms.

The normal upright adult with normal static and dynamic stabilizers exhibits balanced physiologic curves. Loss of the spinal balance produces a position which is at a biomechanical disadvantage. During the acquisition of the standing position, the sacral end-plate becomes more vertical, leading to an increase in the sacral slope (SS) value. However, the SS stabilizes after the acquisition of walking and is not influenced by further growth. The presence of an adequate lumbar lordosis (LL) avoids forward displacement of the center of gravity that may alter the equilibrium of the standing posture (neutral equilibrium). To stand upright and look forward while standing and walking, a person with sagittal plane imbalance causes back muscles to strain in order to successfully or unsuccessfully reduce a person's sideway tilt.[14-18] Static spinal configuration can be considered as "good position (in equilibrium)" if it is an effortless, non-fatiguing posture, painless to the individual who can remain erect for reasonable time period, and present an esthetically acceptable appearance..

Curvature and Low Back Function

Spinal curvature is an important category in assessing lower back function along with range of motion. Because it is demonstrated that sagittal balance is the most important and reliable radiographic predictor of clinical health status. Lumbar lordosis is especially known to be an important and decisive factor in flexibility during lifting, lowering, and other movement.

The level of lumbar lordosis is affected by age and sex, largely by movement in the center of mass from such causes as pregnancy or obesity. In both cases, the center of mass of the trunk is shifted to the front over time, thus increasing moment at the hip joint. When an actual comparison of the hip movement is done in a pregnant woman before and after the pregnancy, there is an eight-fold increase in the magnitude of hip moment due to forward movement of center of mass. Therefore, a reaction occurs to compensate for center of mass by excessively increasing lumbar lordotic angle and pelvic tilt in order to decrease hip moment. This is apparent in those with protruding bellies due to excessive

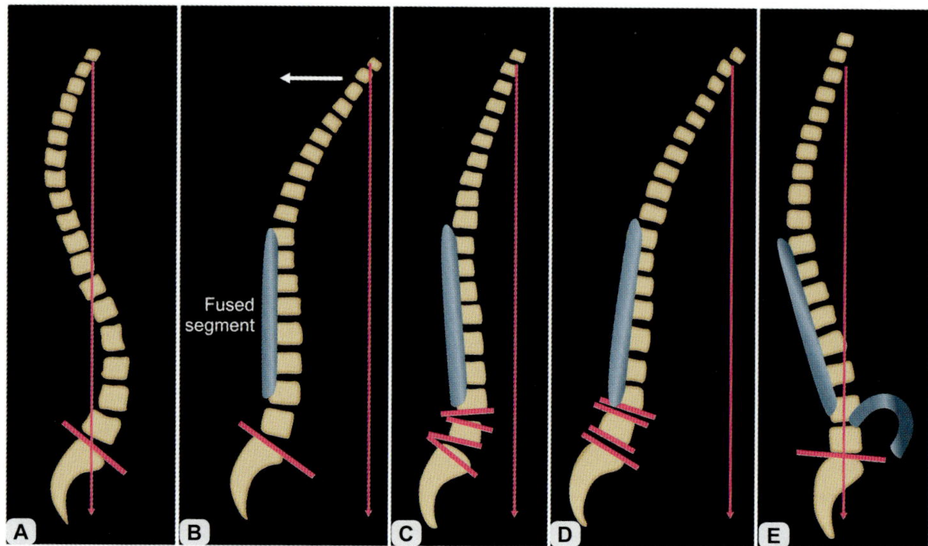

Fig. 28.8 (A) Neutral balance; (B) Positive imbalance; (C) Hyperextended disk; (D) Positive imbalance; (E) Posterior rotation of pelvis. The compensation for sagittal imbalance occurs first at nonfused spinal segments by hyperextending disk. As the patients get older, the degenerative disk change causing loss of lordosis. When the positive imbalance redevelops (D), the pelvis is rotated posteriorly, thereby sagittal balance can be restored (E)

weight or obesity. Also the lifestyle and environmental factors have great impact on lumbar lordosis.

There are mobile and nonmobile (fixed) sagittal imbalance. Also in the fixed sagittal imbalance the primary causes are multilevel disk degeneration and spondylodiskal destructive lesion, such as ankylosing spondylitis. The secondary one is iatrogenic kyphosis (fusion diseases) (Fig. 28.8).

Grobler et al. described the symptom complex of sagittal imbalance with forward thrusting of the trunk as a source of pain and fatigue as in the degenerative lumbar kyphosis and kyphoscoliosis, diffuse idiopathic skeletal hyperostosis, post-traumatic and post-infective kyphosis, and ankylosing spondylitis.[16,18,20,22]

Sagittal Spinal Curve Measurement

Recently, the importance of the normal lumbar lordosis is recognized by the treating physicians.[2-6] One of the examples is the flat back including the degenerative lumbar kyphosis.

The curves are measured by Cobb method. The thoracic kyphosis is measured between upper end-plate of T1 and lower end-plate of T12. However, the measurement is often done between T3 and T12, because identification of T1 is frequently difficult on radiogram. Measurement of lumbar lordosis between upper end-plates of L1 and lower end-plate of L5 or upper end of S1 is most frequently used (Figs 28.5 and 28.6).

The published normal curve data are variable like the measurement data of human face (facial physiognomy). Therefore, spinal curve measurement is called as spinal physiognomy.[16]

The apex of the physiological thoracic kyphosis (normal 36°: range 7°-63°) is located between T5–T8, while that of the lumbar lordosis (normal: 60°: 32°–82°) is located at L3–4 disk level (Figs 28.5 and 28.6).

The thoracic spine should exhibit approximately 10°–40° of kyphosis, and the lumbar spine should have approximately 40°–60° of lordosis (Figs 28.5 and 28.6). The thoracic kyphosis over 45° is considered abnormal.[8] In the cervical spine 5° or more of the fixed posterior angulation is defined as kyphosis. Lumbar hyperlordosis is defined when it is over 70°, and lumbar kyphosis is defined when it is less than 5° (10° by some others). Hypolordosis is in the range 6°–30° (11°–30° by some).[18-20]

The percentile contribution of each segment of lumbar spine in making lumbar lordosis are 5% at L1–2, 10% at L2–3, 20% at L3–4, 30% at L4–5, and 40% at L5–S1, and in the lumbar spine 9° of flexion on an average occurs at each segment until 45° flexion (Figs 28.6).[24]

Factors Affecting the Alignment

The criteria of normalcy of spinal alignment must be considered in ascertaining the cause of painful states and the factors demanding correction. Significant deviations from physiologic static spinal curves can cause discomfort and disability.[19-21,24-28] There are many factors that influence posture, but three factors (i) familial-hereditary, (ii) structural abnormalities, and (iii) posture of habit and training) supersede all others in their prevalence and frequency. Among the three factors, structural abnormalities influence posture most.[21,29] In a person with a congenital or an acquired spinal deformity regardless of skeletal, muscular or neurogenic and either maybe static or progressive, the additional energy expenditure associated with standing and walking leads to the reduced functional capacity. Because postural abnormalities change the weight-bearing axis of the spine, and some muscles, ligaments and discs will be overloaded. However, the abnormal posture can be merely functional and be corrected passively or actively, or it can be irreversible. Postural abnormalities can provoke weakening or shortening of certain muscle groups, shortening of some ligaments and loosening of others, and ultimately accelerate degenerative changes. Also orthosis gives influence.

Posture and Spinal Diseases

The standing balance is considered one of the important physical factors in walking and falling.

In recent years acquired kyphosis, such as tuberculous and post-traumatic ones has drawn clinical attention in the young,[22] while till end of 1980 the spinal deformities in the elderly population have been thought to be the natural process of ageing and not to be the disease.[21]

There are three frequent nontraumatic causes of stooped posture: dorsal round back secondary to the osteoporotic vertebral compression fracture, late sequence of post-infective and Scheuermann's kyphosis, and *de novo* degenerative lumbar kyphosis (DLK).[21,22,24]

The severe spinal deformities are cosmetically unacceptable to the patients, and can cause psychosocial problems especially in the young, though the physical functions are not impaired.[21,22,24–26]

However, restoration of physiological spinal alignment is important by any reasons, because it reduces the motion and load transfer to the adjacent motion segments and provides the most economical standing phase.

The aged populations have high frequency of the crooked backs, such as the dorsal round back secondary to osteoporotic vertebral collapse, and *de novo* degenerative lumbar scoliosis and kyphosis secondary to the advanced disk degeneration associated with segmental flexion instability and back muscle weakness. Degenerative lumbar kyphosis is more commonly seen in the Oriental women who have had different home living style and squatted working in the farm.[26,27] It is a very important message that the weakened erector spinae muscles are the primary cause of DLK. Takemitsu et al. discovered that DLK is the byproduct of erector spinae muscle atrophy. Lee et al. found the secondary atrophy of gluteal and hamstring muscles in addition to atrophy of erector spinae in group II DLK which contributed the postsurgical (postcorrection) persistent stooping.[16]

As mentioned above, DLS and DLK in the past were sorted out as deformities which did not need the management, though those were functionally and aesthetically unacceptable.

Luckily *de novo* lumbar kyphosis in the elderly drew the physician's attention in Japan and Korea since mid-1980s.[12,16,21,26,27]

Abnormal Sagittal Curve and Function

The definition and scope of spinal alignment associated with deformity have continued to evolve. There are two types of abnormal sagittal curves of the skeletal and non-skeletal origins; balanced and unbalanced (decompensated or maladjusted) ones.

When the sagittal curve exceeds the normal curve in the thoracic spine, it is called hyperkyphosis; while the decreased kyphosis is called hypokyphosis. In the lumbar spine the increased lordotic curve is called hyperlordosis or swayback, while the decreased lumbar sagittal curve is called lumbar kyphosis or flat back (Figs 28.5, 28.9 to 28.12).

As regards the positive sagittal balance, Glassman et al. demonstrated that sagittal balance is the most important and reliable radiographic predictor of clinical health status.[5] Their study included the cases with prior fusion or non-fusion. They reported the worse self-assessment in pain, function and self-image domains with a positive sagittal balance. Another study on patients with positive sagittal balance showed that even the mildly positive sagittal imbalance was detrimental. The severity of symptoms increased in a linear fashion with progressive sagittal imbalance (Fig. 28.5).

Postural abnormalities can change the weight-bearing axis of the spine (Figs 28.4 to 28.7). Postural abnormalities or weak trunk muscles (neuromuscular diseases, muscular dystrophy) are frequently found to be the cause of vertebral

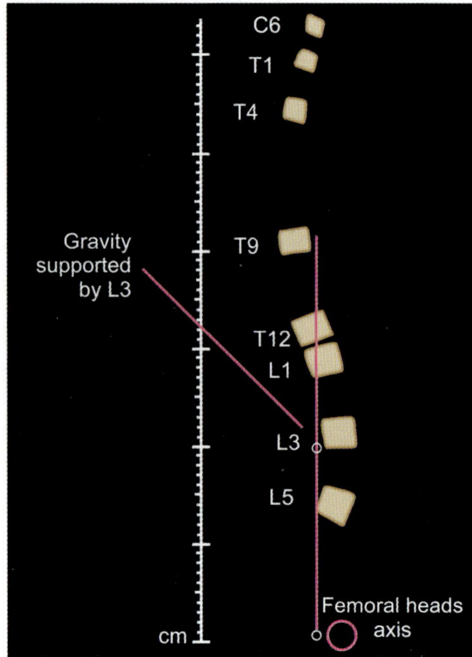

Fig. 28.9 Graphic expression of the result of the Similibary for a normal subject: down projection of gravity supported by L3 facing this vertebral level

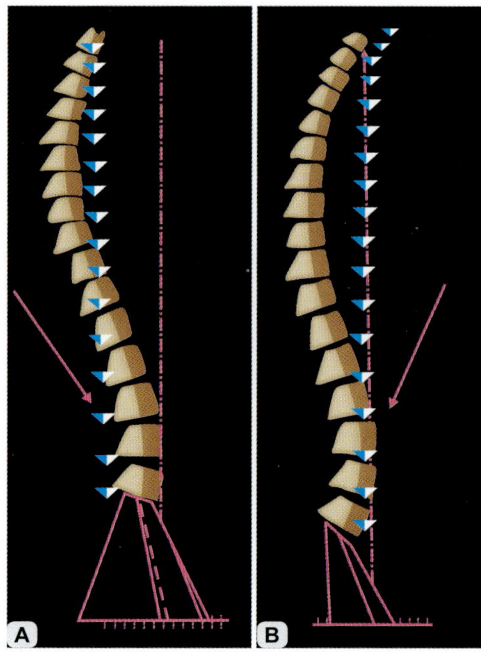

Fig. 28.10 Legaye et al. barycentrimetrical diagram expressing the sagittal shape of the spine and the application points of the gravity supported by each vertebral segment. Vertical arrows in (A) and (B) indicate the gravity lines and the relationship with vertebrae and hip joints, while the oblique arrows indicate the application point of the gravity at the level of L3 vertebra; (A) Economically steady sagittal shape: the gravity is projecting behind the lumbar vertebral structures and the femoral heads; (B) A non-economical sagittal shape: the gravity is projecting in front of the lumbar structures and the femoral heads

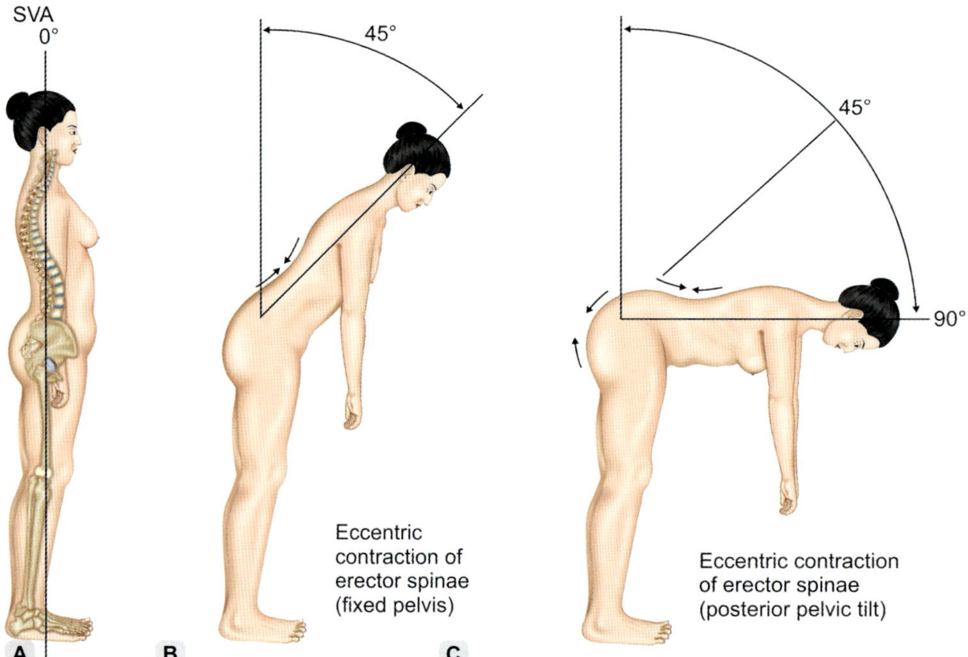

Fig. 28.11 Muscle contraction: Eccentric contraction—accompanying its lengthening. Concentric contraction—accompanying its shortening. Isotonic: contraction with constant tension regardless of its length. Isometric: constant length with tension change. "Lumbopelvic rhythm"

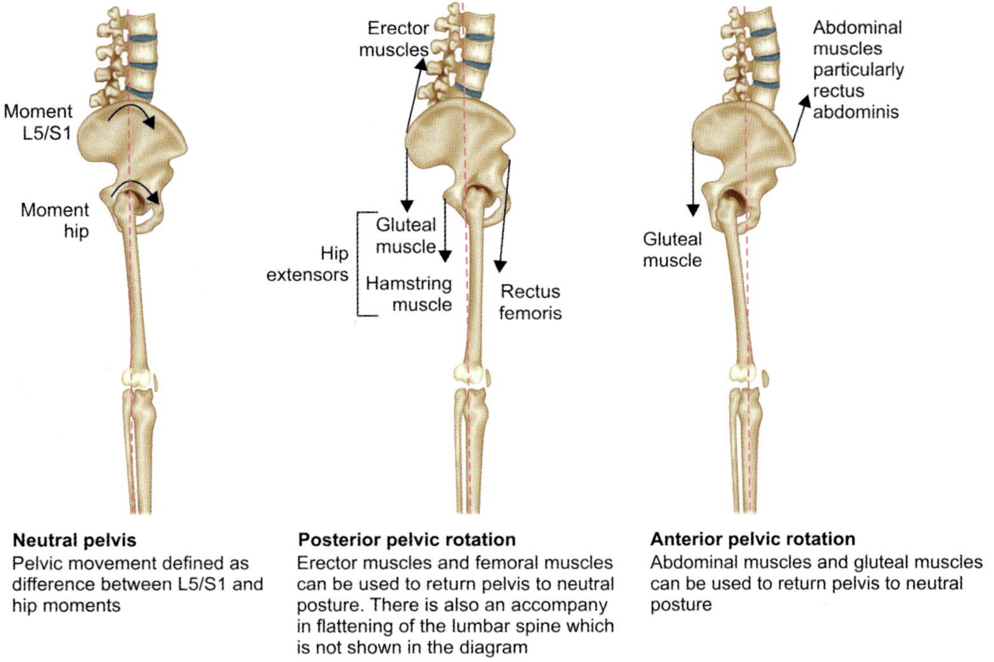

Fig. 28.12 Pelvic rotational freedom about the neutral posture

or pseudoradicular symptoms. In any posture which deviates from the normal one, some muscles, ligaments and disks will be overloaded. Dorsal kyperkyphosis (round back), flat back, hyperlordosis and scoliosis are the most common abnormal postures.

In general for the balanced spine, lumbar lordotic curve must be at least over 30° larger than the thoracic kyphosis.[2,24]

Adolescent scoliosis is only the cosmetic problem clinically, while the degenerative lumbar scoliosis (DLS) is only a pain-provoking condition without cosmetic complaints. The degenerative lumbar kyphosis (DLK) is not only a cosmetic but also a functional one.[14,15,19-22,24,25]

DLK is caused primarily by degenerative disk wedging or disk degeneration associating with or without segmental instability and the erector spinae muscle atrophy, and also the deformity by wedge collapse of the osteoporotic vertebral body in the elderly, and the combined causes.[18,19,21,24,26] That is, clinically lumbar kyphosis is classified into two: pure diskogenic and nondiskogenic (osteopathic), and compensatory and noncompensatory (maladjusted) ones.

Definition and Measurement of Balanced Sagittal Alignment

The spinal balance was assessed by measuring the distance from the posterior-superior corner of S1 or anterior-superior corner of S2 to C7 plumb line (Figs 28.4 to 7).

There are several different assessment methodologies in defining the normalcy of the sagittal spinal alignment by the various authors, based on the 3 different assessing approaches, though those three methods are based on the relation of the sacrum to the C7 plumb line. Several authors measured the distance between the plumb line and measuring points in S1 or S2 (Table 28.1). The aforementioned starting point of the plumb line and sacral measurement point give the different numerical data.

One definition is that the spine is balanced when the plumb line passes within 2 cm of the sacrum, while the spine is imbalanced when the plumb line passes 2 cm away from the sacrum. Another definition is that sagittal alignment is normal when the plumb line passes 5 cm anteriorly from the posterosuperior corner of S1 and 2 cm posteriorly from that corner.[23] In summary, all measured data seem to be arbitrary, because there are no EMG data and tissue compliance meter or tenometer data supporting the each authors' data.

However, Berthonnaud et al., Dubousset, Schwab et al, Joseph et al. reported that the C7 plumb line should pass within a few millimeters of the posterior-superior corner of S1.[2-12,21,22,24-26] Thus, there are wide discrepancy of normal range between the numerical data in defining the normalcy by the various authors (Table 28.1). A maladjusted sacral slope and/or lumbar lordotic curve lead to questioning the location of gravitational force.

To maintain the normal spinal function the curves at each level should be in balance. If the curve loses its balance by the degenerative segmental rigidity, the spine becomes

Table 28.1 Normal ranges of distances between C_7 plumb line and S_1 or S_2 in defining the balanced and unbalanced spines by the various authors

Measurement point at S_1 and S_2	*Authors*	*Distance between C_7 plumb line and S1 or S2 (cm)*	*Remarks*
Anterior-superior corner of S1	Gelb et al.	−3.2 ± 3.2 (−10.1 ~ 7.7)	
	Vedantam et al.	−5.6 ± 3.5 (−13.4 ~ 1.8)	−5.6 cm in adolescents −3.2 cm in middle-aged
Posterior-superior corner of S1	Jackson and McManus	−0.08 ± 2.5 (−6 ~ 6.5)	>2.5 cm anterior or posterior - abnormal
	Peterson et al.	0.38 ± 2.1 (−5.7 ~ 5.2)	
	Berthonnaud et al. Dubousset Swab et al. Joseph et al.	A few millimeters	
S2	Suk et al.	2 inches anterior to S2	Textbook of spine surgery, Korea

the state of imbalance or decompensation. Also certain type of spinosacral and pelvic morphology is poorly adapted to the standing posture, and fail to stand or is prone to more severe listhesis in case of dysplastic spondylolisthesis (spondyloptosis) by increased PI.[2,13]

Assessment Methodology and Clinical Significance of Spinal Alignment

Vedantam et al. indicated that the radiographic assessing method with arms at 90° of flexion at the shoulder may have caused the underestimation of the shift in the sagittal spinal balance.[24] Therefore, it was recommended to take the posture such as fists-on-clavicle or cross-arm position with extended hip and knee during taking whole spine, hip and knee X-rays.

When the balanced spine in standing posture is assessed in coronal plane, the plumb line from external occipital protuberance must pass the intergluteal fold, while C7 plumb line in the sagittal plane in standing posture should pass posterosuperior aspect of S1.

Anteriorly displaced C7 plumb line denotes the positive balance, while the posteriorly displaced C7 plumb line denotes the negative balance (Figs 28.3 to 28.5). Positive balance means the forward trunk tilt, and negative balance means the posteriorly inclined trunk.

In the patients with positive balance, the forward truncal tilt is expressed by the measured distance of the anteriorly displaced C7 plumb line from postero-superior corner of S1.

In case of decompensated spine, C7 plumb line displaces anteriorly (over 5 cm) or posteriorly (over 2cm) from the posterior-superior corner of S1.[2,14,20,25]

The grand mom with forwardly stooped trunk has positive balance. Most of the elderly with DLK has positive balance, but in stage 2 of the DLK patients infrequently show negative balance.[2,21,22,24–26]

Muscles Controlling the Spine and Pelvis

The human body is built around a complex of bone lever whose position and movement are controlled by the muscles. For this purpose each individual is provided with a quarter billion striated muscle fibers actually assembled into muscles and attached to the skeleton levers in strategic positions. Motion is coordinated through the nervous system which can devise programs for complicated activities, store them for later use, and modulate their performance under no influence of feedback signals.

Many muscles contribute towards producing and controlling the spinal movements. The concerned muscles have the following properties. Their length may vary considerably. Some are one joint muscles and the others are multijoint muscles spanning many joints. They may be superficial or deep; the deeper muscle (multifidus) are shorter. The more superficial longer muscles tend to provide a coarse adjustment, whereas the shorter deep muscles provide for fine adjustment and segmental stability. The leverage of the deeper muscles will tend to be less because of its lines of pull at the short distance.[22]

In two-joint muscles, such as the hamstrings, the fiber length is too short for the muscles to accommodate themselves completely to the change in length which should accompany maximum movement in the associated joints. If a person standing with his hip joints fully extended uses the hamstrings to flex one knee, he will feel the tension decreasing before the knee is completely flexed. The muscles are then in a state of active insufficiency. The opposite condition, passive insufficiency, can be illustrated by keeping the knee fully extended and then attempting hip flexion; under these conditions stretching of the connective-tissue element will bring about passive insufficiency long before the hip joint reaches its limit of movements.

The muscles producing movements exist in bilateral pairs. They are placed generally in a plane anterior or posterior to the spine, although some, namely quadratus lumborum and psoas major, are placed laterally. Lumbar spine and pelvis do the afore-mentioned coupled motion, known as lumbopelvic rhythm.

The balanced posture of the body reduces to a minimum the work done by the muscles in maintaining the body in an erect position.

In summary, it is important to know the contribution of the active stabilizers of the lumbar spine and pelvis in management of malaligned lumbosacral spine such as DLK; lumbar, gluteal, and hip extensor muscles.

On bending forwards, two major factors contribute towards supporting the spine. Tension in the steering soft structures behind the spine acts to prevent it from collapsing forward. Under the active contraction of the erector spinae muscle which control the flexion movement being brought about by gravity. As full flexion is reached, the activity in the erector spinae muscle abruptly ceases, so that at full flexion the spine is being supported from behind by the passive tension provided by the ligaments alone. As a consequence, the spine is vulnerable at full flexion because of its posterior support mechanisms—active control by the muscles—shuts down.

There are another opinion for this lumbar flexion movement. In forward trunk bending from 0° to 45° in standing posture, erector spinae (iliocostalis, longissimus, spinalis) muscles participate actively to stabilize the spinal column and it occurs mainly at lumbar spine. Further forward flexion from 45° to 90° muscles fascia of the erector spinae and ligament become tight which does not allow further flexion at low back (Fig. 28.12).[21]

Movement of the Spine and Pelvis

The spinal curves can alter their shape depending on their movement being performed. There may be even a complete reversal of the shape of the curve as it occurs in the lumbar spine during flexion and extension.

When a man is upright the presence of these curves allows the spine to withstand greater compressive forces than if it is just a straight sustaining rod alone.

Most spinal movements are often a combination of movements from each of the three groups of directional movement rather than the pure single directional movement alone. The shape and direction of the facets in the different regions of the spine contribute towards guiding and limiting motion.

In forward trunk bending, 9° of flexion occurs on an average at each segment of lumbar spine until 45° flexion, and then anterior pelvic tilt allows further flexion from 45° to 90° (Fig. 28.12).[19-22, 24-25]

The connection between the sacrum and the iliac bones is so firm so that a change in position of the pelvis leads automatically to a realignment of the spine, particularly in the lumbar region (Fig. 28.13). In forward truncal flexion from 0° to 45° pelvis does not move due to isometric contraction (constant muscle length) of pelvic extensor muscles (gluteus maximus and hamstring muscles). When further flexion continues from 45° to 90°, the pelvis begins to tilt anteriorly to stabilize the lumbosacral joint by the pelvic extensor and hamstring muscles' eccentric contraction (isotonic muscle contraction with lengthening).[13] At 90° flexion, tightened pelvic extensor and hamstring muscles and ligament around pelvis do not allow further forward flexion.

In normal spine by maximum forward flexion, vertebral end-plates of each segment in the sagittal plane become parallel, and by further forward flexion additional angulatory motion does not occur.[21]

Obviously, when there is limitation of motion in the lumbar spine as a result of pain or degeneration, this will have a marked effect on the possible posture adjustments available.

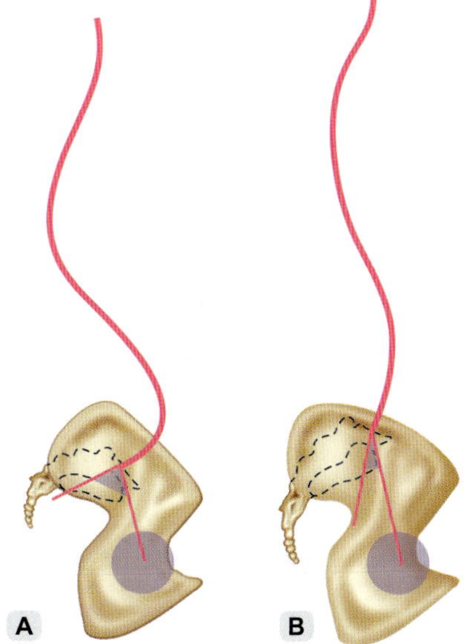

Fig. 28.13 Normal individual variation in the harmony of the sagittal shape of the spine in the presence of dynamic stabilizers (theoretical draws); (A) A large pelvic incidence associated with a greatly tilted upper sacral plate and a pronounced lumbar lordosis; (B) A low pelvic incidence associated with a more horizontal upper sacral plate and flatter sagittal curves

By passively increasing tension build-up in the posterior ligaments, the ligaments become more stretched as full flexion is approached, and thus the neutral zone of normal ROM can be widened. During trunk flexion, there is a transfer of tension from muscular to ligamentous support. When the trunk is raised from the fully flexed position, the movement is initiated by the hip extensor which becomes activated before the back extensors.[19]

When the pelvis tilts anteriorly in the balanced spine, the lumbar lordosis is increased. This is counter-balanced by the contraction of the extensor muscles of the hip. When these muscles contract they tend to tilt the pelvis posteriorly. In this movement these muscles can be actively aided by the abdominals. So, both the hip extensors and abdominalis create a force couple to tilt the pelvis backward (the force couple of abdominalis and hip extensors) and thereby flatten the lumbar spine (Fig. 28.14).

It was reported that sacral inclination decreased significantly in standing in the case with flexed knee, and that it caused low back pain more frequently.[30,31]

The shear force acting across the lumbosacral joint in standing is approximately 50% of the body weight. If one flexes to what the sacral angle increase to 50°, the shear force can increase to as much as 75% of the body weight above the joint.[1]

Lumbosacral Angle and Pelvic Tilt, Sacral Inclination (Sacral Slope), and Pelvic Incidence

The knowledge of lumbosacrocoxal parameters is very important in the management of various spinal deformities including DLK. Lumbosacrocoxal relation is expressed by 5 terms: angle, tilt, inclination, pelvic incidence, and overhang of S1 (Figs 28.15 and 28.16). In surgical management of lumbosacral disorders these parameters should be seriously considered.

Lumbosacral angle (sacral slope angle; SS) is formed by the upper end-plate of the sacrum and the horizontal line. Sacral inclination has similar significance with lumbosacral angle. This angle is formed by line along the posterior sacral surface and the vertical line. According to pelvic tilt the slope of the upper surface of the sacrum changes. There are anterior and posterior pelvic tilt. Sacrocoxal relation is expressed by pelvic incidence. Pelvic incidence is the angle formed by the perpendicular line to the center of the sacral plateau and the line connecting this center to the bicoxofemoral axis. There are close association of pelvic incidence (PI), pelvis tilt (PT), and sacral slope (SS) where a change in one parameter affects the other measurement and the overall alignment of the sacropelvic foundation (Figs 28.13 and 28.14).

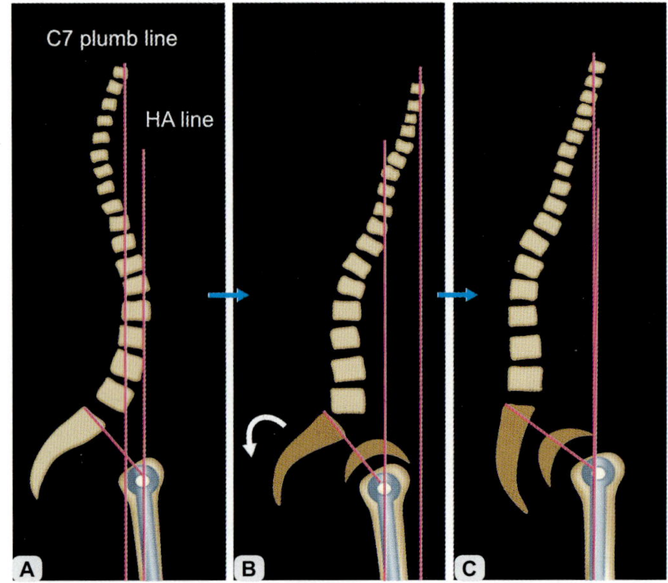

Fig. 28.14 When osteoarthritis of the hip occurs because of insufficient acetabular coverage, the HA shifted to the anterior side. To compensate for the anteriorly shifted center of the hips, the lumbar spine loses normal lordosis and lumbar kyphosis is accelerated. (A) Normal; (B) Lumbar kyphotic change; (C) Compensation of the hip

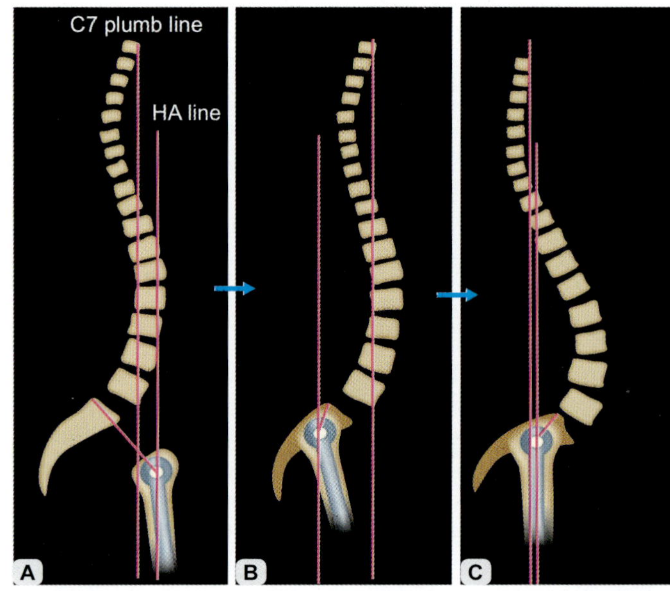

Fig. 28.15 Following congenital hip dislocation, the HA shifted to the posterior side. To compensate for the posteriorly shifted center of the hips, the lumbar spine shows hyperlordosis (A) Normal (B) Hip dislocation; (C) Compensation of the spine

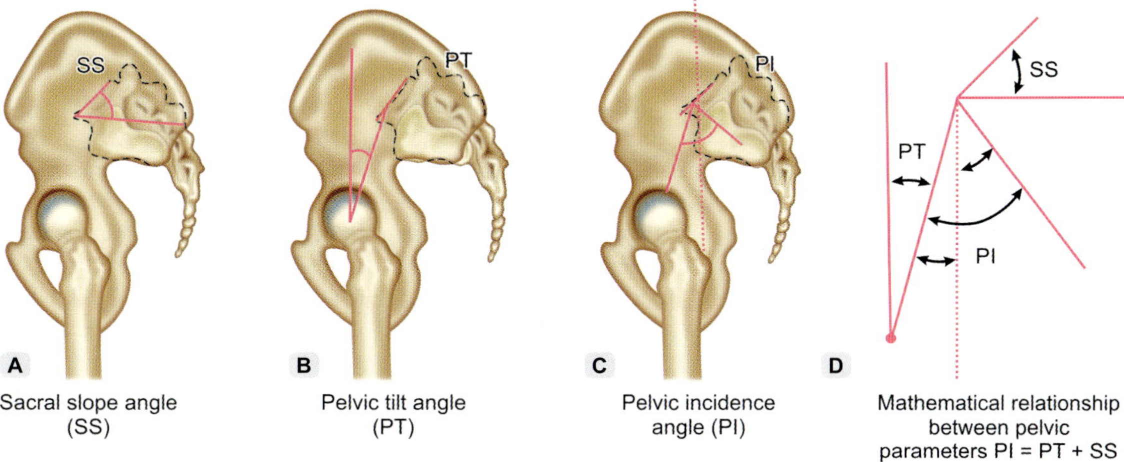

Fig. 28.16 Various pelvic and hip parameters. Pelvic incidence is the sum of the pelvic tilt and sacral slope, and is fixed after maturity in normal person. PI and pelvic thickness are the morphological parameters, while sacral slope, sacrofemoral tilting and overhang are the positional parameters. The term sacral inclination (SI) is also used to define the angle between the vertical plane and the tangential line to the sacral dorsum. The overhang of S1 is to define the horizontal distance between the center of the sacral plateau and the bicoxofemoral axis

The sum of the pelvic tilt and sacral slope is the pelvic incidence.[4-9,17,18]

PI = PT + SS (53.2° ± 10.3° in man and 48.2° ± 7° in women)

PI is a useful descriptor of the global shape of the pelvis as well as of the position of the sacrum within the pelvic unit.

In normal state, pelvic incidence value is found to increase slightly during growth as do pelvic tilt and lumbar lordosis. PI becomes stable at age 10 and remains unchanged throughout an indivicual's adolescent and adulthood. That is, PI becomes fixed even in case of the severely anteverted pelvis after maturity, because sacrum and ilia moves as a unit. This PI change in the growing period probably occur to avoid significant anterior displacement of the body's center of gravity.[4]

Pelvic incidence remains unchanged despite adaptive morphologic changes that occur with increasing severity of spondylolisthesis.

Spondylolisthesis patients with relatively low pelvic tilt (PT) and high sacral slope (SS) were given the term "balanced pelvic version" spondylolisthesis as pelvic spatial orientation was similar to asymptomatic control.

In the well-balanced flexible spinopelvic apparatus a large PI associates with a greatly tilted upper sacral plate and a pronounced lumbar lordosis, while a low PI associates with a more horizontal upper sacral plate and flatter lumbar sagittal curve. However, rigid lumbar curve cannot respond to the PI change (Fig. 28.17).[1]

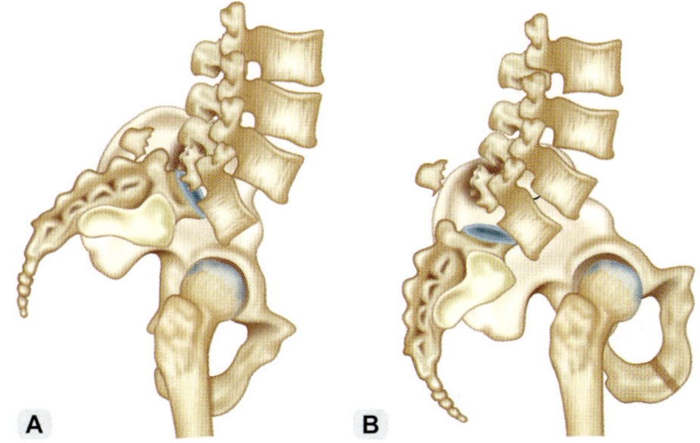

Fig. 28.17 High grade spondylolisthesis. (A) Balanced pelvis; (B) Unbalanced pelvis. Sagittal view of spinopelvic alignment in high-grade spondylolisthesis: Hresko's balanced and unbalanced pelvis. There is no numerical data defining the balanced and unbalanced pelvis. Hresko et al. defined that a high pelvic tilt (PT) indicates a retroverted pelvis, whereas a low PT tends to be associated with an anteverted pelvis. Patients with relatively low PT and high sacral slope (SS) were given the term "balanced pelvic version" spondylolisthesis as pelvic spatial orientation was similar to asymptomatic control. Spondylolisthesis patients with a retroverted pelvis (relatively high PT and low SS) were given the term "unbalanced pelvic version" as this pelvis spatial orientation was not found in the asymptomatic control group. In the unbalanced pelvis of the, high-grade spondylolisthesis with low lumbosacral angle (LSA), the increasing PT (retroverted pelvis) may compensate for the lumbosacral kyphosis which moves the center of mass posterior. The clinical factors that influence the lumbosacral balance have not yet been determined. The overhang of S1 (horizontal distance between the center of the sacral plateau and the bicoxofemoral axis) of the unbalanced pelvis is larger than the balanced pelvis.[4,17] However, in both situation, balanced and unbalanced pelvis, the patient can stand upright unaided regardless of the different energy consumption of the dynamic stabilizers.

Geiger et al. proposed another parameter to correlate the sacral slope (SS), and sacral inclination (SI) with the overhang of S1. The overhang of S_1 is the horizontal distance between the center of the sacral plateau and the bicoxofemoral axis, measured in millimeters. It is negative when the hips are anterior to the sacral plateau, and positive when the hips are posterior to it. This fact contradicts Hresko et al.'s definition of the unbalanced pelvis.[15]

Pelvic tilt occurs only at the lumbosacral joint. Therefore, there is a limitation in compensatory work if the ligament creep does not occur or if lumbar spine does not participate in compensatory curve formation.

Only the hypermobile sacroiliac joints in the certain very rare conditions can produce change in PI in the adult. That is, sole rotation of the sacrum inside the pelvic ring through sacroiliac joint dissociation changes PI. Such incidence is very rare.

A high PT indicates a retroverted pelvis which uncovers the femoral head by the acetabulum, whereas a low PT tends to be associated with an anteverted pelvis in which acetabulum covers the femoral head fully. Dynamic stabilizers function normally in either situation, though energy consumption is increased.

Hresko et al. defined the "balanced and unbalanced pelvic version" without indicating numerical data, based on the static standstill radiograph in interpretation of asymptomatic and symptomatic dysplastic spondylolisthesis.[7] Patients with relatively low pelvic tilt and high sacral slope were given the term "balanced pelvic version" spondylolisthesis as pelvic spatial orientation was similar to asymptomatic control, while spondylolisthesis patients with a retroverted pelvis with relatively high PT and low SS were given the term "unbalanced pelvic version" as the pelvic spatial orientation was not found in the asymptomatic control group (Fig. 28.17). The "unbalanced pelvic version" spondylolisthesis patients had even greater variance from normalcy in sagittal spine balance with more kyphotic lumbosacral angle (LSA), high L5 incidence (L5I), larger lumbar lordosis (LL) with more vertebrae in the lordotic curve, and a less kyphotic thoracic spine (Figs 28.16 to 28.18). Hresko et al. stated that it may be useful to consider the retroverted pelvis with high PT as an adaptation to the local lumbosacral kyphosis as represented by low lumbosacral angle (LSA). In unbalanced high-grade spondylolisthesis with low LSA, the increasing PT (retroversion of pelvis) may compensate for the lumbosacral kyphosis which moves the center of mass posterior. When LSA and L5 incidence are closer to normal values, the PT is less important and the pelvis remains in a more anterverted position. However, even the patients with socalled Hresko's unbalanced pelvis can stand unsupportedly. For this issue a question has been raised what clinical problem will be caused by the socalled Hresko's unbalanced pelvis. Phalen-Dickson sign seen in spondyloptosis patient is an attitude to make trunk balanced, to reduce the hamstring spasm, and thus to make standing possible. In general, the existence of the pelvic compensatory mechanism is expressed by sacral angle that is associated with lumbar lordosis only in cases of the intact pelvic extensor mechanism.

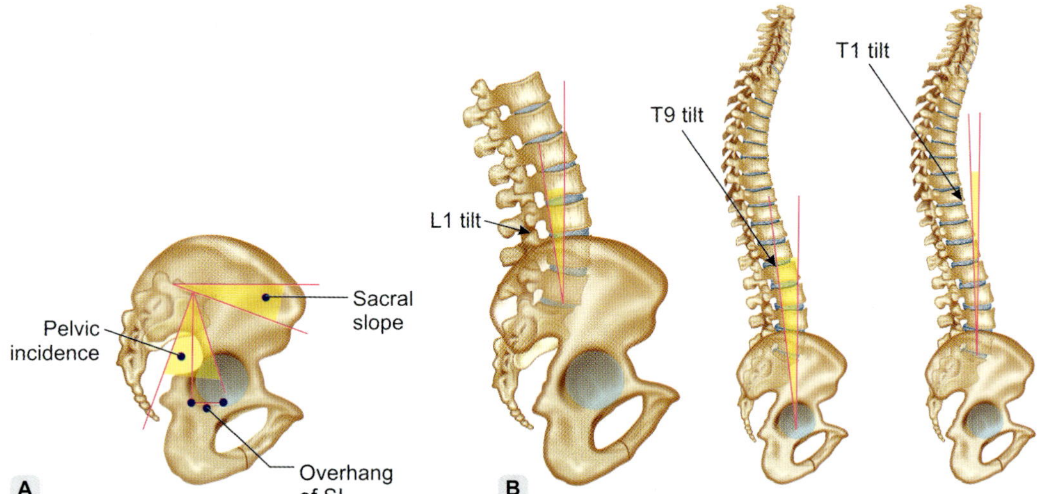

Fig. 28.18 The variables used for the analysis of T1, T9 and L1 tilt on pelvic tilt and overhang of S1. (A) The pelvis variables are shown: the pelvic incidence, the sacral slope, the overhang of S1 on the femoral heads; (B) The spinal variables: the L1 tilt, the T9 tilt, the T1 tilt. The overhang of S1 is the horizontal distance between the center of the sacral plateau and the bicoxofemoral axis, measured in millimeters. It is negative when the hips are anterior to the sacral plateau, and positive when the hips are posterior to it. These statement contradict Labelle et al's definition of the unbalanced pelvis[13]

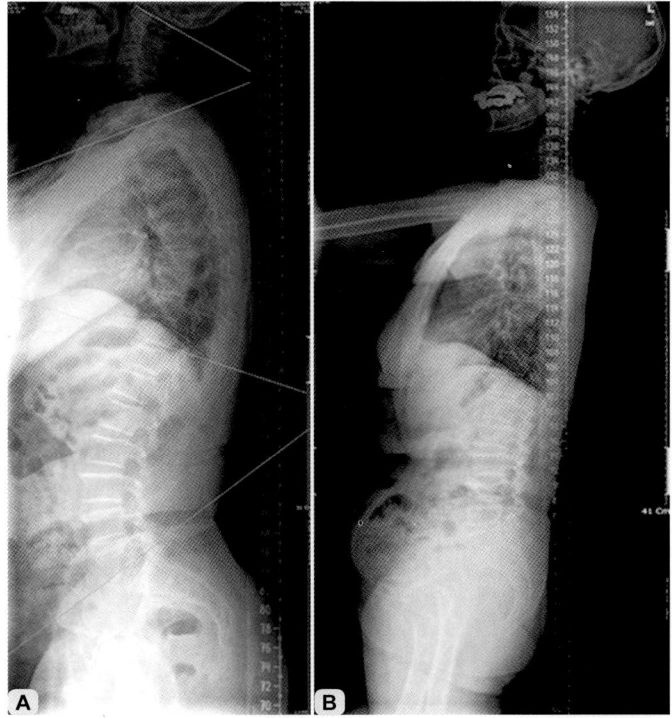

Fig. 28.19 (A) Sagittal radiograph of the spine and pelvis; (B) An example of Takemitsu's type 2 and Lee's group 1 DLK

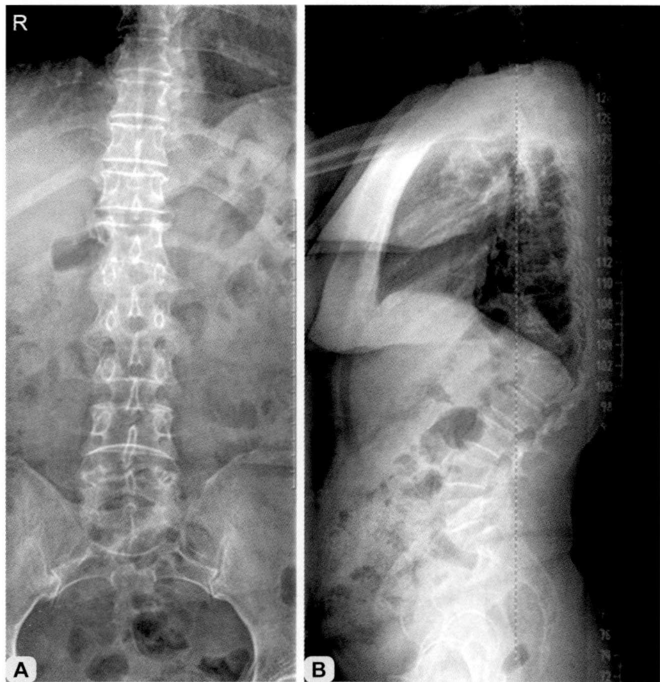

Fig. 28.20 An example of well compensated lumbar lordotic curve against the sagittal wedged T12–L1 block vertebra with negative sagittal balance

In the unbalanced high-grade spondylolisthesis with low lumbosacral angle (LSA), the increasing PT (retroversion of the pelvis) may compensate for the lumbosacral kyphosis which moves the center of mass posterior.

The current authors are rather confused by their definition on the "balanced and unbalanced pelvic version. There were no clear numerical data demarcating the two extreme pelvic versions, and its clinical significance was not mentioned. They illustrated the two extreme sacral versions; horizontal and vertical.[7] In degenerative lumbar kyphosis vertical sacrum in dynamic state (walking) means the relatively good gluteal and hip extensor muscles, while horizontal sacrum denotes the gluteal and hip extensor muscle deficiency resulting in restooping of trunk after corrective surgery. Also it is not clear whether the two terms, "balanced and unbalanced" pelvis is synonymous with the terms, "compensated or decompensated pelvis". The clinical presentation of the unbalanced pelvis is not shown. The unbalanced pelvis in their Figure 28.17 seems wrongly sketched and explained. Hip displaced too far anteriorly from the lumbar spine.[7] Because the pelvic ring moves as a unit, and not separately from sacrum. Only sacroiliac dissociation can allow such a radiographic finding. It is the current authors' view that the concept of dynamic and static imbalance should be brought in interpretation of spinopelvic alignment.

In normal condition pelvic tilt directly develops the compensatory lumbar lordosis in the mobile spine, and also indirectly gives influence on the femoral head coverage by the acetabulum. The influence of the total sagittal alignment of the spine on pathologic state of the hip joint was first recognized as hip-spine syndrome by Offerski and MacNab.[28] Posterior pelvic tilt decreases the femoral head coverage by the acetabulum which leads to the coxarthrosis. Goto demonstrated that when sacral inclination angle change from 35° to 10° femoral head coverage by acetabulum (DLK hip) decreased by 21%.[34] It was also confirmed that pelvic inclination index (PII) approximately correlated with pelvic angle of Jackson.[26,28]

Following congenital hip dislocation, the hip axis (HA) shifted to the posterior side. To compensate for the posterior shifted center of hips, the lumbar spine shows hyperlordosis.[26] The flexed knee also gives influence on hip and lumbar spine.[30-37]

In DLK postoperatively when a patient can decrease the pelvic tilt by gluteal muscles (posterior pelvic tilt), and extend the hips the patient can stand upright without truncal restooping. In case of the remarkable anterior pelvic tilt secondary to the weakened or absent gluteal and hip extensor muscles, the patient can stand only in static standstill shortly, but soon develops truncal stooping without external support or on walking. Lee et al. grouped these two situations; the former one as group I and the latter as group II.[16]

In summary, to maintain the mechanically balanced upright standing position, to conform to the stressing gravity, to permit locomotion and to assist in purposeful movement with minimal muscular activity (with least energy-consumption) are the most desirable and healthy one, though there are permissible range of shift of C7 plumb line and pelvic tilt. Treatment of the unbalanced spine, pelvis and hips in the presence of dynamic stabilizers aims not only at the restoration of the normal sagittal vertical axis but also cosmesis by any means (Figs 28.19 to 28.22).

Acknowledgments

We would like to thank Mr Seog In Moon for his active assistance in the secretariat work in preparation of this article, and to acknowledge Prof Y Takemitsu's and Prof. CS Lee's advice and comments and their help in obtaining the valuable references..

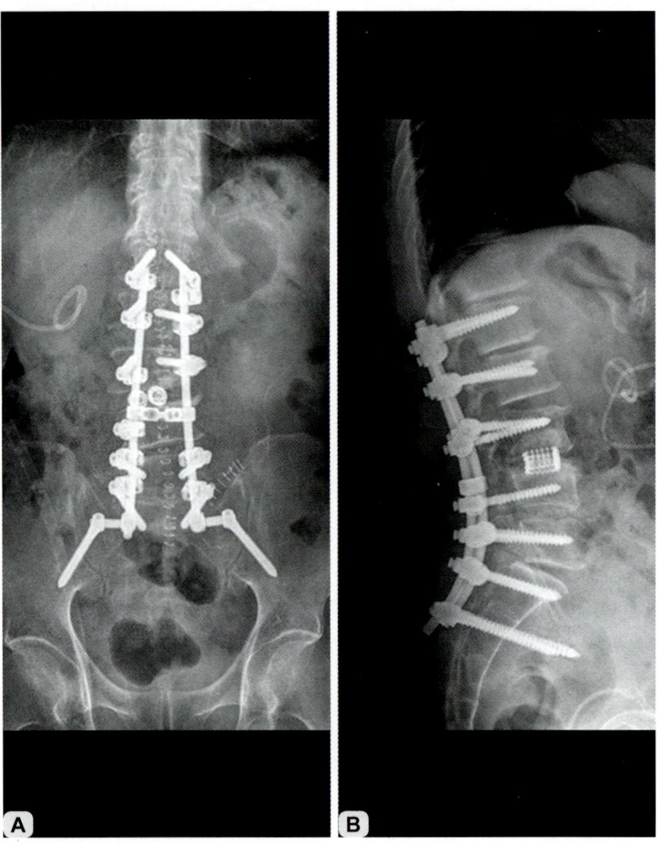

Fig. 28.21 This is an example of good lumbar lordotization in instrumented posterior stabilization and fusion to restore the normal sagittal balance and to prevent postoperative restooping in a 68-year-old lady, though the high rate of the adjacent segment disease at T12–L1 maay complicate sooner or later

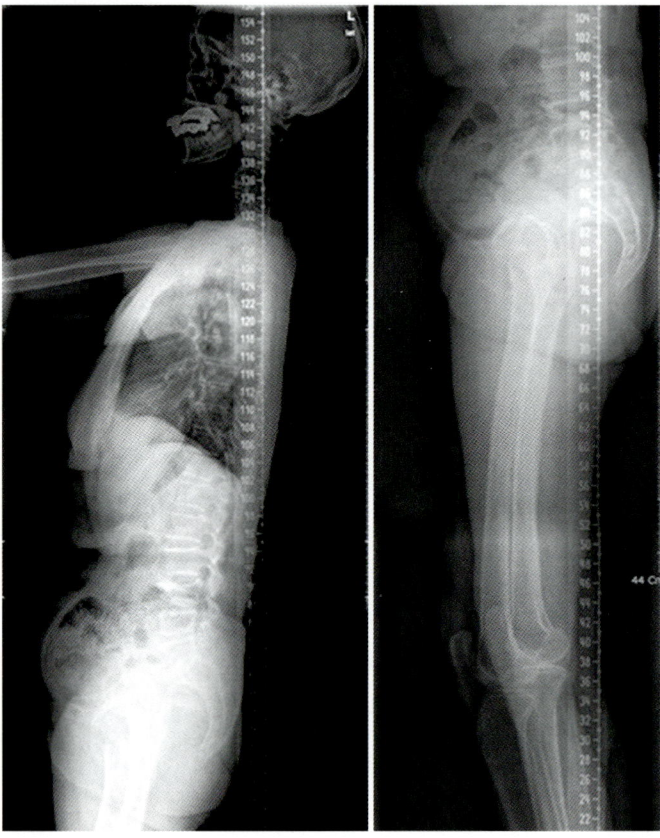

Fig. 28.22A This is a whole spine AP and lateral view in a 65 year-old lady with lower type 2 – group 1 DLK. Flattened whole spine sagittally with posterior tilted pelvis

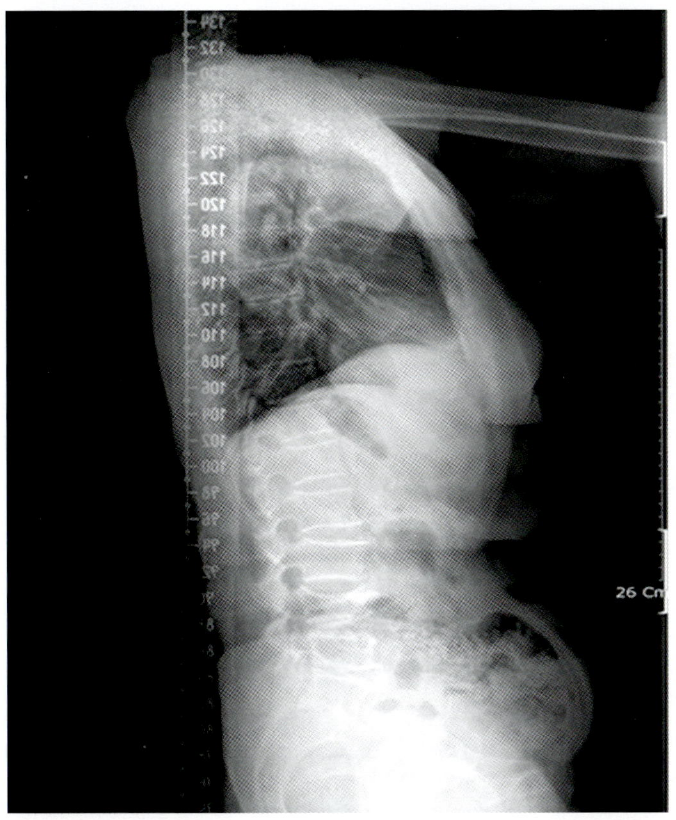

Fig. 28.22B Sagittal spinal view from C5 to sacrum hip. Collapsed L4 vertebral body is shown with vertically situated sacrum (posterior pelvic tilt)

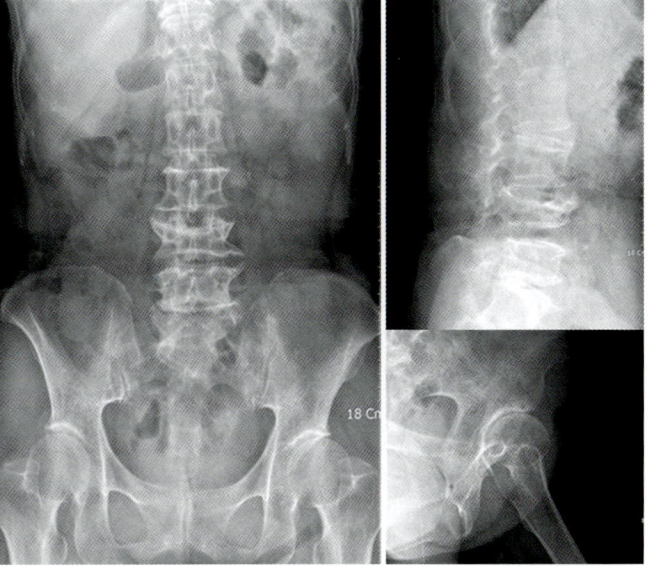

Fig. 28.22C Lumbar spine (AP and lateral views) and an arthritic hip are shown together with uncover anterior part of the femoral head. Posterior pelvic tilt uncovers the femoral head by acetabulum, though posterior pelvic tilt stabilize the lumbosacral joint in standing when the gluteal muscles are intact while it gives ill-effect on hips

References

1. Bae TS, Mun MS. Effect of lumbar lordotic angle on lumbosacral joint during isokinetic exercise: A simulation study. Clin Biomech. 2010; 25: 628-35.
2. Curylo LJ, Edwards C, Dewald RW. Radiographic markers in spondyloptosis—Implications for spondylolisthesis progression. Spine. 2002; 27(18): 2021-25.
3. Dubousett J. Three-dimensional analysis of the scoliotic deformity. In Weinstein SL (ed): The pediatric spine: principles and practice. New York, NY: Ravin Press; 1994. pp 479-96.
4. Geiger EW, Mueller GO, Niemeyer T, Kluba T. Adjustment of pelvispinal parameters preserves the constant gravity line position. Int Orthop. 2007; 31: 253-8.
5. Glassman SD, Bridwell KH, Dimar JR, Horton W, Berven S, Schwab F. The impact of positive sagittal balance in adult spine deformity. Spine 2005; 30: 2024-9.
6. Hanson DS, Bridwell KH, Rhee JM, Lenke LG. Correlation of pelvic incidence with low- and high-grade isthmic spondylolisthesis. Spine. 2002; 27(18): 2026-9.
7. Hresko MT, Labelle H, Roussouly P, Berthonnaud E Classification of high grade spondylolisthesis based on pelvic version and spine balance. Spine. 2007; 32(20); 2208-13.
8. Jackson RP, McManus AC. Radiographic analysis of sagittal plane alignment and balance in standing volunteers and patients with low back pain and matched for age, sex and size. A prospective controlled clinical study. Spine. 1994:19: 1617-8.
9. Jackson RP. Spinal balance, lumboplevic alignments around the hip axis, and positioning for surgery. Spine. State Art Rev. 1997; 11: 33-58.
10. Jackson RP, Peterson MD, McManus AC, et al. Compensatory spinopelvic balance over the hip axis and better reliability in measuring lordosis to the pelvic radius on standing lateral radiographs of adult volunteers and patients. Spine. 1998; 23: 1750-67.
11. Jackson RP, Hales C. Congruent spinopelvic alignment on standing lateral radiographs of adult volunteers. Spine. 2000; 25(21): 2808-15.
12. Jang J-S, Lee S-H, Min J-H, Han K-M. Lumbar degenerative kyphosis – Radiologic analysis and classification. Spine. 2007; 32(24): 2694-9.

13. Jones TR, Rao RD. Adult isthmic spondylolisthesis. J Am Acad Orthop Surg. 2009; 17: 609-17.
14. Joseph SA Jr, Moreno AP, Brandoff J, Casden AC, Kuflik P, Neuwirth MG. Sagittal plane deformity in the adult patient. J Am Acad Orthop Surg. 2009; 17: 378-88.
15. Labelle H, Roussoluly P, Berthonnaud E, Dimnet J, O'Brien M. The importance of spino-pelvic balance in L5-S1 developmental spondylolisthesis. Spine. 2005; 30(65): S27-S34.
16. Lee CS, Lee CK, Kim YT, Hong YM, Yoo JH. Dynamic imbalance of the spine in degenerative flat back. Spine. 2001; 26: 2029-35.
17. Legayo J. Duval-Beaupere G. Gravitational forces and sagittal shape of the spine – clinical estimation of their relations. Int Orthop. 2008; 32: 809-16.
18. Legaye J: Influence of the sagittal balance of the spine on the anterior pelvic plane and on the acetabular orientation. Int Orthop 2009; 33: 1695-700.
19. Mac-Thiong JM, Berthonnaud E, Dimar JR, Betz RR, Labelle H. Sagittal alignment of the spine and pelvis during growth. Spine. 2004; 27: 1642-7.
20. McClure PW, Esola M, Schreier R, Sielger S. Kinamatic analysis of lumbar and hip motion while rising from a forward, flexed position in patients with and without a history of low back pain. Spine. 1997; 22: 552-8.
21. Moon MS, Lee BJ, Kim SS, Lin JF. Evolution of management of spinal deformity: controversial issues and current concepts review. J Spinal Surg. 2010; 2(1): 295-305.
22. Moon MS, Kim SS, Lee BJ, Moon JL, Moon YW. Surgical management of severe rigid tuberculous kyphosis of dorsolumbar spine. Int Orthop 2011; 35: 75-81.
23. Aita K, Yonekura Y, Morimoto T, Hotokebuchi T et al: Hip-spine syndrome: investigations measurement of pelvic inclination at standing position (in Japanese) Seikeigeka to Saigaigeka (Orthop and Traumatol) 2004; 53(4): 867-73.
24. Schwab F, Lafage V, Boyee R, Skalli W, Farcy JP. Gravity line analysis in adult volunteers: Age-relatged correlation with spinal parameters, pelvic parameters, and foot position. Spine. 2006; 31: E959-67.
25. Takeda N, Kobayashi T, Atsuda Y, Matsuno T, Shirado O, Minami A. Changes in the sagittal spinal alignment of the elderly without vertebral fracture: a minimum 10-year longitudinal study. J Orthop Sci. 2009; 14: 748-53.
26. Takemitsu Y, Harada Y, Iwahara T, Miyamoto M, Miyatake Y. Lumbar degenerative kyphosis—clinical, radiological and epidemiological studies. Spine. 1988;306: 64-72.
27. Takemitsu Y, Harada Y, Atsuta Y, et al. Degenerative lumbar kyphosis in the middle-aged and elderly. Orthop Surg. 1987; 12(suppl): 18-21.
28. Iwahara T, Takemitsu Y, Watakabe M, Goto E, et al. Roentgenologic and biomechanical study of lumbar degenerative kyphosis with special reference to effect of sacral inclination and hip joint (in Japan). Rinshho Seikei Geka (Clin Orthop.) 1988; 23(7): 811-9.
29. Vedantam R, Lenke LG, Keenley JA, Bridwell KH: Comparison of standing sagittal alignment in asymptomatic adolescent and adults. Spine 1998; 23: 211-5.
30. Konishi N, Mieno T. Determination of acetabular coverage of the femoral head with use of a single anteroposterior radiography. J Bone Joint Surg. 1993; 75A: 1318-32.
31. Tsuji DI, Matsuyama SH, Koto M, et al. Knee-spine syndrome: correlation between sacral inclination and patellofemoral joint pain. J Orthop Sci. 2002; 7(5): 519-23.
32. Doiguchi Y, Iwasaki K. Radiological investigation of pelvic inlet form and pelvis inclination (in Japanese). Seikei Saigia Geka (Orthop and Traumatol). 1992; 41(2): 641-5.
33. Murata Y, Takahashi K, Yamagata M, Hanaoka E, Moriya H. The knee-spine syndrome. J Bone Joint Surg. 2003; 85B: 95-9.
34. Matsuyama Y, Hasegawa Y, Yoshihara H, Tsuji T, Sakai Y, Nakamura H, et al. Hip-spine syndrome. Spine. 2004; 29(21): 2432-7.
35. Goto E. Biomechanical effects of lumbar degenerative kyphosis on the hip joint – study of electromyography of the muscles around hip joint in patients with lumbar kyphosis (in Japanese). J Joint Surg. 2004; 23(4): 56-61.
36. Doigichi Y, Iwasaki K. Change of pelvic inclination after total hip arthroplasty for osteoarthritis of the hip (in Japanese). Hip Joint. 2004; 30: 450-3.
37. Aita K, Hotokebuchi T: Relation between low back pain and pelvic inclination in patients with hip disease (in Japanese) Kanstsugeka 2004; 23(4): 102-9.

CHAPTER

29

Instability of Lumbar Spine—Diagnosis, Assessment, and Management

Myung-Sang Moon, Sung-Soo Kim, Jeong-Lim Moon, Sung-Sim Kim, Hanlim Moon

When lumbar spine does its work without causing clinical symptom even under the overload, the back is labeled as strong back by the layman, while when the other back fails to bear such same amount of load, the back is labeled as weak back. Of course, it is true that there are great individual differences in the worker's back capacity. A person with strong back is known as a man of muscle who has more strong skeletal and muscular structures and joints than the others with the weak back. The weak back is also known to be associated with the unstable back. The structural defects can be found as the factors of weak or unstable back in any individual regardless of their back strength.

It is true, of course, that the individual physical fitness for a certain work is influenced by the body build and training if a person does not have any basic structural defective weakness. All backs have the physiologically given range of motion at each segment. If the segmental motion becomes wider at any segment, it is the nonphysiological motion which can lead gradually to the symptomatic and failed back. The back with such an abnormally wider motion is labeled biomechanically as unstable back. Thus, it is not simple to define the spinal stability in the clinical sense in a word.

The term "spinal flexibility" is used by some to express the spinal mobility. Also the term "stiff or rigid back" has been used to express the reduced mobility of spine, and the term "unstable" or "weak back" has been used to express the increased mobility. However, the term "weak back" is the layman's term and is not synonymous with unstable back. One says that he or she has "weak back" when he or she cannot tolerates even the nonfatiguing work which is accompanied by aching.

The stiff and rigid back denotes less mobile spine, while the unstable back denotes the unsteady and hypermobile spine which leads to failure of spinal stability. The two conditions can cause clinical symptoms at the certain stage of their development. However, unstable back causes clinical symptoms more frequently than the stiff one.

Segmental spinal instability is a clinical concept which is not closely related to mechanical definitions of stability.[1-5,7,15,19-22] Segmental instability clinically implies excessive or inappropriate movements (wobble) of a motion segment under load, either within a normal range of movement or beyond such a range, despite normal ligamentous constraints to the full range of movement. Instability may also be defined as an abnormally increased joint deformation with stress.[19,21] Newman defined the instability as "a loss of integrity of soft tissue intersegmental control, causing potential weakness and liability to yield[17]".

Clinical instability is not a diagnostic *per se*, and a scale is used to confirm the presence of it. In effect, the motion segment has an enlarged "neutral zone" [Zone of ligamentous laxity (LZ)] within which the intervertebral disk and ligaments offer little resistance to movement. [1,4,15,17,19,22]

This kind of instability could be caused by injury to the disk or vertebral body increasing the size of the neutral zone; for example, a motion segment resistance to bending, shear and torsion is reduced directly by injury to the annulus fibrosus, and indirectly by damage to an adjacent vertebral body end-plate which decompresses the nucleus pulposus and allows more slack to the annulus. Water loss from the nucleus, either as a result of sustained loading or degenerative change, also decompress the nucleus, slackens the annulus and reduces rotational stiffness, even in presence of normal skeletal stability. This may explain why repetitive loading in shear and compression causes a vertebra to creep forwards relative to the one below, and to rotate slightly.[19,22]

Also the motion segments become gradually unstable when there are skeletal defect in spite of presence of the normal ligamentous and muscular structures.[15,19]

The paraspinal muscles are suitably positioned to provide stability within the neutral zone, but only as far as angular rotations are concerned. The back muscles are poorly oriented to prevent small translations. However, muscle could affect translational stability indirectly by changing the compressive force acting on the spine: an abnormally low compressive preload arising from impaired muscle action would reduce impaction of the adjacent neural arches, and thereby reduce the spine's resistance to bending and axial rotation. Inadequate local muscle tone may similarly allow greater translational movement, especially if the disk is degenerated.[19]

As for the age-related spinal flexibility, normally the young people have more flexible spines which are represented by wider range of motion because of more elastic natures of the soft tissue and the normal joint structures.[15] Because of the greater flexibility of the pediatric spinal column, the cervical spinal column is capable of up to 2 inches of elongation whereas the cervical spinal cord with rupture with only 0.25 inch of stretch.

The elderly people have less flexible spine because of age-related joint stiffness due to gradual loss of elasticity of the stabilizing spinal structures. Of course, in addition to the afore-mentioned fact, it is true that the changes of the joint proper also contribute to the spinal flexibility.[15]

In recent years, maintenance of segmental stability of the spine has been frequently overemphasized, because the instability has been one of the most important factors closely related with the causation of the low back disorders.[2,6,15] As yet, its clinical relevance is debated for the low back disorders of non-Charcot's spine. The patient with Charcot's neuropathic spine presents clinically only the mild symptoms, though it has severe instability, which is difficult to manage.

In summary, joint instability can be developed by various causes and is represented by angular difference (tilt) and/or translational displacement on radiograms (Tables 29.1 and 29.2).[1-5,7,15,17,19]

It is essential to discuss the joint stabilizing structures to make the better understanding of the stability of the motion segments.

Table 29.1 Excessive range of movement and structural defects/damages

Excessive range of movement	*Causative structural defects/damages*
Hyperflexion	• Posterior osseous-ligamentous injury/defect
Hyperextension	• Damage to the anterior ligaments • Neural arch damage/defect (including the apophyseal joint, articular surface and capsular ligament)
Excessive lateral bending	• Gross neural arch fracture/severe tear in the anterolateral annulus
Excessive axial rotation	• Neural arch damage/defect (including the apophyseal joint, articular surface and capsular ligament) • Gross neural arch fracture/severe tear in the anterolateral annulus

Table 29.2 Patterns of hypermobile instability

Abnormal motion (displacement)	*Plane of motion*	*Degree of displacement*
Translation • Anterior • Posterior • Lateral (rotatory)	Horizontal	>2–3 mm*
Angulation (angle of disk space or 'tilt') • Forward (flexion) • Backward (extension) • Lateral right • Left	Sagittal Coronal	>9°** L2–L3 ≥ 14.3°† L3–L4 ≥ 15.5°† L4–L5 ≥ 18°†
Rotation • Right • Left	Axial	Facet joint gapping

*Wiltse and Winter; **Graf, †Dvorak

Pathogenesis

Excess axial rotation and translation of lumbar spine may follow injury to the bony neural arch, including pedicle and facet joint, and also can occur in the absence and/or asymmetry of the facet joints. If once the degenerative changes in the disks occur, smooth action is lost, and the movement between the adjacent segments becomes uneven, excessive, and irregular. This is the stage of segmental instability.

Normally on forward bending of the lumbar spine, the diskal borders of the vertebral bodies become parallel on sagittal plane above the fifth lumbar vertebra. So, it is important to look for the causes of the segmental instability for each case, although it is not easy in *per se* to find those out.

Causative Elements of Non-neural Origin

1. Bony element: Skeletal anomaly and defects (bony contour, joint proper, facet shape, facet asymmetry, congenital or iatrogenic absence of facet and lamina (Fig. 29.1), isthmic defect (Figs 29.2 to 29.4), pedicle defect (Fig. 29.5), and other bony defects)
2. Soft tissue (Non-skeletal elements):
   basic (static) stabilizers (ligaments, joint capsules)
   active stabilizer (muscles)
   Neural element (neuropathy)
3. Acquired Charcot joint.
4. Congenital insensitivity.

Enlarged Range of Movement and Structural Defects

- Hyperflexion (forward bending) by posterior ligamento-osseous injury or defect.
- Hyperextension (backward bending) instability:
  1. Damage of anterior ligaments (annular ligament, anterior longitudinal ligament).
  2. Neural arch damage and defect and/or anomaly including apophyseal joint.
- Articular surface.
- Excessive lateral bending by (3) gross neural arch fracture or severe tear of anterolateral annulus.
- Excessive axial rotation by (2) + (3).

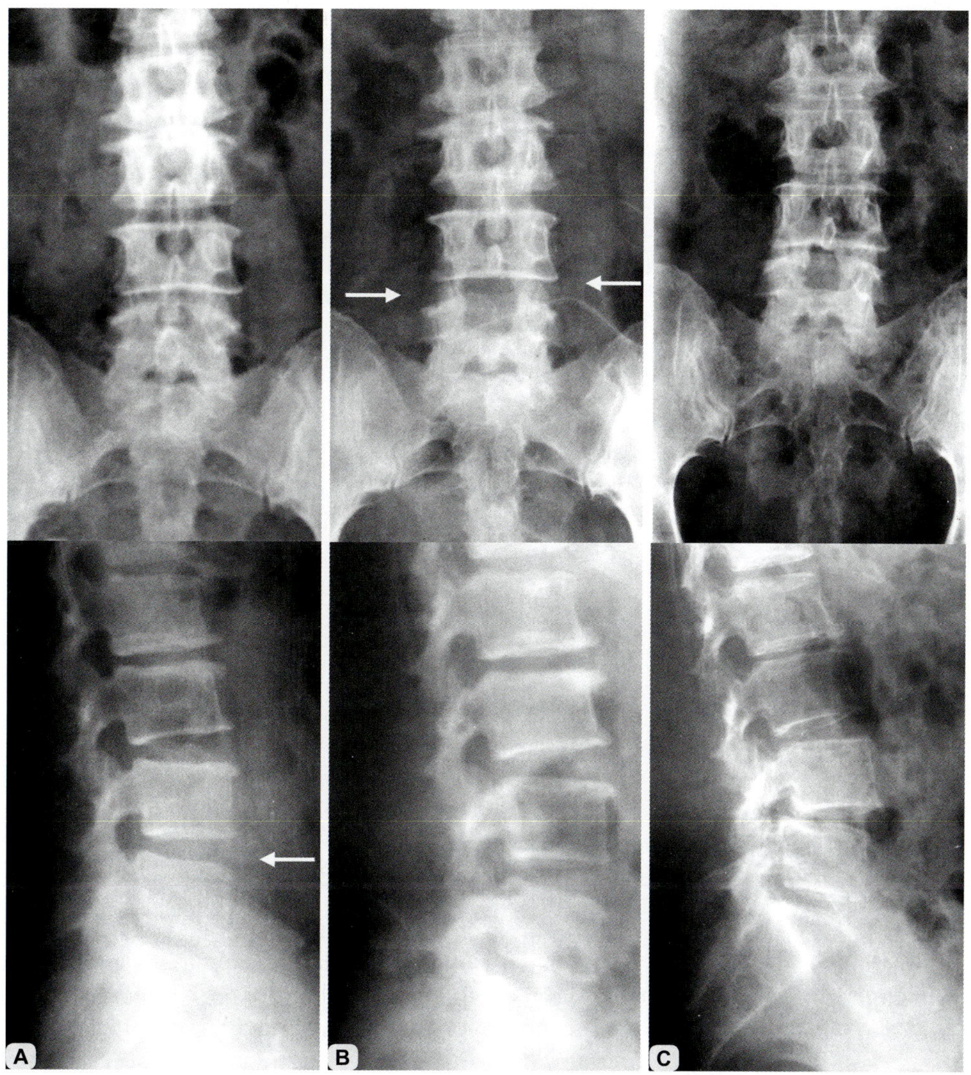

Fig. 29.1 An example of postlaminectomy spondylolisthesis of L4. Extension angular instability with anterior slip is seen: (A) Initial (spinal stenosis); (B) Immediate postoperative radiograms; (C) Postoperative 6 years and 7 months

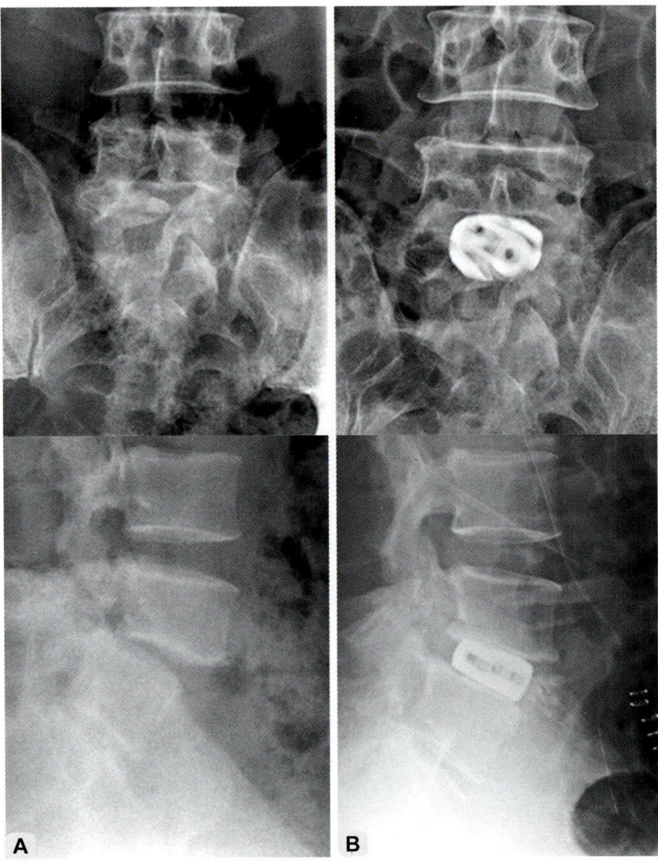

Fig. 29.2 Grade 1 isthmic spondylolisthesis of L4 in a 54 year-old man without neurological involvement; (A) Preoperative; (B) After anterior interbody fusion with Stabilis cage

Assessment of Clinical Instability

The sagittal instability was assessed by the degrees of the vertebral body translation over 2 mm by Wiltse and Winter,[25] and the angular instability by Dvorak:[1] 14.3° ≥ at L2–L3, 15.5° ≥ at L3–4 and 18° ≥ at L4–5 (Table 29.1).

For the instability in coronal plane, numerical clinical data were not presented in spite of the presence of the excessive lateral angular and/or translational instabilities. True lateral translation in spite of its presence has never been reported in clinical situation, while the rotatory lateral olisthesis has been frequently encountered in the elderly patients with degenerative lumbar scoliosis. Also no pure rotatory instability without lateral listhesis could be induced in clinical situation (Table 29.1),[1,2,19] while pure vertical instability could be induced. However, in this paper those were not dealt with.

Classification

Theoretically, in the angulatory and translational instabilities, there are seven types consisting of pure five basic ones (anterior, posterior, lateral, vertical and rotational) and combined forms. However, clinically, there are no pure lateral listhesis and rotational instability without lateral translation as mentioned above (Figs 29.6 to 29.12).[15,16]

1. Angulation only without horizontal translation:
   a. Forward
   b. Backward
2. Translation only
   - Forward (antelisthesis)
   - Backward (retrolisthesis)
3. Translation and angulation :
   a. Forward or backward translation and angulation (ante- or retrolisthesis).
   b. Lateral angulation and translation (scoliosis with lateral rotatory olisthesis).
4. Lateral rotatory translation (lateral olisthesis) (Figs 29.13 and 29.14)
5. Lateral angulation (tilt) and lateral rotatory translation (scoliosis and lateral olisthesis).
6. Vertical translation.[7]
7. Other combined forms.[15]

Among those seven types, the angulatory, translational, and combined angulatory–translational instabilities in sagittal and coronal planes are the most frequent clinical forms (Figs 29.6 to 29.10)[1,13,15].

Also these conditions are classified further into two major groups clinically by associating stenotic symptoms.

1. Instability without stenosis
2. Instability with stenosis.

The translational instability associating stenotic sympotoms and signs again can be subdivided by postures into two clinical forms: reducible and nonreducible types (Figs 29.2 and 29.15), and dynamic and static stenosis types, respectively.[11,12,14,15]

It is considered that the nonreducible type is one of nonhypermobile patterns of instability, and that nonhypermobile instability is the manifestation of the near end stage of the instability which reached static equilibrium between the degenerative and reparative processes. Any disturbance in this equilibrium will result in the perpetuation of hypermobile instability.

If the instability classification is too simplified, it cannot provide enough information in making diagnosis and selection of the surgical procedures for unstable lumbar and lumbosacral spines. Therefore, the current authors attempted a new practical clinical classification which

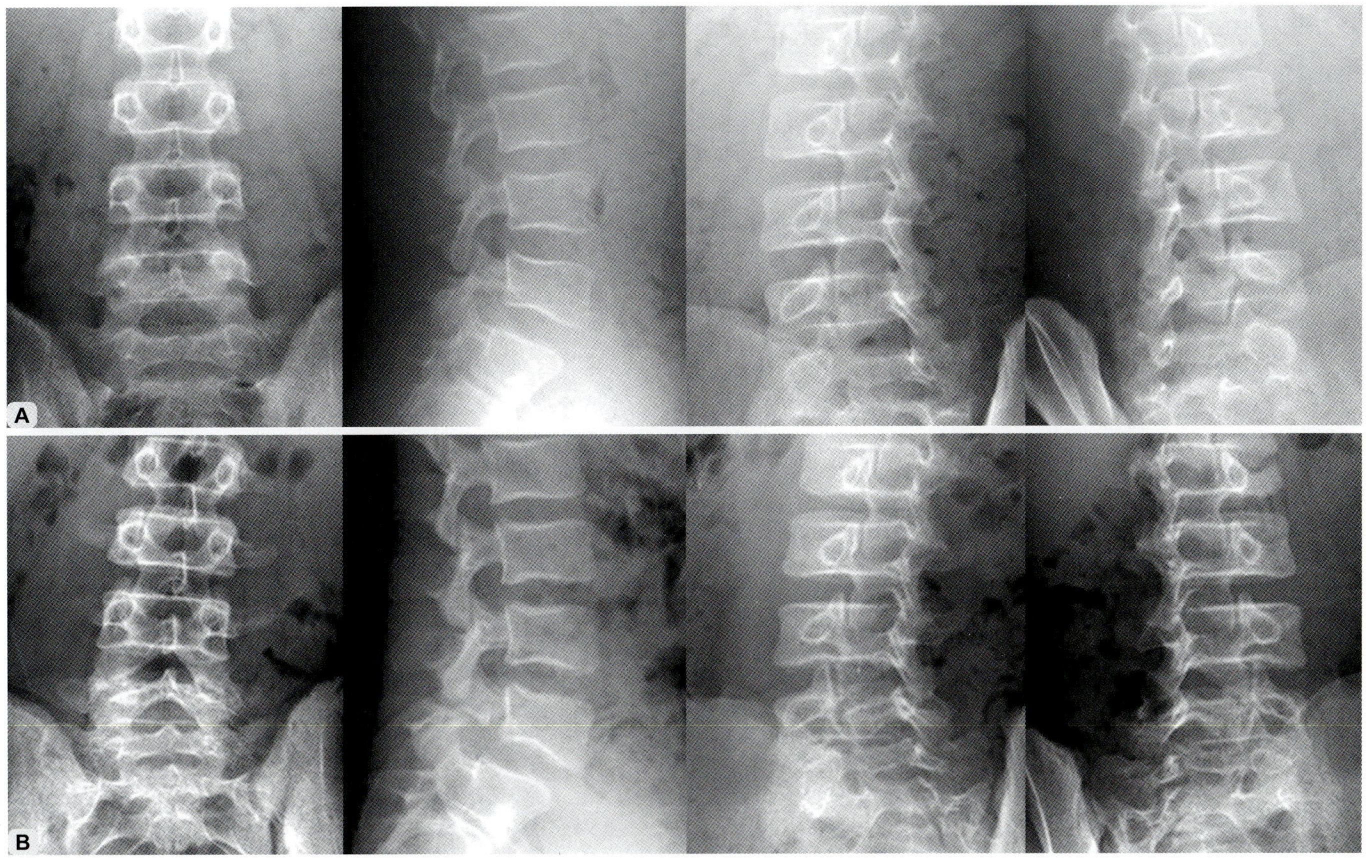

Fig. 29.3 An example of isthmic spondylolisthesis in a 12 year-old boy. (A) On initial radiograms of A-P, lateral and both oblique views, isthmic defect is seen without slip; (B) On radiograms of A-P, lateral and both oblique views, taken 6 months later, show slight anterior slip of L5

was thought to be more plausible in understanding the unstable spine. There are two patterns of abnormal motion: hypomobile and hypermobile.

Thus, theoretically, lumbar instability can be classified or grouped into many clinical types according to the severity of instability and clinical symptoms and signs, i.e.

1. By severity of angulation, translation, and rotation.
2. By the presence or absence of postural central stenotic symptoms and signs—dynamic and static, and
3. By postural reducibility.

In some cases of dynamic central stenosis symptoms could be relieved by flexion, while in others symptoms could be relieved by extension with reduction or without reduction of the slipped vertebral body (Fig. 29.16).[15]

Pope and Frymoyer, Pope and Panjabs have classified the segmental instability in 2 major types: primary and secondary ones which were again subclassified into several subgroups.[21,22]

A. The primary (non-iatrogenic) instabilities were subclassified into 5 types:
   1. Axial rotational instability
   2. Translational instabilities
   3. Retrolisthetic instability
   4. Progressing degenerative scoliosis
   5. (?) Disk disruption syndrome
B. Secondary (iatrogenic) instabilities were subclassified into 3 types :
   1. Postdisk excision
   2. Postdecompression laminectomy
   3. Postspinal fusion
      a. Above or below a spinal fusion (junctional instability)
      b. Pseudoarthrosis.

Clinical Symptoms and Signs

Patients' complaints are mostly low back pain, sciatica and/ or claudication, and patients may experience frequent episode of so-called "catching pain" (known as the "instability catch") or acute asymmetrical low back pain against a background of chronic pain with or without leg pain. This pain is automatically accompanied by an asymmetrical muscle contraction.

Pain is the most common and early clinical symptom, although pain can arise from a number of structures within

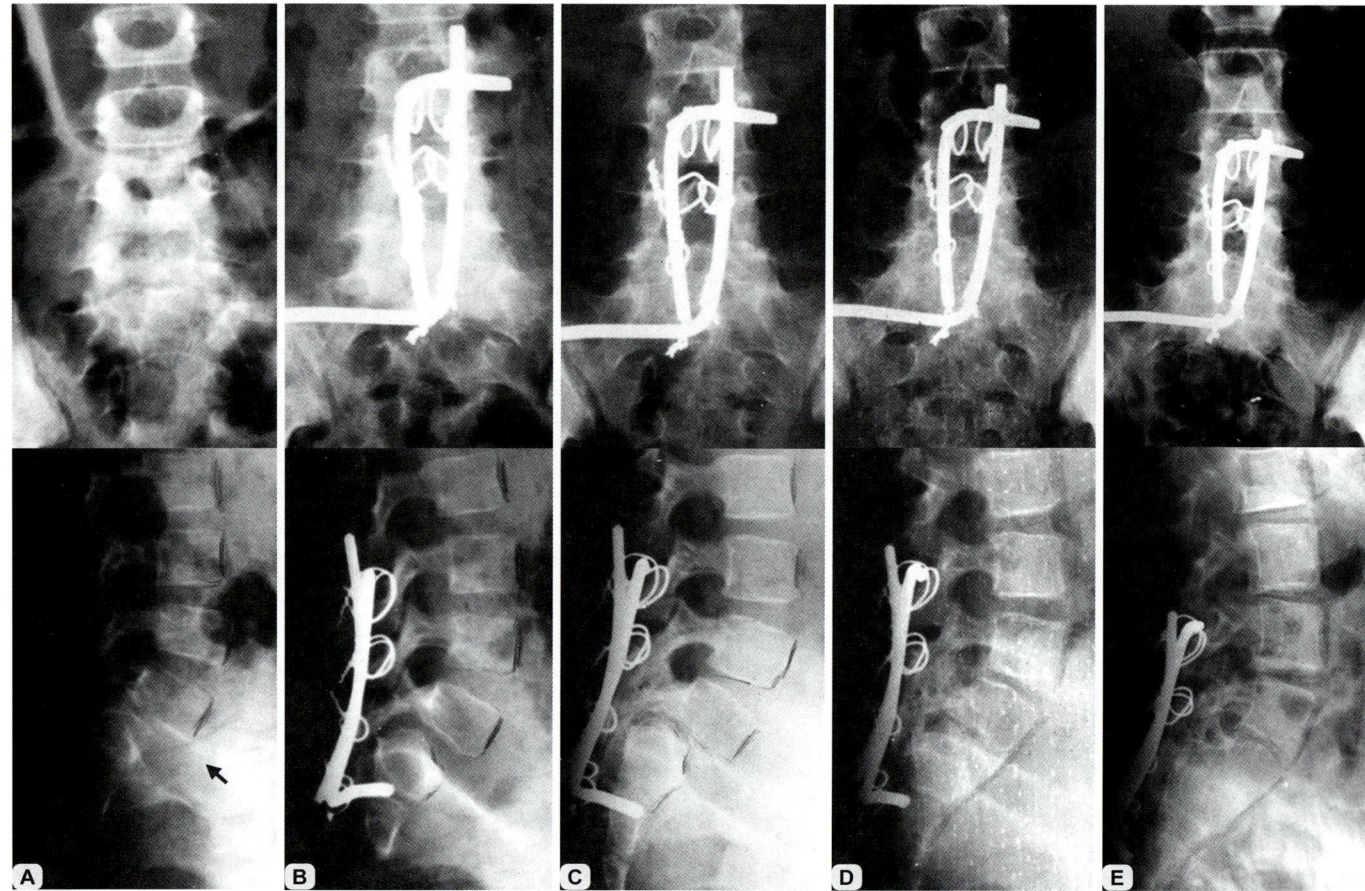

Fig. 29.4 An example of isthmic spondyloptosis of L5 in a 13 year-old girl with severe back muscle spasm and markedly limited straight leg raising; (A) Initial; (B) Immediate after posterior stabilization; (C) After anterior interbody fusion of L5–S1; (D and E) Postoperative 1 and 6 years. Solid anterior fusion of L5–S1 is seen

or adjacent to the spinal column. The structures include the intervertebral disc, zygoapophyseal joints, vertebral bodies, and surrounding ligaments and muscles. In addition to the musculoskeletal elements, pain also may arise from compression and damage to nerve roots exiting from the spinal canal and damage to the spinal cord itself.

Diagnosis

Before treatment, we have to look for the true cause of unstable back with pain, though there is still disagreement as to what pathology gives rise to pain.

Thus, the low back pain is largely grouped into 4 due to their probable origins: group 1, radiculopathy and spinal stenosis: group II, anterior column origin or diskogenic pain associated with degenerative disk disease or spondylolisthesis: group III, posterior column pain, including the facet joints: group IV, back pain of soft tissue origin. The last one is generally the nonsurgical condition[15,16] (Table 29.3).

Table 29.3 Classification of low back pain

Group I	Radiculopathy and spinal stenosis
Group II	Anterior column origin or diskogenic pain associated with degenerative disk disease or spondylolisthesis
Group III	Posterior column pain, including the facet joints
Group IV	Back pain of soft tissue origin*

*Generally a nonsurgical condition

To provide the better treatment for patients with unstable back, accurate diagnosis should be made before treatment by utilizing all the available modern modalities.[1,3,5,6,15,24-26] However, it is emphasized that the plain roentgenograms, including stress X-rays are the basic key for diagnosis. Therefore, the current authors suggest to have simple and stress X-rays as first step of diagnosis, when a patient has complaints seemingly being originated from the unstable back.[15]

To make a conclusive diagnosis, the causes have to be searched; basic anatomical defects in bones and

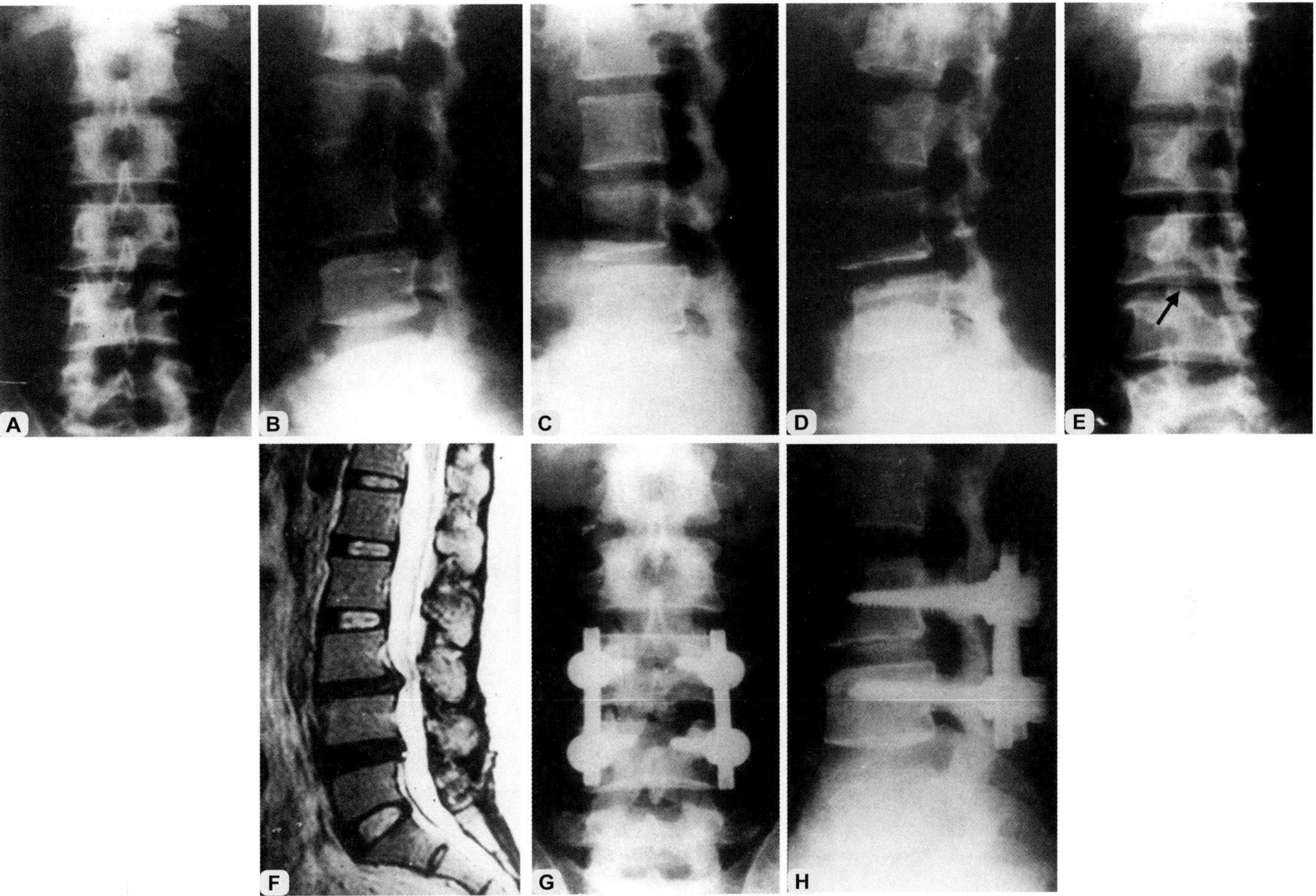

Fig. 29.5 Spondylolisthesis of L3 due to congenital pedicle absence. (A to E) Initial radiograms: (A) Anteroposterior; (B) Neutral lateral; (C) Forward flexion; (D) Extension; (E) Oblique. (F) MRI; (G and H) Postoperative (pedicle screw fixation)

ligaments. Plain radiograms at least should show the following findings: angulatory and/or translational displacement of the vertebral body against the apposing vertebral body, Hadley's lazy S sign[3], traction spur, facet joint fluid, and the Knuttson's vacuum sign in the disk (Fig. 29.17).[5] According to Lin and Moon, the detection rate of the Knuttson's sign was higher in extension lateral radiogram and computed tomogram than the plain flexion and neutral lateral radiograms.[6] They stated that the unstable segment with vacuum sign was the main site causing back pain, and therefore, they strongly recommended the fusion to eradicate the pain source.[6] Also, it was disclosed that vacuum sign disappeared gradually after the posterior instrumented stabilization of the unstable segment. The reason is that normal intra-articular pressure is negative, and consequently, the joint becomes stable. Joint, filled with fluid and/or air becomes unstable, because the joint pressure converts from negative to positive pressure.

If any evidence of segmental instability is not shown by simple and stress X-rays, diagnosis of unstable back cannot be made. Because the modern medicine has been known as the evidence-based medicine.

Diagnosis of clinical instability of a spinal motion segment can be established when pain is caused by demonstrable hypermobility, such as increased abnormal angular, translational and axial motions at the disk, i.e. abnormal movement or abnormal alignment of one vertebral body to another are thought to indicate instability. Angulatory instability is most difficult to assess, and also it is very difficult to establish when pain is caused by non-hypermobile abnormal motion and/or abnormal biomechanical response of structures to a physiologic loading situation.

It should be known that even an unstable segment with a small isthmic osseous defect can cause 3 different olisthetic conditions (antelisthesis, pure lateral listhesis, and rotatory lateral listhesis), and scoliotic tilt.

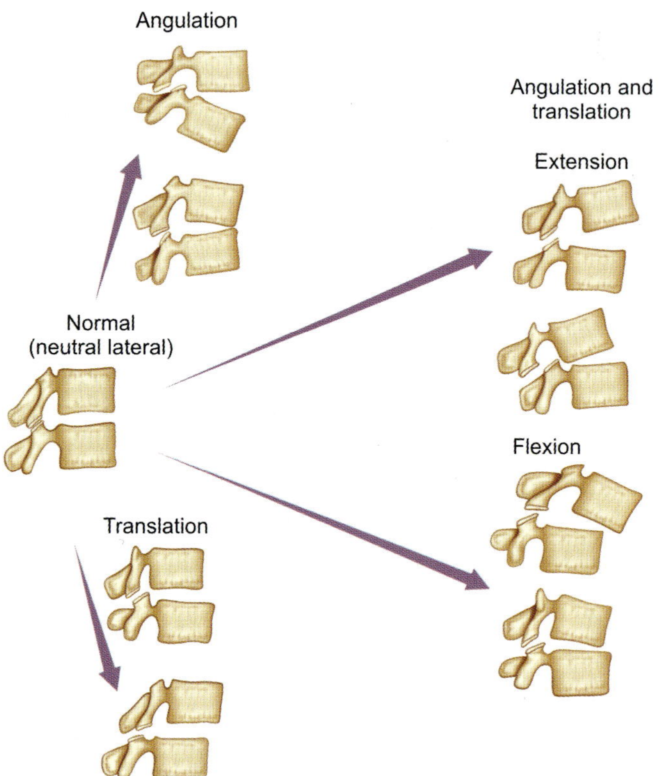

Fig. 29.6 Schematic illustration of the various developmental phases and types of sagittal spinal instability

Presently, there is no reliable diagnostic test to identify rotational instability in its earlier phase, although the manifestation of pain on axial rotation is highly suggestive of this condition. Again, it is known that dynamic CT scans under truncal twist are useful in the diagnosis of the rotational instability(gapping signs of facet joint), and it is mandatory to have bending and twist X-rays of the unstressed and stressed lumbar spine[2]. During surgery, it can also be measured by using a measuring gauge such as A-P and lateral angular motions and rotatory motion.

The diagnosis of stenosis in the unstable spine depends mainly on clinical symptoms, and it can be further proven by myelogram, CT myelogram and MRI.

A CT scan in rotation (twist test) demonstrates opening of one posterior facet joint (gapping) with dynamic recurrent spinal nerve entrapment.[2]

MRI of the lumbar spine demonstrates (i) the state of discal hydration (discal involution), (ii) subchondral marrow changes adjacent to a degenerative disk, and (iii) facets joint fluid. That is, signs of diskal dehydration at T2 indicate discal involution. An oblong white mirror image in the subchondral marrow at T1 image indicates fat degeneration, and a hyperclear band in the subchondral area at T2 indicates the presence of hydrated inflammatory elements. It is reported that 20% of discal involutions are accompanied by the afore-mentioned MRI signs, and that

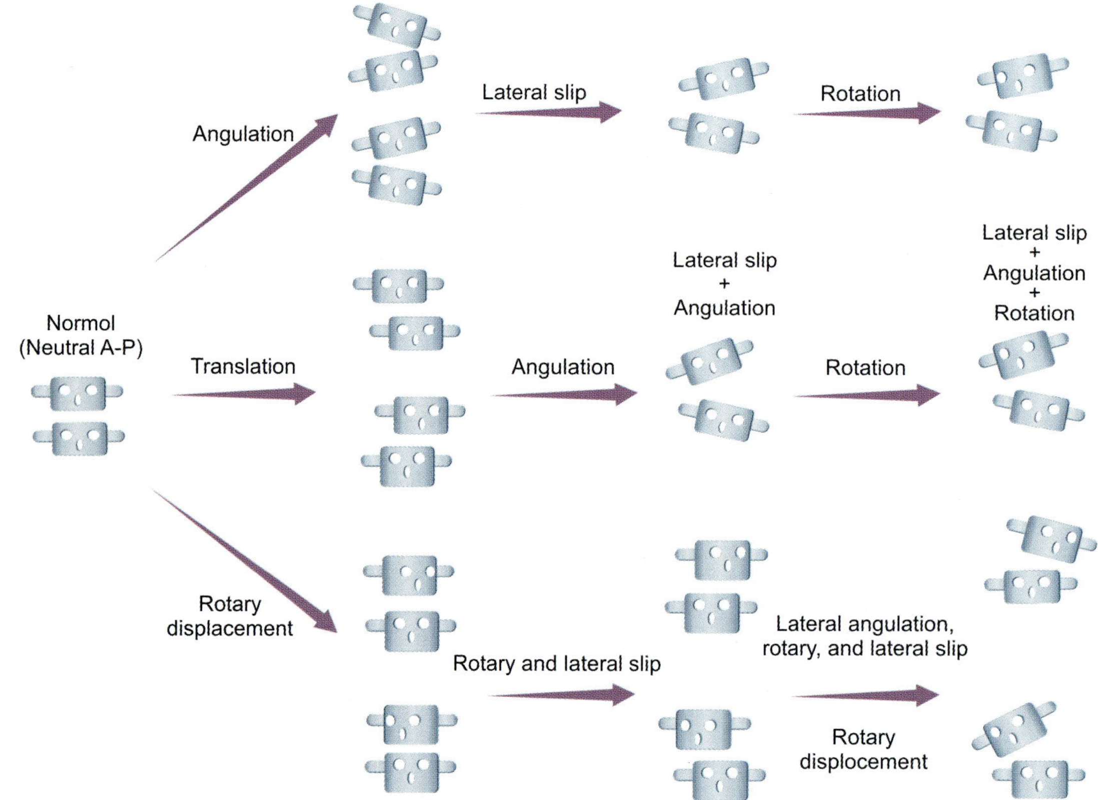

Fig. 29.7 Evolutional processes of segmental spinal instability in coronal plane

Rotatory displacement		Rotatory and lateral slip		Rotatory and lateral angulation and lateral slip	
Right	Left	Right	Left	Right	Left

Fig. 29.8 Various types of angular, rotatory, translational, and combined vertebral displacements in coronal plane

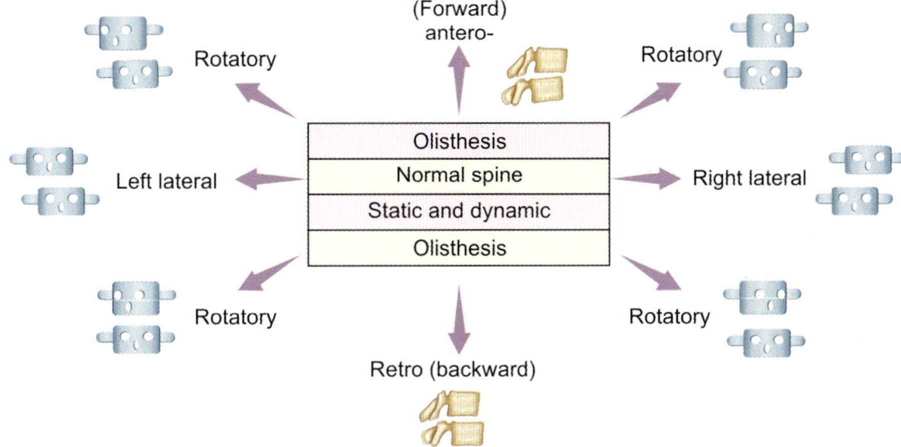

Fig. 29.9 Various types of dynamic and static olisthesis in sagittal and coronal planes

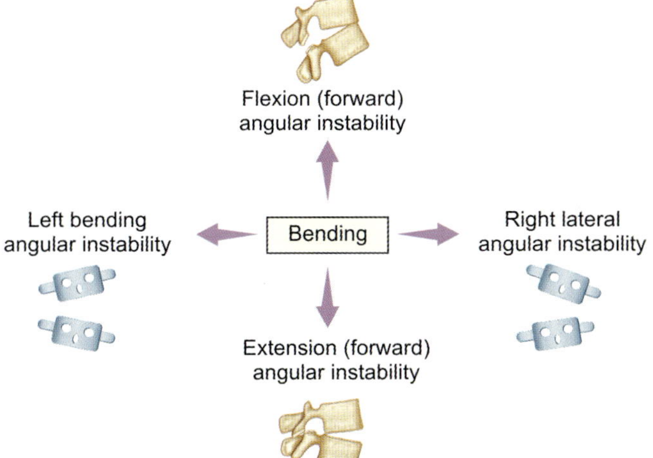

Fig. 29.10 Various types of angular instability in sagittal and coronal planes

for patients with these signs, instability was accompanied. However, when these signs were not accompanied with discal involution, gapping of the facets were not noted. Thus, changes on MRI may accompany spinal instability, but are not conclusive because these abnormal findings are the secondary products of instability, and change with time.[15]

Prognosticating Factors of Instability

Prognosis of instability depends on its natural course. Prognosis is generally good if signs of symptom relief and radiological improvement can be observed during the natural course of stabilization. Clinical symptoms should gradually subside towards the end stage of instability when the static equilibrium is reached. Radiologically, gradural decrease of motion should be demonstrated with the stress test, with no further collapse of disk height. Formation of anterior or lateral bony buttress should be seen in the upper margin of the lower vertebral body. If hypermobile segment is spontaneously stabilized by static equilibrium at the end stage of instability, prognosis will be good. But prognosis will be poor if it is not stabilized. Moreover, prognosis depends generally on age and sex, severity of disk degeneration, bony and facet configuration and defect, shape of spurs (traction and claw), lumbosacral angle, height of L4 in regards to the intercrestal line, and pelvic incidence.

In summary, the stabilizing symptoms and signs of the unstable segment can be listed as follows;

1. Gradual spontaneous relief of clinical symptom is experienced.
2. As radiological stabilizing signs: (i) gradual decrease of motion by stress test, (ii) no further collapse of disk height or body, (iii) growth of anterior or lateral bony spurs (buttress formation) in the upper margin of lower body can be listed.[15]

The above listed clinical symptom relief and radiological signs suggest the spontaneous or natural stabilization of the persistent symptomatic unstable motion segment.

Treatment

In general the treatment of a person with painful unstable back remains poorly defined, and also there is still disagreement as to when surgery is indicated in the management of pain that is thought to be arising from spinal structures. Stabilization surgery should not be done to treat low back pain of unproven origin under the diagnosis of unstable low back (Figs 29.11, 29.12, and 29.18).

In the unstable lumbar spine, if there is persistent disabling low back pain, or any evidence of deteriorating instability and/or no signs of spontaneous stabilization, the segment should be stabilized by brace or through mobility restriction or elimination surgery. Nonoperative treatment must last a sufficient time to determine adequately the course of treatment and the patient's clinical response (Fig. 29.11).[9-11,16,17,25]

Any types of conservative treatment of the unstable lumbar spine without stenotic signs should be directed at decreasing the stress on the unstable segment with the desired outcome of preventing deterioration and reducing pain. Time alone will reduce hypermobility, and contribute in providing lasting stability. The most harmful motion appears to be rotation, since it produces both compression and shear. The patient should reduce such activities as shoveling, lifting, gardening and playing sports such as handball, squash, tennis, and cycling. Posture should be improved (Table 29.4).

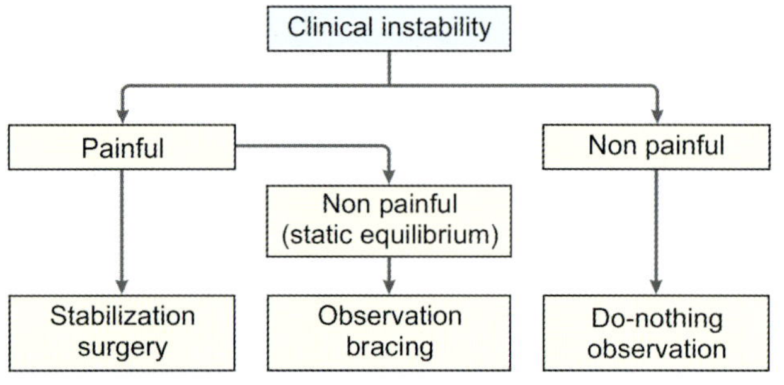

Fig. 29.11 Treatment chart of clinical instability

Table 29.4 Posture and exercise suggestions for patients without stenotic symptoms

- Avoid activities, such as shoveling, lifting and gardening
- Avoid sports, such as handball, squash, tennis, and cycling
- Avoid standing on one leg, as it produces asymmetrical stress on the pelvis and spine
- Isometric, abdominal and low back exercise that work primarily on the 'deep muscles of the back/the multifidus' stabilize the back and improve balance. These exercises are best done on exercise mats
- Physiotherapy with a back muscle training program and lifting technique training are beneficial.

Standing on one leg should be discouraged because it produces asymmetrical stress on the pelvis and spine. Obesity generally occurs about the abdomen, thus increasing the lordotic strain in men, whereas in women increased weight is more evenly distributed.

Isometric abdominal and low back exercises work primarily on the "the deep muscles of back multifidus" which stabilize the back to maintain balance. These exercises for multifidus are best done on exercise mats.

The athlete with weak back should improve his technique or change his working posture in order to relieve the clinical symptoms, and also should improve his back muscles by comprehensive training which should be included in all training programs.

The doctor may prescribe physiotherapy with a back muscle program, and give advice on lifting technique, and so on.

Surgical Management

Surgery is indicated whenever a program of active nonoperative treatment fails.

Facet rhizotomy to relieve back pain is contraindicated because it denervates the multifidus and increases the hypermobility and instability. Stabilization surgery for the symptomatic unstable spine is solely directed towards restoration to a normal spine. However, surgery should be based on the normalization of the spine-spinal nerve relationships: stabilization of the spinal unit in addition to the restoration of normal alignment (correction of deformity), and/or nerve decompression (Fig. 29.12).

Stabilization surgery consists of three categories: (i) mobility maintenance, (ii) mobility restriction, and (iii) motion eradication surgeries.

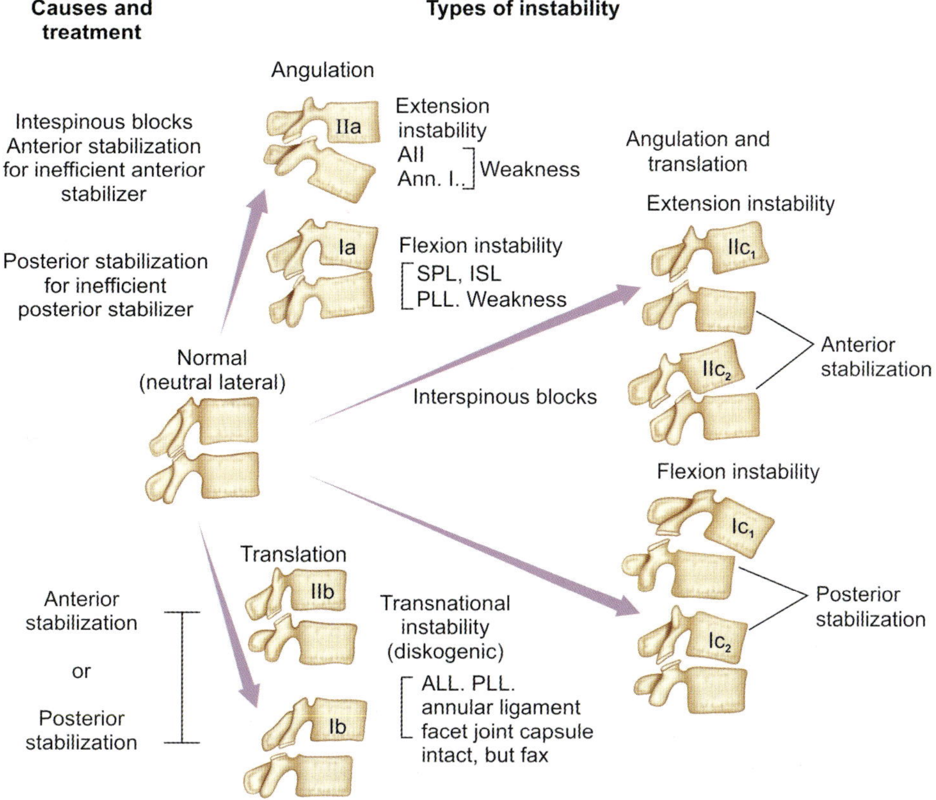

Fig. 29.12 Various types of sagittal instability; its progress and treatment.
- "I" indicates the flexion instability, and "II" indicates the extension instability.
- "a" indicates angular difference, while "b" indicates the pure translational instability.
- "c" indicates the combined angular and translational instability: "c_1" indicates anterior slip, while "c_2" indicates posterior slip

The first one is the normal mobility maintenance surgery such as repairing the isthmic defect. Second one is the motion restriction surgery utilizing the tension band dynamic pedicle screw system [ligamentoplasty (Graf's procedure), Dynamic Neutralization System for the Spine (Dynesys), Fulcrum Assissted Soft Stabilization System (FASS), or Mochida et al. osseous Keio-Leed's ligamentoplasty (Tokai University)] (Figs 29.12 and 29.18).[9-11] Also, recently, the following devices, such as semi-rigid Rod Dynamic Pedicle Screw Systems {(Isobon TTL, AccuFlex, CS-Horizon Agile, Stabilimax NZ, Bioflex Spring Rod pedicle screw system, Truedyne PDS, Cosmic posterior Dynamic system, Dynamic Stabilization system (DSS), NFlip)} (Fig. 29.18) are introduced. The third one is the rigid stabilization— osseous fusion (Figs 29.2, 29.4, 29.5, 29.19, and 29.20).[15]

In patients having unstable back with symptomatic stenosis the symptoms should be relieved by any means — conservatively or surgically. Nerve decompression surgery consists of laminotomy, foramenotomy, the combined extensive laminectomy and foramenotomy and facetectomy, laminoplasty, and finally, *in situ* or post-reduction fusion.

In cases of instability associating the stenosis regardless of its cause, treatment of stenosis should be done prior to the management of instability. The sites of root compression in isthmic and degenerative spondylolisthesis are different; the exiting spinal root is compressed beneath the isthmus in isthmic spondylolisthesis, and the root is compressed at the central canal in degenerative spondylolisthesis. Thus, in isthmic spondylolisthesis L4 root is compressed at L4–5 and L5 root at L5–S1 disk level, while in degenerative spondylolisthesis L5 root at L4–5 and S1 root at L5–S1 disk level.

For dynamic stenosis the distraction–flexion or distraction-extension fusion without decompressive laminectomy can theoretically relieve stenotic symptoms (Fig. 29.16). However, flexion–distraction fusion is not preferred, because it malaligns the sagittal lumbar curvature (flat back).

In static stenosis, decompressive foramenotomy, laminotomy, laminectomy, and combined laminectomy and facetectomy should be done first, and then stabilization surgery should be followed. In cases of nonhypermobile instability with steonsis, extensive decompressive laminectomy and/or

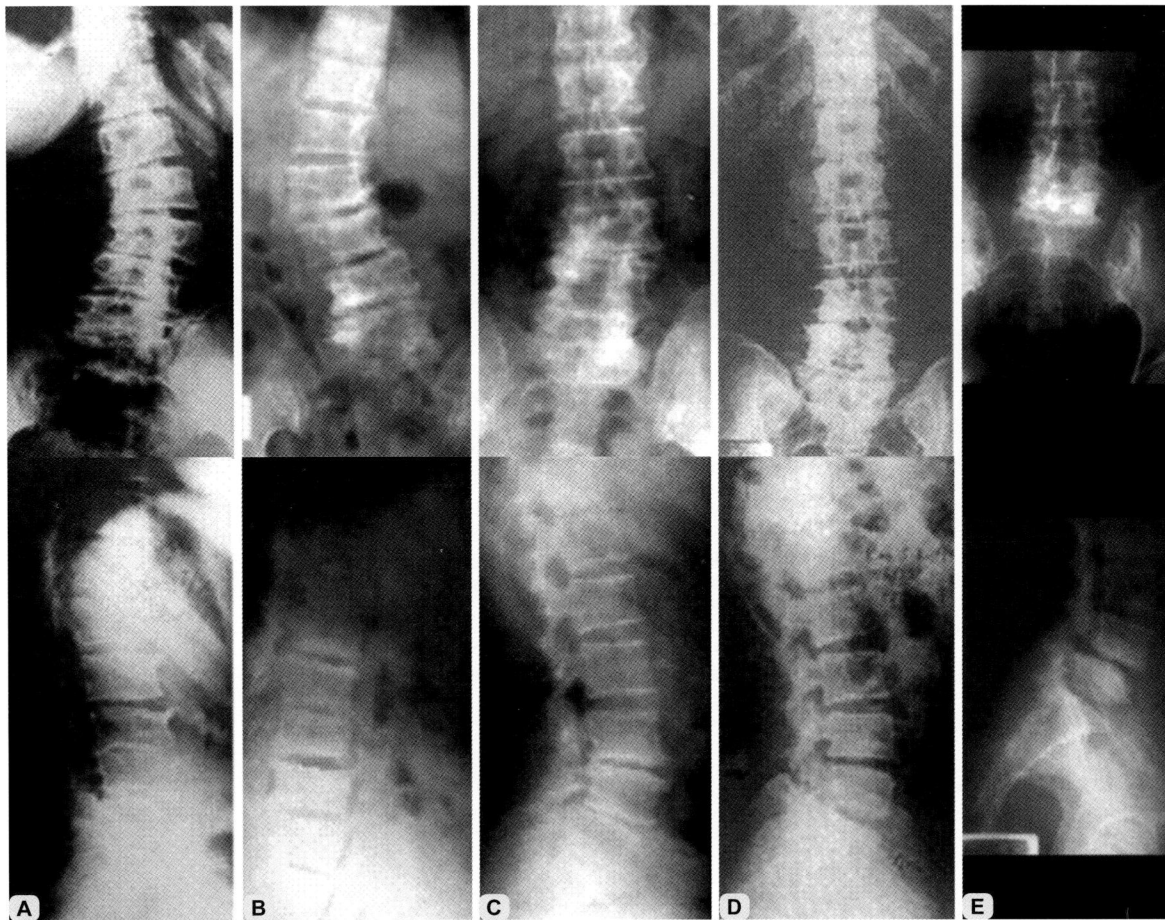

Fig. 29.13 Examples of different types of lumbar scoliosis with lateral rotatory slips. (A) Idiopathic scoliosis with hyperlordosis and L3 lateral rotatory slip; (B) Degenerative scoliosis with L3 lateral rotatory slip with loss of lordosis; (C) Post-laminectomy mono-segmental scoliosis with advanced disk degeneration at L3–4 and L4–5, and anterior slip of L4; (D) A case of isthmic spondylolisthesis showing mono-segment (L4–5) degenerative scoliosis with pure left lateral slip of L4. There is no vertebral rotation; (E) A case of grade I L4 isthmic spondylolisthesis showing scoliosis with vertebral rotation

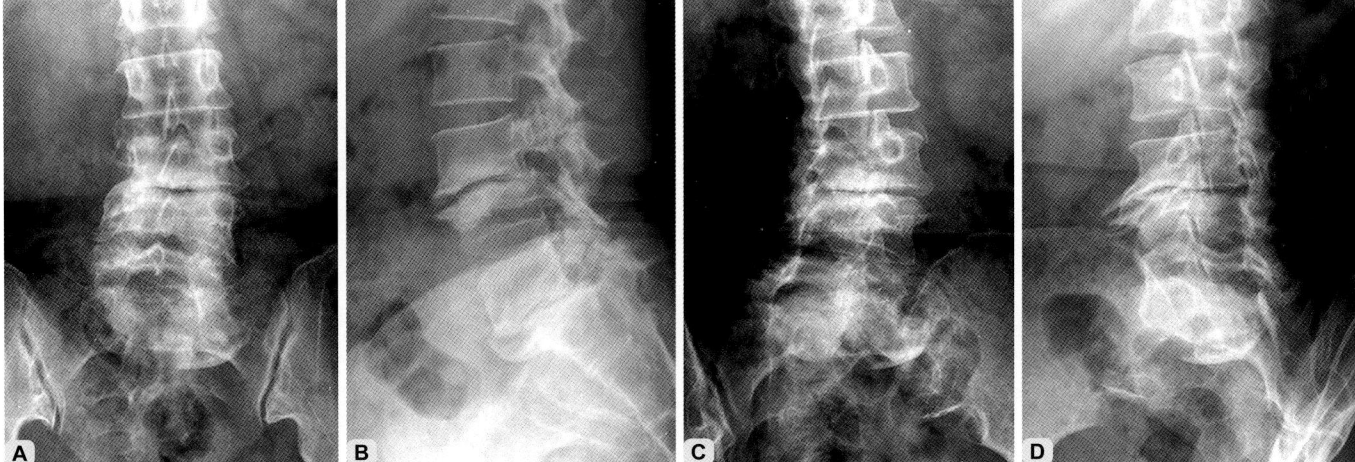

Fig. 29.14 Degenerative lumbar scoliosis associating with isthmic spondylolisthesis at L3–4 and L5–S1 in a 62 year-old lady. Well-formed anterior bony buttress on the anterosuperior margin of S1, indicating the stability of the segment. Advanced disk degeneration and spur formation are seen at L3–4

facetectomy should be combined with stabilization surgery, because extensive decompressive surgery destabilizes further the unstable segment.

Stabilization Surgery

Instrument-aided stabilization of the symptomatic unstable spine alone cannot relieve pain completely in every case, though stabilization is generally expected to relieve pain completely. Also it is difficult to treat preexisting neuropathic pain by spinal stabilization surgery alone, though trauma-related unstable back with musculoskeletal pain can be relieved by it.

Stabilization Surgery for Sagittal Instability

Motion Preservation Surgery

This is a surgical procedure to repair the isthmic defect by direct osteosynthesis with screwing and/or wiring and bone grafts (Table 29.5).

Motion Restriction Surgery (Nonfusion stabilization)

Restriction surgery reduces normal range of motion of the affected segment (Table 29.6).

Forward Flexion Instability

Since last two decades for the dynamic lumbar instability two categories of stabilizing devices were introduced; (i) tension band dynamic pedicle screw system and (ii) semi-rigid rod dynamic pedicle screw systems.

Table 29.5 Motion-preserving stabilization surgeries

1. Direct osteosynthesis of lytic isthmus with screwing and bone graft
2. Scott wiring for direct repair
3. Combined stabilization surgery

Table 29.6 Motion-restriction surgeries

Type of instability	*Procedure*
Flexion instability	Ligamentoplasty 1. Graf's procedure 2. Mochida's procedure
Extention instability	1. Interspinous process decompression devices extension block spacer (Coflex, Wallis, Diam, X-stop) 2. Dynessy dynamic stabilizer

a. *Ligamentoplasty procedures:* There are two ligamentoplasty procedures:
   i. *Graf's ligamentoplasty procedure:* Graf's band fixation procedure is the re-enforcement surgery for inefficient posterior stabilizer and serves as tension band (Table 29.6, Figs 29.12 and 29.18).[2,13,23] It aims to suppress firstly excess flexion, and secondly rotation by apposing the facet joints in lordosis. Complete unroofing of the lateral canal in case of lateral canal stenosis is mandatory, because bandaging causes extension and compression of the applied segment, and again makes the neural foramen narrower. As an ideal band application pressure, Graf recommended 75 Newtons of pressure. This Graf procedure should be indicated only for the pure forward flexion instability, and should not be indicated in the presence of extension instability secondary to anterior stabilizer inefficiency or failure, and facet defect.
      This posterior stabilization by the pre-stressed flexible ring ligaments makes gapping of facet joints

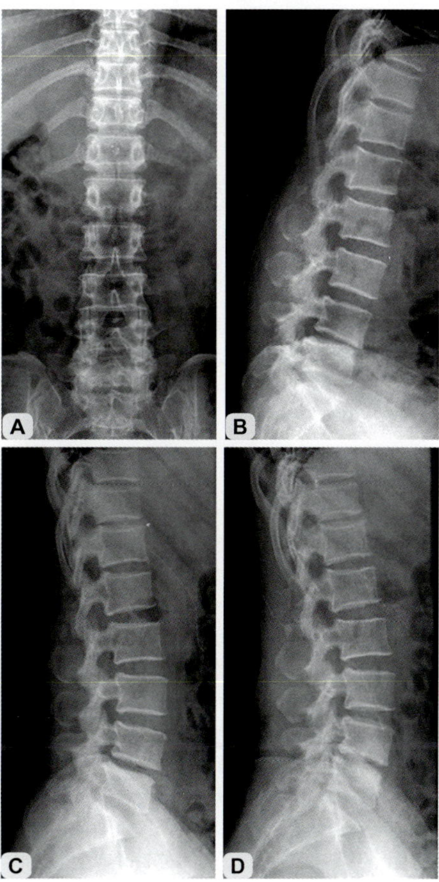

Fig. 29.15 An example of reducible degenerative antelisthesis of 4–5, grade I (flexion angular and forward translational instability)

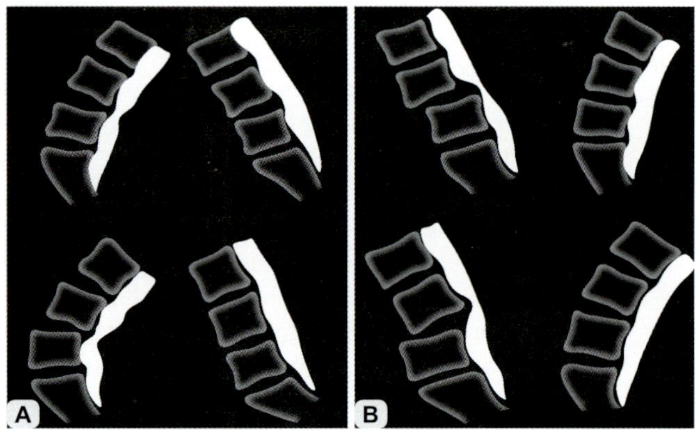

Fig. 29.16 Simple extension/flexion radiograms showing reducible anterolisthesis, and extension/flexion myelograms showing dynamic stenosis. (A) Dynamic stenosis in extension; (B) Dynamic stenosis in flexion

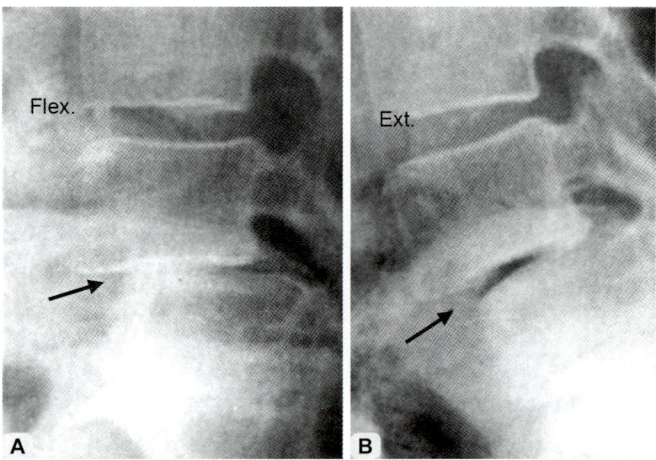

Fig. 29.17 An example of Knuttson sign. Vacuum disappears (A) on flexion, and (B) appears on extension

impossible which is the source of most of the pain felt by the patients. It also restores lumbar lordosis which repositions the stabilized joint away from rotative mechanical aggression, but at the present time, the main concern must be the long-term fate of the ligaments. It is again stressed that Graf's ring ligament fixation should not be indicated for cases which present anterior, posterior and rotatory corporal translation with posterior angulation.[14,16]

ii. *Mochida et al. posterior ligamentoplasty:* Artificial (Keio-Leed) ligaments are used instead of instruments to stabilize the posterior element through the iatrogenically made bony tunnel in the posterior part of vertebral body just in front of the posterior wall and both pedicle holes.[9,10] In the procedure the ligament fixation area is too close to the spinal flexion axis, and provision of proper ligament tension is also a problem. Therefore, it is believed that it does not help much in reinforcing the inefficient posterior stabilizer. Also material creep may be a problem in providing the long-lasting posterior stability without failure as in the Graf's band ligamentoplasty.[2,11,16,23]

b. *Semirigid rod dynamic pedicle screw systems:* In this system, rigid rods with associated hinge, springs or bumpers are used to allow for longitudinal component (rod) movement.

Backward Extension Instability

For extension instability in sagittal plane causing extension dynamic stenosis, interspinous decompression devices (Coflex, Wallis, Diam and X-stop) are now available for stabilization (Fig. 29.16).[8,14,16,24,26] However, this surgery is indicated only when the posterior spinal elements are maintained intact. Dynessy dynamic posterior stabilization (fulcrum assisted soft stabilization) system is also available to replace the interspinous implants in cases of the posterior element defect. These devices prevent further extension of the instrumented segment from its neutral position in the sagittal plane. This helps maintain a wider foraminal space and prevent the development of symptoms secondary to dynamic extension stenosis of the affected segment, but almost does not give effect in flexion, lateral bending and axial rotation. However, the inclusion criteria for this technique, proposed by Zuckerman et al. are that pain had to be relieved during flexion and the patients had to be able to walk fifty feet (15.2 meters).[26] It is as yet a matter of debate which patients with spinal claudication can be managed with this technique as opposed to requiring foraminal decompression. As yet there exist three unanswered questions for this technique: time-related clinical outcome, survivorship of the device, and chronological effect of the device on the disk of the implanted segment.

Motion Elimination Surgery (Fusion) for Sagittal Instability

In stabilization surgery, the basic principle should be considered (Table 29.7). There are two mobile columns in the spine: anterior and posterior columns. In the anterior column, the movement is transferred through the disk in relation to its elastic deformity, while in the posterior column the movement is transferred through the facet joints. Thus, both elements serve together to maintain the spinal integrity by load-sharing.

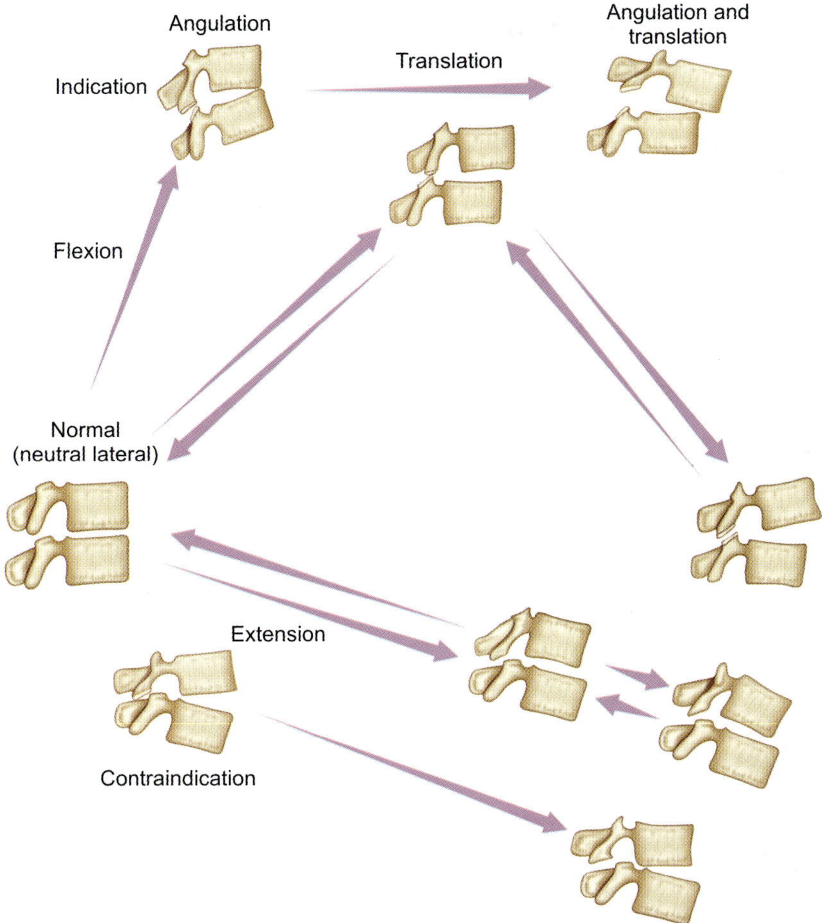

Fig. 29.18 Indications and contraindication of Graf ring ligament stabilization

The architecture of the spine is constructed so as to resist anteriorly against compression and torque forces, and posteriorly against tension force.

The muscles and ligaments act posteriorly in the sense of compression. This means that posterior instrumentation has to act as a compressive device (tension band). Therefore, recently it is suggested by some surgeons that a secure fusion requires a combined anterior and posterior instrumented stabilization (Table 29.7).[18]

Table 29.7 Motion-elimination surgeries

1. Posterior stabilization surgery
   - Posterior fusion (± posterior instrumentation)
   - Posterolateral fusion (± posterior instrumentation)
   - Posterior interbody fusion
   - Transforaminal interbody fusion
2. Anterior stabilization surgery
   - Anterior interbody fusion ± anterior instrumentation
3. Combined anterior and posterior fusion ± anterior and/or posterior instrumentation.

a. *Posterior procedures:*
   1. Posterior fusion (PF).
   2. Posterolateral fusion (PLF) with or without posterior instrumentation.
   3. Posterior lumbar interbody fusion (PLIF) or posterior transforaminal lumbar interbody fusion (TLIF) with or without posterior instrumentation

   Posterolateral fusion (PLF) and posterior lumbar interbody fusion with or without posterior instrumentation are the most popular procedures (Figs 29.4, 29.5, 29.19, and 29.20). Derotation facet fusion (Farfan) is indicated for the axial rotatory instability.[16]

b. *Anterior procedure* (anterior lumbar interbody fusion (ALIF) with or without instrumentation): Both *insitu* and post-reduction fusions are the well accepted procedure for the oligosegmental spinal disorders with instability[12]. In cases of sagittal translational instability without neurological symptoms, ALIF is one of the methods (Fig. 29.2).

Axial rotatory instability: Derotation facet fusion is enough because derotation alone may decompress the nerve roots. However, now there are trends to stabilize the unstable segment by derotation facet fusion which is

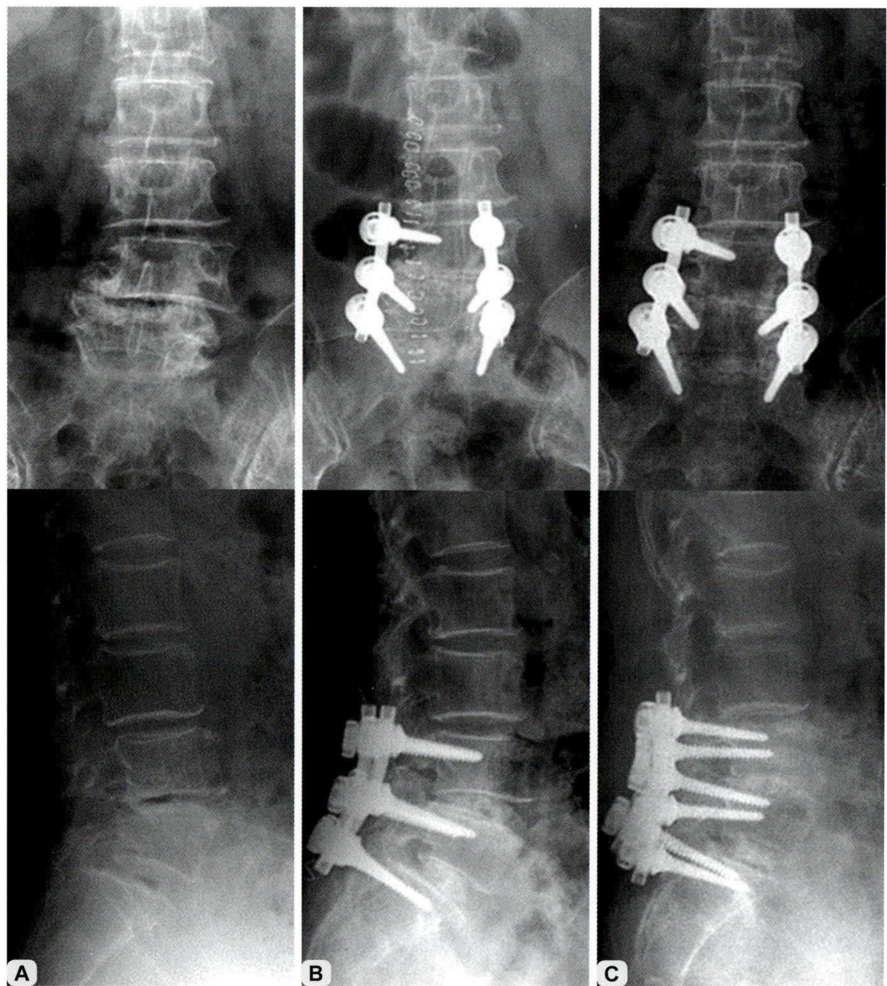

Fig. 29.19 An example of symptomatic oligosegmental degenerative scoliosis of lower lumbar type with lateral rotatory slip of L4. (A) Initial; (B) Immediate postoperatively; (C) Postoperatively one month

usually supplemented by transverse process fusion and instrumented stabilization.

Stabilization Surgery for Degenerative Lumbar Kyphosis with Instability

Degenerative lumbar kyphosis infrequently associates the spondylolisthesis. However, stabilization surgery confined only to the olisthetic segment is contraindicated. The instrument-aided surgery should aim primarily to restore the sagittally malaligned lumbar spine to normal (>35° lordosis), and the olisthetic segment should be included in the instrument-aided deformity correction and stabilization.

Stabilization Surgery for Coronal Instability

Coronal instability is frequently seen in patients with degenerative lumbar scoliosis (DLS), and less frequently in the other spinal disorders (Figs 29.7 to 29.10, 29.13, 29.14, and 29.19)

The DLS differs from adult idiopathic scoliosis, because there is minimal structural vertebral deformity, advanced degenerative change, and a lower lumbar curve. Radiologically, there are two main types—oligosegmental and polysegmental. Those patients present clinically back pain, spinal deformity with body tilt and rotatory vertebral slip and/or stenotic symptoms. Treatment of DLS aims primarily at alleviation of symptoms such as radicular pain by any means—conservative or surgical. The primary aims of surgery are to relieve pain by decompression of the compressed nerve root and secondly to stabilize the unstable segments after curve correction, and finally to improve spinal function.

There are two types of fusion operation according to the clinical types—multisegmental and oligosegmental fusion procedures.

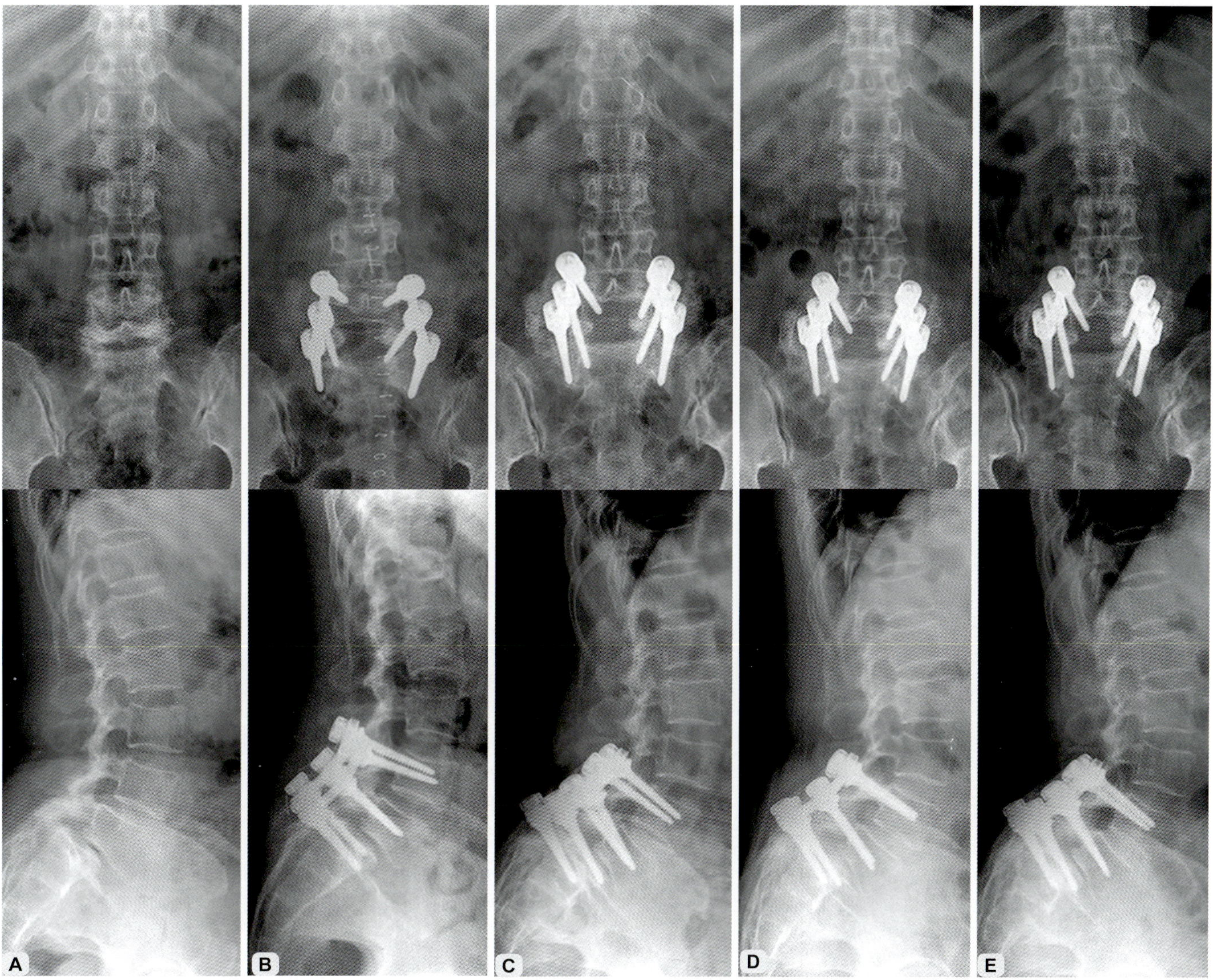

Fig. 29.20 An example of two level degenerative spondylolisthesis of L4–5 and L5–S1 which was treated by posterior pedicle screw *in-situ* stabilization and PLF

In case of symptomatic progressive DLS without stenotic symptoms, fusion supplemented by internal fixation after complete correction of coronal deformity together with the sagittal alignment is most appropriate. Fusion of the scoliotic spine without deformity correction is not recommended, because undercorrection of coronal deformity complicates the early development of junctional instability in most of the cases.

In summary, for the painful oligosegmental DLS without rotation and stenotic symptoms (localized to lower one or two joints), ALIF is preferably recommended.[16] For stable nonprogressive polysegmental DLS with stenotic symptoms decompression surgery alone is recommended, while for the unstable DLS with stenotic symptoms instrumented stabilization of the entire scoliotic segment after complete decompression and deformity correction is essential. The current clinical issue in DLS surgery is the extent of stabilization surgery; upto L1, T10, T6 and/or down to S1 (Fig. 29.21).

Nerve Decompression Surgery for Stenosis

I. Extension instability and extension dynamic stenosis: For this condition interspinous decompression devices and Dynesys dynamic neutralization system are now available (Table 29.8 and Fig. 29.19).[8]

II. Posterior decompression involving the posterior unroofing of central and/or lateral canal:

Table 29.8 Nerve decompression procedures

- Interspinous process decompression devices
- Laminotomy
- Foraminotomy
- Combined extensive laminectomy and foraminotomy
- Facetectomy
- *In situ* or post-reduction fusion

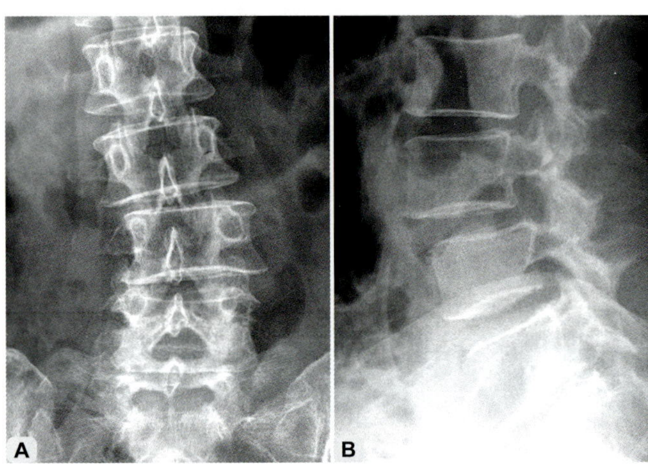

Fig. 29.21 An example of degenerative lumbar scoliosis with multi-segment involvement in a 53 year-old lady. Lateral rotatory slip of L2 and anterior slip of L3 are seen

As yet it is the procedure of choice for unstable degenerative lumbar spine with stenotic symptoms regardless of the associating deformity. However, since this procedure destabilizes the spine further, it should be combined with stabilization surgery.

III. Anterior decompressive corpectomy: This procedure is generally not indicated in the treatment of unstable lumbar spine with stenosis. However, even for the static stenosis anterior lumbar interbody fusion alone can reduce and realign the slipped vertebra, and restore the stability and finally relieve stenotic symptoms (Fig. 29.2).[12] Recently anterior fusion cage with screw fixation system is available for this condition.[16]

IV. Posterior instrument-aided reduction: For the lateral and vertical displacements (migration) this procedure restores the central canal size and spinal alignment, thereby effectively decompress the entrapped nerves. However, decompression may not always be achieved completely with this procedure.

V. Fusion in distraction-flexion or in distraction-extension: This procedure effectively relieves the symptoms of dynamic stenosis and also provides stability.[14] The position of fusion is important in relieving symptoms. In cases of L5 retrolisthetic instability, which is frequently associated with symptoms of central canal stenosis affecting S1 nerve root, fusion in flexion (distraction rods or pedicle fixation devices and facet fusion) is the most logical approach to this lesion. In general, as adjuncts to spinal fusion, an internal fixation system should be used to stabilize the fusion segment and to maintain the fusion position.

Conclusion

Unstable segment should be stabilized surgically if conservative management fails. Stabilization surgery should aim at the alleviation of pain. Assessment of type of instability is essential for surgical management. However, the effort should be paid to preserve the motion if possible. Selection of stabilization surgery should be based on the type of clinical instability and its clinical symptoms and signs.

Stabilization surgery can be categorized into three:

1. Motion preservation (full motion maintenance) surgery,
2. Motion restriction surgery, and
3. Motion elimination surgery.

References

1. Dvorak J. Panjabi M, Chang D. Functional radiographic diagnosis of the lumbar spine - Flexion, extension and lateral bending. Spine. 1991;165:562-71.
2. Graf H. Instabilite vertebrale. Treatment a 1'aide d'un system soule. Rachis;1992.
3. Hadley L. Apophyseal subluxation. J. Bone Joint Surg. 1936; 18:428.
4. Kirkaldy-Willis WH, Farfan HF. Instability of the lumbar spine. Clin Orthop. 1982; 165:110-23.
5. Knuttson F. The instability associated with disk degeneration in the lumbar spine. Acta Radiol. 1944;25:593.
6. Lin JF, MS Moon. Symptomatic vacuum phenomenon of the lumbar disc. In: Bhave A (Ed): Emerging techniques in spine surgery. New Delhi, Jaypee Brothers; pp. 240-9.
7. Luk KDK, Chow DHK, Halmes A. Vertical instability in spondylolisthesis: a traction radiographic assessment technique and the principle of management. Spine. 2003; 28:819-27.
8. Minns RJ, Walsh WK: Preliminary design and experimental studies of a novel soft implant for correcting sagittal plane instability in the lumbar spine. Spine 1977; 22(16): 1819-25.
9. Mochida J, Toh E, Suzuki K, et al. An innovative method using the Leeds-Keio artificial ligament in the unstable spine. Orthop. 1997; 20(1):17-23.
10. Mochida J. Suzuki K, Chiba M. How to stabilize a single level lesion of degenerative lumbar spondylolisthesis. Clin Orthop. 1999;308:126-34.
11. Moon MS: Treatment of unstable lumbar spine with Graf band system. presented at 19th World Congress, SICOT, 1993.

12. Moon MS, Kim SS, Sun DH, Moon YW. Anterior spondylodesis for spondylolisthesis; isthmic and degenerative type. European Spine J.1994;3:172-6.
13. Moon MS, Moon YW, Moon JL, Kim SS, Shim YS. Treatment of flexion instability of lumbar spine with Graf band. J. Musculoskelet Res. 1999; 3(1):49-63.
14. Moon MS, Moon JL, Kim KW: Letter to editor 25:1739-41. 2000; for Minns RJ, Walsh WK, Spine, 1997;22:1819-25.
15. Moon MS: Unstable lumbar spine : Diagnosis and assessment. Med, Progress. 2006;386-9.
16. Moon MS. Unstable lumbar spine: Management. Med Progress. 2006;390-4.
17. Newman PH. Surgical management of derangement of the lumbar spine. J Bone Joint Surg Br. 1973; 55(1):7-19.
18. Oda I, Abumi K, Yu BS, Sudo H, Minami A. Type of spinal instability that require interbody support in posterior lumbar reconstruction – An in vitro biomechanical investigation. Spine 2003; 28:1573-80.
19. Panjabi MM, Goel RK, Takata K. Physiologic strains in the lumbar spinal ligaments : an in vitro biomechanical study. Spine. 1982;7:192.
20. Pearcy M and Sheperd J. Is there instability in spondylolisthesis. Spine. 1985;10: 175.
21. Pope M, Panjab M. Biomechanical definitions of spinal instability. Spine. 1985; 10:255-6.
22. Pope M, Frymoyer JW, Krag MH. Diagnosing instability. Clin Orthop. 1992; 279: 60-7.
23. Strauss PJ, Novotmy JE, Wilder DG, Grosler LJ, Pope MH. Multidirectional stability of the Graf system. Spine. 1994; 19: 965-972.
24. Wilke HJ, Drumm J, Haussler K, Mack C, Steuolel WI, Kettleer A. Biomechanical effect of different lumbar interspinous implants on flexibility and intradiscal pressure. Eur. Spine J. 2008; 17: 1049-56.
25. Wiltse LL, Winter RB. Terminology and measurement of spondylolisthesis. J Bone Joint Surg. 1983; 65A: 768.
26. Zucherman JF, Hsu KY, Hartjen CA, Mehalic TF, Implicito DA, Martin MJ, et al. A multicentre, prospective, randomized trial evaluating the x-stop interspinous process decompression system for the treatment of neurogenic intermittent claudication: two-year follow-up results. Spine. 2005; 30: 1355-58.

CHAPTER

30

Lateral Access to the L5–S1 and Adjacent Disks by Retracting the Psoas Muscle

Jin-Fu Lin

Introduction

Lateral access for lumbar interbody fusion becomes popular recently due to claimed advantages of less traumatic feature by accessing the lumbar discs between the important posterior (muscles, nerves) and anterior (vessels) structures, when compared to posterior and anterior lumbar interbody fusion (PLIF and ALIF).[1] Nowadays, lateral access usually uses trans-psoas route by piercing through, dissecting, and dilating the psoas muscle to expose the lateral disk. Several terminologies have been used by different investigators to describe the same method: extreme lateral interbody fusion (XLIF),[2] lateral lumbar interbody fusion (LLIF),[4] lateral trans-psoas interbody fusion (LTIF) and direct lateral interbody fusion (DLIF).[5]

Despite the increasing popularity of lateral trans-psoas access (LTA), but it has two major shortcomings. First, trans-psoas has the potential risk of injuring the lumbar nerves, which reside inside the psoas muscle and neuromonitoring is required to avoid the insult;[6-12] second, trans-psoas cannot access the L5–S1 level laterally, one of the most common disks needs fusion, due to obstruction by the pelvis,[13-16] and requires a traditional access.

In this report, we describe our method of lateral access to the lumbar disks, including the L5–S1 level by retracting instead of piercing the psoas muscle; the specific anatomical issues and complications for accessing the L5–S1 level are also discussed.

Materials and Methods

We reviewed the medical records in patients who underwent lateral lumbar interbody fusion between 2002 and 2010, and there were 55 patients receiving 1- to 3-level lateral fusion including the L5–S1 level; those without L5–S1 level fusion were excluded. There were 15 males and 40 females with a mean age 61.7 years (range 28–82), and with a mean follow-up period of 24.6 months (range 10–54 months). Among them, 38 patients were of one level (L5–S1) and 17 patients were either 2- or 3-level fusion (L4–5 and L5–S1, or L3–4 to L5–S1). The surgical indications were degenerative disorders (n = 51), pyogenic L5–S1 diskitis (n = 2), and failed prior L5–S1 ALIF (n = 2).

Twenty eight patients (50.9%) required posterior decompression, and singlestand- alone rectangular titanium cage was used in 53 patients (using graft only in 2 cases of diskitis). A mean of 7.5 mL bone graft (auto- or allograft, range, 5–16 mL) was used for one disc level. Left flank approach was used in 50 patients (90.9%) and right approach in 5 patients (9.1%).

Surgical Technique

Long-handle and blunt-tipped tools are used; suction pressure and electrical current for thermal coagulation are reduced to a minimal working level. After general anesthesia, the patient is placed on prone position for decompression when indicated and autograft is harvested from the posterior iliac crest. The patient is then turned to true lateral decubitus position and firmly fixed.

Patient Positioning and Incision (Fig. 30.1)

The operating table is flexed at the lumbopelvic junction to open up the lateral disk space. The ipsilateral thigh is flexed to relax the psoas muscle. Before draping, the L4–5 and L5–S1 disk levels are marked on the skin using a lateral fluoscopic view.

After draping, the operator is standing in front of the patient. An oblique incision about 6–10 cm long is made, started from the anterior axilla line and about one-inch anterior to the iliac crest, then the abdominal muscles (external and internal) are bluntly dissected.

Entering the Retroperitoneal Cavity

The retroperitoneal cavity is entered by penetrating the posterior end of the third layer of abdominal muscle (transversus abdominis) which attaches to the quadratus lumborum. After entering the cavity, the psoas muscle is identified by sweeping away the covering retroperitoneal fat and then identifies the psoas and its anterior margin.

A malleable retractor is placed against the anterior longitudinal ligament (ALL) to separate and protect the soft organs (ureter, great vessels). The disk is searched by using the sucker head to palpate the vertebral column along the anterior margin of the psoas. After the protruded contour of the disc is palpated, a 2 mm Kirschner wire (K-wire) is hammered into the adjacent vertebra and the exact disk level is checked by taking a lateral fluoscopic view.

Identifying and Handling the Iliolumbar Vein (Fig. 30.2A)

The psoas muscle covering the cortex of L5 vertebra is then carefully dissected and retracted backward from the L4–5 disk and preceded distally to look for the iliolumbar vein (ILV) which tethering the common iliac vein (CIV). The tethered CIV usually traverses over the anterolateral aspect of the L5–S1 disk and renders lateral accessing to the disk impossible. Once the ILV has been divided the tethered CIV thereby can be mobilized away from the disk.

The ILV is usually located at the waist of the L5 vertebral body; once it is found, the vein is isolated by fixing the retracted the psoas with 2 K-wires, one above and one below the vein, to expose the whole length of ILV. Bipolar diathermy is preferred to coagulate the vein rather than suture-ligation because of convenience and safety. Before coagulating the ILV, a sucker head is gently pressing at the junction of ILV and CIV to stretch the ILV a little longer and also to shrink the ILV slightly narrower by reducing venous blood return from the CIV. The sucker head is also used to protect the CIV during bipolar coagulation. The mid-portion of the exposed ILV is then coagulated and divided using a No. 15 scalpel, and leaves a safe length of ILV stump connecting the CIV.

Protecting the Common Iliac Vein and Lateral Diskectomy (Fig. 30.2B)

After the ILV is divided, the big and thin-walled CIV is then carefully mobilized away from the L5 vertebral body and until the lower margin of the L5–S1 disk. The CIV is then protected by placing a malleable retractor against the ALL at the L5–S1 level. The lateral L5–S1 annulus is exposed by retracting the covering psoas and fixed *in situ* using two K-wires above the below the disk, and then starts lateral discectomy (Fig. 30.3).

L5 Lateral Wedge Osteotomy (Fig. 30.4)

Lateral distal L5 wedge osteotomy is a useful maneuver to improve working fields which are hindered by the overhang pelvis and in cases of narrowed disk or with osteophyte. However, sometimes the opposite 1/3 of disk space may

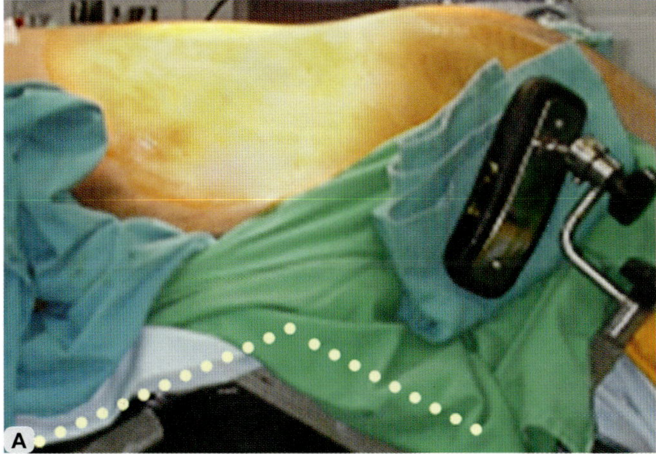

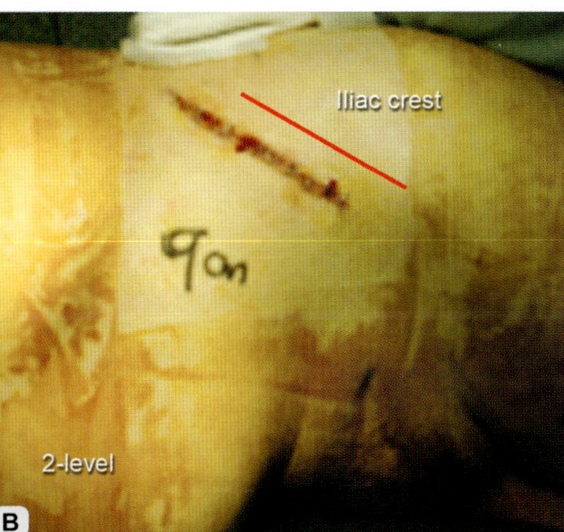

Fig. 30.1 (A) True lateral and table bended; (B) Oblique incision and 1 inch anterior to the iliac crest; 9 cm incision for 2 levels

not be approachable by the long-handle and angled tools due to obliquity of the L5–S1 disk space attributed by the overhang pelvis.

Hemostasis is performed after completing fusion procedure, venous bleeding usually can be stopped by compression using Gelfoam or Surgicel. After removing the K-wires, the wound is closed and no drainage is used.

In simultaneous 2- or 3-level fusion (Fig. 30.5), the L5–S1 fusion is usually performed firstly, because bleeding from other level may obscure the working field of L5–S1 level. L3–4 and L4–5 fusion is substantially easier and straightforward because there is no need to handle the venous system and the possible hindrance by the pelvis.

The sympathetic chain running at the anterolateral side of the lumbar column usually has to be severed in order to do lateral diskectomy.

After Care

Postoperatively, the oozed blood in the retroperitoneal cavity is estimated to be about 400 mL and hemoglobin level is routinely checked on the next morning. Paralytic ileus is expected to last 1–3 days. The patient is encouraged to ambulate using a walker as long as the wound pain is tolerable and wearing the lumbar brace is optional.

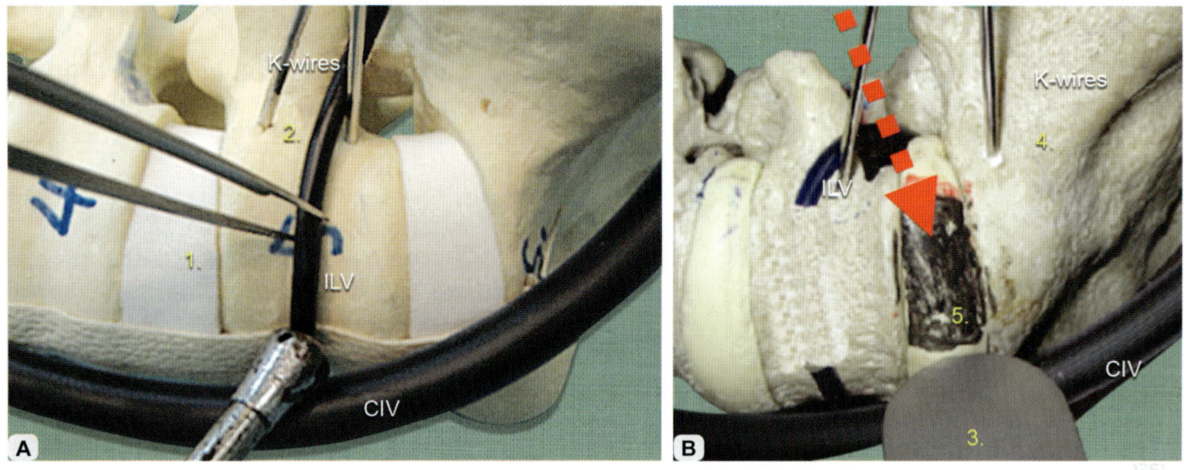

Fig. 30.2 (A) 1. Retract the psoa from L4–5 disk and fixed using K-wires. 2. The iliolumbar vein (ILV) is coagulated using bipolar diathermy at the portion well above the common iliac vein (CIV) then divided; (B) 3. Mobilize the CIV away from the disk. 4. Distal psoas is retracted and fixed. 5. Diskectomy behind the ALL while protecting the CIV (Red broken arrow indicates the direction of diskectomy)

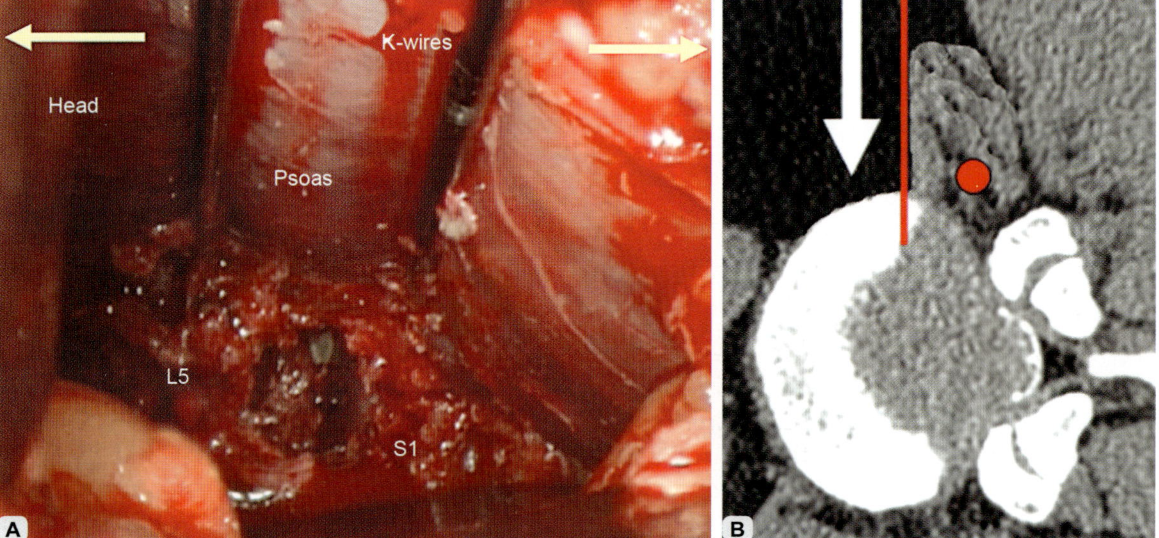

Fig. 30.3 (A) The L5–S1 level after diskectomy; the psoas has been retracted posteriorly and fixed using two K-wires (Yellow arrows indicate the directions of head and legs); (B) The white arrow indicates the direction of lateral access; the red line symbolizes as the K-wire used to fixed the retracted psoas; red dot indicates the lumbar plexus, which resides inside the psoas muscle

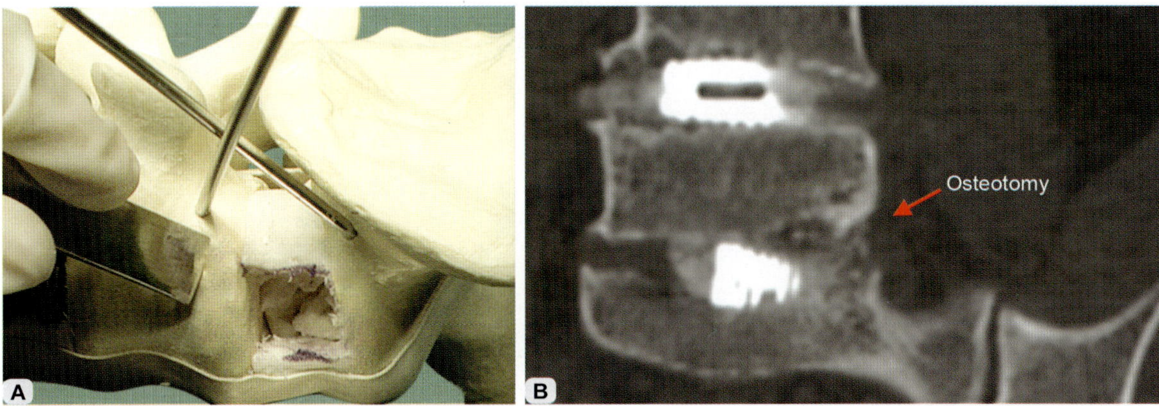

Fig. 30.4 (A) L5 lateral distal osteotomy to improve working field, also used for narrowed disk with osteophyte; note that the crisscrossed K-wires at the margins of L5 and sacrum vertebrae; (B) Reformatted CT AP image shows the osteotomized L5 vertebra

Results

The major perioperative complication rate was 7.3% (n = 4), including two cases of L5 nerve incomplete injury in single-level access to the L5–S1 disk, in both cases the nerve palsy was resolved 6 months later. Two cases suffered from venous injury during accessing the L5–1 disk; one had ILV injury and resulting in blood of 400 mL, the other was of CIV injury and had 700 mL blood loss. In both cases, massive venous bleeding was stopped by prolonged (>30 minutes) massive gauze compression. In both cases no attempt had been made to repair the venous wall tear. While there was no neurovascular injury occurred in accessing the cranial discs.

The mean blood loss and operating time were 250 mL and 100 minutes, respectively; the mean hospital stay was six days (range, 4–10 days); and the estimated mean length of incision was 8.6 cm (range, 4–12).

Anatomical Variations during Accessing the L5–S1 Disc

There were five anatomical variations which affected the access to the L5–S1 disk. The degrees of access difficulty in these 55 patients varied individually, depending upon the presence of one or more of the five anatomical variations, which are listed in order of difficulty:

1. Short and big ILV (diameter >10 mm; 40%, n = 22). Short and big diameter ILV was difficult to coagulate and the coagulating site was very close to the CIV as well.
2. Tight CIV (14.5%, n = 8). Despite the ILV had been divided, in some cases with tight CIV that the vein was difficult to be mobilized away from the anterolateral side of the L5–S1 disk.
3. Low-seated disk (58.2%, n = 32) (Fig. 30.5B). This was referred to the distance of the disk in the pelvis relative to the intercristal line (ICL), the disk located lower than the ICL and usually required L5 lateral wedge osteotomy to obtain a workable surgical field; in contrast, in some cases their L5–S1 disks were near parallel to the ICL and these discs were relatively easy to access.
4. Bulky psoas muscle (36.4%, n = 20). In senile patients, the atrophied psoas was easy to retract, but in young muscular male the bulky psoas required sequential muscle retraction.
5. Absence of the ILV (18.2%, n = 10). In the absence of ILV, lateral access to the L5–S1 disc became much easier.

In comparison, lateral accesses to the L3–4, L4–5 levels were much easier because there was no need to manage the great veins which was technically demanding. There was not much technical difference between left and right approach for L5–S1 disk, except that in right access to L4–5 or L3–4 levels, the vena cava was very close to the disks.

Ipsilateral warm leg was found in all 55 patients due to sympathectomy. Most patients were asymptomatic and the warm leg was resolved 6 months later due to cross-innervation; 19 patients (34.5%) had temporary anterior thigh paresthesia or pain which was resolved within 2 months. No retrograde ejaculation, deep vein thrombosis, infection had occurred at latest follow-up.

Discussion

The disadvantages of conventional approaches, such as anterior, posterior, and transforaminal, for lumbar interbody fusion are well known. Minimal lateral trans-psoas access (LTA) by dilating the psoas muscle is an attractive alternative and minimizes approach-related issues. However, there are two major limitations of LTA: risk of lumbar plexus injury and inaccessible to the L5–S1 disk. Nerves at risk include lumbar nerve roots, ilioinguinal nerves, and genitofemoral

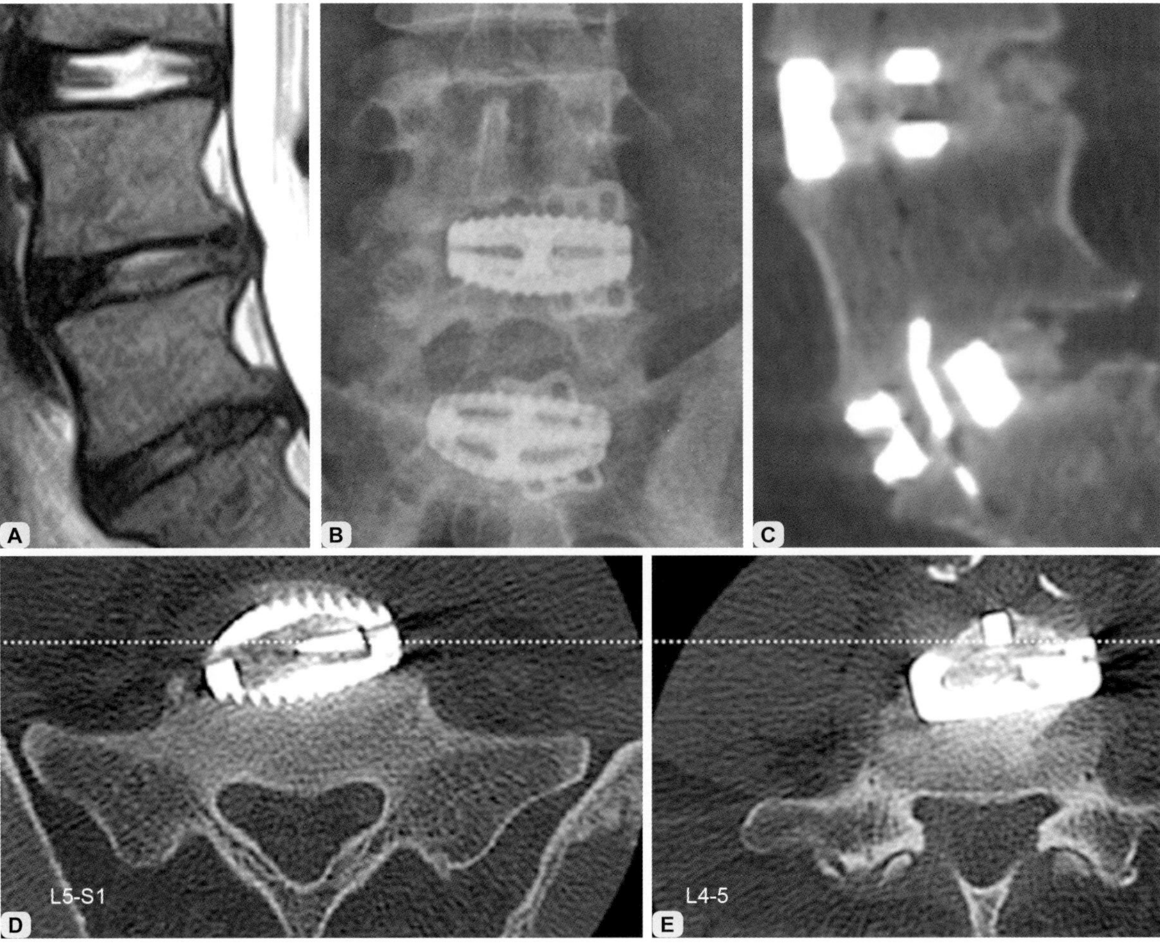

Fig. 30.5 (A) Lumbar MRI T2-weighted sagittal image, a 35 years old female with 2-level discogenic pain; (B) Postoperative lumbar AP radiograph shows L4–5 and L5–S1 fusion; note that the pelvis crest (intercristal line) is above the L5–S1 level; (C) Reformatted sagittal CT image at 3-month follow-up; The axial views of (D) L5–S1 and (E) L4–5 levels. The cages was implanted from lateral side and seated in transverse direction

nerves, and neuromonitoring is therefore recommended to reduce the potential risk of nerve injury in LTA. Several anatomical studies intended to define the safe working zones during LTA to prevent nerve injury. One cadaveric study tried to map the nerves during LTA and concluded that there is no zone of absolute safety and the authors recommended direct visualization of the roots and/or use neuromonitoring [10]. But neuromonitoring is not always foolproof that nerve injury still occurred particularly at the L4–5 level,[6] and one author suggested using conventional approaches of ALIF, TLIF, or PLIF when accessing this level.[11]

In our method, the lumbar nerves are protected inside the retracted psoas and no permanent nerve injury has occurred in this series. There were two cases of incomplete L5 nerve injury which resolved later and the presumed cause of nerve injury was due to tension from the retracted muscle. The same cause may be contributed to some case who suffered from transient paresthesia or pain of anterior thigh postoperatively. The most common temporary neurological deficit in our series is asymptomatic ipsilateral warm leg due to severing the sympathetic chain on the same operative side. Because we prefer to do discectomy just behind the ALL, the sacrificing of nearby sympathetic chain seems unavoidable; fortunately, the warm legs in most cases were gradually resolved after 6 months due to reinnervation. By retracting the psoas, not only the underlying nerves are protected, the muscle itself remains intact and not disrupted.

Lateral access to the L5–S1 disk has long been considered impossible due to obstruction by the pelvis. However in our series, the pelvis is thought to be annoying rather than obstructive. The results showed that there were combinations of anatomical variations among individual patients, including the venous system,[17,18] the relative distance of the disk to the pelvic rim or ICL,[19] and the muscle mass of psoas.

Access difficulties varied among the patients depending upon the presence of the anatomical variations. The highly variable venous system is considered the major access issue because it requires a steep learning curve to manage the friable veins. Our solutions included: (1) Place the mini-open incision more anteriorly; (2) Manage the great veins: isolate, coagulate and divide the iliolumbar and then mobilize the common iliac vein away from the anterolateral side of the L5–S1 disk; (3) Perform L5 distal lateral wedge osteotomy, this maneuver also can be used in other disk levels with narrow height and osteophyte. There were two venous injures resulting in profuse bleeding and fortunately they were stopped by prolonged (>30 minutes) and massive gauze compression. For vascular issue, consulting an access surgeon preoperatively is recommended, and a basic skill in handling the venous injury is preferable, particularly when the access surgeon is unavailable.

Compared to the L5–S1 disk, accessing the cranial level becomes relatively easy and safe because there is no vein nearby and usually above the intercristal line. But it should be noted that the great veins in vicinity should always be watched for and protected, especially during right-side access.

In this series, there were only two cases having prior anterior L5–S1 procedure. Therefore the experience in managing the scarred tissue was limited despite that there was no neurovascular injury occurred. In the other 2 cases with pyogenic L5–S1 diskitis, it was found useful to use finger-dissection to separate the disc from the surrounding dense granulation tissue caused by infection.

In conclusion, we used a mini-open lateral access to the lumbar disks by retracting the psoas muscle, and the retracted muscle also protects the nerves when compared to trans-psoas method which has potential risk of nerve injury. We accessed the L5–S1 disks laterally which had been considered not possible by handling the great veins. Our method of lateral access to the lumbar disk seems to a safer alternative than transpsoas approach.

References

1. Heth JA, Hitchon PW, Goel VK, et al. A biomechanical comparison between anterior and transverse interbody fusion cages. Spine. 2001;26(12):E261-7.
2. Ozgur BM, Aryan HE, Pimenta L, Taylor WR. Extreme Lateral Interbody Fusion (XLIF): a novel surgical technique for anterior lumbar interbody fusion. Spine J. 2006; 6(4):435-43.
3. Sharma AK, Kepler CK, Girardi FP, Cammisa FP, Huang RC, Sama AA. Lateral lumbar interbody fusion: clinical and radiographic outcomes at 1 year: a preliminary report. J Spinal Disord Tech. 2011;24(4):242-50.
4. Kepler CK, Sharma AK, Huang RC. Lateral transpsoas interbody fusion (LTIF) with plate fixation and unilateral pedicle screws: a preliminary report. J Spinal Disord Tech. 2011;24(6):363-7.
5. Knight RQ, Schwaegler P, Hanscom D, Roh J. Direct lateral lumbar interbody fusion for degenerative conditions: early complication profile. J Spinal Disord Tech. 2009;22(1):34-7.
6. Houten JK, Alexandre LC, Nasser R, Wollowick AL. Nerve injury during the transpsoas approach for lumbar fusion. J Neurosurg Spine. 2011;15(3):280-4. Epub 2011 May 27.
7. Benglis DM, Vanni S, Levi AD. An anatomical study of the lumbosacral plexus as related to the minimally invasive transpsoas approach to the lumbar spine. J Neurosurg Spine 2009; 10(2):139-44.
8. Uribe JS, Arredondo N, Dakwar E, Vale FL. Defining the safe working zones using the minimally invasive lateral retroperitoneal transpsoas approach: an anatomical study. J Neurosurg Spine. 2010;13(2):260-6.
9. Kepler CK, Bogner EA, Herzog RJ, Huang RC. Anatomy of the psoas muscle and lumbar plexus with respect to the surgical approach for lateral transpsoas interbody fusion. Eur Spine J. 2011;20(4):550-6. Epub 2010. Oct 13.
10. Banagan K, Gelb D, Poelstra K, Ludwig S. Anatomic mapping of lumbar nerve roots during a direct lateral transpsoas approach to the spine: a cadaveric study. Spine (Phila Pa 1976). 2011;36(11):E687-91.
11. Guérin P, Obeid I, Bourghli A, Masquefa T, Luc S, Gille O, et al. The lumbosacral plexus: anatomic considerations for minimally invasive retroperitoneal transpsoas approach. Surg Radiol Anat. 2011. Oct 5.
12. Davis TT, Bae HW, Mok MJ, Rasouli A, Delamarter RB. Lumbar plexus anatomy within the psoas muscle: implications for the transpsoas lateral approach to the L4-L5 disc. J Bone Joint Surg Am. 2011;93(16):1482-7.
13. Peretti F, Hovorka I, Fabiani P, et al. New possibilities in L2-L5 lumbar arthrodesis using a lateral retroperitoneal approach assisted by laparoscopy: preliminary results. Eur Spine J. 1996;5(3):210-6.
14. McAfee PC, Regan JJ, Geis WP, et al. Minimally invasive anterior retroperitoneal approach to the lumbar spine. Emphasis on the lateral BAK. Spine. 1998;23(13):1476-84.
15. Wolfla CE, Maiman DJ, Coufal FJ, et al. Retroperitoneal lateral lumbar interbody fusion with titanium threaded fusion cages. J Neurosurg. 2002;96:50-5.
16. Bergey DL, Villavicencio AT, Goldstein, et al. Endoscopic lateral transpsoas approach to the lumbar spine. Spine. 2004;29(15):1681-8.
17. Jasani V, Jaffray D. The anatomy of the iliolumbar vein. A cadaver study. J Bone Joint Surg Br. 2002;84(7):1046-9.
18. Kiray A, Akcali O, Guvencer M, Tetik S, et al. Iliolumbar veins have a high frequency of variations. Clin Orthop Relat Res. 2004;(425):252-7.
19. MacGibbon, Farfan HF. A radiologic survey of various configurations of the lumbar spine. Spine 1979;4(3):258-66.

CHAPTER

31

Lumbar Spinal Stenosis—Current View

Myung-Sang Moon, Sung-Soo Kim, Jeong-Lim Moon, Jang-Cheol Sihn

Introduction

Spinal stenosis is the neural compression disorder in the spinal canal and is a common acquired spinal disorder usually in the elderly patients, though some of the patients have had congenital narrowness of the bony canal and foramens of the mobile cervical and lumbar spines in the third or fourth decade.[1-12] An example is the spine of the achondroplasia and another short-stature syndromes in which the low Pavlov ratio is demonstrated.[1] Stenosis is caused primarily by the disk degeneration under the narrowed bony canal (short pedicles, thickened lamina, hypertrophic facet osteoarthropathy) and hypertrophic soft tissue (ligamentum flavum). The lumbar spine stenosis (LSS) is classified by its etiology (Table 31.1 and Fig. 31.1).

The symptoms of the lumbar spinal canal stenosis are elicited by the constriction neuropathy of the compressed neural elements, such as the cauda equina and nerve roots. The dynamic factors, such as posture and spinal instability participate in inducing the symptoms, and further increased compression makes the symptoms worse. The severity of the symptoms is not necessarily associated with the magnitude of the compression seen on the imaging studies. Vascular impairment is also thought to participate in precipitating the symptoms.

Many different terminologies are used in expressing the stenosis, based on the anatomical site of compression; central canal stenosis, lateral recess stenosis, subarticular stenosis, subpedicular stenosis, lateral gutter stenosis, foraminal stenosis, intervertebral foraminal stenosis. These terms have confused the readers.

Table 31.1 Classification of lumbar spine stenosis

I. Congenital or developmental (primary canal narrowing)
A. Idiopathic
B. Achondroplastic
C. Osteopetrosis
II. Acquired (secondary canal narrowing)
A. Degenerative
1. Central
2. Lateral recess and foraminal
3. Degenerative spondylolisthesis
B. Iatrogenic
1. After laminectomy
2. After arthrodesis
3. After diskectomy
C. Miscellaneous disorders
1. Acromegaly
2. Paget's disease
3. Fluorosis
4. Ankylosing spondylitis
D. Traumatic
III. Combined: any combination of congenital, developmental, or acquired stenosis

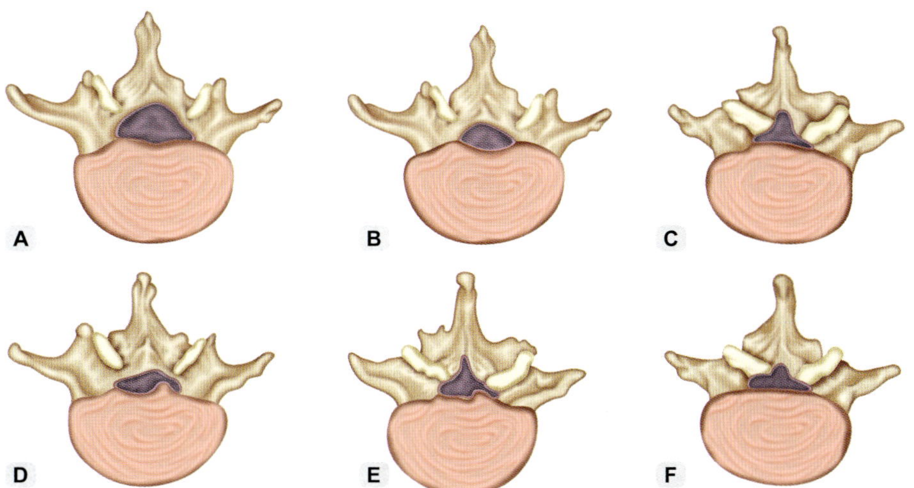

Fig. 31.1 Various types of spinal canal stenosis by Arnold et al. in 1976. (A) Normal canal; (B) Congenital/developed stenosis; (C) Degenerative stenosis; (D) Congenital/development stenosis with disk herniation; (E) Degenerative stenosis with disk herniation; (F) Congenital/development stenosis with superimposed degenerative stenosis

Regional Anatomy and Amplitude

The ranges of the amplitude of the lumbar spine are presented in Table 31.2.

The lumbar spinal canal can be divided into two: static and dynamic. The static segment is the osseous canal between the disks, and the dynamic (mobile) segment corresponds the distribution of the ligamentum flavum (Fig. 31.2). The stenotic segments, which cause the symptoms is the dynamic segment, which is related to the branched level of the spinal root.

Table 31.2 Amplitude of lumbar spine

Disk level	*ROM (degrees)*			*Remarks*
	Begg & Falconer	*Allbrook*	*Louis R*	
L_1 (L1–2)	10°	6°	11°	
L_2 (L2–3)	12°	8°	12°	
L_3 (L3–4)	14°	13°	18°	
L_4 (L4–5)	15°	19°	24°	Hallinshead L4 > L5
L_5 (L5–S1)	15°	18°	18°	
Total	60°	64°	83° (30°/53°)	Forward: 3 V Backward: 1

- Ratio of lateral bending: forward-backward bending; 2:3
- Total axial rotation: 16° (Rt/Lt: 8°/8°)
- Rotation at L5–S1 { 5 – 6°; 1.5° in normal walking }
- (/): extension/flexion
- Lateral bending: 40° (Rt/Lt: 20°/20°)

The cauda equina is surrounded anteriorly by the disk, posterior longitudinal ligament, and vertebral bodies, and laterally by the pedicles and the lateral extension of the ligamentum flavum. The ligamentum flavum, laminae, and the facet joints form the posterior element (Fig. 31.3).

The spinal nerve root canal (neural foramen) are bounded anteriorly by the disks, the vertebral bodies, posteriorly by the facet joints, and superiorly and inferiorly by the pedicles.

The mean A-P diameter of the spinal canal of 12 mm, and minimum cross-sectional area at least of 77 ± 13 mm^3 are essential to accommodate the average-sized neural element.

The normal intervertebral foraminal height is 16–19 mm and the foraminal dimensional area is 40–160 mm.[2] The height ≤15 mm is defined to be pathologic.

According to Mayoux-Benhamon et al. in 1989, foraminal width is 5–6 mm at minimum, and superior width is 7–8 mm. Forward flexion increases 12% in foraminal area (30% of foraminal width) and 15% decrease (narrower) in extension. 13% increase of superior width in forward flexion, and 9% decrease in extension. However, there is more leeway present for the nerve root and more leeway of the spinal nerve in the lumbar foramina than in the cervical area. The reason is that the ratio of size of nerve root and foramen in the cervical spine is 1:2, while in the lumbar spine it is 1:5 (30% by Jenis and An; 10–30% by Hayland et al.).

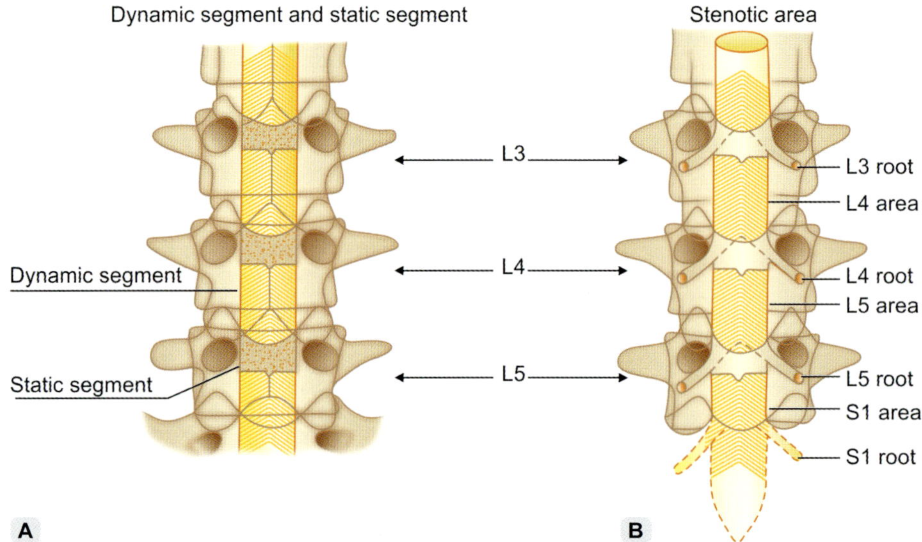

Fig. 31.2 (A) The lumbar spinal canal is divided into a static segment, the osseous spinal canal, and a dynamic segment corresponding to the distribution of the yellow ligament; (B) Since the stenotic area in the lumbar spinal canal related to symptoms is a dynamic segment, we have regarded the existence of stenosis in such a dynamic segment as being the stenotic area which is related to the branched level of the root

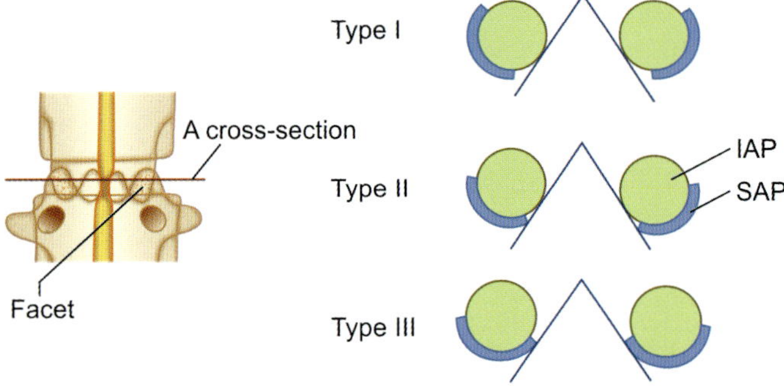

Fig. 31.3 A cross-section at level of the facets showing the relationship of IAP and SAP.

IAP, inferior articular process; SAP, superior articular process; type I, sagittally aligned facet joints; type II, semisagittally aligned facet joints; type III, coronally aligned facet joints

Anatomy of Neural Element (Intra- and Extradural Nerve Root Orientation in the Central Canal and Neural Foramens)

Within the cauda equina, the neural elements inside the dura are organized in a well-defined orientation pattern (Figs 31.4 and 31.5). The most posteriorly oriented neural element within the thecal sac are the fifth sacral nerve roots, which progress anteriorly from the fourth through the first sacral vertebra between the fifth lumbar and first sacral disk level. The most anterior element at the fifth lumbar and first sacral disk level is the first sacral nerve root. Between the 4th and 5th lumbar vertebra, the 4th lumbar nerve root enter anterolaterally, displacing the first sacral nerve root more posteriorly. This arrangement progresses symmetrically and regularly with one root being added in the cephalad direction at each disk level. Nerve root branching from dural sheath is shown in Figure 31.4.

Lateral spinal canal is divided in 3 zones: entrance zone, mid (middle) zone, and exit zone. It connects the intraspinal space to extraspinal space.

Entrance zone is most cephalad part of the lateral canal and is located medial to or underneath the superior articular process. Its anterior wall is the disk and posterior wall is the facet joints. Medial and lateral aspects are open.

Mid-zone is located under pars interarticularis, part of the lamina and the pedicle below. In this zone dorsal root ganglia (DRG) and ventral motor nerve root (funiculus) are covered by dura mater with cerebrospinal fluid. Anterior border is the posterior aspect of the vertebral body, posterior border is the pars interarticularis, and medial border is open to central canal.

The motor fiber components are located anteromedially, and the larger sensory components are located posterolaterally. Root-specific sensory and motor fibers are contiguous and oriented in an oblique fashion. Within the neuroforamen lies the dorsal root ganglia (DRG) containing neural fibers and cell bodies, which consists of a small motor component anteriorly and a larger sensory component posteriorly. The dorsal root ganglia are almost always within the confines of the neuroforamen and frequently is situated adjacent to the disk space at the level of the pedicles.

DRG normally occupies approximately 23–30% of the area of the foramen and lies within the superolateral portion

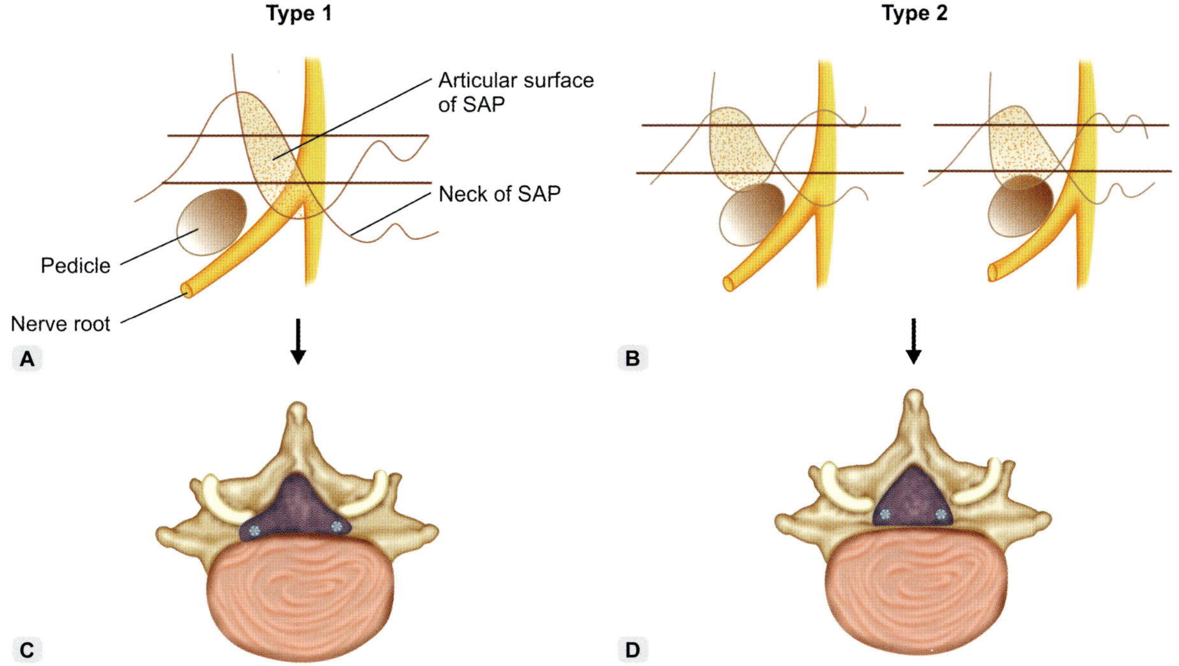

Fig. 31.4 Type 1: (A) Nerve root branches off from dural sheath or runs under the articular surface of SAP; (B) Nerve root branches off from dural sheath and runs under the neck of SAP; (C) Diagram showing a cross section of the type 1; (D) Diagram showing a cross section of the type 2

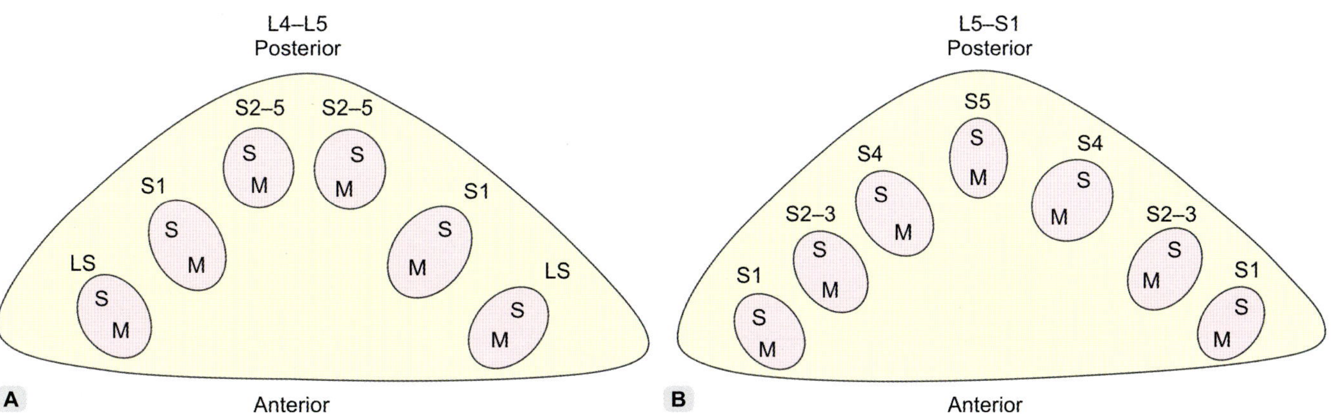

Fig. 31.5 Drawings showing neural organization within the thecal sac at the fourth and fifth lumbar and first sacral disk levels. M, motor components; S, sensory components

of lumbar foramen, and directly below the pedicle in 90% of lumbar level.

Exit zone is the area surrounding the intervertebral foramen; posteriorly bordered by the lateral aspect of facet joint one level below the entrance zone of same segmental nerve, anteriorly bordered by disk of one level below the disk of entrance zone. Its neural content is the peripheral nerve with perineurium.

Narrowing of the intervertebral neural foramen by itself and in association with vibration would stimulate the mechanosensitive DRG. Vibration affects the synthesis and transport of two dorsal root ganglia neuropeptides; substance P (VP) and vasoactive intestinal peptide (VIP). Substance P associated with the development of degenerative arthritis, probably through stimulation of synthesis of collagenase and PGE2, while VP increases bone resorption via a cAMP-dependent mechanism.

The causes of high incidence of stenosis at L4–5 and L5–S1, are the smaller foramen/root area ratio due to larger diameter of the lower lumbar and sacral root and DRG

(7 mm in diameter); more oblique root course throughout the lateral canal increases susceptibility to effect of pedicular kinking and foraminal stenosis; higher incidence of disk degeneration and spondylosis.

The reported potential incidences of foraminal stenosis in the lumbar spine by An et al. are 4.0% in 2nd root, 5.3% in 3rd root, 15% in 4th root, and 75% in 5th root.

Spinal Motion

Amplitude of motion in the lumbar spine is shown in Table 31.2. The total range of flexion/extension of lumbar spine is approximately 60°–83° (50°/30°). Segmental range of motion (ROM) becomes gradually wider from L1–2 to L4–5. The lateral bending reaches up to 40° (right/left: 20°/20°). The total axial rotation is 16° (right/left: 8°/8°). The ratio of lateral bending and forward-backward bending is 2:3. Rotation ranges at L5–S1 is 5°–6° and 1.5° rotation at L5–S1 occurs on walking.

Nerve Root Pathophysiology

Cauda equina and the proximal portion of the nerve roots within the subarachnoid space in the dural sleeve, are suspended in cerebral spinal fluid. Nerve root sheath is very thin, and lacks a diffusion barrier corresponding to the perineurium of peripheral nerve and so the endoneural space is continuous with the subarachnoid space. Accordingly, the diffusion barrier is found deeper in the arachnoid membrane at the inner wall of the dura matter and the dural sleeve. Owing to such specific feature, the mechanism involved in the development of cauda equina and radicular symptoms in lumbar canal stenosis is somewhat different from that related to the development of peripheral nerve symptoms.

Endoneurial fluid pressure of the diffusion barrier of the free nerve root shows no increase if the subarachnoid space is open. However, when lumbar lordosis increases on standing and walking, subarachnoid obstruction can occur and the nerve root becomes surrounded by the diffusion barrier of the arachnoid. Subsequently, diffusion of edema into the subarachnoid space becomes impaired, resulting in an increase of endoneurial fluid pressure and occurrence of the so-called "compartment syndrome".

Compression neuropathy denotes the nerve affection, caused primarily by the passive mechanical compression. Therefore, the nerve will be affected in various manner by the different compression force patterns:

1. Rapidity: acute (sudden) vs. gradual (chronic progressive); continuous or intermittent).
2. Size of the load (force).
3. Area size of compression: small vs. wide area with same size of load.
4. Duration: [short period or long period / frequency of compression]
5. Structural compressors: soft vs. hard (no resiliency) tissue: disk vs. bony spicule.

The five above listed factors affect the compressed nerve in various ways.

By compression the circulation to the nerve is impaired: arterial and/or venous circulation. Impaired arterial circulation results in ischemia and the impaired venous circulation results in blood pooling (stasis) and finally compartment syndrome by edema. Also axon by compression is directly or indirectly damaged. Also by compression nutritional impairment in nerve can be complicated.

Compression exceeding the arterial pressure in the nerve is known to be 200 mm Hg (22.66 kilopascals).[19] Sudden high compression shuts down arterial circulation, while the gradual compression initially induces venous blood pooling (stasis) and neural edema, and finally reduces arterial circulation.

Pathology of the Stenotic Segment

The biomechanical and biochemical alteration of the disk by aging process leads to decrease in disk height, annular bulging, disk herniation, early osteophyte formation in the body margin and facet joint arthropathy. Occasionally instability of the affected segments can be complicated. As the disk collapse by degeneration, the cephalocaudal foraminal space narrowing progresses, and nerve–root entrapment can occur. Thus, the stenosis results in the central canal and lateral recess. Retrolisthesis occurs when the rate of disc degeneration exceeds that of alteration in the facet joints, while if the rate of facet joint alteration exceeds that of the disk degeneration anterolisthesis can occur. This is true when the facet joints are in a sagittal plane.

Nerve Compression Effect: (Compression Force, Rate and Duration and Blood Flow on Nerve Function)

It is a known fact that compression load, duration, and rate give direct effect on the compressed nerve. According to Garfin et al.[3,10,11] and Rydevik et al.[19], nerve root compression at 200 mm Hg (26.55 kilopascals) which was greater than the mean arterial pressure, caused a rapid decrease in conduction with almost no recovery in the afferent fibers and only a 30–40% improvement in the efferent fibers after removal of the compression. Increasing the compression time from 2 to 4 hours has an effect on the nerve's ability to recover. Although the initial deterioration was the same, the recovery was remarkably prolonged, particularly at 100 mm Hg (13.33 kilopascals), when the duration of the compression was doubled. These changes were greater in the afferent than in the efferent pathways.

The compression rate and its effect on the nerve function may be the prognosticating factors. Edema and nutritional deficits are related to the magnitude of the pressure and the rate of its symptom onset. The higher the pressure the onset was more rapid, and the greater the edema more loss of nutritional support.

Clinical Symptoms

Early symptoms are often insidious in onset because of its slow relentless degenerative process. Clinical symptoms are neurogenic claudication, low back pain with bizarre unilateral, leg pain (sciatic type), numbness, muscle weakness, and sensory disturbance (Tables 31.3 to 31.5).

a. Low back pain: It cannot be the major symptoms, but it can be exacerbated by activity and often are relieved by rest.

Table 31.3 Physical findings in three conditions for differential diagnosis of symptoms

Findings	*Neurogenic claudication*	*Vascular claudication*	*Lumbar spondylosis*
Pain			
Type	Vague cramping, aching, sharp burning in lower extremities	Tightness, cramping (usually in calf)	Dull aching in low back
Location	Back, buttock, lower	Calf	Back
Radiation	Proximal to distal	Localized to lower extremities	Localized to back
Exacerbation	With standing, particularly with trunk extended: less with walking: rare with bicycling unless trunk is extended	With walking and bicycling (activities involving lower extremities)	With general activity, bending, standing, twisting and lifting
Improvement	With sitting, flexion and squatting	With sitting and cessation of muscular activity	With decreased activity and rest
Time to relief	Prolonged	Rapid	Prolonged
Walking uphill	More or less pain	Pain	More or less pain
Walking downhill	Pain (with lumbar hyperextension)	Pain	More or less pain
Back pain	Common	Uncommon	Common
Limitation of spinal movement	Common	Uncommon	Common
Physical findings			
Neurological examination	Occasional findings, usually asymmetrical	Findings rare, symmetrical if present	Negative
Straight-leg-raising test	Usually negative	Negative	Negative
Femoral stretch test	Usually negative	Negative	Negative
Pulses	Present or symmetrically diminished	Diminished or absent, often asymmetrical	
Skin	Normal	Hair loss, atrophy	Normal
Bicycle test	Positive with lumbar hyperextension	Positive with the spine in any position	Negative

Table 31.4 Characteristic clinical features of two different claudication and lumbar spondylosis

Findings	*Neurogenic claudication*	*Vascular claudication*	*Mixed type*	*Lumbar spondylosis*
Neurological examination	Occasional findings, usually asymmetrical	Findings rare, symmetrical if present	Symmetrical if present	Negative
Straight-leg-raising test	Usually negative	Negative	Usually negative	Negative
Femoral stretch test	Usually negative	Negative	Negative	Negative
Pulse	Present or symmetrically diminished	Diminished or absent, often asymmetrical	Diminished symmetrically	Symmetrical
Skin	Normal	Hair loss, atrophy	Hair loss, atrophy	Normal
Bicycle test	Positive with lumbar hyperextension	Positive with the spine in any position	Positive in any spinal position	Negative
Ankle-brachial pressure index (ABPI)			<0.9 (coexistance: 25%)	

Table 31.5 Physical Findings in spinal stenosis (LSCS) and vascular insufficiency (PAOD)

	LSCS	*PAOD*
Pain:		
Standing load test:		
Walking	+	+ (stop walking → –)
Forward bending	–	–
Backward bending	++	–
Sitting	–	–
Lying	–	–
Posture		
Stooping	–	–
Sensory march	+	–
Paralysis	+ or –	–
Muscle power ↓	+ or –	–
Thermography (right/left) difference	+ or –	+
ABPI: <0.9	–	+
Dorsal pedal arterial pulse	+	+ or –
Localized calf pain	–	+

PAOD: peripheral arterial occlusive disease

b. Cauda equina type intermittent claudication: The symptoms arise due to chronic root constriction and ischemia. Bilateral lower limb numbness (sensory disturbance) which becomes worse on walking and impossible to continue walking. The symptoms relieves on forward trunk flexion and rest which allows to walk again. The tingling which starts from the sole and spreads upwards with increased severity (sensory march) is the characteristic feature. Worsening of the low back pain is rare. The limb weakness follows the tingling, but not remarkable.
c. Unilateral limb pain and weakness complicate sometimes, but rare. This condition, due to the complicated severe lateral recess stenosis or disk herniation suggests the presence of the mechanically and inflammatorily stimulated lumbar and sacral nerve roots.
d. In the severe cases, limb tingling can be induced by standing and/or trunk dorsiflexion (postural factors), and perineal paresthesia, difficult urination, intolerable limb tingling on supine bed posture (restless leg syndrome) are complained.
e. Walking distance inducing intermittent claudication: The most distinctive symptom is neurogenic claudication which should be distinguished not only from arteriosclerosis obliterans but also from other vascular diseases (Table 31.3). It depends on the age and local disease severity, and the walking distance chronologically becomes short by several meters though there is individual difference.

Double Crush Phenomenon of the Compressed Root

The root compression at two levels has more than an additive effect on compromise of nerve function, even if both areas of compression are of relatively low pressure. This is the so-called double crush phenomenon. This may be due to the production of a region of the nerve with venous stasis.

The compressed dorsal root ganglion can cause release of inflammatory mediators (neuropeptides); substance P (SP) and vasoactive intestinal peptide (VIP): Thus, the mediators have effect of producing pain and also worsening the compression by increasing vascular permeability and therefore edema.

The ever-unsolved pending question is how does walking produce the symptomatic worsening. One of the possible theories is that there is vascular dilatation associated with the nerve roots causing a reduction in available space. In claudicants this may involve an increase in venous pooling with impairment of arteriolar inflow.

Neurological Characteristics

a. *Tendon reflex*: Loss or remarkable decrease of Achilles tendon reflex in case of nerve root impairment, while the increased reflex indicates the pyramidal tract impairment in which the cervical and thoracic cord lesion must be searched.
b. *Asymptomatic phase in sitting*: Superficial sensory disturbance is usually not recognized. Sometimes, calf muscle (triceps) and quadriceps tension decrease and atrophies are recognized at the end stage.
c. *Toe gait, heel gait*: Abnormality is seen.
d. *Laseque test*: Almost negative in the aged in spite of the complicated disc disease.
e. Neurological analysis disclosed the polyradicular disturbances in the most of the cases.

The double crush phenomenon of the compressed root:

The root compression at two levels has more than an addictive effect on compromise of neural function, even if both areas of compression are of relatively low pressure. This is the so-called double crush phenomenon. This may be due to the production of a region of the nerve with venous stasis.

The compressed dorsal root ganglion can cause release of inflammatory mediators (neuropeptides); substance P (SP) and vasoactive intestinal peptide (VIP): Thus, the mediators have effect of producing pain and also worsening the compression by increasing vascular permeability and therefore edema.

The ever-unsolved pending question is how does walking produce the symptomatic worsening. One of the possible theories is that there is vascular dilatation associated with the nerve roots causing a reduction in available space. In claudicants this may involve an increase in venous pooling with impairment of arterial inflow.

Image Findings

Clinical diagnosis should be basically supplemented by the image study.

a. *Simple two dimensional radiograms*: Bulbous hypertrophy of the facet joints, inwardly deviated sagittally aligned facet surface, "W"-shaped facets of the lower vertebra, disk space narrowing and bony spur, thickened lamina, foraminal narrowing, degenerative scoliosis, olisthesis are seen. For the developmental stenosis in the young, canal measurement is important.
b. *Radiculography and recording of sensory nerve action potentials (SNAPs)*: They are useful as examination of foraminal stenosis. In radiculography, it is important to examine whether the root sleeve is constricted or interrupted, and particularly to determine the site of interruption of the contrast medium. When the contrast medium is interrupted near the exit of the intervertebral foramen, an approach from outside the spinal canal is necessary. When laterality is observed in saphenous (L4), superficial peroneal (L5), and sural (S1) nerves, constrictive disturbance at the dorsal root ganglion or the more distal site is suspected.
c. *Myelography*: This is nowadays rarely done, because the MRI replaced its clinical significance. In the past, myelogram was thought to provide the most accurate definitive diagnosis (Figs 31.6 to 31.8). On AP myelogram picture of various degree of multiple tapering or incomplete or complete stasis, defective root figure, narrowed image column, remarkable streaking and serpentine configuration of cauda equina (redundant nerve roots) were seen. On lateral myelograms, disk bulge, posterior compression at each spinal level were seen.
d. *CT scans*: Spinal canal shape, degenerative changes of the intervertebral joints, bony spurs, intracanal ligament and its ossification. CT myelogram could demonstrate the deviation of dural sac (Fig. 31.9).
e. *Magnetic resonance imaging*: It should be reserved for planning the operation, assessing the number of levels involved, and evaluating the spine for the other diseases.

   Central stenosis and stenosis of the lateral recess can be well visualized. Also abnormalities of the facet joints, osteophytes, disc herniations or protrusions, invaginated thickened ligamentum flavum are seen (Fig. 31.10).

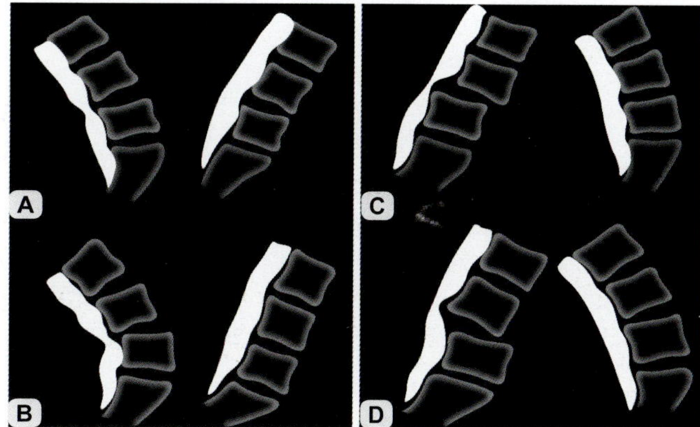

Fig. 31.6 Myelogram provides the two different patterns of stenosis: (A and B) Dynamic stenosis in extension; (C and D) Dynamic stenosis in flexion. Extension dynamic stenosis is more frequently seen: stenotic symptoms are relieved on forward declined walking, while the symptoms become worse on posteriorly declined walking

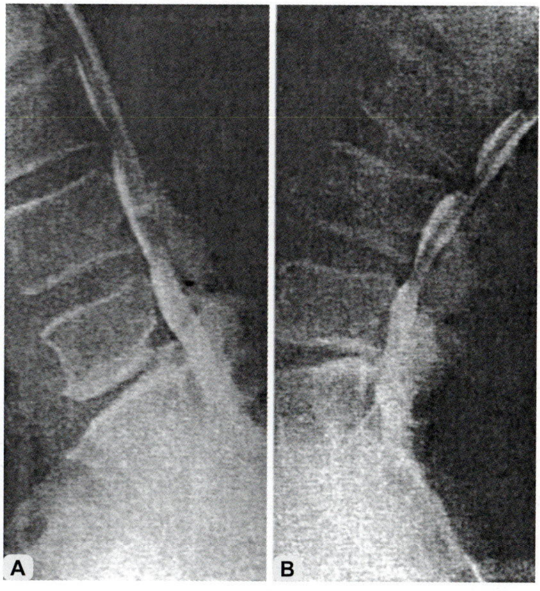

Fig. 31.7 Dynamic myelography. In the extended position, lumbar spinal canal stenosis becomes more severe and the dural tube is compressed more strongly

Diagnosis

Generally it has been thought that it is easy to make diagnosis by the characteristic clinical symptoms. But it is not true, though the diagnostic accuracy is around 90%. Diagnosis of stenosis is not easy for the general physicians.

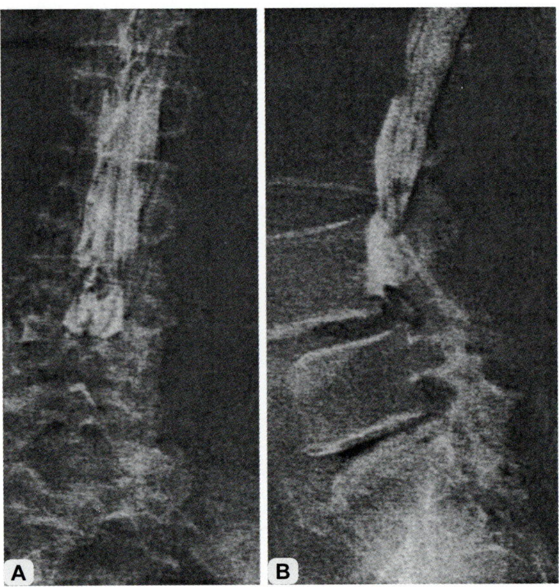

Fig. 31.8 Serpentine myelographic defect (redundant nerve root) observed on the central side of the stenosis

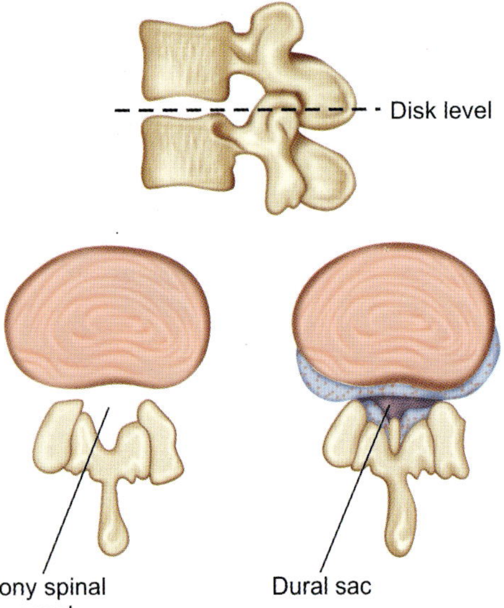

Fig. 31.9 Tracings of a CT showing the discrepancy between the size of the dural sac and the size of the bony canal. The dotted areas represent the soft tissues, the disk and the ligamentum flavum. In the majority of the cases, the maximum stenosis is at a level corresponding to the picture on the top. Diagnostic value of CT is that the condition of the bony spinal canal, especially the lateral spinal canal, can be determined. The severity of dural tube stenosis can also be determined by special methods

The disease cannot be diagnosed by the image findings alone, such as myelography, CT myelography, and MRI. Because asymptomatic patients often display abnormal

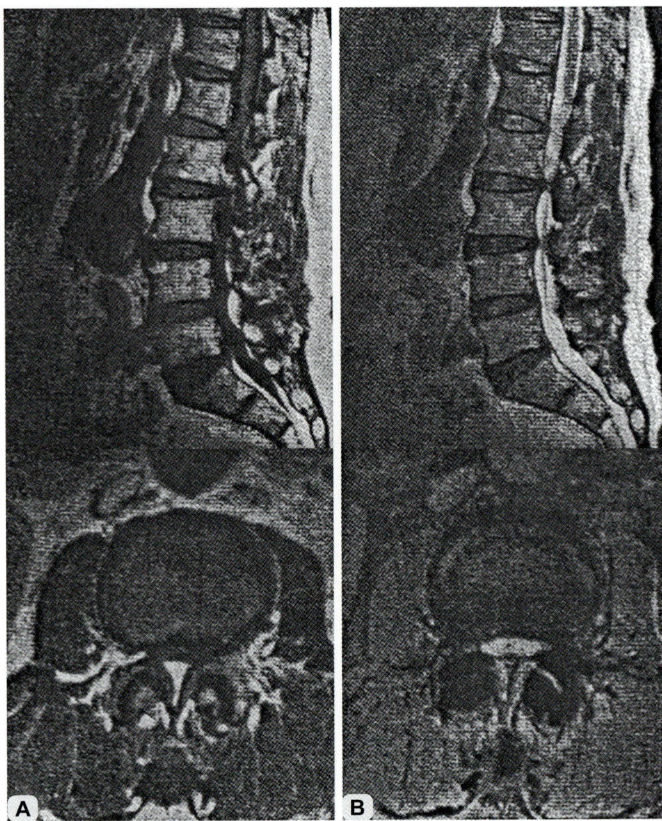

Fig. 31.10 Characteristic MRI findings of lumbar spinal canal stenosis are that constriction of the dural sac, and abnormal intrathecal enhancement on gadolinium-enhanced MRI. MRI of symptomatic lumbar spinal canal stenosis due to spondylosis. (A) T1-weighted image; (B) T2-weighted image. The sagittal image (top) showing the most severe canal stenosis at L2–3 level and the axial view (bottom) at the top of the intervertebral disk (facet joint level)

image findings. Also the clinical symptoms are not limited only to the stenosis especially in the aged patients.

It is frequently seen in the elderly males with degenerative spine over age of 60 years, while the developmental stenosis is seen in the age group over 30 years. The differential diagnosis includes vascular claudication, peripheral neuropathy, and lumbar spondylolisthesis. Electromyography and nerve-conduction studies are useful.

Root block at the time of radiculography is a helpful diagnostic procedure (Figs 31.11 and 31.12).

Adjuncts to Diagnosis of Lateral Stenosis

To confirm the lateral stenosis, epidural infusion of anesthetics and also root block (L5, S1) are carried out. By these needle procedures, stenosis, block or abnormal location of the epiradicular space can be assessed by nerve block and periduro- and perineurographies. Symptomatic improvement of radicular symptoms can be assessed by anesthetic injection.

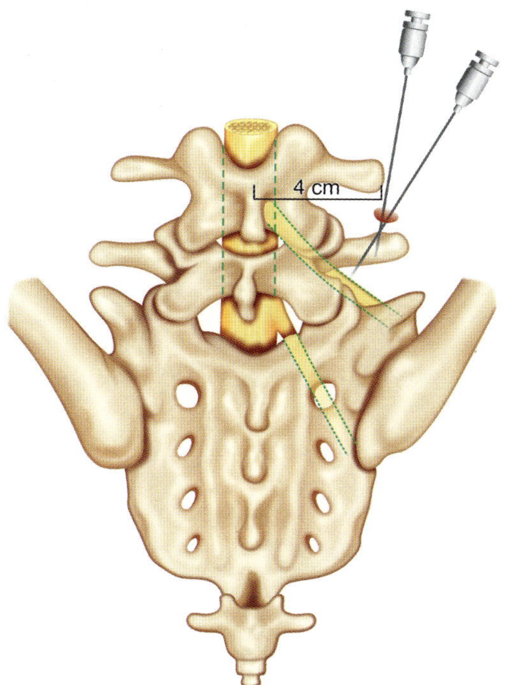

Fig. 31.11 Approach to the L5 root block

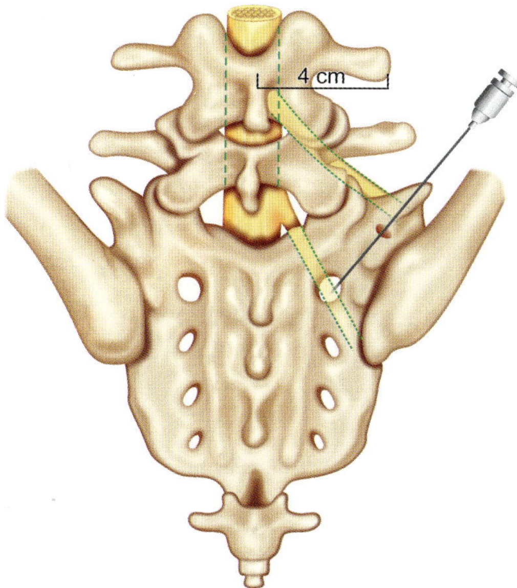

Fig. 31.12 Approach to the S1 root block

A diagnostic tool, the so-called "clinical diagnosis support tool (CDST)" was developed to assist the general physicians by the Japanese Society for Spinal Surgery and Related research.[30]

Management

It is apparent that complete resolution of the symptoms by the conservative management is unusual, although it can occur infrequently. A similar percentage of patients have worsening symptoms. The surgical decision on a patient who has stenosis should be based more on the decrease in the patients' quality of life and an increase in symptoms rather than on the subtle neurological findings and a positive MRI scan. An additional reasoning of the operative treatment in an effort is to alleviate the neurological signs and to improve the quality of life. However, it is strongly suggested to the patients and their supporters that decompression surgery cannot routinely be expected to reverse the neurological deficits in all the patients.

As the first step of therapeutic measures, conservative treatment must be basically provided. Surgical management must be finalized by the patient and her or his supporters after the informed consent, when the conservative management fails.

Conservative Treatment

It should be started with primary modalities such as patient education, reassurance, analgesics non-steroidal anti-inflammatory drugs, and narcotics. Exercise to build-up muscle strength and tolerance is prescribed. Physical therapy is also helpful, but is not curative. Physical therapist educates the exercise program for the patients self-treatment.

Corset-type brace (flexion orthosis) is helpful, but should not be worn over long period to avoid additional muscle weakness (Fig. 31.13).

Epidural and Nerve Root Blocks

It is selected according to the pathologic condition (Figs 31.11, 31.12, and 31.14). Local anesthetics such as lidocaine, mepivacaine, and bupivacaine are used. Steroid reduces inflammation. However, as yet controversy exists.

Surgical Management

The primary goal is to decompress the compressed roots at the level and anatomic site of the compression: central canal, lateral recess, foramen, and extraforamen.

According to the individual differences in severity, chronicity and the stenotic area, the type of decompression should be selected. No one procedure can solve all types of stenosis. The principles of surgery are to achieve neural decompression. It is easy to underestimate the extent of the decompression required. In general, it is better to decompress more than less. However, when the decompressed segment is destabilized, it must be stabilized by fusion. However, surgical treatment has become progressively less invasive. Several techniques of minimally

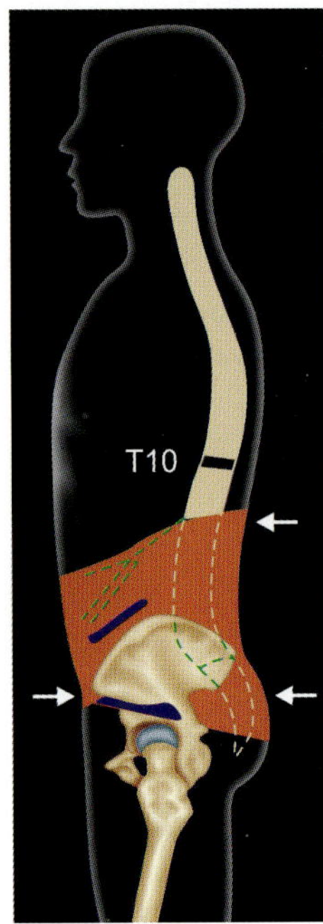

Fig. 31.13 Williams flexion orthosis

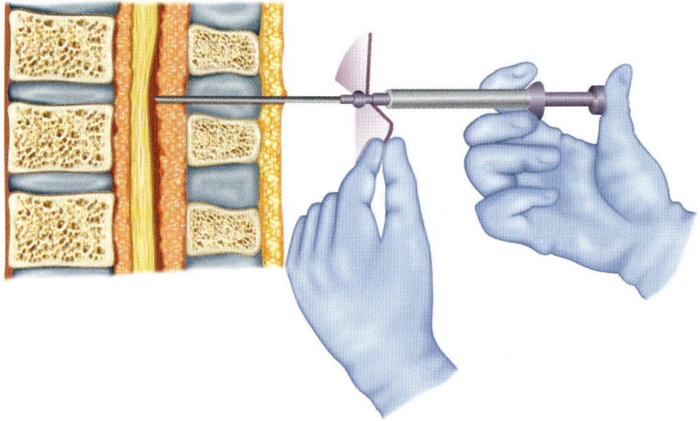

Fig. 31.14 Infusion method of the anesthetic into the epidural space to treat the radicular symptoms

invasive decompressive surgery, such as microscopic and microendoscopic techniques had been reported, and their results have been favorable. The recent rising popularity of the minimally or less invasive surgical technique had been based on the promising goal of minimization of structural destruction of the unaffected tissues and optimization of the maintenance of stability of the decompressed site, avoidance of instrumentation and cosmetic results. The surgical goal should be to achieve decompression completely and safely.

The following prognostic indications help provide the surgeons with realistic expectations of the results of decompression so that the surgeon can advise the patient appropriately.

Good prognosis are expected to be obtained: (i) adequate decompression is carried out, (ii) facet joint stability is maintained, (iii) early decompression surgery is performed, and (iv) postoperative corset is worn and exercise can be done.

Poor prognosis is indicated by (i) persistence of postoperative predominating back pain, (ii) multi-level decompression, (iii) preoperative prolonged delay, and (iv) preoperative presence of significant neurological deficit including sudden difficult urination.

The sooner the cauda equina is decompressed after the onset of symptoms, the more likely it is that the patient will not be left with residual neurologic deficit: decompression should be done as early as possible within 48 hours.

Decompression by Interspinous Process Distraction Devices

The procedure is best indicated for the extension dynamic stenosis: evidence of relief of symptoms with flexion and worsening of symptoms with extension.

Decompression

The ultimate surgical goal is adequate decompression of the neural structures including both cauda equina and exiting nerve roots (Figs 31.15 and 31.16). Preservation of postoperative stability of the decompressed segment is also an important issues; however, complete decompression of the neural structures should always be the primary concern because failure of surgery is more commonly due to inadequate decompression rather than excessive decompression. Whenever postoperative instability is anticipated after posterior decompression, fusion should be considered, though post-surgical instability is not as common as is expected.

Fenestration

It denotes the procedure which makes a small bony window to decompress: The procedure consists of laminectomy and resection of the medial portion (1/3) of the articular facet joints, preserving the joints as much as possible, and complete removal of the ligamentum flavum, is a method of choice for the majority of patients with LSS, because it preserves better spinal stability than total laminectomy.

When decompression is complete, dural sac pulsation returns, and venous refilling of the nerve roots is noted, and the nerve root becomes mobile. A highly selective spinal decompression is preferred, which speeds recovery, preserves canal height. Because, spinal stenosis involves in most cases only the motion segment (dynamic level; disk and facet joint level) and not the fixed segment (static

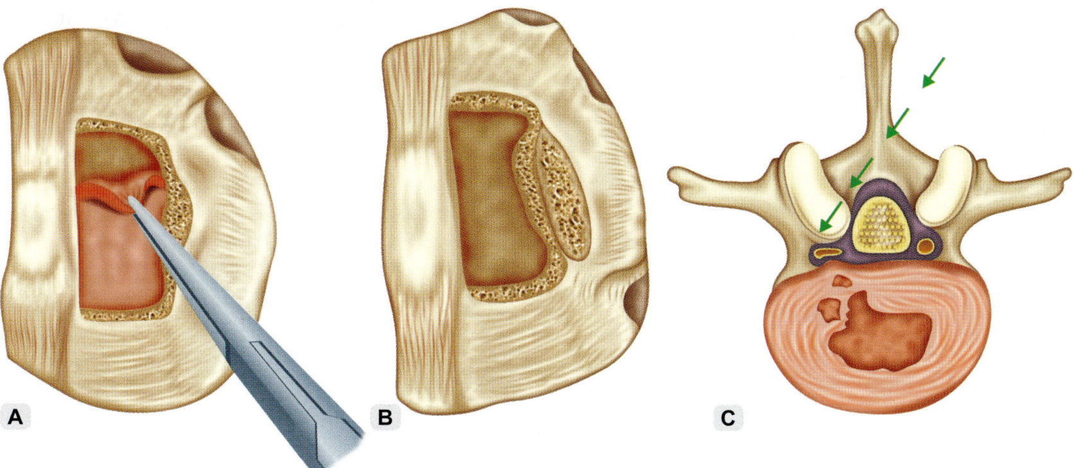

Fig. 31.15 These drawings show the technique for segmental spinal decompression. (A) After removing the ligamentum flavum bony overgrowth is visualized and can be removed carefully; (B). After removal of the medial third of the inferior facet laterally, the superior facet osteophyte can be seen intruding into the lateral recess of the spinal canal; (C). The osteophyte can be removed using an osteotome or sharp curette

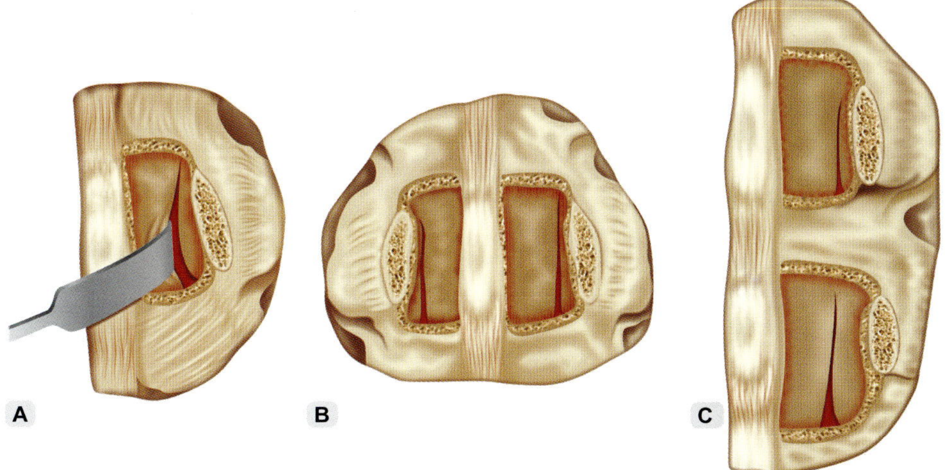

Fig. 31.16 (A) The nerve root previously trapped deep to the superior facet osteophyte will become visible following removal of this osteophyte; (B). The selective decompression can be repeated on the other side of the canal preserving the important midline ligamento-osseous to maintain stability structures; (C). The level above can be decompressed, if necessary

level; vertebral body, pedicle and laminar level). This makes it possible to decompress the stenotic segment while preserving the structural bony arch (Fig. 31.2). Fenestration should always be converted to laminectomy when the procedure does not provide adequate decompression of the central canal. When the radicular symptoms is associated with central canal stenosis, sufficient unroofing of the lateral recess must be supplemented.

Laminectomy

Laminectomy is the more extensive decompression surgery which sacrifices a part or whole of the laminae and facets in one or multisegments, particularly in elderly. It warrants decompression of the central canal alone, and must therefore be supplemented with sufficient unroofing of the lateral recess if associated radicular symptoms are to be addressed.

The position of the dorsal root ganglion must be determined by MRI. The compressed dorsal root ganglion, located in the spinal canal must be decompressed inside the spinal canal, while if it locates in the intervertebral foramen decompression from outside of the spinal canal.

Laminoplasty

Enbloc expansive laminoplasty is introduced by Tsuji. But it is rarely indicated. This procedure is similar to the cervical laminoplasty for the cervical myelopathy.[31]

The result of decompression surgery for spinal stenosis are reported to be good in high rates between 77–85% and low in 20%. Residual back pain or sciatica are common. Post-decompression instability is reported to develop in wide range (0–100%), though in general it is in range 10–12%. Reoperation rates was reported to be 16.6% (Hopp & Tsou) because of Olisthy in 4.6% disk herniation in 4.3% and intractable in 8%.

Conclusion

In conclusion what we have learnt are as follow:

Accurate diagnosis is essential in management. Differential diagnosis of central canal stenosis and foraminal stenosis is essential together with dynamic and static stenosis. Compressed root should be decompressed sufficiently, while the surgical destabilization should be minimized if possible.

References

1. Verbiest H. Aradicular syndrome from developmental narrowing of the lumbar vertebral canal. J Bone Joint Surg. 1954; 36B:230-7.
2. Epstein JA, Epstein BS, Lavine L. Nerve root compression associated with narrowing of the lumbar spinal canal. J Neurol Neurosurg Psychiat. 1962;25:165-76.
3. Garfin SR, Herkowitz HN, Mirkovic S. Spinal stenosis. J Bone Joint Surg. 1999; 81A: 572-86.
4. Arnoldi CC, Brodsky AE, Cauchoix J, Crock H, et al. Lumbar spinal stenosis and nerve root entrapment syndromes. Definition and classification. Clin Orthop. 1976;115:4-5.
5. Ciol MA, Deyo RA, Howell E, Krief S. An assessment of surgery for spinal stenosis: time trends, geographic variations, complications, and reoperations. J Am Geriat Soc. 1996; 44:285-90.
6. Cohen MS, Wall EJ, Brown RA, Rydervik B, Garfin SR. 1990 Acromed Award in basic science. Cauda equina anatomy II: extrathecal nerve roots and dorsal root ganglia. Spine. 1990; 15:1245-51.
7. Cohen MS, Wall EJ, Kerber CW, Abitbol JJ, Garfin SR. The anatomy of the cauda equina on CT scans and MRI. J Bone Joint Surg. 1991; 73(B): 381-4.
8. Cornefjord M, Takahashi K, Matsui H, Olmarker K, Holon S, Rydevik B. Impairment of nutritional transport at double level cauda equina compression. Neuro-ortho. 1992; 13:107-2.
9. Dodge LD, Bohlman HH, Rhodes RS. Concurrent lumbar spinal stenosis and peripheral vascular disease. A report of nine patients. Clin Orthop. 1988; 230:141-8.
10. Garfin SR, Cohen MS, Massie JB, Abitbol JJ, Swenson MR, Myers RR, Rydervik BI. Nerve-root of the cauda equina. The effect of hypotension and acute graded compression on function. J Bone Joint Surg. 1990;72(A):1185-92.
11. Garfin SR, Rydevik BL, Brown RA. Compressive neuropathy of spinal nerve roots. A mechanical or a biological problem? Spine. 1991;16:162-6.
12. Grob D, Humke T, Dvorak J. Degenerative lumbar spinal stenosis: decompression with and without arthrodesis. J Bone Joint Surg. 1995;77A:1036-41.
13. Hawkes CH, Roberts GM. Neurogenic and vacular claudication. J Neurol Sci. 1978; 38:337-45.
14. An HS, Butler JP. Lumbar spinal stenosis: historical perspectives, classification, and pathoanatomy. Semin Spine Surg. 1999;11:184.
15. Herkowitz KZ, Garfin SR. Decompressive surgery for spinal stenosis. Semin Spinal Surg. 1989;1:163-7.
16. Johnsson KZ, Rosen I, Uden A. The natural course of lumbar spinal stenosis. Clin Orthop. 1992;279:82-6.
17. Olmarker K, Rydevik B, Holm S, Bagge U. Effects of experimental graded compression on blood flow in spinal nerve roots. A vital microscopic study on the porcine cauda equina. J Orthop Res. 1989;7:817-23.
18. Postacchini F: Management of lumbar spinal stenosis. J Bone Joint Surg. 1996; 75B(1):154-64.
19. Rydevik B, Lundborg G: Permeability of intraneural microvessels and perineurium following acute, graded experimental nerve compression. Scan J Plast and Reconstr Surg. 1977;11:179-87.
20. Wall EJ, Cohen MS, Abitol JJ, Garfin SR: Organization of intrathecal nerve roots at the level of the conus medullaris. J Bone Joint Surg. 1990; 72A:1495-9.
21. Wall EJ, Cohen MS, Massie JB, Rydevik B, Garfin SR. Cauda equina anatomy I: Intrathecal nerve root organization. Spine. 1990; 15:1244-7.
22. Yoshizawa H, Kobayashi S, Hachiya Y. Blood supply of nerve roots and dorsal root ganglia. Orthop Clin North America. 1991; 22:195-211.
23. Ikuda K, Arima J, Tanaka T. Short-term result of microscopic posterior decompression for lumbar spinal stenosis. J Neurosurg. 2005; 40:624-33.
24. Gelalis ID, Stafilas KS, Korompilias AV, Zacharis KC, Beris AE, Xenakix TA. Decompressive surgery for degenerative lumbar spinal stenosis: long-term results. Int Orthop. 2006; 30:59-63.
25. Takaso M, Nakazawa T, Imura T, Okada T, et al. Less invasive and less technically demanding decompression procedure

for lumbar spinal stenosis – appropriate for general orthopedic surgeons? Int Orthop. 2011;35:67-73.
26. Schatzker J, Pennel GF: Spinal stenosis, a cause of cauda equina compression. J Bone Joint Surg. 1968;50B:606-18.
27. Jones RAC, Thompson JLG. The narrow lumbar canal, a clinical and radiolgical review. J Bone Joint Surg. 1968; 50B:595-605.
28. Arnold CC, et al. Lumbar spinal stenosis and nerve root entrapment syndromes. Definition and classification. Clin Orthop. 1976;115:4-5.
29. Spurling RG: Hypertrophy of the ligamenta flava as a cause of low back pain. JAMA. 1937;109:928-33.
30. Takoso M, Nakazawa T, Imura T, et al. Less invasive and less technically demanding decompression procedure for lumbar spinal stenosis – appropriate for general orthopedic surgeons? Int Orthop. 2011; 35: 67-73.
31. Tsuji H et al: Expansive laminoplasty for lumbar spinal stenosis. Int Orthop. 1990;14:307-14.

CHAPTER

32

Combined Lumbosacral Fusion in One Stage Using Anterior Then Posterior Approach: Surgical Technique and Results

Cédric Barrey, Boissiere L, D'acunzi G, Perrin G

Introduction

Lumbosacral arthrodesis is one of the most common surgical procedures performed for the management of lumbar degenerative disease. The objectives of lumbosacral fusion are to stabilize the spinal segment, to restore lordosis, to obtain intervertebral fusion end to perform decompression of the neurological structures when required. Different techniques have been proposed to achieve these goals. Each technique has its own advantages and disadvantages. With recent progress of anterior instrumentation and surgical technique, the anterior approach of the lumbar spine has become more popular.

We propose in this chapter to report our personal experience with the combined approach using anterior then posterior approach in only one stage and to discuss the advantages of this technique in comparison with the others types of arthrodesis.

Case Series

The aim of this chapter is to report clinical and radiographic results at 1 year through a prospective series of 62 patients undergoing combined 360° lumbosacral fusion (1 or 2 levels) in a single step. The surgical technique is also described in details.

Material and Methods

Sixty-two patients underwent surgery between June 2008 and December 2010 and were consecutively included in the study.

The mean age was 44 ± 11 years and the series consisted of 39 women and 23 men. Pre- and postoperative clinical (VAS, Oswestry Disability Index) and radiological (segmental and global lordosis) data, the surgical technique used and all complications were recorded. A CT scan was systematically performed at 1 year to assess the fusion quality (according to the Spine Interbody Research Group Criteria).

Indications for surgery included degenerative disk disease in 36 cases (isolated n = 6; associated with MODIC 1 changes n = 4; post-diskectomy n = 9; L5–S1 retrolisthesis n = 11; transitional lumbosacral anomaly n = 6) and low-grade (I or II) isthmic spondylolisthesis in 26 cases. All patients presented with low back pain and/or radicular pain for more than 6 months.

All patients underwent surgery involving a combined approach: anterior retroperitoneal route (A) with PEEK cage and BMP then posterior route (P) with pedicular screws under the same general anesthesia session.

Surgical Technique

The two steps (anterior then posterior) are performed under only one general anesthesia.

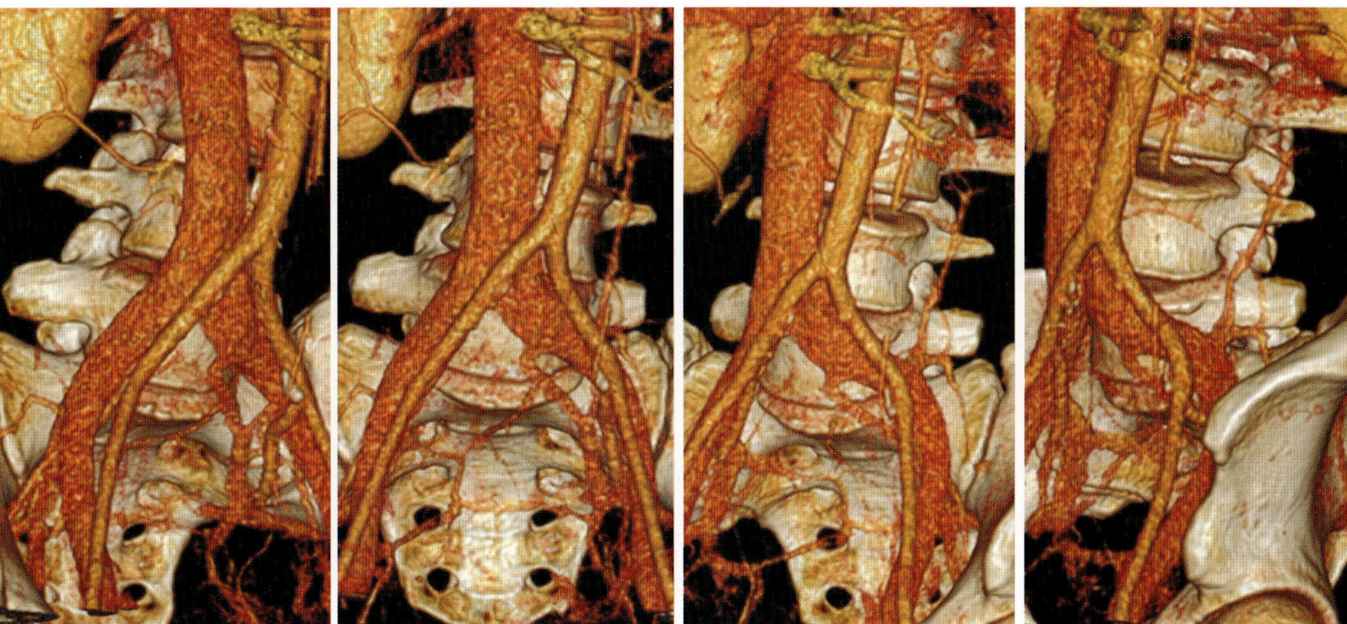

Fig. 32.1 Preoperative assessment of vascular anatomy in the lumbar spine using 3D CT angiography

Anterior Step

The morphology and location of prevertebral vascular structures, arteries and veins, are preoperatively analysed by realizing a 3D angio-CT scan (Fig. 32.1), with a special interest on relationships between iliac veins and intervertebral disks. 3D reconstructions of prevertebral vessels provide easier information to fully understand the vascular anatomy in the lumbar spine.

To facilitate lumbosacral area access, urinary catheter, which allows bladder emptying, is systematically placed preoperatively. Otherwise, oxymeter is bilaterally placed at the foot to verify pulse during the procedure and thus avoid excessive vessels retraction or vessels compromise by retractor blades.

Positioning

We routinely use the French position with the patient supine, legs in abduction and the lumbar spine slightly hyperextended.

X-rays

Once the patient is installed, disk projection and disk angulation are marked onto the skin by using antero-posterior and lateral radiographs. Although, in general, L4–L5 disk projects at umbilicus and L5–S1 at midway from umbilicus to pubis symphysis, significant variations can be observed and preoperative X-rays are strongly recommended.

Exposure of the Retroperitoneal Space

A paramedian vertical skin incision is performed, on the right side for L5-S1 and on the left side for L4–L5. Horizontal incision can be realized at L5–S1. After exposure of the anterior rectus sheath, this one is cut vertically and then the rectus muscle is divided away from the under surface of the anterior sheath by using two Kocher clamps. The rectus muscle is retracted laterally permitting exposure of the posterior rectus sheath and retroperitoneal fat. At this time of the procedure the arcuate ligament, which limits inferiorly the posterior rectus sheath, has to be identified. The arcuate ligament extends from the midline to the lateral wall of abdomen and marks laterally the point of entrance to the retroperitoneal space.

We recommend starting dissection of the retroperitoneal fat from the lateral abdominal wall approximately at the area of the anterior iliac crest. The retroperitoneal fat is gently retracted from the fascia and from iliac muscle with a sweeping motion from lateral to medial. Packing some abdominal wet compresses on the inner surface of iliac fossa may be helpful for the dissection. Inferior epigastric vessels are left intact on the deep surface of the rectus muscle.

To facilitate medial retraction of the peritoneum and its contents, the arcuate ligament could be cut vertically. At this stage the purpose is to progressively expose the psoas muscle. Care must be taken to avoid injury of the genito-femoral nerve running onto the surface of the muscle. In females further exposure of iliopsoas muscle may require division for the round ligament which extends from the lateral border of the uterus to the deep inguinal ring and may limit exposure in some cases.

Exposure of the Prevertebral Space

Once iliopsoas muscle is exposed, progressive lateromedial retraction of the peritoneum and its contents allows

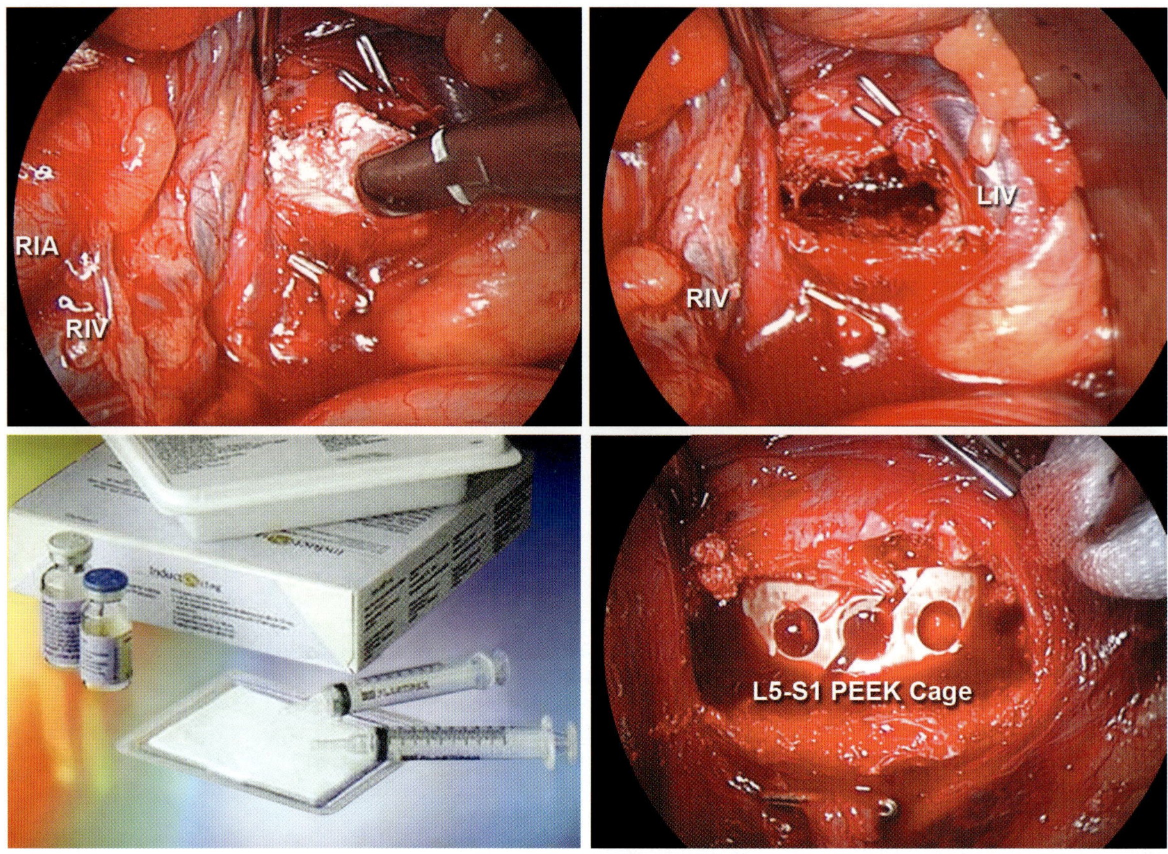

Fig. 32.2 The anterior procedure consisted of retroperitoneal approach, complete diskectomy, clearing the endplates and insertion of large and lordotic PEEK cage filled with bone morphogenic protein (BMP)

identification of iliac vessels, arteries and veins, and then of the left ureter. Fat tissue closely related with iliac vessels often contains lymphatics which injury could lead to a chronic retroperitoneal lymphocele and has not to be further divided. The ureter and vas deferens are gently displaced medially without separation from the peritoneal contents. In general ureter is adherent to the peritoneum. At this stage digital palpation can be helpful to locate the promontory which exposure is typically performed between the left common iliac vein and the right common iliac artery. Optimal exposure is obtained with the help of a self-retaining retractor by placing 3 blades: medial, lateral and third one at the cephalad area of the field. In order to avoid any damage of the sympathetic hypogastric plexus, which almost 80% of ramifications are located on the left side of the aorta and across the left common iliac artery before crossing the pelvis brim, only bipolar coagulation is used in the area just front of the promontory.

In most cases no retraction of iliac vessels is necessary to expose L5–S1 disk but middle sacral vessels need to be divided.

Diskectomy and Stabilization Stage

After division of the anterior longitudinal ligament, complete diskectomy is carried out (Fig. 32.2). In general, all disk material is removed in front of the posterior longitudinal ligament which one is respected**.** The quality of diskectomy is verified by introducing the endoscope through the disk place.

Then a large and lordotic Peek cage, filled with bone marrow harvested from the iliac crest and mixed with porous biphasic ceramic, permits to stabilize the spinal segment**.** One or two anterior plate is systematically associated in order to increase construct stiffness and enhance rates of interbody fusion.

Closure

In most cases retroperitoneal drainage is not necessary. Closure of arcuate ligament is usually realized, especially when division was more than 2.5 cm. Meticulous closure of the anterior rectus sheath is then performed by a running suture.

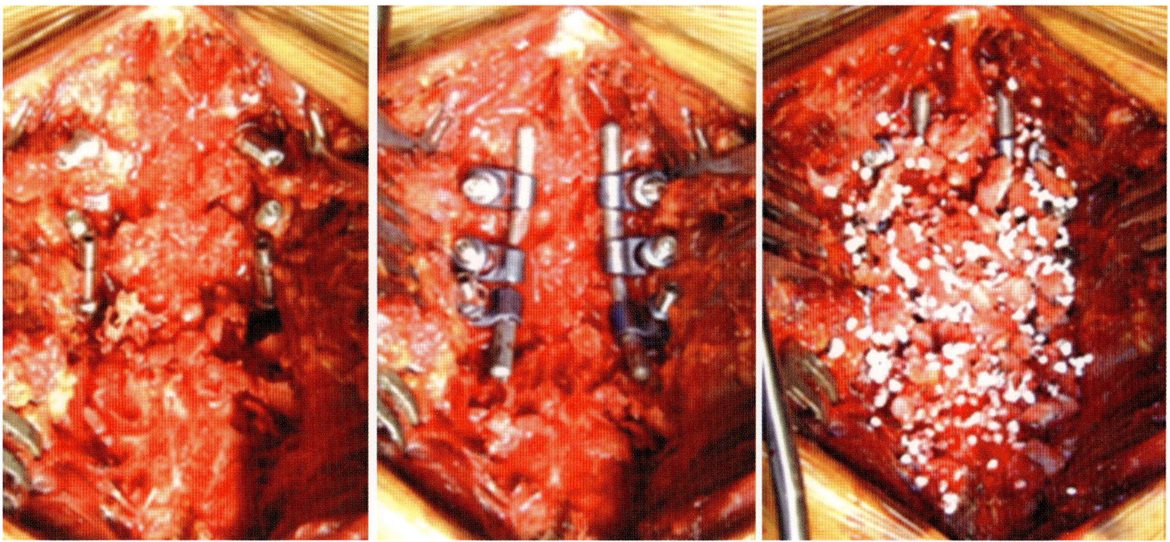

Fig. 32.3 Posterior step with pedicle screw-based stabilization and posteromedian bone graft

L4–L5 Approach

When consider L4–L5 approach, it appeared to us that five points differ from the L5–S1 approach:

- Left side approach is almost always used because of the cavoiliac bifurcation on the right side
- Exposure is carried out laterally to the left common iliac artery and not between iliac bifurcation
- We almost always need to divide the arcuate ligament
- Dissection of the iliolumbar ascending vein can be required. We advise double hemoclip on each side of the vessel to secure haemostasis which failure could lead to catastrophic bleeding. In cases of low origin of the ascending branch, this one can be left intact but great care must be taken to avoid any excessive traction.
- Finally mobilization of iliac vessels, especially the left iliac vein, is usually necessary to achieve appropriate exposure of the L4–L5 disk space.

L4–L5/L5–S1 Approach

When L4-S1 segment is required, we recommend exposing one level at a time rather than exposing both levels at the same time, thus avoiding excessive traction on visceral and vascular structures.

Posterior Step

The patient was then placed in prone position. After standard posterior midline approach, partial arthrectomy were systematically performed. According to preoperative clinical and radiological data, limited decompression could be done via lamino-foraminotomy. Pedicle screws were then implanted and stabilization was obtained using mono and polyaxial hemispherical screws-clamps system. Specific care was achieved for the binding of the rod. Finally, decortication was carried out and posteromedian graft interlaminar and interfacet) was realized using autologous bone graft mixed with phospho-calcic bone substitutes (Fig. 32.3).

Finally, 360° arthrodesis was obtained with optimal biomechanical stabilization of the spinal segment (Fig. 32.4).

Results

The levels involved were as follows: L5–S1 for 42 patients, L4–S1 for 12 patients and L4–L5 for 8 patients (Fig. 32.5).

Mean operative time was 185 min and mean blood loss was 315 mL (including anterior and posterior approaches) (Table 32.1).

No serious complication was encountered in this series. We observed 1 per-operative vascular injury (iliac vein) without sequelae, 2 abdominal wall hematoma and 2 deep vein thrombosis.

Table 32.1 Perioperative data

n = 62	*Operative time*	*blood loss*	
		Per-operative	Drains
Anterior	87 ± 15 min [63–119]	70 ± 80 mL [0–600]	40 ± 22 mL [0–50]
Posterior	96 ± 30 min [78–175]	245 ± 102 mL [100–500]	280 ± 72 mL [100–550]

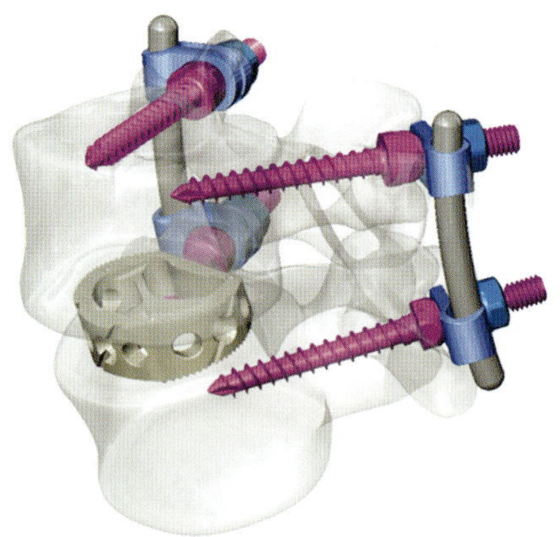

Fig. 32.4 Oblique view of the construct demonstrating anterior interbody cage associated with pedicle screw-based posterior stabilization (from ScientX-Alphatec™ Spine, Carlsbad, USA)

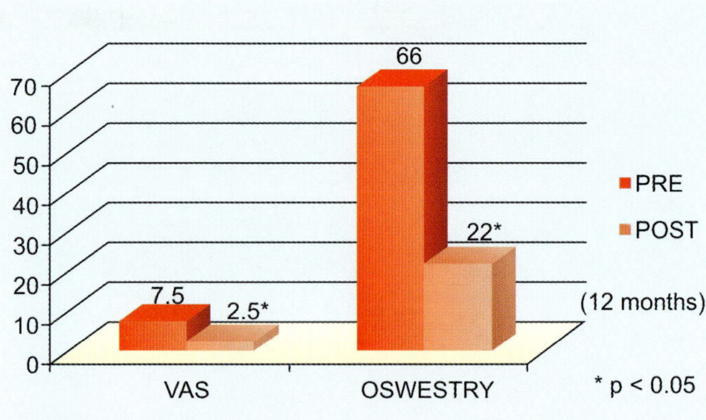

Fig. 32.6 Clinical results for pain and functional status at 1 year

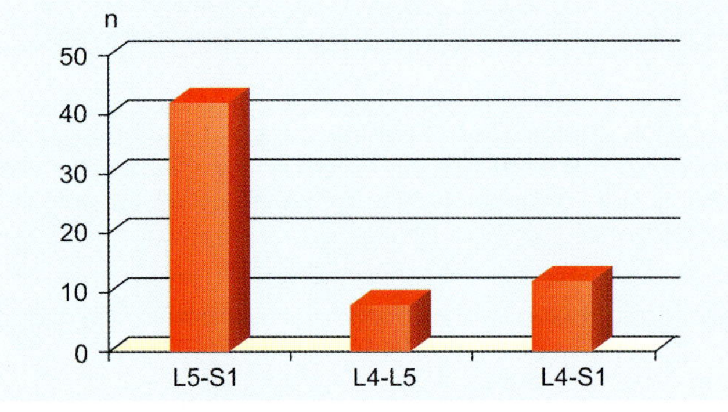

Fig. 32.5 Levels involved

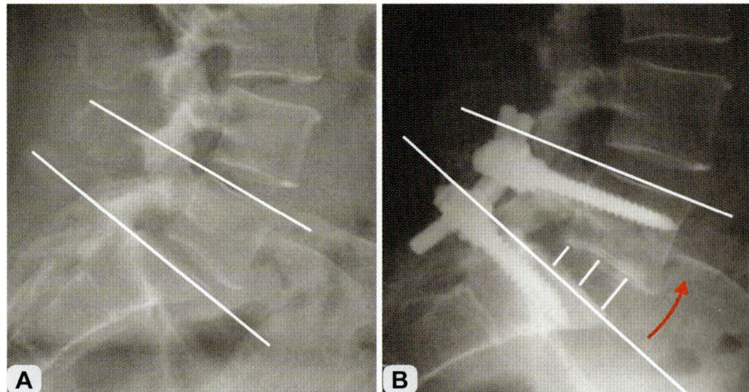

Fig. 32.7 Grade I isthmic spondylolisthésis treated by combined anterior then posterior approach. Segmental lordosis significantly increased postoperatively at the index level. (A) Preoperative; (B) Postoperative 1 year

At the final follow-up, the Oswestry Disability Index had fallen from 66 preoperatively to 22 postoperatively and the VAS had fallen from 7.5 to 2.5 respectively, $p < 0.01$ (Fig. 32.6).

Segmental lordosis was a mean 5° preoperatively versus 13.5° postoperatively, $p < 0.01$ (Figs 32.7 and 32.8).

No pseudarthrosis was evident in the routine control scan at 1 year; however the quality of fusion appeared to vary from one patient to another. Otherwise, we observed neither mechanical complication neither implant migration (Fig. 32.9).

Discussion

The advantages of the combined technique, in comparison with isolated anterior or isolated posterior approach, are represented by:

- The quality of the discectomy (source of pain) and of the endplates clearing (promoting fusion) during the anterior approach
- The opportunity to insert large and lordotic PEEK cages with a great surface of contact between the bone graft and the endplates (Fig. 32.10)
- The biomechanical quality of stabilization provided by the pedicle screw-based stabilization (Fig. 32.11)
- The avoidance of nerve roots manipulation.

The surgical sequence is also very important to consider. The concept of the anterior then posterior combined arthrodesis is to realign the spine during the anterior step then just stabilize during the posterior one. With the patient supine and the lumbar spine slightly in extension, realignment and restoration of lordosis is optimally achieved in most cases during the anterior procedure. This facilitates strongly the posterior procedure in which the goal is simply to stabilize a spine already realigned and reduced in terms of lordosis.

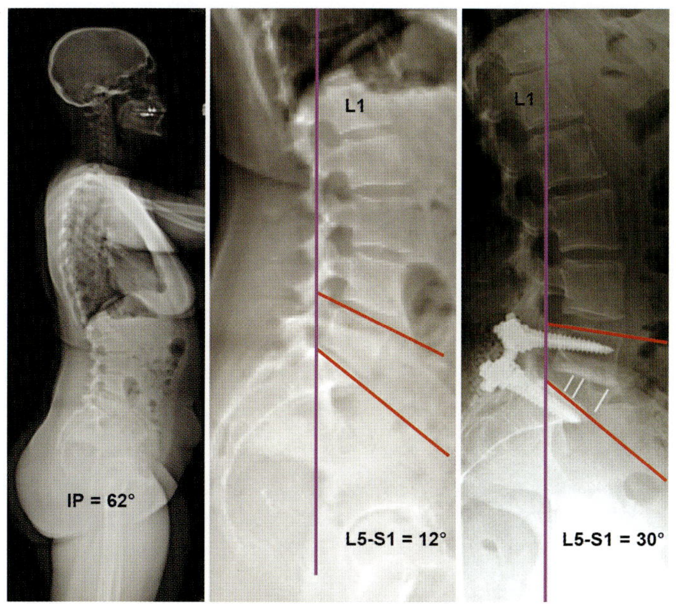

Fig. 32.8 The amount of lordosis restored during the surgical procedure was adapted to the spinopelvic parameters and especially to the value of pelvic incidence. This is the case of a woman with a high value of PI (more than 60°). Theoretical lumbar lordosis is approximately 70° (theoretical PI is calculated according to the classes of pelvic incidence), meaning that L5–S1 segment requires between 25° and 30° of lordosis (corresponding to 40% of the global lordosis). This objective could be satisfied using the combined anterior then posterior strategy for fusion.

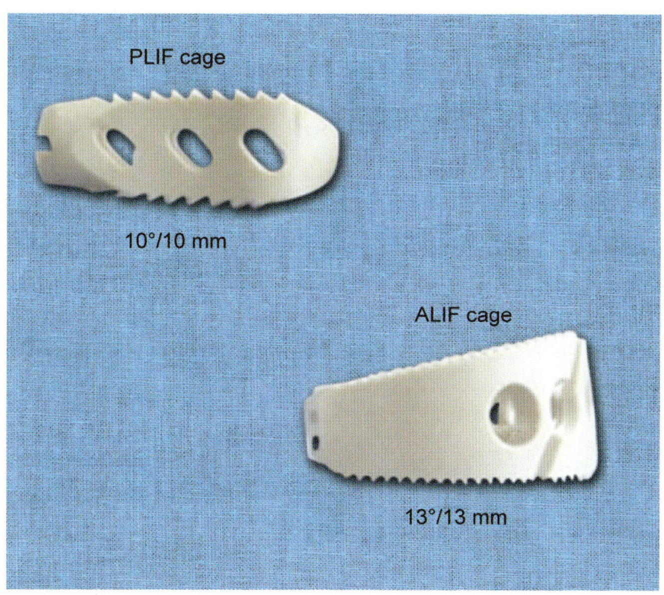

Fig. 32.10 Comparison of interbody cages usually implanted during posterior technique (PLIF) versus anterior approach (ALIF). Typical cages implanted by PLIF technique correspond to 10° of lordosis and 10 mm of height versus 13°/13 mm, respectively, by ALIF technique. This underlies the advantages of the combined approach in terms of lordosis and disk height restoration and volume bone graft.

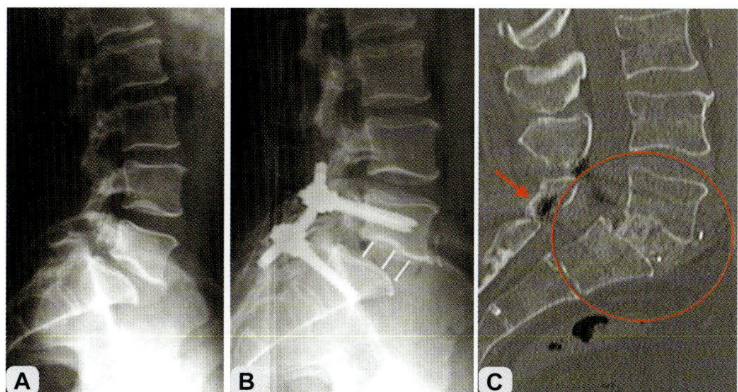

Fig. 32.9 Combined approach permits to obtain a 360° intervertebral fusion in a very high percentage of cases with a large interbody and posteromedian (i.e. interlaminar and interfacet) bone mass fusion as illustrated in this case. (A) Preoperative; (B) 4 months; (C) 12 months

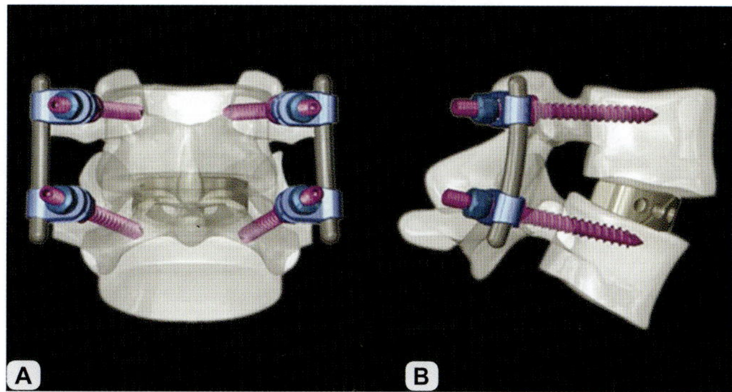

Fig. 32.11 (A) Posterior and lateral views of combined arthrodesis with large and lordotic ALIF cage and (B) posterior pedicle screw-based stabilization (from ScientX-Alphatec^{TM} Spine, Carlsbad, USA)

In addition, concerning the fusion rates, it is well established in the literature that more circumferential the fusion is, higher is the fusion rates.

Limitations of the combined procedure are represented by:

- The requirement of two approaches
- Higher rates of complications
- And increased operative time

Conclusion

In conclusion, lumbosacral fusion by a combined approach in one stage is safe and successfully meets the requisite criteria in terms of clinical and functional results, of fusion rates and of restoration of segmental lordosis.

Bibliography

1. Barrey C, Jund J, Noseda O, Roussouly P. Sagittal balance of the pelvis-spine complex and lumbar degenerative diseases. A comparative study about 85 cases. European Spine Journal. 2007;16:1459-67.
2. Barrey C, Ene B, Louis-Tisserand G, Montagna P, Perrin G, Simon E. Vascular anatomy in the lumbar spine investigated by 3D CT angiography: the concept of vascular window. World Neurosurgery. 2012. In Press.
3. Bianchi C, Ballard JL, Abou-Zamzam AM, Teruya TH, Abu-Assal ML. Anterior retroperitoneal lumbosacral spine exposure: operative technique and results. Annals of Vascular Surgery. 2003;17:137-42.
4. Leufven C, Nordwall A. Management of chronic disabling low back pain with 360 degrees fusion: Results from pain provocation test and concurrent posterior lumbar interbody fusion, posterolateral fusion, and pedicle screw instrumentation in patients with chronic disabling low back pain. Spine. 1999;24:2042-5.
5. Mayer HM, Wiechert K. Microsurgical anterior approaches to the lumbar spine for interbody fusion and total disc replacement. Neurosurgery. 2002;51:S159-64.
6. Vaccaro AR. Core knowledge in orthopedics. In Spine, Surgical management of low back pain, Elsevier; 2005. pp 98-115.

CHAPTER

33

Surgical Results of Dynamic Nonfusion Stabilization with the Segmental Spinal Correction System for Degenerative Lumbar Spinal Diseases with Instability: Minimum 2-year Follow-up

Hideki Ohta, Yoshiyuki Matsumoto, Yuichirou Morishita, Tsubasa Sakai, George Huang, Hirotaka Kida, Yoshiharu Takemitsu

Introduction

There has long been a conflict of opinions regarding whether the best treatment for unstable degenerative lumbar disease is spinal fusion or decompression surgery. Despite good results with fusion, adjacent segment disease remains a long-term issue. With decompression surgery, on the other hand, revision surgery may be required in many cases because of recurrence of spinal canal stenosis caused by increased instability on operated segments. We applied nonfusion stabilization with the segmental spinal correction system (SSCS) (Ulrich Medical, Ulm, Germany) and decompression to mitigate the disadvantages of both procedures.

The disadvantages of conventional spinal fusion are the requirement for bone grafting, potential adjacent segment disease (fusion disease), and the relatively invasive approach. Adjacent segment disease is obviously a major issue. To address it, instruments have been actively developed (mainly in Europe), primarily motion-preserving devices whose purpose is to restore physiologic motion and provide prophylaxis for adjacent segment disease while allowing for decompression. Devices for lumbar spine artificial disk replacement are in the review stage, but posterior motion preservation techniques remain in development.

The SSCS was developed by Professor Archibald H. von Strempel in 1989.[1] It is a unique system with a solid rod and a pedicle screw that has mobility in its screw head. The screw controls lateral bending, rotation, and translation completely and allows some motion in flexion and extension (sagittal plane) (Fig. 33.1). The SSCS was originally used together with posterolateral fusion. However, von Strempel realized that patients were asymptomatic and no SSCS implant failure occurred even with occurrence of pseudarthrosis. A multicenter study of nonfusion stabilization without bone grafts was started in 2004 with the concept of motion preservation.[2] The dynamized pedicle screw is available elsewhere under the Cosmic System (Ulrich Medical, Ulm, Germany)1 with bioactive calcium phosphate coating. (The Japanese Ministry of Health, Labor and Welfare has not approved the bioactive coated screw for use yet in Japan, hence the use of the uncoated screw.) Although hinge breakage is of concern, no failure has been reported.

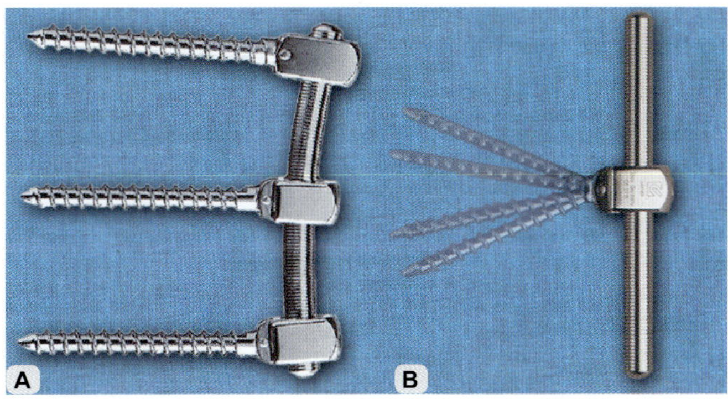

Fig. 33.1 (A) Segmental spinal correction system controls rotation and translation and allows flexion and extension. The screw has 20° of mobility in both the cranial and caudal directions; (B) The hinged screw allows motion

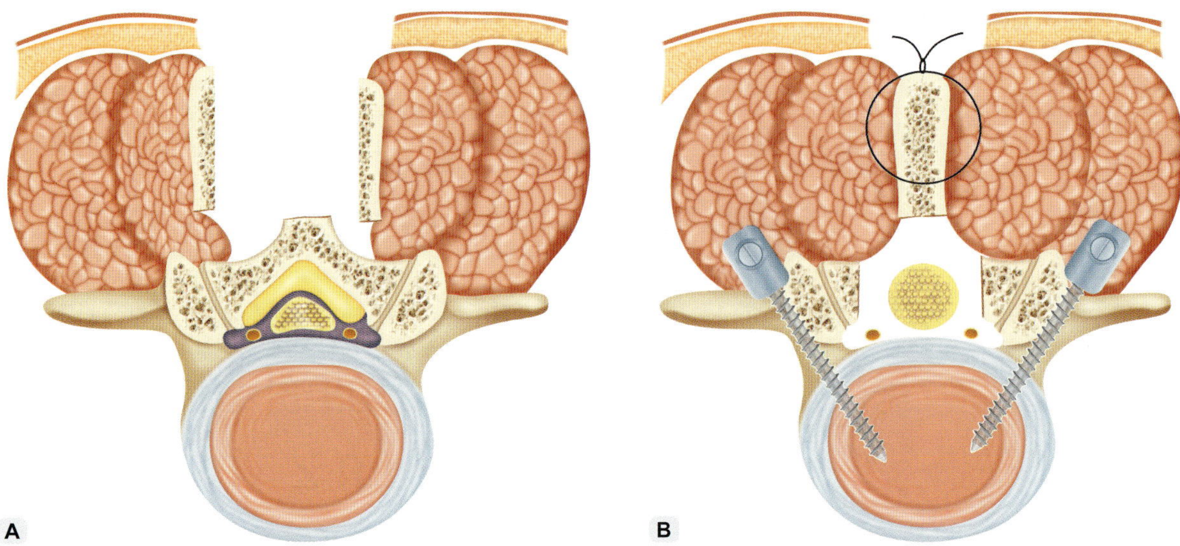

Fig. 33.2 Spinous process splitting approach. The advantages of the spinous process splitting laminectomy include minimizing damage to the posterior supporting structure, less dead space and less blood loss, and the prevention of muscular atrophy because nerves and vessels on the paraspinal muscle remain undamaged. (A) Split the spinous process longitudinally in the middle; (B) Suture the split spinous process after decompression and insertion of the pedicle screw

We used SSCS nonfusion stabilization combined with spinous process splitting laminectomy for unstable degenerative lumbar disease. A less invasive spinous process splitting[3] allows for SSCS implantation (Fig. 33.2).

The surgical results of SSCS for unstable degenerative lumbar disease with a minimum 2-year follow-up are presented. The purpose of this study was to determine the clinical results and the incidence of adjacent segment disease as well as instrument failure.

Methods

We performed SSCS nonfusion stabilization in 214 patients from June 2005 to September 2009. We chose 52 patients (35 men and 17 women) with a minimum 2-year follow-up. The mean age was 64.3 years (range, 21–82 years), with a mean follow-up of 35 months (range, 24–46 months). The operative indications were as follows: degenerative spondylolisthesis (20 patients), lumbar spinal canal stenosis (10 patients), disk herniation (6 patients), lumbar canal stenosis with disk herniation (15 patients), and lumbar discopathy (1 patient). In all cases instability was observed by use of plain radiographs. We defined instability as more than 5° of posterior angulation, more than 3 mm of anterolisthesis, or sagittalization of facet joints. Positioning the patients in the prone position on the 4-point frame maintains the lumbar spine in a neutral or mildly lordotic position. Decompression was achieved by spinous process splitting followed by pedicle screw insertion. The screws were then tightened with rods *in situ* without correction, followed by split spinous process suturing to complete the procedure. No bone graft was used. Postoperatively, a soft corset was applied to the patients with no activity restriction.

The investigational items are as follows: (i) changes in clinical symptoms based on the Japanese Orthopaedic Association (JOA) score, which correlates to Oswestry Disability Index and Roland-Morris Disability Questionnaire,[4] (ii) Cobb angle (maximum flexion-extension) of operated segments preoperatively and at final follow-up, (iii) range of motion (ROM) of the operated segments preoperatively and at final follow-up, and (iv) occurrence of adjacent segment disorders and instrumentation failure.

Results

The JOA score was 14.4 ± 5.3 preoperatively, and it improved to 25.5 ± 2.8 postoperatively. The Hirabayashi recovery rate was 76.0%. The preoperative Cobb angle was –2.8° ± 4.8° (maximum flexion) and 6.8° ± 4.8° (maximum extension), and ROM was 9.6° ± 4.2°. The postoperative Cobb angle was 3.2° ± 3.7° (maximum flexion) and 5.1° ± 3.9° (maximum extension), and ROM was 2.0° ± 1.8°. The posterior angulation (flexion instability) disappeared, and the ROM was decreased statistically ($P < 0.001$, paired "t" test). Adjacent segment disease appeared in 3 patients (5.7%). One patient had pain in the lower extremity at 1 year after surgery, when falling during a walk. Disk herniation was observed in the upper adjacent segment, and discectomy and posterolateral lumbar fusion were performed because the patient did not agree to undergo conservative treatment. Two other patients had low-grade spinal canal stenosis in both upper and lower adjacent segments after surgery, but they have been followed up closely with conservative treatment because the symptoms were very mild. Loss of disk height at the lower adjacent segment was observed in 2 cases but produced no symptoms. There was 1 implant screw breakage; thus, the failure rate was 0.47% (1 of 214 screws). Screw loosening was observed in a 3-level stabilization asymptomatic patient.

Case Presentation

A 74-year-old man was diagnosed with lumbar spinal canal stenosis. Symptoms included low-back pain for 2 years, pain and paralysis in the right lower extremity, and intermittent claudication. Stenosis in L4–5 was observed by myelography. A disk angle of –8° in flexion (posterior angulation) and +4° in extension was observed on radiographs. Surgery was performed for spinal canal stenosis with instability. The technique used was spinous process splitting laminectomy at L4–5 and stabilization with the SSCS in neutral position. The operation time was 79 minutes. Blood loss was 52 mL. Thirty-four months after surgery, 2° of motion remained in the disk (Fig. 33.3), and the JOA score had improved from 13 to 28.

Discussion

Proponents of spinal fusion and nonfusion have not yet reached consensus regarding degenerative disk disease treatment. Spinal fusion immediately stabilizes diseased segments in terms of pain relief while enhancing nerve recovery. Adjacent segment disease remains a midterm/long-term drawback with conventional spinal fusion. Ghiselli et al.[5] reported revision surgery rates of 16.5% (5 years) and 36.1% (10 years) after lumbar posterior fusion (Kaplan-Meier method). Motion preservation technology with the purpose of achieving decompression and physiologic reconstruction with preservation of the physiologic spine motion has received attention.

Spinal motion preservation techniques include intradiskal stabilization by artificial disk and extradiskal stabilization that stabilizes segments outside of the disk. Lumbar artificial disks have been actively used mainly in Europe and the United States, but they are being reviewed because of complications. Extradiskal stabilization can be achieved in 2 ways. One is a flexible rod with a pedicle screw, and the other is an interspinous process spacer. There are many implants available in the European market, but only the Isobar TTL (Alphatec Spine, Carlsbad, California) and the Graf system (SEM, Co., Mountrouge, France) are available for use in Japan. For the Graf system, the revision surgery rate because of adjacent segment disease was 7% at 10-year minimum follow-up, and this system is considered to have less effect on adjacent segments.[6] The Graf system has less control for lateral bending and rotation.[7] Facet joint fusion due to strong posterior compression forces has been reported;[7] therefore, it may be a less-than-ideal motion preservation system.

The SSCS differs from the previously mentioned implants. It is a pedicle screw–based system with a rigid rod, but the unique structure of having a hinge in the screw head allows for micromotion.[8] The screw hinges 20° in the sagittal plane and is rigid in the coronal plane and for rotational movement and rotational direction. The SSCS does not allow for lateral bending, rotation, or translation except for sagittal plane motion. Dynamic compression testing showed no implant failure after 10 million cycles (a 30-year lifetime)[9]; the screw hinges remained intact, showing no macroscopic signs of wear debris or loosening. Wear debris was not observed during revision surgery for 1 patient. Hinged posterior fixation has been reported to reduce load to the screw and may reduce breakage risk.[8,10] von Strempel et al.[2] in a multicenter study reported breakage in 2 of 1,604 screws (0.12%) and 1 of 658 rods (0.15%). We found screw breakage in 1 of 214 screws, or a 0.47% implant failure rate. The implant failure rate was low for this nonfusion stabilization and avoided the morbidity associated with bone grafts. This hinged screw is more physiologic than a rigid screw and shares load moderately with vertebral motion segments[8,10] while reducing load to the device. The instantaneous axis of rotation[11] of flexion and extension is located in the dorsal half of the disk on the superior vertebral body. With flexion instability, the disk has posterior (kyphotic) angulation centering on the instantaneous axis of rotation in flexion and the facet joint slides greatly. Neutral-position tightening of the SSCS rod and screw head controls facet joint slide and removes flexion instability. Thus, flexion instability (instability in the sagittal plane direction) is removed. This allows 2° – 3° of micromotion in the disk through a hinge mechanism. This micromotion function prevents adjacent segment disease (Fig. 33.4). One root cause for adjacent segment disease is increased intradiscal pressure[12] in adjacent disks of operated segments, which can also occur with nonfusion stabilization.[13] Nonfusion stabilization compensates for some ROM in adjacent disks, which may be forced to increase by spinal fusion. In our study ROM in patients' discs was largely reduced, from 9.6° preoperatively to 2.0° postoperatively. Further consideration is necessary to find out whether the mean motion of 2° is enough to prevent adjacent segment disease.

Case 1: Male, 74 years old Lumbar spinal canal stenosis
· Low back pain, right lower extremity-based paralysis and pain over 2 years
· Intermittent claudication for 10 minutes

L4/5 Spinous Process Splitting Laminectomy + SSCS
2 years and 10 months Post OP, the patient is doing well JOA score 13 ® 28

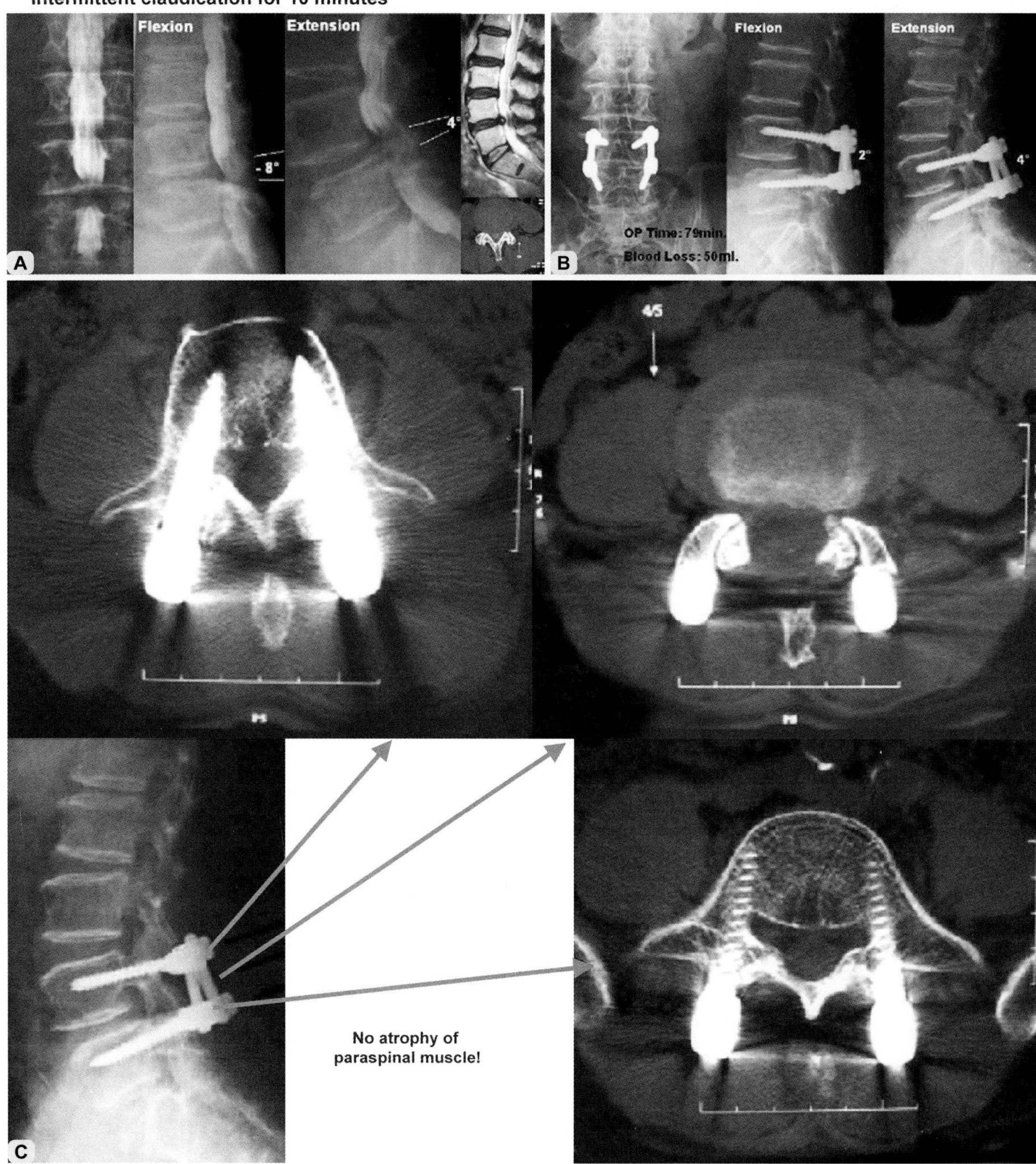

Fig. 33.3 Case presentation: (A) Preoperative radiograph; (B) Postoperative radiograph; (C) Postoperative radiograph and computed tomograph. Post OP, postoperative; OP time, operation time; JOA, Japanes Orthopedic Association

Revision surgery was required in 1 case (1.9%) because of adjacent segment disease at less than 5 years. Although further long-term follow-up is necessary, short-term results are good with maintained stability of the spine. Using spinous process splitting laminectomy for decompression minimized the damage to the paraspinal muscle, which may lead to less lower-back discomfort after surgery.

The indications for the SSCS are (i) mild degenerative spondylolisthesis, (ii) preserved anterior column support, (iii) posterior angulation in the flexion position (flexion

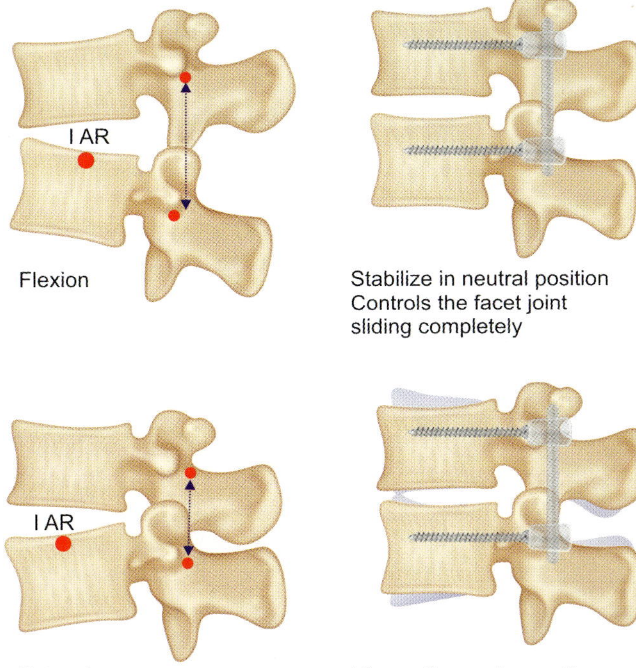

Fig. 33.4 Mechanism of SSCS stabilization. The instantaneous axis of rotation (IAR) of flexion and extension is located dorsal to the disk on the superior part of the vertebral body. If there is flexion instability, the disk would have posterior angulation centering on the IAR in flexion, with facet joint sliding. With the SSCS, the rod and the screw head are tightened in neutral position. Therefore facet joint sliding is controlled while still allowing micromotion of the disc because of the hinge between the screw head and the screw thread. It is thought that the micromotion works as a shock absorber, like a car suspension, and prevents adjacent segment disorder.

instability), and (iv) sagittalization of facet joints. Instability was defined as the presence of more than 5° of posterior angulation, more than 3 mm of anterolisthesis, or sagittalization of facet joints. Further evaluation is necessary to determine the level of instability best managed by the SSCS (maximum instability in this study was 12° posterior angulation and 15 mm of anterolisthesis). We have no experience with the SSCS in patients with severe instability.

The contraindications are severe instability, degenerative scoliosis, foraminal stenosis, isthmic spondylolisthesis, trauma, and infection. Hinge motion is asymmetrically restricted in degenerative scoliosis, increasing the risk of screw breakage. Short disk height with foraminal stenosis restricts SSCS application. In short, the SSCS is not suitable if correction for alignment is required. In case of isthmic spondylolisthesis, there is a risk of breakage because the facet joint is destroyed and the load to the device will be excessive.

Spinal fusion with instrumentation was developed for the purpose of scoliosis correction. In the early 1980s, the technique was applied to degenerative lumbar disease, and the application became frequently used. Is it necessary to correct the malalignment of the lumbar spine excessively? The concept of the motion preservation technology is to provide spinal decompression and stabilize physiologic instability.

Worldwide, companies are competing to develop marketable implants for spinal fusion with the aim of achieving bony fusion in alignment. The SSCS was originally developed to be used in conjunction with bone grafts. However, it was later found that with pseudarthrosis, the implant failure rate was low and patients were asymptomatic. Thus the SSCS has also become a nonfusion stabilization system. Long-term follow-up data are pending. There is room for modification of the SSCS device in that it only allows motion in the sagittal plane. Lumbar artificial disk revision has a potential high risk, given anatomic concerns. On the other hand, motion preservation technology with a posterior approach has expected growth potential because of surgeon familiarity and ease of revision. We expect further development of ideal instrumentation facilitated by advancements in technology.

Conclusion

The results of SSCS nonfusion stabilization for 52 patients with unstable degenerative lumbar disease with a minimum 2-year follow-up found improved JOA scores and a Hirabayashi recovery rate of 76%. ROM was significantly controlled, from 9.6° ± 4.2° preoperatively to 2.0° ± 1.8° postoperatively. There was screw breakage in 1 case, but stability of the spine was maintained. Long-term follow-up focusing on adjacent segment disorder is required.

References

1. von Strempel A, Stoss C, Moosmann D, Martin A. Non-fusion stabilization of the lumbar spine in the case of degenerative disease with A dynamic pedicle screw rod. Coluna/Columna. 2006;5:27-34
2. von Strempel A, Schiavone MA, Ozer F, et al. Non fusion stabilization with a non rigid but stable pedicle screw system-results of a multicentre study, Presented at Spine Arthroplasty Society - 7th Annual Conference, Berlin, Germany. 2007;May 1-5.
3. Watanabe K, Hosoya T, Shiraishi T, Matsumoto M, Chiba K, Toyama Y. Lumbar spinous process-splitting laminectomy for lumbar canal stenosis. Technical note. J Neurosurg Spine. 2005;3:405-8.
4. Fujiwara A, Kobayashi N, Saiki K, Kitagawa T, Tamai K, Saotome K. Association of the Japanese Orthopaedic Association score

with the Oswestry Disability Index, Roland-Morris Disability Questionnaire, and short-form 36. Spine. 2003;28:1601-7.

5. Ghiselli G, Wang JC, Bhatia NN, Hsu WK, Dawson EG. Adjacent segment degeneration in the lumbar spine. J Bone Joint Surg Am. 2004;86:1497-503.
6. Kanayama M, Hashimoto T, Shigenobu K, Togawa D, Oha F. A minimum 10-year follow-up of posterior dynamic stabilization using Graf artificial ligament. Spine. 2007;32:1992-6.
7. Hadlow SV, Fagan AB, Hillier TM, Fraser RD. The Graf ligamentoplasty procedure (Comparison with posterolateral fusion in the management of low back pain). Spine. 1998;23:1172-9.
8. Scifert JL, Sairyo K, Goel VK, Grobler LJ, Grosland NM, Spratt KF, et al. Stability analysis of an enhanced load sharing posterior fixation device and its equivalent conventional device in a calf spine model. Spine. 1999;24:2206-13.
9. von Strempel A, Sukopp C, Basso S. Non-fusion versus fusion technique for the stabilization of the lumbar spine, Presented at Spine Arthroplasty Society - 4th Annual Conference, Vienna, Austria. 2004;May 4-7.
10. Goel VK, Konz RJ, Grosland NM, et al. Hinged-dynamic posterior device permits greater loads on the graft and similar stability as compared with its equivalent rigid device: a three-dimensional assessment. JPO. 2001;13:1-6.
11. White AA, Panjabi MM. Clinical Biomechanics of the Spine. In: 2nd ed.. Philadelphia: Lippincott; 1990; p.88-9.
12. Weinhoffer SL, Guyer RD, Herbert M, Griffith SL. Intradiscal pressure measurements above an instrumented fusion (A cadaveric study). Spine. 2005;20:526-31.
13. Kitahara K, Takano K, Hara T, et al. Effects of lumbar spinal instrumentation on the adjacent intradiscal pressure [in Japanese]. J Soc Biomechanisms. 2005;26:121-6.

CHAPTER

34

Pyogenic Spinal Infection—Current Views in Diagnosis and Management

Myung-Sang Moon, Sung-Soo Kim, Bong-Jin Lee, Young-Wan Moon, Jeong-Lim Moon

Introduction

Pyogenic spinal infection can be thought as a spectrum of disease comprising spondylitis, diskitis, spondylodiskitis, pyogenic facet arthropathy, and epidural abscess.

In spinal infections there are two main clinical types by its origin; hematogenous and nonhematogenous so-called trauma- and/or needle intervention- or surgery-related ones. In the past hematogenous infection was the main clinical problelm.[1-27] A high mortality rate of approximately 20% was once reported. Hematogenous spinal infection is uncommon in developed countries, while in developing countries the disease is still a major and common problem. Also in this decade spinal infections associated with various epidural and intradiscal needle and surgical procedures became another thread, whether the implants were used or not to both patients and the surgeons.[3,4,6,9,23,28-31] The current issues are its prevalence and difficulties in treatment even in the era of the increasing armamentarium of antimicrobial agents.[10-13,32-40]

On this occasion three forms of spinal infections—hematogenous pyogenic spondylitis, infectious discitis in children, trauma-related, and surgical site infections, including biomaterial-centered infection after implantation surgery—will be presented. The granulomatous infections of the spine, such as tuberculous, mycotic and brucellar spondylodiscitis will not be dealt in this review (Table 34.1).

Regardless of the causes of the infection, initial bacterial inoculation is followed by a complex interaction between the inoculated microorganisms and the local and systemic host environment. Development of the infection is facilitated by the virulence of the microbe, the suboptimal condition of the local environment and systemic compromise of the host.

As a first step the vascular anatomy of spine will be explained briefly because of its significance with regards to the establishment of hematogenous infections. Because generally non-iatrogenic infections of the spine are

Table 34.1 Infections of spine

1. Hematogenous
   a. Spondylitis
      - In adults
      - In children
   b. Diskitis in children
2. Nonhematogenous
   a. Iatrogenic diskitis after
      - Diskography
      - Chemonucleolysis
      - Epidural anesthesia and other
      - Procedures:
        Diskectomy
        - Open
        - Percutaneous (Micro- or endoscopic)
   b. Facet joint procedure
   c. Infections after surgery (surgical site infection)
      1. Noninstrumented fusion
         - AIF*
         - PLF*
         - PLIF*
         - TLIF*
      2. Instrumented fusions : (biomaterial-centered infection):
         - Posterior
         - Anterior
         graft (bone, substitute and/or cage) :
      3. Artificial disk
   d. Trauma-related direct or indirect infection

* AIF: anterior interbody fusion
PLF: posterolateral fusion
PLIF: posterior interbody fusion
TLIF: posterior transforaminal interbody fusion

secondary to blood-borne spread. In the spine small arterial vessels penetrate the disk early in life, but by the third decade these vascular channels disappear. Thus, in the child the disk can be primarily involved because of the presence of nutrient arterioles. In adults these vessels are absent, and infection will involve the body first and the disk second by direct extension.[24,41] Due to the common blood supply of two adjacent vertebrae by the same segmental artery, the infection commonly affects two adjacent vertebrae and the intervertebral disk. The intervertebral disk lacks vasculature. Thus, it is initially spared and is affected after destruction of the adjacent vertebra, which occurs later. The paraspinal venous plexus may additionally contribute to the spread of the infection.

Now for the clinical, laboratory, and radiological findings, bone scans, CT and MRI findings, diagnosis, and treatment will be presented in order.

Pathogenesis

If the host resistance is low or the focal resistance in bone has been impaired, a virulent organism may find a situation suitable to its reproduction and a site of infection becomes established. Also minor trauma causes a minute hemorrhage that lowers the resistance of a bony focus. If there happens to be a bacteremia and the organisms are carried to this exact area, they are able to multiply because bactericidal factors are inhibited. Bone that suffers from the lower oxygen tension of sickle cell disease is prone to develop one or more foci of osteomyelitis.

Clinical Manifestations

Manifestations of the spinal infection can be varied, and patients with the disease will present it in a variety of ways. Many patients with pyogenic infections have major associated diseases, such as diabetes mellitus, malignancies, chronic alcoholism, drug addiction, Mannose-binding lactin (MLB) deficiency, and acquired immunosuppression.[18,34,39,42-45] The immune suppression masks the early presentation of the clinical symptoms and signs. Thus, the disease can present perplexing diagnostic problems.

Pain is the major complaint, and is centered over the involved area. The pain may be referred to various site in the body. Temperature elevation is one of the most consistent complaints, and decreased range of spinal motions, muscle spasm and rigidity are generally present. Percussion tenderness may be noted over the involved vertebrae.

The "hip syndrome" by the psoas irritation and abdominal pain may develop.[8,39] Straight leg-raising is limited due to severe back pain, rigidity, and meningeal syndrome.[7] Different degrees of neurological loss can be found in these infections.[45,46] The onset of paraplegia may be quite sudden in pyogenic spondylitis, while in tuberculosis and other nontuberculous granulomatous infections it is rather slow and gradual in the development.[37,47-50] An abscess may develop, but sinus formation is rare.[1,32,47,48]

Laboratory Studies

Complete Blood Counts and Inflammatory Markers

Complete blood counts including erythrocyte sedimentation rates (ESR)[33] and C-reactive protein (CRP)[51] are the key study. Also there is usually a relative neutrophilia. The level of neutrophil CD64 expression is helpful in confirming the presence of infection.[52] Although the administration of antibiotics before its measurement reduces its negative predictive value, it still appears to be a better predictor of local infection than CRP, ESR, and/or the WBC count.[52] Lymphopenia and decreased serum albumin represent immunosuppression status, thus indicating the increased susceptibility to infection. The percentage and number of lymphocytes decrease to 10% or less, and 1,000/µL or less.[18,31]

In spinal infection patients' immune state should be studied, because the incidence of the infection is high in the immunosuppressed patients, particularly the elderly people. Also, it is a very important information for the clinicians that iatrogenically induced bone marrow suppression relates with humoral immunity (bone marrow dependent), while HIV disease relates with thymus-dependent cellular immunity (cell bound processes, T-lymphocytes). The two systems interact in complex ways. If one or more defects whether congenital or acquired are present in a person's specific or nonspecific immune defenses, a diversity of disorders arise that are characterized by increased susceptibility to a wide range of infections and whose consequences often include severe acute, recurrent, and chronic diseases. It seems wise to do the immune study in the infected patients.

Imaging Studies

Radiographic Features

Classic concepts of pyogenic infections of the spine have come to be associated with fairly definite descriptions of the radiographic appearances, but X-ray appearances are of limited value in distinguishing pyogenic from non-pyogenic lesions.[1,2,4] In our experiences, spinal infection in adults is frequently a problem in differential diagnosis[4,49] (Fig. 34.1).

While it is usually apparent from the radiographs that the lesions are infective rather than neoplastic or degenerative, we have found it difficult on this basis to distinguish pyogenic spondylitis from the other infections. Because there are two different forms of pyogenic spondylitis (osteogenic and osteolytic) which are easily misdiagnosed as spinal tuberculosis.[47] Therefore, in many instances it has been necessary to resort to biopsy and even then the diagnosis has not always been established. In some cases, a conclusion has been reached only in retrospect, based on the natural course of condition together with the response to treatment.[47,48]

Three areas in the spine must be examined individually on X-ray films: (i) the vertebral body, (ii) the disk space, and (iii) the adjacent soft tissues.

Radiographic findings are divided into early and late findings (Tables 34.2 and 34.3).

Generally in pyogenic spondylitis there are osteolytic and reactive osteoblastic activities. Rapid new bone formation in the early infection helps distinguish pyogenic spondylitis from tuberculosis. Localized rarefaction and some collapse of vertebral bodies are seen. Narrowing of a disk space more rapidly occurs in high proportion of pyogenic spondylitis (2–4 weeks) and sometimes in both disks above and below the infected body. The reason is that disk destruction in pyogenic spondylitis is caused by enzyme and in tuberculosis it is due to mechanical cause. In general the paraspinal soft tissue swelling tends to be smaller, but is seen earlier (2 weeks) in pyogenic infection (Fig. 34.1). Speckled calcification is not seen in pyogenic infection.

In early stage of disk space infection in children normal space is maintained, and it gradually becomes narrower with irregularity and haziness of the affected end-plate as in the pyogenic (Figs 34.2 and 34.3). However, bone destruction without sclerosis of the end-plate and spinal deformity are seen (Tables 34.2 and 34.3).

Table 34.2 Early X-ray changes in pyogenic spinal infections

Paravertebral soft tissue shadow (edema and swelling)	2 weeks (1/3 cases)
Disk space narrowing	3-4 weeks
Rarefaction or eroded area on the adjacent body margins	6 weeks

Table 34.3 Late X-ray changes in pyogenic spinal infections

Progressive destruction	8 weeks
Deformity (displacement or kyphosis)	8–10 weeks
Reactive sclerosis	8–10 weeks
New bone formation and bony bridge	12 weeks
Fusion	<6 months

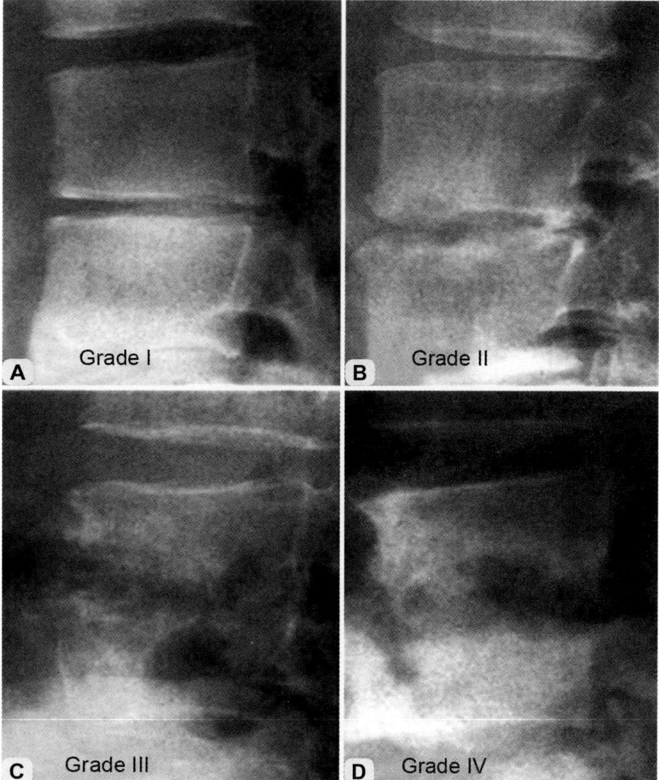

Fig. 34.1 Kulowski's radiological classification of pyogenic spondylitis. (A) Grade I: Only disk space narrowing; (B) II: Bony destruction limited only in the end-plate; (C) III: Vertebral body destruction of less than 50% of vertebral height; (D) IV: Vertebral body destruction over 50% of vertebral height

Kulowski classified the pyogenic spondylodiskitis into 4 stages, based on the radiographic stage of the disease progression[49] (Fig. 34.4).

Bone Scintigraphy

In scintigraphic manifestations, there are only minor differential features between pyogenic and tuberculous spondylitis, because those two manifestations vary according to the disease stage.[2,43,47] Radionuclide imaging may detect the lesion at pre-radiologic stage, but is nonspecific.

However, pin-hole scintigraphy of pyogenic spondylitis can clearly localize the uptake in the end-plates of the affected vertebrae, and visualize the photogenic disk space (Fig. 34.5). In the acute and subacute stages, tracer distribution is typically asymmetric between end-plates.

Antibiofilm antibodies can be tagged with specific "opacity markers" for various types of scans. Antibody based imaging could help localization and clinical treatment.[53-55]

CT Findings

CT provides better informations regarding the extent of the bony lesion including the endplate, posterior element, and bony canal.

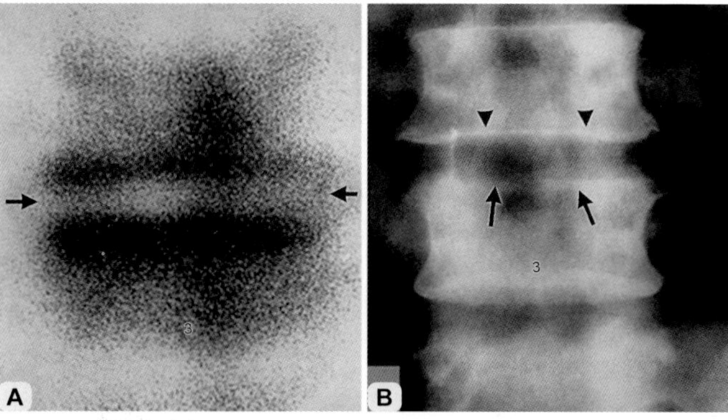

Fig. 34.2 Asymmetric end-plate involvement in acute hematogenous pyogenic spondylitis. (A) Posterior pinhole scintigram of L2–3; (B) Lysis in the initial infection site of L3 vertebra (open arrow) and mild shagginess in the secondarily involved L2 vertebra (arrow head)

MRI Findings

The number of involved vertebral bodies is less in pyogenic spondylitis than in tuberculous spondylitis, and the paravertebral abscess in pyogenic one is smaller.[20,56-58] MRI is useful for the early diagnosis of hematogenous pyogenic spondylitis, because it clearly demonstrates edema and inflammatory changes. MRI with gadolinium showing enhancement of the disk space is indicative of infection. Type 2 marrow changes, high signal on T2-weighted MRI scans and low signal on T1-weighted scans are typical but nonspecific. It may be about two weeks after the onset that the lesion of the pyogenic spondylitis can be detected by MRI. The magnetic resonance intensity of the involved vertebral bodies is more homogenous in pyogenic spondylitis than that in tuberculous spondylitis.

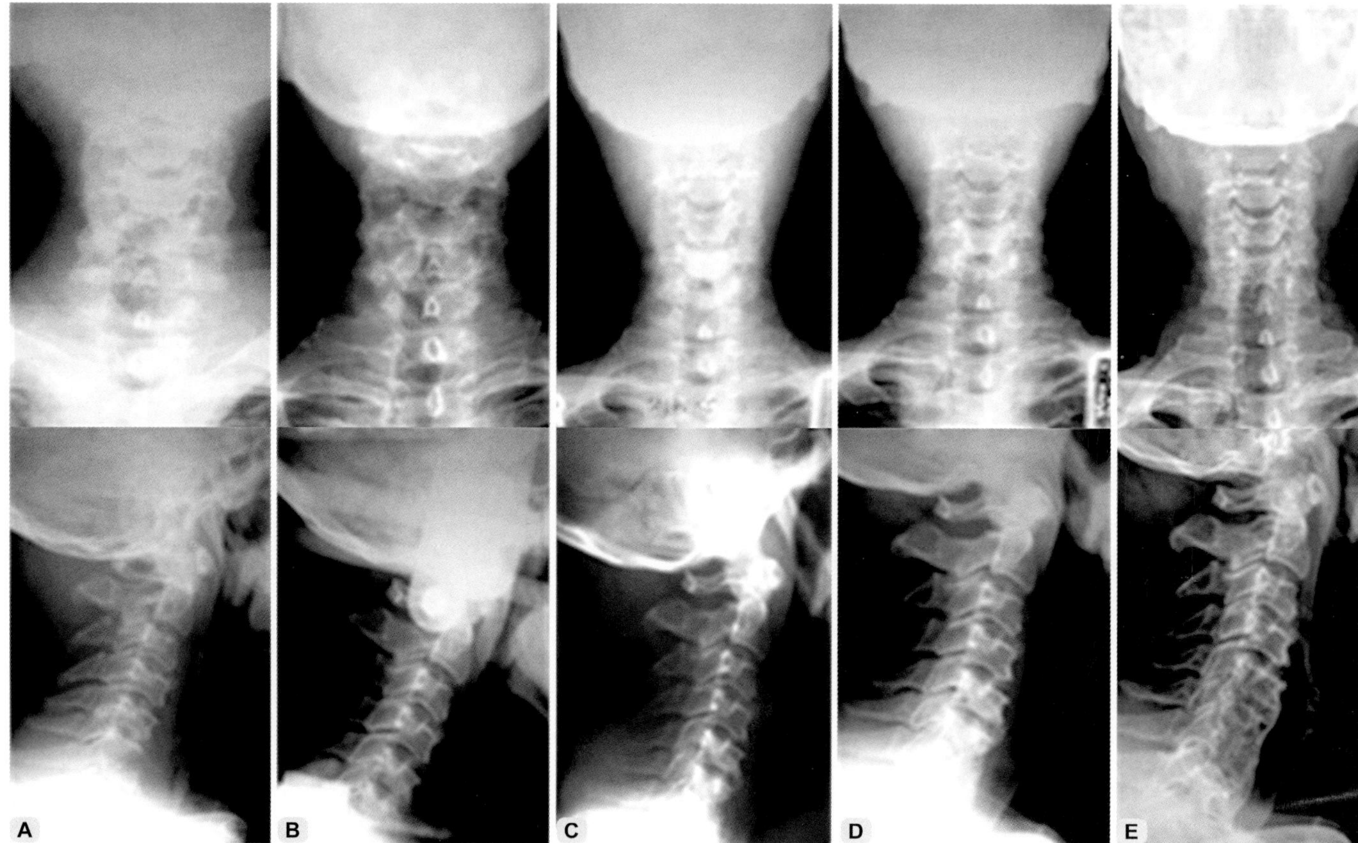

Fig. 34.3 Post-traumatic hematogenous pyogenic spondylitis in a 53-year-old male (Ahn, H-S). This man sustained whiplash injury in the neck a month ago for which conservative treatment was given at a local hospital without successful cure. The patient was referred for further treatment because of gradual worsening of clinical symptoms and sign; pain greatly aggravated with stiffened neck. Also the patient had fever. Laboratory examination disclosed the leukocytosis, elevated ESR and CRP. Finally diagnosis of pyogenic infection of C5–7 was made. (A) Initial radiograms of the cervical spine show the straight spine, but there was no evidence of fracture and/or dislocation or bone and disk lesion; (B) Narrowing of C5–6 and C6–7 disk spaces was seen a month later; (C) Further disk space narrowing and end-plate irregularity were seen on radiograms, taken 5 months later. Clinically symptoms and signs were completely disappeared; (D) C6–7 disk was almost destroyed, and further narrowing of C5–6 disk space is seen; (E) Completely fused C5–7 is seen on radiograms, taken 2 years and 9 months after injury

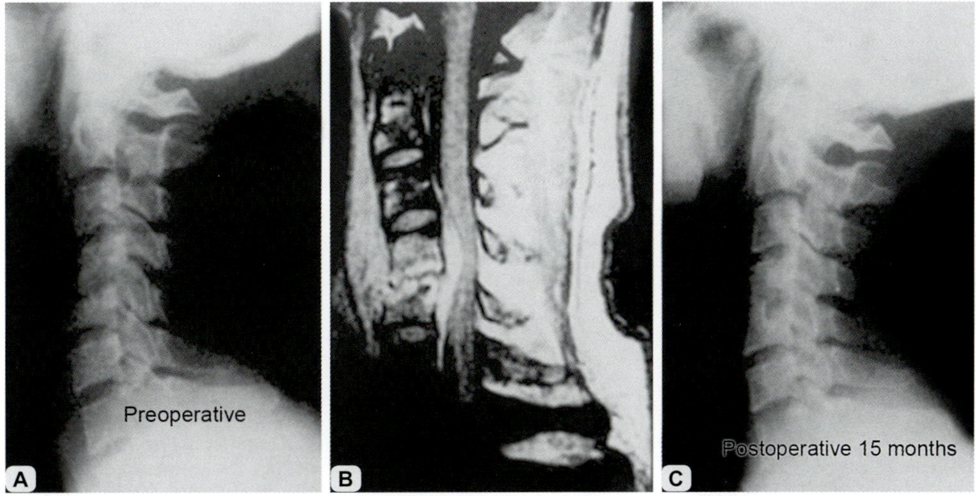

Fig. 34.4 Infected lesion at C4–5 in a 32 year-old man: Anterior interbody fusion and 4 pillar brace management under cover of antibiotic therapy was given. (A) Preoperative lateral X-ray of the cervical spine: The patient developed gradually worsening quadriparesis, Frankel's grade D. Initial lateral radiogram showed the destructed C4–5 disk and endplates; (B) The T2-sagittal MRI, showing moderately destroyed C4 and C5 bodies with kyphosis and retropharyngeal and epidural abscess compressing the cord anteriorly; (C) The X ray, taken 15 months after anterior radical surgery shows the solid fusion of C4–5 with restored lordosis

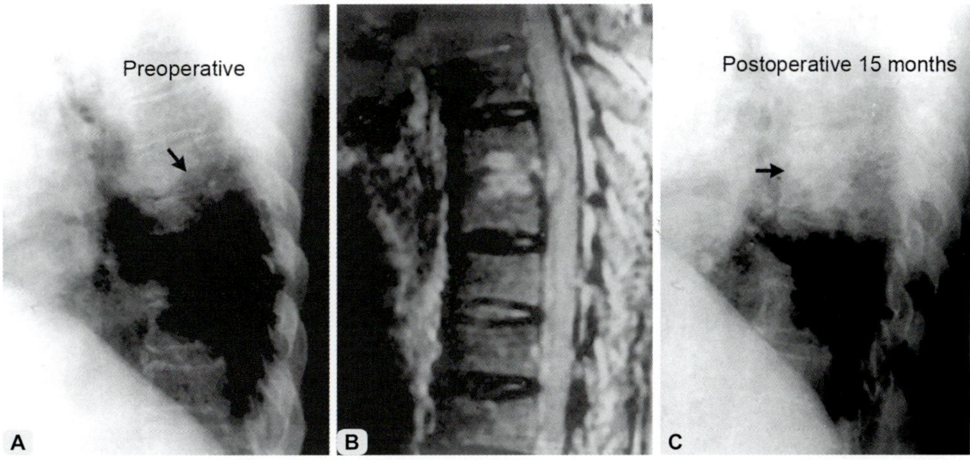

Fig. 34.5 (A) Lateral radiogram of a 60-year-old gentleman with Frankel's C paralysis showing destructive lesion in T7–8; (B) MRI showing scanty epidural abscess compressing cord in front; (C) Lateral radiogram, taken at 15 months after anterior decompressive radical surgery showing solid fusion. Complete neurological recovery and cure of the disease were followed

Rim enhancement with gadolinium-DTPA is less frequent in pyogenic spondylitis. MRI also provides better informations regarding the compressed cord[56,57] (Figs 34.6 and 34.7).

Bacteriology

Culture will be positive in less than 50% of patients.[4,59-62] The bacteria in the blood cultures will be occasionally different to those in the disk space infection. Bacterium initially presents in free floating form (planktonic), and by division becomes biofilm-producing sessile form.

Biofilm formation is the key in the development and persistence of infection.[9,16,37,55,63,64] The biofilm is an aggregation of microbe colonies enclosed within an extracellular polysaccharide matrix (glycocalyx) that adheres to the surface of implants or devitalized bone. Gristina and Costerton reported that 59% of orthopedic

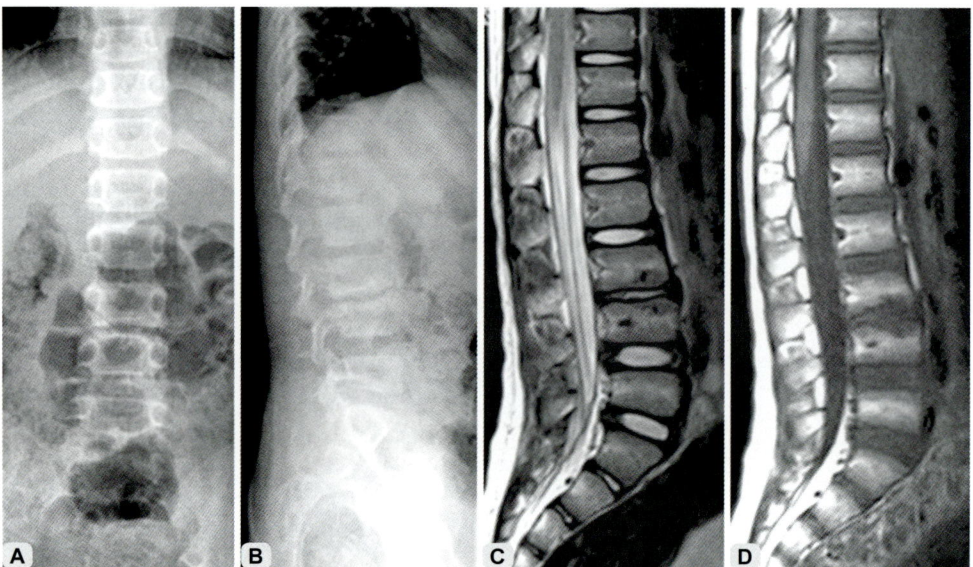

Fig. 34.6 A case of subacute pyogenic spondylitis of L3–4 in a 9-year-old boy, treated by 6 weeks of intravenous antibiotic administration. (A and B) Simple radiograms show only the narrowed L3–5 disk space with loss of lumbar lordosis; (C and D) MRI (T1 and T2 weighted images) showing the narrowed disk space and irregular endplates. However no abscess image is seen

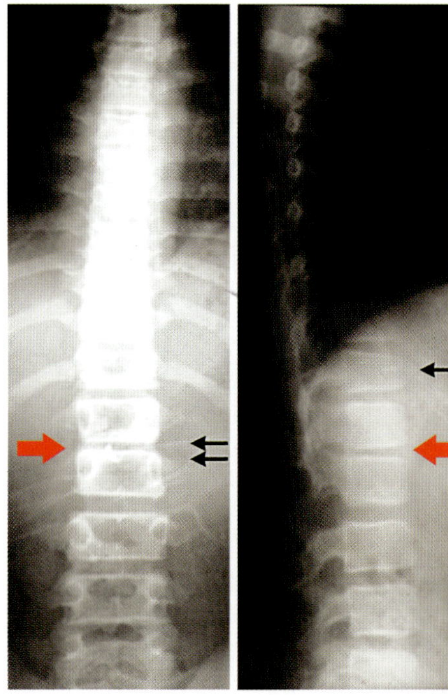

Fig. 34.7 Hematogenous pyogenic spondylodiskitis of L1–2 in a 11-year-old boy who was treated conservatively by 4 weeks of intravenous and 2 weeks of oral antibiotic administration. Infection was well controlled. Only L1–2 disk space narrowing is seen at final

biomaterial-related infection had positive findings of glycocalyx-enclosed organisms on electron microscopy.[42-44]

Presence of implants promotes both adherence of microbes and biofilm formation.[3-7,9,11-12,16] It adversely affects phagocytosis, thereby facilitating development of infection. Biofilm protects the organism from antibiotics and host defense mechanisms, such as antibody formation and phagocytosis. It also allows infections to exist in a subclinical state and recur.[22,25,37,42,43,55,64]

A genetic profile of the glycocalyx-producing bacteria is currently being identified.[55] Certain bacterial DNA gene sequences have been identified, such as the intracellular adhesion (ICA) complex. Bacteria that have these genes may possess the ability to produce more virulent infections associated with orthopedic hardware.[16,42,43,53,55,72] In the future, detecting these genes by molecular diagnostics may assist the clinician with regard to planning a strategy for infection control.

Methicillin-resistant staphylococci can be differentiated from methicillin-sensitive staphylococci based on the detection of the mecA gene, which is only present in methicillin-resistant staphylococci.[42,63,65] This gene encodes for a cell wall protein termed penicillin binding protein 2a(PBP2a) which has a low affinity for binding all beta-lactam antibiotics.[65,66]

Chronic infections are associated with bacterial biofilms which are characterized by microcolonies of bacteria encased in a protective extracellular polymeric matrix. The biofilm also can produce periodic planktonic showers of bacteria (i.e. bacteria shedding from the biofilm) into the bloodstream.[66] Bacteria have a life cycle just as many eukaryotes do.

Existence within a biofilm represents a basic survival mechanism of microorganisms in which microorganisms are protected through mechanisms that are in the process of being defended from environmental influences including host immune responses (e.g. opsonization, phagocytosis, and complement-mediated lysis) and normal levels of conventional antimicrobial agents.[7,9,16,66]

Polymerase Chain Reaction

Since the introduction of polymerase chain reaction (PCR) into the area of diagnostic microbiology, the test has been extensively used in the diagnosis of many viral, bacterial, fungal and parasitic infections such as cytomegalovirus (CMV), *M. tuberculosis*, the Whipple's disease agent, *Pneumocystis carinii*, *Toxoplasma gondii*, which are either slow-growing, difficult to culture or non-culture.[53,67] Using the enzymatic amplification technique, PCR, more than a million copies of a segment of gene sequence flanked by two primer sequences specific to the microbe can be generated in a few hours. At present, however, a few laboratories would use PCR for the routine detection of slowly and rapidly growing bacteria. Due to its exquisite sensitivity, the test has been utilized as a marker for monitoring the response to treatment, for determination of the duration of therapy and possibly for prediction of relapse of the infection. Moreover, by using evolutionary conserved areas of 16s risosomal DNA, PCR has enabled scientists to discover the existence of previously unknown and nonculturable bacteria.

PCR has opened up another exciting era in the diagnosis and treatment of infectious disease. Through PCR technique (i) identification of causative organism possible, and also (ii) analysis of multidrug resistant bacteria is possible.

For detection of biofilm infections molecular methods [PCR and fluorescence *in situ* hybridization (FISH)] are more suitable because of lack of sensitivity of conventional microbiologic methods.[67] Also positive enzyme-linked immunosorbent assay (ELISA) tests could be informative as a diagnostic tool.[53,67,68]

Diagnosis

If the clinical manifestations, the X-ray changes, cultures of blood and/or percutaneous vertebral aspirate, still do not provide an etiologic diagnosis, bone biopsy (either by an open or percutaneous) procedure should be strongly considered in any forms of spinal osteomyelitis.[20,47,56-58]

Treatment in General (Table 34.4)

Treatment is directed at obtaining a firm diagnosis, controlling and eradicating the infection, and limiting damage to local tissue, including the neural elements.[15,37,69-73] Immunocompromised patients are much more difficult to manage clinically.[18]

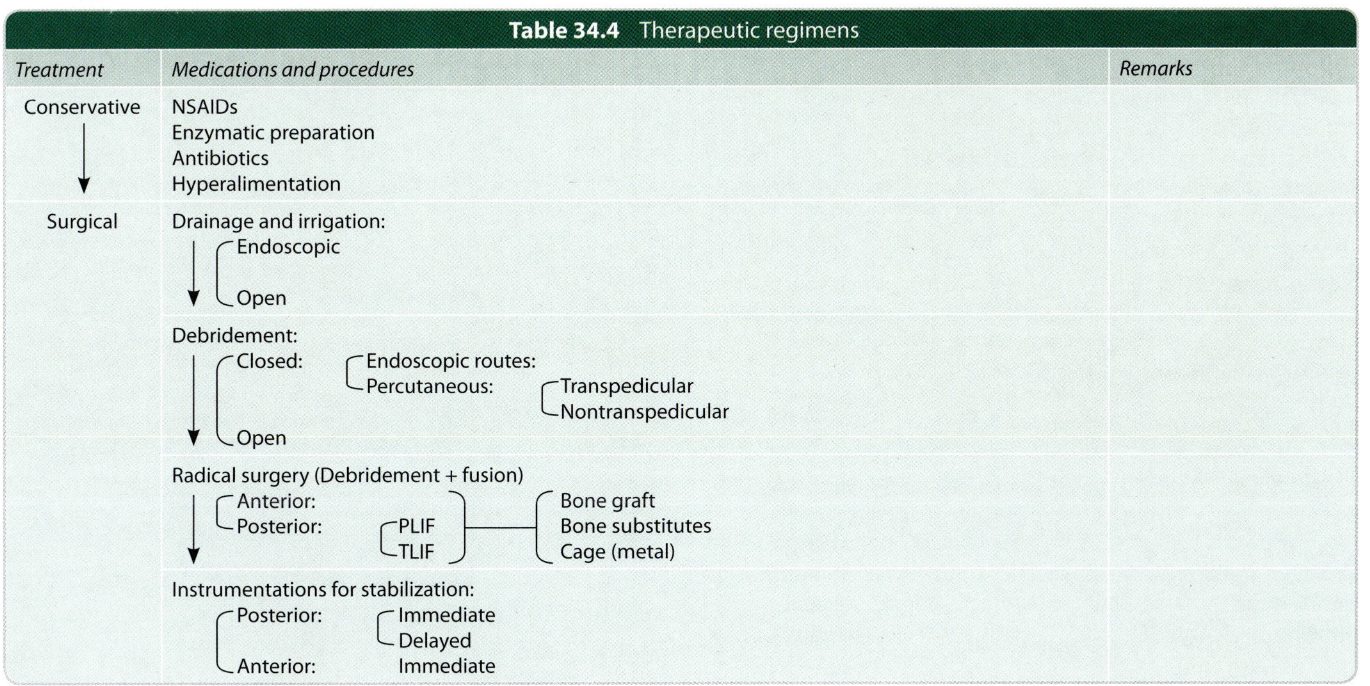

Table 34.4 Therapeutic regimens

Treatment	*Medications and procedures*	*Remarks*
Conservative ↓	NSAIDs Enzymatic preparation Antibiotics Hyperalimentation	
Surgical	Drainage and irrigation: ↓ Endoscopic Open	
	Debridement: ↓ Closed: Endoscopic routes: Percutaneous: Transpedicular / Nontranspedicular Open	
	Radical surgery (Debridement + fusion) ↓ Anterior: Posterior: PLIF / TLIF — Bone graft / Bone substitutes / Cage (metal)	
	Instrumentations for stabilization: Posterior: Immediate / Delayed Anterior: Immediate	

Present thoughts on treatment have varied a good deal from the conservative to the complicated surgery (Table 34.4), though the antibiotic therapy was the key (Table 34.5). Two methods of treatment are advocated; conservative and operative.[74-80] Free floating (i.e. planktonic) bacteria are easily eliminated or controlled by antibiotics. Early appropriate

Table 34.5 Causative organisms and the recommended antibiotics

Gram (+)		
Methicilline-sensitive	First choice	Second choice
Staphylococcus aureus	Nafcilline or clindamycin	Cefazoline or vancomycin
Coagulase-negative *Staphylococcus aureus*	Nafcillin or clindamycin	Cefazoline or vancomycin
Methicilline-resistant		
Staphylococcus aureus	Vancomycin or linezolid	Bactrim or Minocycline c/o rifampin
Coagulase-negative *Staphylococcus aureus*	Vancomycin or linezolid	Bactrim or minocycline c/o rifampin Clindamycin
Group-A *Streptococcus* or *Streptococcus pyogenes*	Penicillin G or ampicillin	Clindamycin, cephalosporin or vancomycin
Group-B *Streptococcus* or *Streptococcus agalactiae*	Penicillin G or ampicillin	Clindamycin, cephalosporin or vancomycin
Sensitive		
Streptococcus pneumoniae	Penicillin G	Clindamycin or erythromycin
Intermediate		
Streptococcus pneumoniae	Cefotaxime	Clindamycin or Erythromycin
Resistant		
Streptococcus pneumoniae	Vancomycin or levofloxacin	Quinopristin/dalfopristin or linezolid
Sensitive		
Enterococcus species	Ampicillin or vancomycin	Ampicillin-sulbactam linezolid
Resistant		
Enterococcus faecium	Quinopristin/dalfopristin or linezolid	Chloramphenicol and rifampin
Gram (–)		
Acinetobacter species	Ceftazidime and levofloxacin or imipenem	Ampicillin-sulbactam
Enterobacter species	Cefotaxime or imipenem	Levofloxacin, meziocillin or ticarcillin-clavulanate
Escherichia coli	Ampicillin-sulbactam	Cefazolin, levofloxacin, gentamicin or azithromycin
Haemophilus influenza	Cefotaxime or ampicillin-sulbactam	Levofloxacin, bactrim, ampicillin or azithromycin
Proteus mirabilis	Ampicillin or levofloxacin	Cefazolin, bactrim or gentamicin
Proteus vulgaris, Proteus rettgeri or *Morganella morgani*	Cefotaxime or imipenem or levofloxacin	Bactrim, amikacin or imipenem
Pseudomonas aeruginosa	Cefepime or piperacillin or imipenem	Ticarcillin-clavulanate, tobramycin, amikacin or ciprofloxacin
Serratia macescens	Cefotaxime	Levofloxacin, gentamicin or imipenem

Table 34.6 Suggested methods to prevent bacterial adherence to implant surface

1. Incorporating antibiotics to biomaterials
2. Immobilization of antimicrobial peptide
3. Surfactant coating, such as
   - Salicylic acid
   - Silver
   - Substituted dextrans
   - Polyethylene oxide
   - Serum proteins (fibronectin, albumin)
4. Material property (components)

antibiotic therapy within 3 days after onset of symptoms can abort the infection medically. Lack of improvement of the inflammatory markers after 48 hours of an adequate antibiotic therapy is defined as failure of medical treatment. Surgical intervention must be considered for any patient who has failed medical treatments, and has neurologic findings, and has had spinal instability, or who requires tissue diagnosis.

Surgical management can be very challenging. The principles of treating any infection are equally applicable to the treatment of infection in bone. Any postoperative spine infection, which does not respond to antibiotic treatment or which creates unacceptable deformity or neurologic compromise requires surgical management. The best surgical technique for patients with bacterial spine infection is still a matter of debate. If immediate treatment for any form of pyogenic spondylodiskitis is initiated after early diagnosis, the better outcome will be expected. Debridement surgery is the foundation of osteomyelitis treatment, and should be direct, atraumatic and executed with reconstruction (Table 34.6).

The prognosis is generally good. Patients with spondylodiskitis who were treated nonsurgically reported residual back pain more often (64%) than patients treated surgically (26.3%).[41] In the conservatively treated patients spontaneous intercorporal fusion at the end of treatment is most desirable, and is accepted as the best indication of healing. However, the current authors' personal impression is that spontaneous fusion rates in pyogenic spondylitis were relatively lower than that of tuberculous spondylitis.[82] Therefore, stabilization and fusion of the spine are often necessary as well.

Healing or cure of the infection by antibiotic therapy and spontaneous intercorporal fusion are most desirable. It is speculated by the authors that spontaneous intercorporal fusion occurs by the locally produced BMP and/or the local activities of PGE2, mediated through 4G protein-coupled receptor subtypes, EP1–EP4.[83]

Patients with multiple or resistant organisms with myonecrosis were difficult to manage, and had poor outcomes. If paraplegia once develops, it is a disastrous sequel to pyogenic spondylitis and disk space infection.

Various Forms of Pyogenic Spondylodiskitis

Hematogenous Spondylitis

Hematogenous Pyogenic Spondylitis

It presents a diagnostic and therapeutic challenge. The disease affects all age groups. However, during the last 30 years pyogenic spondylitis was found to be more common in adults, while very early literature disclosed that the disease was more common in adolescence than adults. Waldvogel's summary of 311 out of 348 patients disclosed the adult to children ratio of 262 : 49 (5:1).[41] According to recent papers it is known that the aging spine in the diabetics appears to be more at risk.[8,18,31] Traumatized spine can be a focus of infection[70] (Fig. 34.1).

The infection may present with various clinical pictures, from the septic forms with progressive neurologic disorders to the forms with no septic signs.

Once diagnosis has been made treatment consists primarily of antibiotic therapy, bed-rest, and immobilization of the affected segments by casts or brace. Spinal osteomyelitis can be cured by antibiotics without surgery, provided that the diagnosis is well established, and antibiotics used are appropriate in type, dose and duration. But initial antibiotics should be made on a "best guess" basis before the sensitivity of organisms to antibiotics is determined, and also even for the culture-negative cases. Negative culture does not mean the infected lesion sterile. Unfortunately, duration of therapy is still not clearly defined. The current authors prefer 4–8 weeks of antibiotic therapy including 4 weeks of initial intravenous administration to other methods (Table 34.5, Figs 34.2, 34.3, and 34.8).

The success of nonoperative treatment is predicted by four independent variables: an age of less than sixty years, the immune status, infection with *Staphylococcus aureus*, and a decreasing erythrocyte sedimentation rate and CRP.

Whereas surgery is mandatory for the treatment of complications, such as paraspinal abscess, recurrence of the disease, or progressive paraplegia, its value in the uncomplicated cases is less evident except the undiagnosed and unresponsive cases (Figs 34.6 and 34.7).

Some recommend the anterior radical surgery early on with or without instrumentation.[15,16,19,32,36,38,39,43,48] However, as yet the combined anterior radical surgery and in situ anterior instrumentation are not well accepted by the most surgeons, while the combined anterior surgery

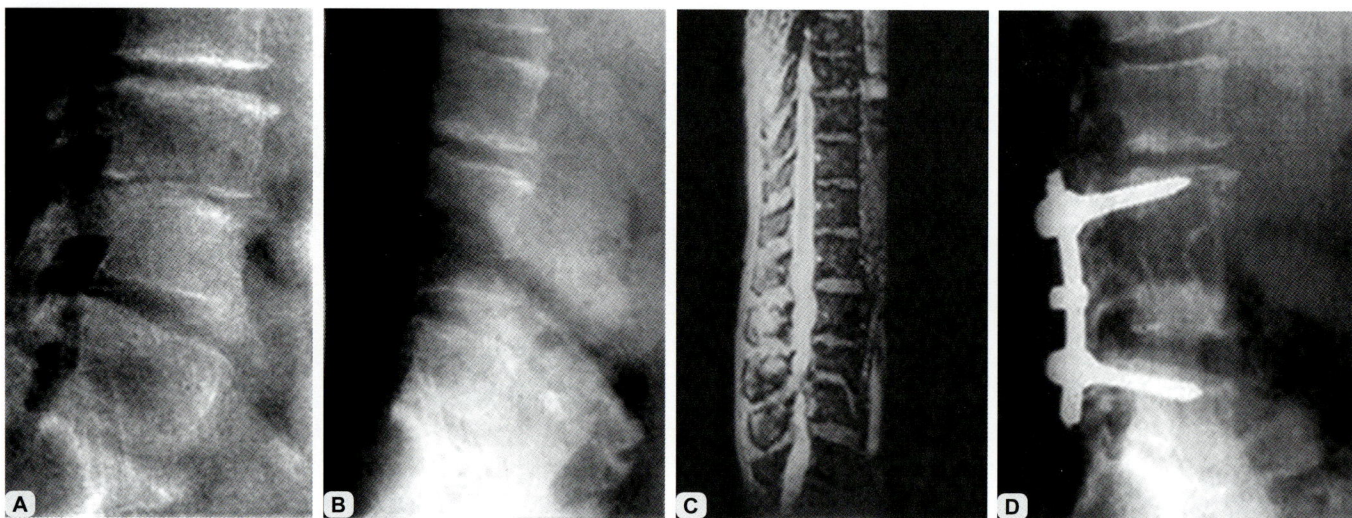

Fig. 34.8 Hematogenous pyogenic spondylodiscitis in L3–4 in a 67-year-old man. (A and B) Preoperative radiograms showing the narrowed L3–4 disc space with endplate irregularity; (C) Preoperative T2-weighted MRI showing narrowed L3–4 disk space and anteriorly compressed dural sac; (D) Postoperative radiogram showing intercorporal bone graft between L3–4 and posterior short segment pedicular screw fixation between L3–5.

and posterior instrumentation away from the lesion may be a accepted procedure (Fig. 34.8). As we mentioned above, implantation of the biomaterial in the infected focus is known to make the infection prolonged, worse and uncontrollable. Because the biomaterials, such as metals, methylmethacrylate, carbon cage, ceramic and titanium cages, and so on serve as the substratum for bacterial adhesion.[5,9,11,13,15,38,42-44,55]

Cord compression is characterized by more rapid development, and its prognosis is worse if the disease is left surgically untreated. There is no perfect clinical means at present to ascertain the degree of presenting irreversible cord damage, even in the era of the advanced MRI technology. Thus, any patient with spinal cord involvement deserves an immediate surgical decompression (Figs 34.6 and 34.7).

Spontaneous Childhood Infectious Diskitis

Diagnosis is often delayed, especially in young children, as the initial symptoms may mimic other processes such as septic arthritis, appendicitis or meningitis. An annual incidence of 0.3 – 0.6 per 10,000 cases was reported. Radioisotope bone scanning has been found particularly useful in the early phase of the disease when the radiographs are still normal.

Treatment consists of bed rest or immobilization of the spine. The use of antibiotics is still controversial, as the course of the disease in all children is notably benign.

Iatrogenic Spinal Infection (Infection after Spinal Procedures)

It is a known fact that any type of external violation of intervertebral disk and vertebral bone by needle and/ or surgical procedure can complicate infection (Table 34.4, Figs 34.9 to 34.12). The two causative factors relate closely with surgical site infection: patient- and surgeon-dependent factors. Diagnosis of early infection after spinal needle or surgical procedures can be readily made with evidence from the history and physical examination, confirmed by simple imaging and laboratory investigations. Ultrasonography is useful to demonstrate the location of an infected hematoma or abscess in case of posterior procedures, and to guide diagnostic aspiration. The CRP level and the level of neutrophil CD64 expression appear to have a higher predictive value for deep sepsis than the ESR and WBC count.[33,51,52] The CRP level falls rapidly after the second postoperative day following uncomplicated spinal surgery: Maintained high levels (over 2.0 mg/dL) at postoperative 2 weeks may indicate possible postoperative infection together with elevated ESR over 50 mm/ hour.[33,51,60] Scintigraphy presently has no important role in this clinical context.

The various prophylactic measures have been taken to prevent or reduce the infection. The prophylactic antimicrobial regimen is one of the measures.[74,79] It is already pointed out that the prophylactic antimicrobial regimens are of proven effectiveness in reducing infection

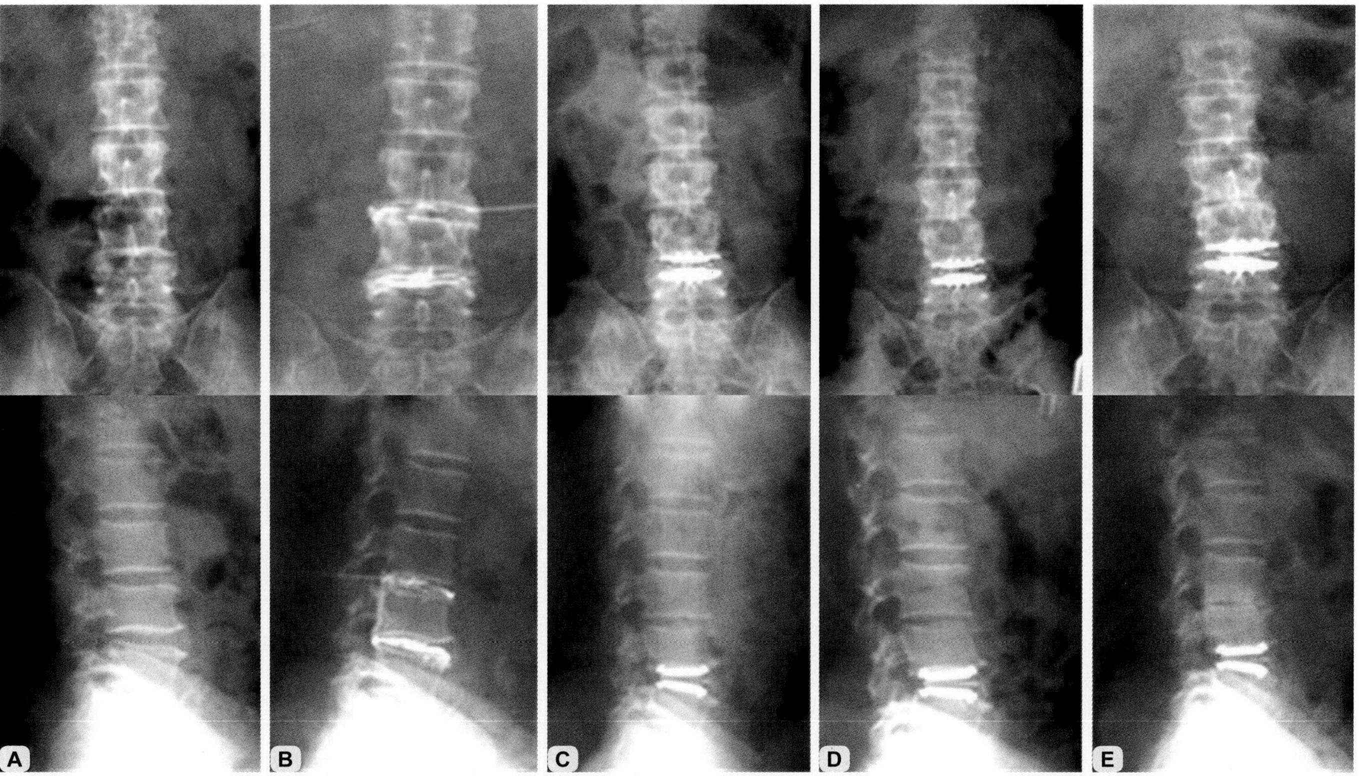

Fig. 34.9 An example of L3–4 disk space infection after diskography: This 65-year-old man suffered from diskogenic low back pain for which artificial disk replacement surgery was planned. Preoperatively diskography of L3–4 and L4–5 was performed which was followed by artificial disk replacement surgery, because there was no evidence of any diskography-related complications at the time. Also he did fine postoperatively, and then was lost for 7 months. At his last visit he stated that he has had persisting low back pain after diskography and disk replacement. (A) Initial radiogram shows mild spondylosis at L4–5; (B) Diskograms show the lobular disk of L3–4 and fissured L4–5 disk; (C) L4–5 disk was replaced with artificial disk (Charitte); (D) Radiograms, taken 2 weeks after arthroplasty showed narrowed disk space of L3–4 which indicated the suspicion of disk space infection, but the surgeon missed to find it; (E) Almost fused L3–4 vertebrae were seen on radiograms taken 7 months after surgery

rates, and that of the regimens administered for as short a period as 24 hours after surgery have been shown to be effective.[15,21,46,74,79]

Infection after Epidural and Intradiskal Procedures

The increased popularity of epidural and various intradiscal procedures, such as diskometry, diskography, chemonucleolysis, percutaneous nucleotomy, and microscopic and conventional diskectomies makes it likely that epidural abscess and diskitis will become more frequent complications.[23,28-30,84] The clinical presentation of epidural abscess and pyogenic diskitis may be variable; an increase in temperature, ESR, and CRP with a few days after epidural or intradiskal procedure is the first signs of infection, and then difficult walking and standing, abdominal pain, back pain or an abnormal spinal posture being followed.

To prevent the infection, it is recommended to use a suitable broad spectrum antibiotics in a single dose whenever the disk is entered. However, when once infection is established, antibiotics rarely can reach the disk and becomes difficult to control the infection. Thus, it was found that the delayed postoperative antibiotic administration failed to arrest or modify the course of diskitis because of the intradiskal multiplication of bacteria which already destroyed the end-plate and disk degeneration.

Spinal infection following epidural anesthesia and steroid injection (retrodiskal infection): Epidural abscess following catheter insertion and epidural injection is a rare complication, but can result in significant long-term morbidity if not recognized and treated early. This infection can also cause spinal osteomyelitis.[31]

It is estimated to occur in between 1: 100,000 and 1: 400,000. It was reported that one out of 45 cases of spinal infection developed following epidural anesthesia.[31]

Selected cases who do not present neurological deficit can be managed successfully with massive antibiotic therapy, or in cases with retrodiskal infection or abscess, revision and evacuation are essential. Persisting pain and/

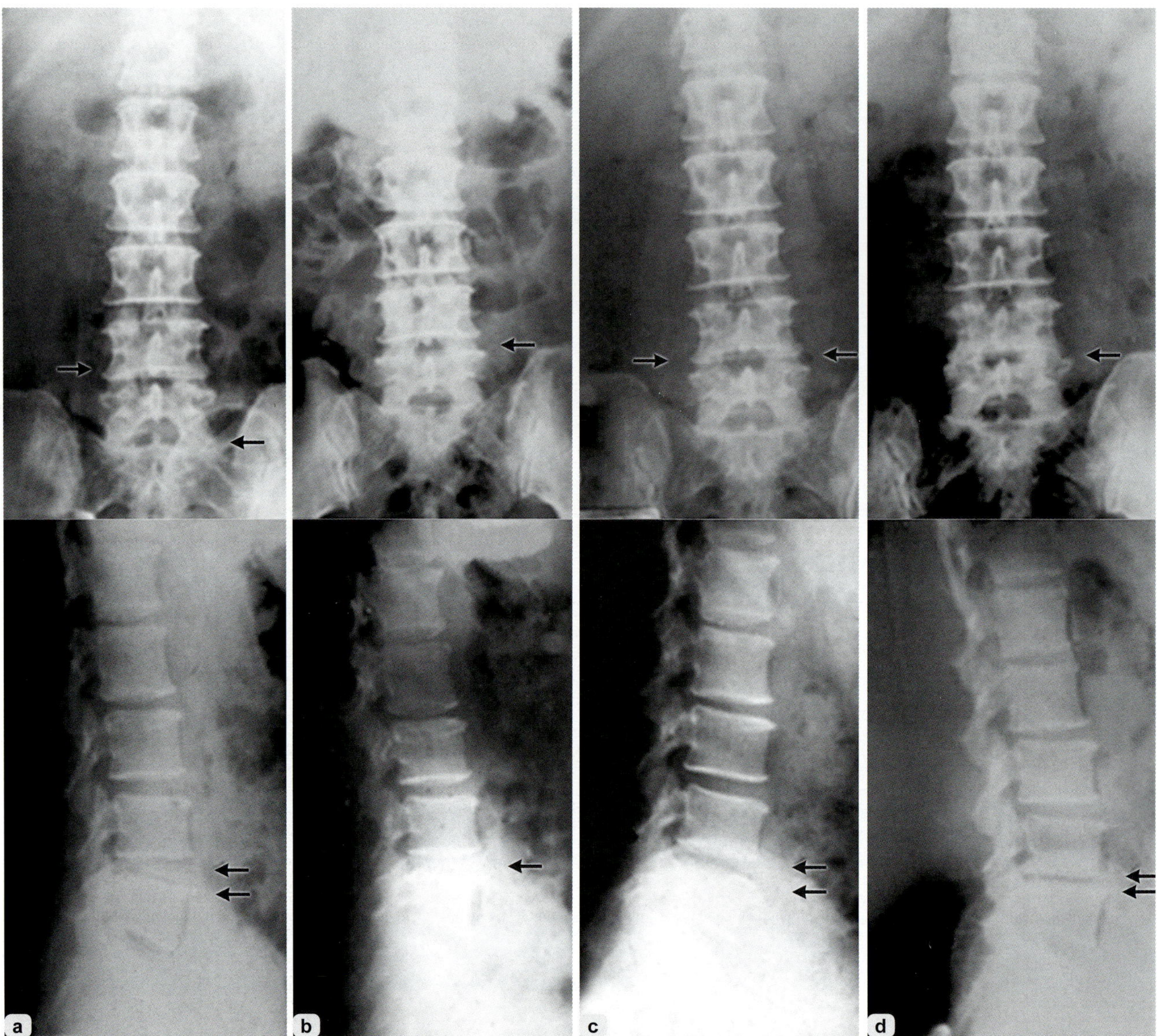

Fig. 34.10A This 47-year-old housewife developed diskitis of L4–5. (a) 7 days after disk surgery; (b to d) Postoperative X-rays taken on (b) 3rd day, (c and d) 4 and 16 months, showed gradual narrowing of disk space. She was successfully treated by conservative means. The involved segment was gradually being stabilized by disk absorption, but did not fuse completely by 2 years

or the development of neurological deficit should prompt surgical intervention and decompression.

Diskitis after intradiskal needle procedures: It is due to bacterial penetration into the intervertebral disk by a contaminated needle, and has an incidence of 0.2–4%. Fraser et al. pointed out that diskitis after diskography (2.3% of patients or 1.3% per disk) has increased.[23,28-30,59,60] To reduce the incidence of diskitis after intradiskal injection, the procedure should only be carried out in a clean room with full aseptic technique. It is recommended that only stiletted needles should be used, and a two-needle technique for each level is recommended. The prophylactic antibiotics at the time of chemonucleolysis and diskography is stressed.[23,28-30] Early detection of infection and early treatment is the key to bring about the medical abortion of the infection, while in the fulminating infection and the lately diagnosed cases surgery is preferably recommended under potential antibiotic coverage.

Surgical Site Infection

Surgical site infections (SSI) were classified into several clinical types on the basis of the disease onset (early and

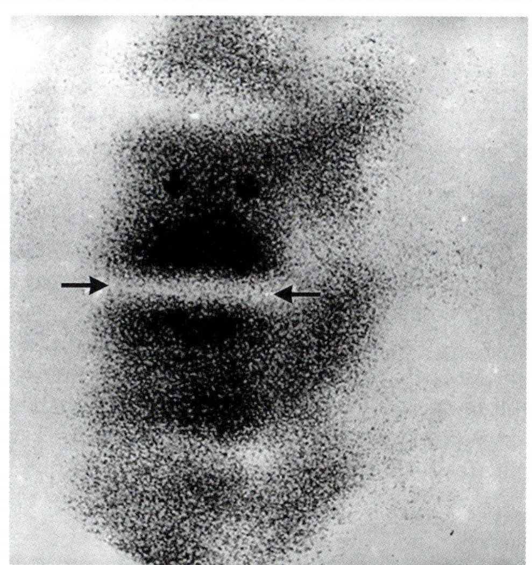

Fig. 34.10B Postoperative spondylitis: lateral pinhole scan. Reversed asymmetry of the endplate involvement; Lateral pinhole scan of the midlumbar spine in a 25-year-old man with post-diskectomy diskitis (L3–4) shows intense, semilunar tracer uptake in the initial focus in the lower L3 vertebral body and less uptake in the apposing upper endplate of L4 body with narrowed disk space

late), sites (superficial and deep), severity and variety of causative organisms (simple, multiorganisms, resistant multi-organisms with myonecrosis), and host characteristics (normal systemic defense, multiple systemic disease, and immunocompromised or severely malnourished).

Surgical wound infection is infrequently and unexpectedly complicated even though the strict aseptic surgical procedures are carried out. However, it is more frequently complicated in the immunocompromised patients.[8] Smoking, obesity, malnutrition, diabetes, long-term steroid use, alcohol abuse, and preoperative irradiation are well documented as risk factors.[18] Preoperative serum glucose level >125 mg/dL and postoperative level >200 mg/dL were listed as risk factor. Irradiated tissue with ischemia cannot tolerate bacterial contamination resulting in SSI because of impaired granulocyte adherence and microangiopathy.[21]

Prophylaxis (Prevention Strategy) and Early Management against Surgical Site Infection

Host characteristics should be carefully studied before surgery whether the patients have risk factors.

With regard to the timing of antimicrobial prophylaxis (AMP) administration, the blood and tissue concentrations of the drug used for AMP must, as a rule, reach adequate levels at the start of the operation.[74] Classen et al. reported that these levels become adequate within 2 hours before the start of the operation, and indicated that the frequency of infection was high when the administration was too early or when the drugs were administered only postoperatively. For surgery of ischemic irradiated tissue, administration of prostaglandin E1 derivative "limaprost alfadex (limaprost)" is recommended to reduce SSI.[21]

Debridement with low-pressure irrigation with 1% soap or povidone solution mixed with detergent solution can be effective for up to 6 hours to remove adherent bacteria from bone after contamination.

Postdiskectomy Diskitis

Diskitis can complicate after any type of disk surgery.[35,46,59-62] Patients are usually pain-free for 1–2 weeks after surgery, and then a patient may present with only increasingly low back pain with an otherwise uneventful postoperative course.

Diskitis after percutaneous endoscopic diskectomy: There are paucity of papers regarding the diskitis following the percutaneous endoscopic diskectomy.[18,35,46,59] The incidence of infection after the procedure is known to be less than 1%, and the clinical symptoms and signs, and laboratory data are same as that of the discitis following the other intradiskal needle procedures. Prophylactic measures and treatment protocol are also same as that of the diskitis following the intradiscal needle procedures.

Diskitis following microdiskectomy: Any operation has the potential of a postoperative wound infection. The incidence is 0.5% or less.[18,35,46] If a disk space infection occurs after surgery, it will be signaled by a sudden increase in pain, which quickly becomes nonmechanical and is present night and day. A significant amount of back muscle spasm, fever, leukocytosis, and high ESR (60 mm/hour) strongly suggest its presence.[33] On plain X-rays significant disk space narrowing is shown in short period of time. Bone scan is helpful for diagnosis.[2] MRI is the most sensitive test.[20,56-58]

It is preferably recommended to use a third generation cephalosporin for *S. aureus* infection. Improvement in the patients' symptoms should be seen within 48 hours. If this does not occur or if the patient maintains any signs of systemic infection beyond 3–5 days or develops an abscess or neurologic compromise, it is essential to reopen and drain the disk space. Fortunately, most postoperative disk space infections respond to nonoperative care if diagnosed early. Once if missed, they can affect the vertebra and become difficult to eradicate. However, in case of disk destruction even after control of infection, secondary osteoarthritis is obviously followed and can cause persistent back.[70,75] In such case the involved segment should be fused anteriorly, because it is difficult to expect spontaneous fusion.

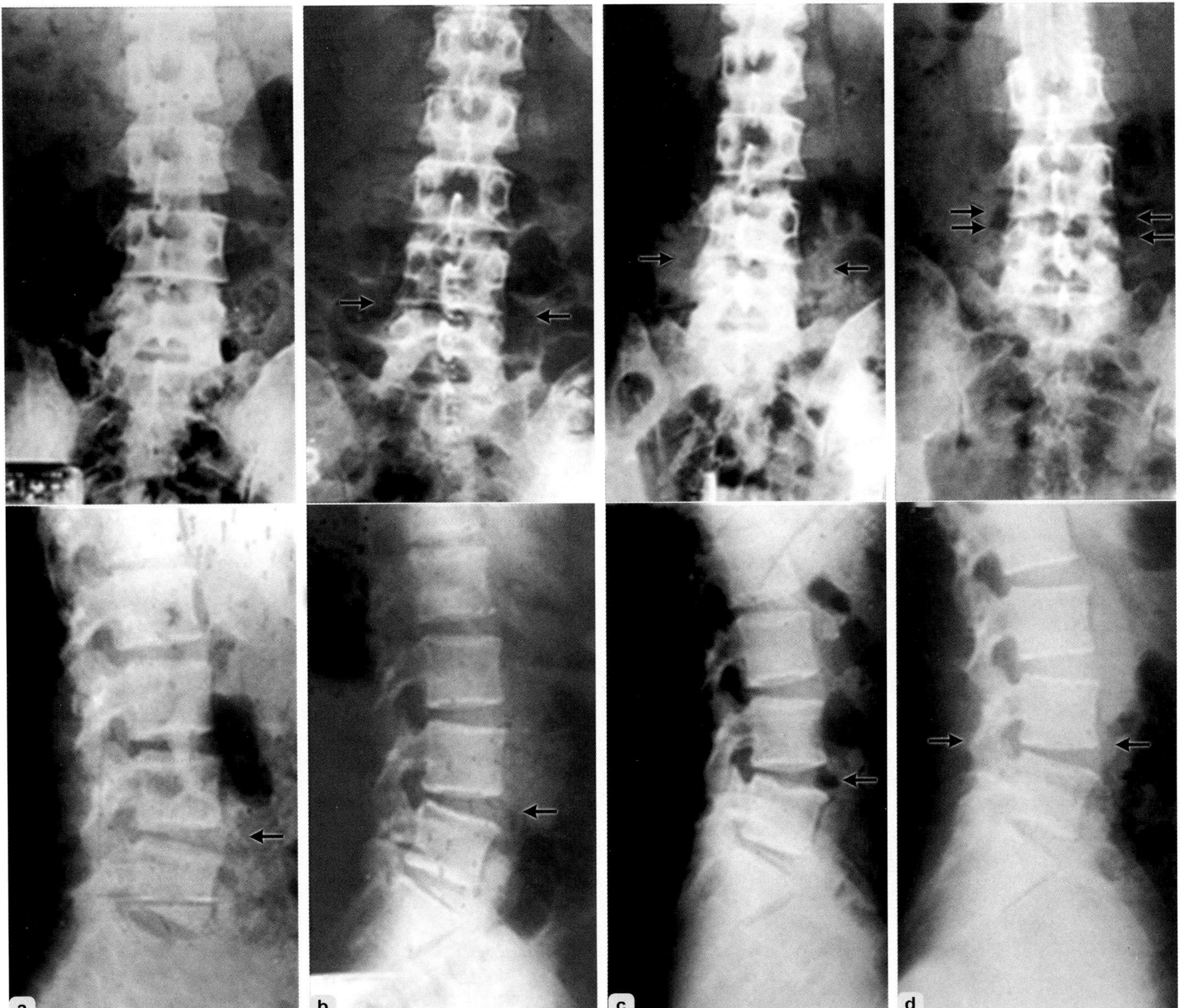

Figs 34.11A (a) A 37-year-old gentleman had diskectomy at L4–L5; (b to d) The radiograms, taken on postoperative (b) 9 days, (c) 3 weeks and 4 days, and (d) one year 2 months show gradual disk space narrowing and extension angular difference

The use of two doses of prophylactic antibiotics is recommended; the first dose is given intravenously at least 30 minutes before the skin incision, and the second dose is given 2 hours after wound closure. Most surgeons would use a first-generation cephalosporin (e.g. cefazolin sodium).

Diskitis after conventional diskectomy: Infection rates after conventional disk surgery is less than 4.0%.[18,35,46,59-62] The standard evaluation for a postoperative wound infection should be performed in the patient with increasing pain even in the presence of a well-healed incision. Disk space infections often present several months after diskectomy, with increasing pain and disability even with a normal appearing wound. Symptoms usually begin 7–12 days postoperatively with an increase in back pain and, most typically, muscle cramping in the legs. The CRP and ESR are found to be consistently elevated.[51,52] In the uncomplicated postoperative course the CRP level on day 6 after surgery drops below that on day 1 after surgery.[51]

Patient is recommended to remain at bed rest until he or she is comfortable. Treatment requires tissue or fluid culture and appropriate antibiotics. That is, antibiotics should be selected, based on the result of a biopsy or aspirates. As in the hematogenous spondylitis, our antibiotic regimen

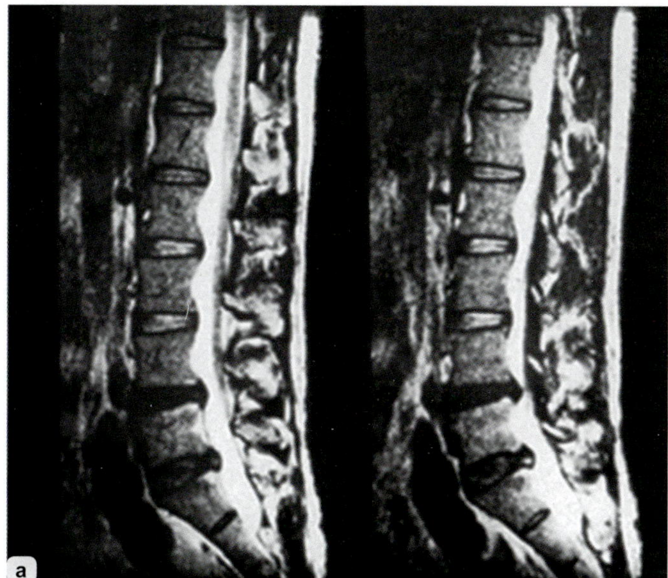

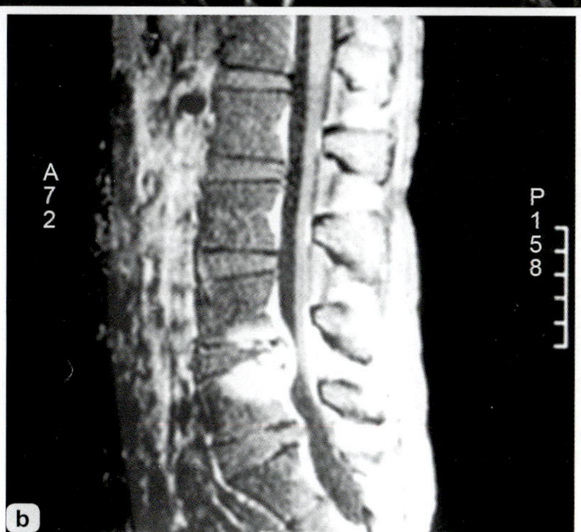

Fig. 34.11B (a) Preoperative MRI show the herniated black disk of L4–5 in a same patient; (b) Sagittal T1-weighted MR image, taken 3 weeks after diskectomy, demonstrating high signal intensity within the disk space and intraosseous high signal in upper half of L4 body is consistent with diskitis. He has had mild low back pain, though the infection was completely controlled

consists of 4 weeks of intravenous antibiotics followed by oral drugs until all signs of infection subside and a normal ESR is reached at least 3 months or longer. The recommended antibiotics are cefazolin, vancomycin, and cloxacillin for staphylococci, ciprofloxacin or ampicillin for E. coli, and cefepime, piperacillin, imipenem, ceftazidine for pseudomonas (Table 34.5)(Figs 34.10 to 34.12).

A paravertebral abscess may require open drainage and debridement. Also if the patients is first seen after advanced destructive changes become apparent, and pain is uncontrollable without resolution, it may be necessary to excise the infected disk and bony tissue, and to fuse the infected segment. For the painful healed lesion with advanced destructive changes, fusion operation is the preferred procedure.

The use of metallic implant anteriorly in the site of infection remains still now a point for controversy. However, despite the concerns of the presence of infection, recent few studies suggested the use of a titanium mesh cage even in vertebral osteomyelitis for reconstruction and maintenance of sagittal spinal profile and achievement of solid fusion. The current authors, however, do not agree with the aforementioned suggestions. The reason is that the implanted biomaterial contributes the perpetuation of infection, particularly in case of the biofilm-forming multiorganism infection.

Generally, the prognosis for resolution of the infectious process within 6–12 months with adequate treatment is excellent. In some patients spontaneous intercorporal fusion takes place together with resolution of the infection by conservative treatment. Placement of gentamicin-containing collagenous sponges in the cleared disk space was recommended to prevent the postoperative spondylodiskitis by the current and other previous authors, and was found effective.[23,29,30,59-62]

Biomaterial-centered Infection after Implantation

Biomaterial-centered infection is also known by various other names such as biofilm-mediated or cryptic infection. Infection rates is 1–2%. Orthopedic implant infection is a devastating disease because of the physical and emotional trauma. The patient encounters a situation that is associated with revision surgery compounded by the long-term postoperative treatment needed.

Comparative colonization study of *Staphylococcus epidermis* and *aureus* disclosed that initial attachment time for *S. epidermis* was significantly lower than *S. aureus* ($P < 0.05$) for all materials (4 hours for *S. epidermis* versus 1 hour for *S. aureus*). Slime production was evident after 4 hours of incubation for both strains.[13-15] Nonliving substrata (biomaterial devices and some tissue transplants) are introduced into mammalian hosts, they may become favored sites for adhesive colonization, especially in the immunocompromised patients.[15]

The main problem in orthopedic infection in the new millenium continues to be bone infection and infection around implants because of its prevalence, clinical and economic importance, and difficulties in treatment. That is, bacterial infection is one of the most serious complications of implantation surgery, and can lead to failure of the implant.[2,5-7]

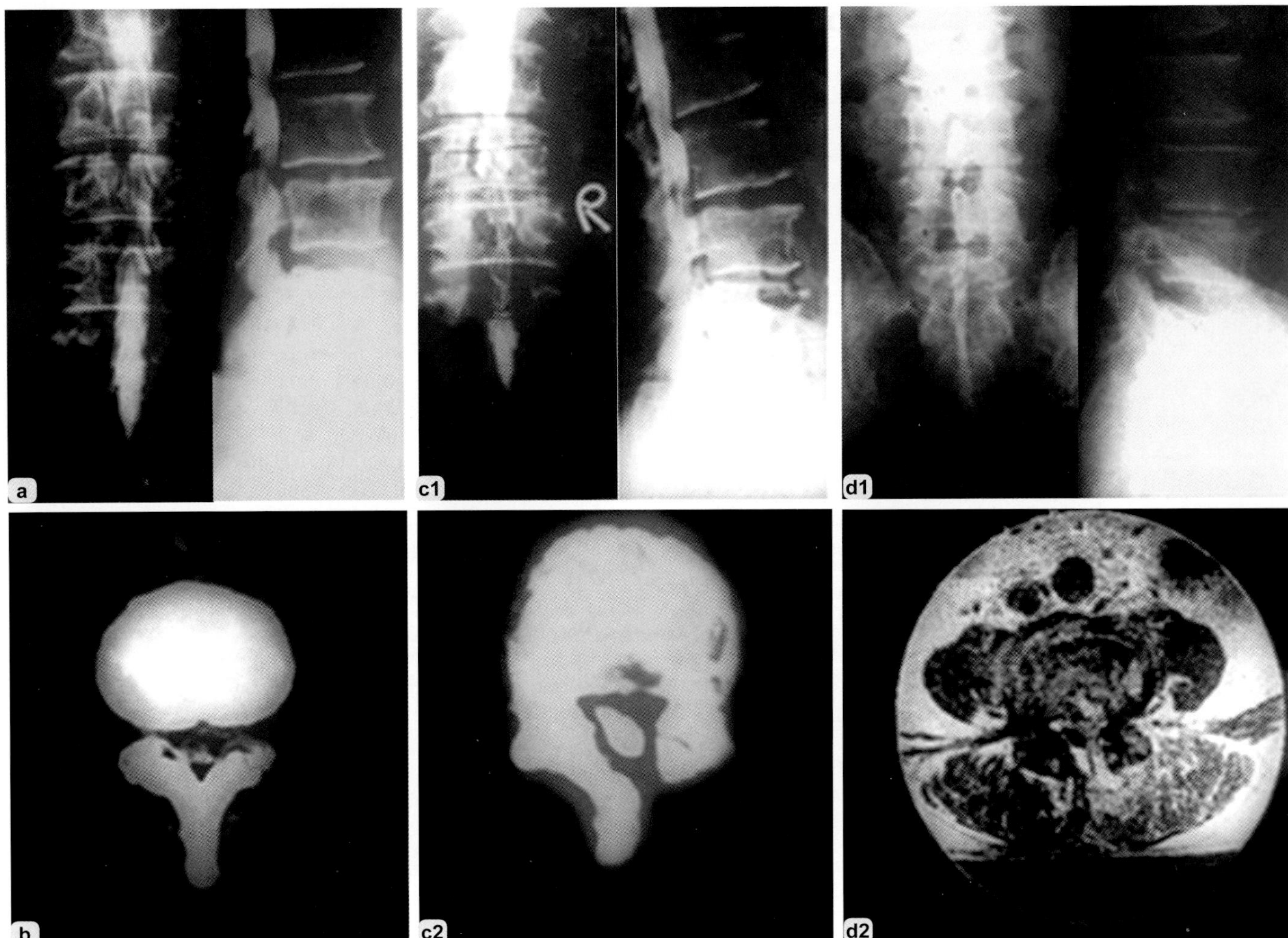

Fig. 34.12A A 62 year-old man had disk herniation at L4–5 [(preoperative myelogram (a) and CT myelogram (b)] for which disk surgery was performed on October 22, 1997. The postdiskectomy myelogram (c1) and CT myelogram (c2), taken two months and one week (December 30, 1997) afterward showed rapid disk space narrowing and the partial reblocking of the central canal at L4–5 disk level, which indicated the possible disk reherniation. The patient was cared continuously under the diagnosis of disk reherniation until he was transferred to authors' spine service. Radiograms (February 2, 1998: (d1) and MRI (February 3, 1998, (d2) disclosed the findings of post-diskectomy spondylodiskitis, which supported the clinical findings and the laboratory data. Disk of L4–5 was almost absorbed and seemed stabilized, though the segment was not fused completely as yet

Prosthetic material generally enhances the postoperative infection rate, although Ti alloys have been reported to yield a lower infection risk. All our infected patients had such implants inserted intraoperatively.[3,6,11-13]

Up to now most clinicians have believed that there is the higher prevalence of infection in implant surgery than in surgery without implants. It is not true. Cordero et al. (1996) showed that with *S. aureus* phage type 94/96, bone without an implant is more susceptible to infection than bone with some metallic implants (polished CrCo or Ti and porous-coated Ti).[13,14] According to him, with *S. aureus* phage 94/96, polymethylmetacrylate is more conducive to infection than polished metal and porous-coated Ti, but less conducive than porous-coated CrCo, bone without an implant, or bone graft.[13,14,42,43]

There have been similar reports. According to Gristina et al. these results could be plausibly explained by the osseous affinity of some bacterial strains, which would adhere more easily to damaged bone tissue than to a metallic implant.[42-44] Chang and Merritt stated that bacterial adherence varied less with the properties of the material than with the properties of the bacteria and the nature of the methods for interaction.[11,12]

Biomaterial-centered infections are causally related to the high adaptive ability of bacteria to colonize the surfaces of "inert" biomaterials or of adjacent damaged

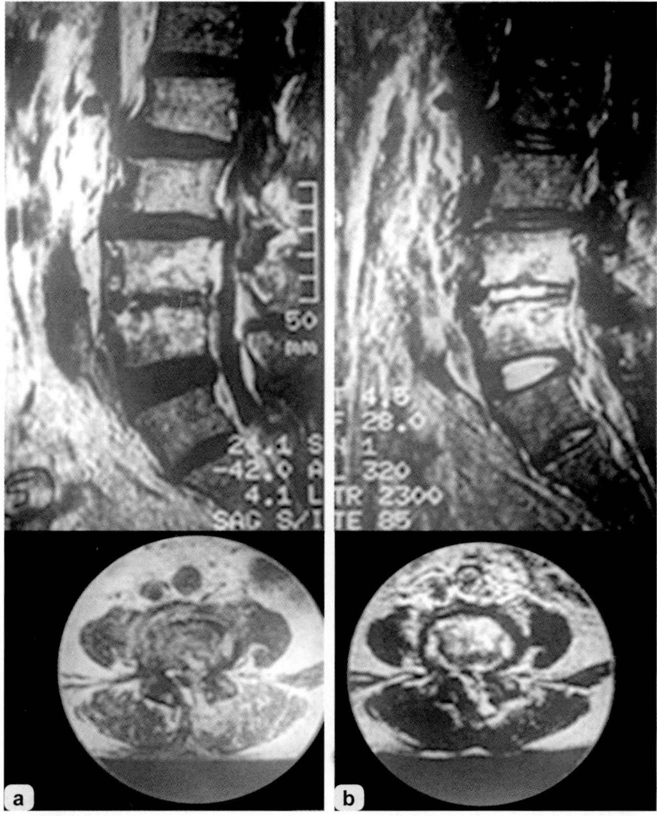

Fig. 34.12B On admission laboratory data, including CBC were Hb. 14.0 g%; Hct, 39.1; WBC, 10,200; ESR, 84 mm/hr; CRP, 3.6 mg/dL. One week after antibiotic therapy, WBC was 7,200, ESR, 75 mm/hr, and CRP, 2.27 mg/dL. Two weeks later, WBC was 6,500, ESR, 60 mm/hr, and CRP, 1.4 mg/dL. Also the patient felt comfortable with subsidence of back muscle spasm and pain. MRI shows high signal intensities in L4 and L5 bodies and disks of L4–5 and L5–S1, with increased epidural signal intensity and compressed dural sac at L4–5 disk level

tissue cells. Its characteristics derive from the adherent and biofilm-mediated mode of bacterial growth. The hydrated poly-anionic bacterial glycocalyx acts as an ion-exchange resin in binding charged antibiotic molecule, and that it thus limits their access to targets within cell and cell envelope.[3,6,13,16,42,43]

Machining techniques can lead to biofilm development. Sterilization kills the bacteria in these biofilms but fails to remove the residue of their matrices. These deposits must be removed before the devices can be implanted.

Clinical reports clearly show that the presence of biomaterials makes adjacent tissue susceptible to both immediate and delayed infections.[3,11,13,26,65]

Recent studies in the composite science and relation between microbial colonization of biomaterials and tissue cell integration of those surfaces are the "races for the surface". It is suggested that the fate of an avoidable surface maybe conceptualized as a race for the surface, which is a contest between tissue cell integration and bacterial adhesion to that same surface.

Host defense systems that are perturbed by biomaterials are a vital factor. If the race is won by tissue, then the surface is occupied and defended, and is thus less available for bacterial colonization.

Many risk factors have been identified for the development of surgical infection following implantation surgery including artificial disk replacement and instrumentation surgery for spinal fractures and diseases; Underlying comorbidities (obesity, malignancy, diabetes mellitus, local irradiation, and rheumatoid arthritis) or interferon (IFN-γ) and Mannose-binding lectin (MBL) deficiencies are listed. It has been known that certain individuals have genetic susceptibility to opportunistic infection. Also recently important role of cytokines, in particular interleukin-6 (IL-6) and the acute phase protein mannose binding lectin (MBL) was reported.[67] MBL (a 96 KDa trimer) is a hepatic derived acute phase protein with an important role in the innate immune system, and its synthesis is induced by IL-6 which is derived from bacterial stimulation of macrophages. It was found that MBL deficient patients are very susceptible to post-arthroplasty infection. MBL has been shown to have high-level binding for *Staphylococcus aureus*, *Candida albicans*, *Aspergillus fumigans*, and *Streptococcus pyogenes*.

Two main barriers to the extended use of implanted biomaterials and complex artificial organ devices are the possibility of biomaterial-centered infection and the lack of successful tissue integration of biomaterial surfaces. These seemingly disparate phenomena are actually similar expression of cell-to-substratum surface interactions.[67,81]

The pathogenesis of adherent infections is related, in part, to preferential colonization of inert substrata whose surfaces are not integrated with healthy tissues composed of living cells and intact extracellular polymers. Even in healthy patients, host defense mechanisms may be perturbed by the presence of biomaterials.

The ability to adhere to surface is a general property of almost all bacteria, and depends on intricate and sometimes exquisitely specific series of events. These events are based on determinants and characteristics of the bacteria, the substratum surface to be colonized, and the intervening ambient fluid milieu.

The most frequently isolated bacteria from the biomaterial surface are *Staphylococcus epidermidis*, *Staphylococcus aureus* (less frequently associated with polymer-sited infection), and additional organisms (*Escherichia coli*, *Peptococcus*, *Pseudomonas aeruginosa*, *Proteus mirabilis*, β-hemolytic streptococci).

Studies of adult osteomyelitis have shown polymicrobial infections were in more than two-thirds of the cases.[88] The most commonly isolated pathogens were *Staphylococcus aureus* and *epidermidis*, *Pseudomonas*, *Enterococcus*, *Streptococcus*, *bacillus*, and *Proteus* species.[15,18,37]

Polymicrobial infections which appear to be an important feature of substratum-induced infections are probably present more often than is realized, and should be regarded as poor prognostic sign for revision surgery.

There has been some extraordinary reports that the use of a titanium mesh cage anteriorly in the site of active infection not only had no negative influence on the eradication of infection, but is additionally corrected and maintained the sagittal profile at the affected segments, positively contributing to an uneventful fusion. There is no increase in the rate of recurrence or persistence of infection related to the implantation of titanium mesh cag es.[36,38,40,42,50,79,81,82,85] Those authors provided the following reason to support their view; Titanium may be more resistant to bacterial infection than stainless steel. Thus, bacteria adhere less to titanium than stainless steel, because titanium has a less electrochemically active oxide surface compared to stainless steel, which has a higher surface free energy (>40 mV/m) and hence more available ligands for binding with cells both bacterial and tissue competing for the biomaterial surface.

It is, however, the current authors' view that the implanted metals and nonmetallic materials serve to promote the infection and making it resistant to antibiotic therapy. That is, it is known that the local effect is similar when compromised tissue such as dead bone or traumatized soft tissue and organs, is present.

Among the orthopedic implants, polymethylmetacrylate is often considered to be the most conducive to septic complication, and bone graft also poses a high risk of infection because they are foreign bodies. Other researchers have disagreed, at least in past, with all these statements. Preferential bacterial adhesion is the surface of the polymer for *Staphycoccus epidermidis*, and metals for *S. aureus*. *Staphylococcus epidermidis* is a factor in polymicrobial infections associated with other substrata, such as metals, and compromised bone and tissue.[11,42-44,79,85,86] As yet there are no clinical reports, which definitely answered to these questions.

Most infections around orthopedic implants (fixation instruments, fusion cages, vertebroplasty cement, artificial joint) are caused by staphylococci, followed in frequency by some gram-negative bacilli (*E. coli*, *Proteus*, *Pseudomonas*, and *Klebsiella/Enterobacter/Serratia*). Two staphylococcal species are important: *Staphylococcus aureus* and *epidermidis*. *S. aureus* has been the most frequently isolated pathogen in implant-related infections. The skin saprophyte, *S. epidermidis*, less aggressive and less sensitive to prophylactic measures, has been the second most frequent isolate in clinical series.[3,11]

The benefit of prophylactic cephosporins in spinal surgery has been proven. Therefore, to prevent wound sepsis after cage fusion, vertebroplasty, joint arthroplasty, and spinal instrumentation, aseptic surgical techniques and the appropriate administration of perioperative antibiotics have been practiced. Perioperative antibiotics (24–48 hours postoperatively is considered the gold standard) have been established as routine in all spinal procedures.[75]

Despite these preventive measures, there remains a subset of patients who appear to acquire prosthetic joint infections without obvious predisposition. This raises the possibility that there may be an underlying genetic immunological component responsible for infection in this vulnerable subgroup. MBL deficiency appears to increase the likelihood and severity of sepsis.[67]

In HIV positive patients the use of biomaterials in the infected foci is inappropriate, because they are susceptible to a variety of other opportunistic infection.[8,18] A good understanding of the bacterial and metal characteristics is vital as is the knowledge of bacterial response to implanted material and chemotherapy.

The challenge still remains for better preventative measures against postoperative infection. In case of bacterial contamination, the measure to control and/or eradicate infection and to prevent bacterial adherence are the key factors.[1,2] It has been established that the adherence of bacteria to material surfaces plays an important role in the pathogenesis of infection of implant surgery. Several methods to prevent bacterial adherence to implant surfaces have been suggested: (i) incorporating antibiotics to biomaterials, (ii) immobilization of antimicrobial peptide, (iii) surfactant coatings, such as salicylic acid, silver, substituted dextrans, or polyethylene oxide, and (iv) serum proteins such as fibronectin and albumin (Table 34.5). Those serum proteins play an important role in the process of bacterial adhesion to biomaterials. An albumin coating on a titanium surface has been shown to have inhibitory effects of bacterial adherence, and additionally prevents platelet adhesion and subsequent thrombus formation.

To control implant-related severe infections, the biomaterials should be assessed from the view point of their resistibility to bacterial adhesions and infections. Petty et al. found no difference between smooth-surface implants (stainless-steel, CrCo, polymethylmetacrylate, and polyethylene) when contaminated with *S. aureus*, but bone implanted with polymethyl-metacrylate became infected more easily when contaminated with *S. epidermidis* or *E. coli* than when implanted with smooth-surface metals.[89] Barth et al. (1989) found that with *S. aureus* metal-implanted bone became infected more easily;[3] however, with *S. epidermidis* bone implanted with polymer (polymethylmetacrylate) was more easily infected. It appeared that *S. aureus* had preferential adherence to metal, and *S. epidermidis* to polymer.

One of most practical strategies for the prevention of colonization biofilm formation is the use of materials and coating that release antibiotics into the surrounding tissues and fluids.

Topography and chemical properties of biomaterial surfaces could be modified to alter the propensity for bacteria adhesion and subsequent biofilm formation. Electropolished titanium or titanium alloy (Ti-6Al-7Nb) may be a solution for avoiding infections associated with intramedullary nailing systems as there are indications that *Staphylococcus* tends to adhere more to standard titanium alloy nails both *in vitro* and *in vivo*. Another possibility is to coat titanium or stainless steel with nitrogen ions which affects the resistivity and chemical topography of the surfaces; titanium nitride coatings induce fibroblast attachment and growth, minimizing the adhesion of *S. aureus*, *S. epidermidis*, *Streptococcus mutans* and *Pseudomonas aeruginosa*.

As other methods protein coatings (heparin or albumin), surface modification by hydrophilic chains, phosphorylchiline-modified polymer coatings and poly (ethylene glycol-based coating) reduce protein absorption, bacterial attachment and biofilm formation on biomaterial surfaces.[5,7,9,80]

Prophylactic measures for the biofilm-mediated infection are already listed (Table 34.5), and pathogenesis of cryptic infection are discussed. The management of biomaterial- and compromised tissue-associated spinal infection will be followed.

Treatment must be centered on identifying and eradicating the infecting organism, while maintaining spinal stability, protecting neurologic status, and producing a nutritional state sufficient to foster healing.

Because different antibiotics behave differently within the biofilm environment, combining two antibiotics with different characteristics may improve efficacy and facilitate the eradication of the infection.

According to Fujimura et al. the combined treatment using clarithromycin (CAM) and vancomycin (VCM) may effectively eradicate staphylococcal biofilms in patient with implant-related infection.[64] It was reported that rifampin eradicated biofilm embedded *Staphylococcus epidermis* colonies in combination with other antibiotics, such as vancomycinin an *in vitro* setting.[90] Also, proteolytic enzyme “serratiopeptidase” (Danzen, Takeda Pharm. Japan), is known effective to lyse the biofilms.[91-95]

Surgical management consists of drainage and focal debridement under cover of antibiotic therapy for the acute cases, but for the chronic infection removal of implanted biomaterials, radical debridement, sequential surfactant irrigation, and reconstructive surgery for defective spinal column have to be carried out.

In conclusion it is confirmed that the susceptibility to infection in orthopedic surgery is not only material dependant but also bacterial dependant. In the presence of foreign bodies and necrotic tissues, infection control is not easy. It is reminded that antibiotics can control infection only by suppression and cannot eliminate it. Because antibiotic therapy in itself cannot kill bacteria inhabiting the biofilm on the implant surface. Once the therapy is discontinued, these bacteria will form a nidus for reinfection of the surrounding tissue.

In early infections after posterior instrumentation, surgical debridement and treatment with antimicrobial agents may allow fixation metals to be preserved to maintain stability during treatment.

A frank peri-implants infection should always be treated by surgery that includes the radical debridement of infected tissues and bone sequestra and the removal of all posterior and anterior implant materials. This is necessary to ensure complete eradication of the biofilm. Implanted anterior fusion cage regardless of implantation approach, it should be removed through anterior or lateral approach for safety reason when it get infected. Therefore, surgeon must adhere to primary principles of minimizing tissue destruction and assuring removal of all "foreign bodies" (biomaterial, dead bone, or diseased tissue) which may act as sites for bacterial adhesion, and potentiate an infection.[16,37,38] In particular when infection is established and fixation metal components are loose, radical surgical debridement is necessary to remove all foreign material and involved bone and soft tissue. In addition to this primary surgical procedure, antibiotic-impregnated acrylic beads may be used to sterilize and temporarily maintain dead space.[19,74] The most commonly used antibiotics in beads are heat-stable vancomycin, tobramycin and gentamicin.

Many questions still need to be answered, especially in the field of optimal therapies for bone infections in the presence of foreign materials in the tissue. When developing a new implant, medical device or biomaterial, not only strength and biocompatibility but also the effect of an anti-biofilm substance should be considered.

Primary Epidural Abscess

Primary epidural abscess should be drained as early as possible, if the patient presents the neurological symptoms under the cover of the antibiotic therapy.[96-99]

References

1. Bonfiglio M, Lange TA, Kim YM. Pyogenic vertebral osteomyelitis. Disk space infections. Clin Orthop. 1973;96:234-47.
2. Bahk YW, Kim OH, Chung SK. Pinhole collimator scintigraphy in differential diagnosis of metastasis, fracture, and infections of the spine. J Nucl Med. 1987;28:447-51.
3. Barth E, Berg E, Gristina AG. Biomaterial specificity of S. Aureus and S. epidermis in orthopedic infections. Trans Orthop Res Soc. 1989;14:558.
4. Buchelt M, Lack W, Kutschera HP, Katterschafka T, Kiss H, Schneider B, Kotz R. Comparison of tuberculous and pyogenic spondylitis- An analysis of 422 cases. Clin Orthop. 1993;296:192-9.
5. An YH, Stuart GW, McDowell SJ, McDaniel SE, Kang Q, Friedman RJ. Prevention of bacterial adherence to implant surfaces with a crosslinked albumin coating in vivo. J Orthop Res. 1996;14:846-9.
6. Arens S, Schlegel U, Printzen G, Ziegler WJ, Perren SM, Hansis M. Influence of materials for fixation implants on local infection: an experimental study of steel versus titanium DCP in rabbits. J. Bone Joint Surg. 1996;78B:647-51.
7. An YH, Bradley J, Powers DL, Friedman RJ. The prevention of prosthetic infection using a cross-linked albumin coating in a rabbit model. J Bone Joint Surg. 1997;79B:816-9.
8. Bono CM: Spectrum of spine infections in patients with HIV. Clin Orthop. 2006;444:83-91.
9. Adachi K, Tsurumoto T, Yonekura A, Nishimura S, Kajiyama S, Hirakata Y, Shindo H. New quantitative image analysis of staphylococcal biofilms on the surfaces of nontranslucent metallic biomaterials. J Orthop Sci. 2007;12:178-85.
10. Cierny G, Mader JT, Pennik JJ. A clinical staging system for adult osteomyelitis. Contemporary Orthopedics. 1985;10:17-37.
11. Chang CC, Merritt K. Effect of Staphylococcus epidermidis on adherence of Pseudomonas aeruginosa and Proteus mirabilis to polymethyl metacrylate (PMMA) and gentamycin-containing PMMA. J Orthop Res. 1991;9:284-8.
12. Chang CC, Merritt K. Infection at the site of implanted materials with and without pre-adhered bacteria. J Orthop Res. 1994;12:526-31.
13. Cordero J, Munuera L, Folgueira MD. Influence of metal implants on infection: an experimental study on rabbits. J. Bone Joint Surg. 1994;76B:717-20.
14. Cordero J, Munuera L, Folgueira MD. Influence of bacterial strains on bone infection. J Ortho Res. 1996;14:663-7.
15. Costerton JW. Biofilm theory can guide the treatment of device-related orthopedic infections. Clin Orthop. 2005;437: 7-11.
16. Dimar JR, Carreon LY, Glassman SD, Campbell MJ, Hartman MJ, Johnson JR. Treatment of pyogenic vertebral osteomyelitis with anterior debridement and fusion followed by delayed posterior spinal fusion. Spine. 2004;29:326-32.
17. Christodoulou AG, Givissis P, Symeonidis PD, Karataglis D, Pournaras J. Reduction of postoperative spinal infections based on an etiological protocol. Clin Orthop. 2006;444:107-13.
18. Cunningham ME, Girardi F, Papadopoulos EC, Cammisa FP. Spinal infections in patients with compromised immune systems. Clin Orthop. 2006;444:73-82.
19. Dairaku K, Tokagi M, Kawaji H, Sakaki K, Ishii M, Ogino T. Antibiotics-impregnated cement spacers in the first step of two-stage revision for infected totally replaced hip joints: report of tentrial cases. Orop Sci. 2009;14:704-10.
20. Cousins JP, Houghton VM. Magnetic response imaging of the spine. J Am Acad Orthop Surg. 2009;17:1:22-30.
21. Demura S, Kawahara N, Murakami H, Nambu K, Kato S, Yoshioka K, et al. Surgical site infection in spinal metastasis. Spine. 2009;34:635-9.
22. Nylor PT, Jennings R, Wbb LX, Gristina AG. Antibiotic sensitivity of biomaterial-adherent Staphylococcus epidermidis and Staphylococcus aureus. Trans Orthop Res Soc. 1989;14:108.
23. Osti OL, Fraser RD, Vernon-Roberts B. Discitis after discography. The role of prophylactic antibiotics. J Bone Joint Surg. 1990;72B:271-4.
24. Norden CW. Bone and Joint infection - an update. Clin Infect Dis. 1997;25:1293-4.
25. Nishimura S, Tsurumoto T, Yonekura A, Adachi K, Shindo H. Antimicrobial susceptibility of Staphylococcus aureus and Staphylococcus epidermidis biofilm isolated from infected total hip arthroplasty cases. J Orthop Sci. 2006;11:46-50.
26. Pappou IP, Papadopoulos EC, Sama AA, Girardi FP, Cammisa FP: Postoperative infections in interbody fusion for degenerative spinal disease. Clin Orthop. 2006;444:120-8.
27. Ozuturk C, Adyinli U, Vural R, Sehirlioglu A, Mutlu M. Simultaneous versus segmental one-stage combined anterior and posterior spinal surgery for spinal infections (outcomes and complications). Int Orthop. 2007;31:363-6.
28. Fraser RD. Chemopapain for the treatment of intervertebral disc herniation. The final report of a double-blind study. Spine. 1984;9:815-8.
29. Fraser RD, Osti OL, Vernon-Roberts B. Discitis following chemonucleolysis: An experimental study. Spine. 1986;11:679-6887.
30. Fraser RD, Osti OL, Vernon-Roberts B. Discitis after discography. J Bone Joint Surg. 1987;69B:26-35.
31. Mahendru V, Bacon DR, Lema MJ. Multiple epidural abscess and spinal anesthesia in a diabetic patient. Reg Anesth. 1994;19:66-8.
32. Carragee EJ. Pyogenic vertebral osteomyelitis. J Bone Joint Surg. 1997;99A:874-80.
33. Carragee EJ, Kim D, Van der Vlugt T, Vittum D. The clinical use of erythrocyte sedimentation rate in pyogenic vertebrae osteomyelitis. Spine. 1997;22:2089-93.
34. Buchholz HW. Antibiotic-loaded acrylic cement; Current concepts. Clin Orthop. 1984;190:96-108.
35. Fernand R, Lee CK. Post-laminectomy disc space infection: A review of the literature and a report of three cases. Clin Orthp. 1986;209:215-8.
36. Eysel P, Hopf C, Vagel I, Rompe JD. Primary stable anterior instrumentation or dorsoventral spondylodesis in spondylodiscitis -- Results of a comparative study. European Spine J. 1997;6:152-7.

37. Ehrlich GD, Stoodley P, Kathju S, et al. Engineering approaches for the detection and control of orthopedic biofilm infections. Clin orthop. 2005;437:59-66.
38. Ha KY, Kim YH. Postoperative spondylitis after posterior lumbar interbody fusion using cages. Eur Spine J. 2004;13:419-24.
39. Ha KY, Shin JH, Kim KW, Na KH. The fate of anterior autogenous bone graft after anterior radical surgery with or without posterior instrumentation in the treatment of pyogenic lumbar spondylodiscitis. Spine (Phila pa 1976). 2007;32:1856-64.
40. Korovessis P, Petsinis G, Koureas G, Iliopoulos P, Zacharatos S. One-stage combined surgery with mesh cages for treatment of septic spondylitis. Clin Orthop. 2006;444:51-9.
41. Waldvogel FA, Vasey H. Osteomyelitis. The past decade. New Engl J Med. 1980;303:360-70.
42. Gristina AG, Costerton JW. Bacterial adherence to biomaterials and tissue. The significance of its role in clinical sepsis. J Bone Joint Surg. 1985;67A:264-73.
43. Gristina AG, Barth E, Webb LX. Microbial adhesion and the pathogenesis of biomaterial- centered infection. In Orthopaedic infection: Diagnosis and treatment. RB Gustilo. RP Cruninger, and DT Tsukayama Eds: Philadelphia: WB Saunders; 1987. p.325.
44. Gristina AG, Naylor PT, Myrvik QN. Mechanisms of musculoskeletal sepsis. Orthop Clin North Am. 1991;22:363-71.
45. Lindholm TS, Pylkk nnen P. Discitis following removal of intervertebral disc. Spine. 1982;7:618-22.
46. Frank AM, Trappe AE. Spondylodiscitis after lumbar spine intervertebral disc surgery. Clinical patterns, diagnosis, treatment. Neurochirurgia. 1988;31:205-9.
47. Keenan TL, Benson DR. Differential diagnosis and conservative treatment of infectious diseases. In: Frymoyer JW, (Ed.): The adult spine: principles and practice. 2nd ed. Philadelphia: Lippincott-Raven; 1997;pp.871-94.
48. Kim YT, Hwang WY, Han BH. Analysis of pyogenic spondylitis in adults. Korea Spine Surg. 1996;3:69-76.
49. Kulowski J. Pyogenic osteomyelitis of the spine. An analysis and discussion of 102 cases. J Bone Joint Surg. 1936;18:343-64.
50. Lee JS, Suh KJ. Posterior lumbar interbody fusion with autogenous iliac crest bone graft in the treatment of pyogenic spondylodiscitis. J Bone Joint Surg. 2006; 88B:765-70.
51. Waleczek H, Hozianka J, Everts H. C-reactive protein in the early diagnosis of postoperative infection following bone surgery. Chirug. 1991;62:866-90.
52. Tanaka S, Nishino J, Matsui T, et al. Neutrophil CD64 expression in the diagnosis of local musculoskeletal infection and the impact of antibiotics. J Bone Joint Surg Br. 2009;91-B:1237-42.
53. Tarkin IS, Dunman PM, Garvin KL. Improving the treatment of musculoskeletal infections with molecular diagnostics. Clin orthop. 2005;437:83-8.
54. Stoodley P, Kathju S, Hu FZ, et al. Molecular and imaging techniques for bacterial biofilms in joint arthroplasty infections. Clin Orthop. 2005;437:31-40.
55. Donlan RM. New approaches for the characterization of prosthetic joint biofilms. Clin orthop. 2005;437:12-9.
56. Frank AM, Trappe AE. The role magnetic resonance imaging (MRI) in the diagnosis of spondylodiscitis. Neurosurg. Rev. 1990;13:279-83.
57. Maiuri F, Laconetta G, Gallicchio B, Manto A, Briganti F. Spondylodiscitis. Clinical and magnetic resonance diagnosis. Spine. 1997;22:1741-6.
58. Yoshikawa T, Maeda M, Ueda Y, Matsuyama E, Kugai A, Tamai S, Ichijima K. Magnetic resonance imaging in the early phase of pyogenic spondylitis : A report of four cases. J Orthop Sci. 1997;2:16-23.
59. Pilgoald S. Discitis (closed space infection) following removal of lumbar intervertebral disc. J Bone Joint Surg. 1969;51A:713.
60. Patgaonkar P, Cuevas G, Moheshwari S, Tampi C. Disc space infection (discitis) following interdiscal ozone therapy for acute low back pain due to prolapsed lumbar intervertebral disc; a case report. J Spinal Surgery. 2010;1:253-6.
61. Puranen J, M Kel J, L HDE S. Postoperative intervertebral discitis. Acta Orthop Scand. 1984;55:461-5.
62. Rohde V, Meyer B, Schaller C, Hassler WE. Spondylodiscitis after lumbar discectomy -- Incidence and a proposal for prophylaxis. Spine. 1998;23(5):615-20.
63. Sasso RC, Garrido BJ. Postoperative spinal wound infections. J Am Acad Orthop Surg. 2008;16:330-7.
64. Fujimura S, Sato T, Kikuchi T, Zaini J, Gomi K, Watanabe A. Efficacy of clarithromycin plus vancomycin in mice with implant-related infection caused by biofilm-forming Staphylococcus aureus. J Orthop Sci. 2009;14:658-61.
65. Patel R: biofilms and antimicrobial resistance. Clin orthop. 2005;437:41-7.
66. Marcotte AL, Trzeccak MA. Community-acquired methicilline-resistant Staphylococcus aureus: An emerging pathogen in orthopedics. J Am Acad Orhop Surg. 2008;16:98-106.
67. Longley RJ, Rowley DI. Is infection inevitable in some arthroplasty patients? Orthop and Trauma. 2008;23:2:117-21.
68. Uchida K, Yayama T, Kokubo Y, et al. Direct detection of pathogens in osteoarticular infections by polymerase chain reaction amplification and microarray hybridization. J Orthop Sci. 2009;14:475-83.
69. Tsiodras S, Falagas ME. Clinical assessment and medical treatment of spine infections. Clin Orthop. 2006;444:38-50.
70. Hadjipavlon AG, Mader JT, Necessary JT, Muffoletto AJ. Hematogenous pyogenic spinal infections and their surgical managements. Spine. 2000;25:1668-79.
71. Lin MR, Lee JY, Vaccaro AR. Surgical infections in the traumatized spine. Clin Orthop. 2006;444:114-9.
72. Matsui H, Hirano N, Sakaguchi Y. Vertebral osteomyelitis: an analysis of 38 surgically treated cases. Eur Spine J. 1998;7:50-4.
73. Nade S. Infection after joint replacement: Current Orthop. 1997;11:129-33.
74. Jeong ST, Kim JY, Park YJ, Koo KH, Song HR, Cho SH. Treatment of wound infection using antibiotics-mixed bone cement beads as complication of spine surgery. J. Korea Spine Surg. 1996;3:225-31.
75. Takahashi H, Wade A, Iida Y, et al. Antimicrobial prophylaxis for spinal surgery. J Orthop Sci. 2009;14:40-4.

76. Swanson AN, Pappou IP, Cammisa FP, Girardi FP. Chronic infection of the spine – surgical indication and treatments. Clin Orthop. 2006;444:100-6.
77. Viola RW, King HA, Adler SM, Wilson CB. Delayed infection after elective spinal instrumentation and fusion. A retrospective analysis of eight cases. Spine. 1997;22:2444-51.
78. Yang S-C, Fu T-S, Chen L-H, Niu C-C, Lai P-L, Chen W-J. Percutaneous endoscopic discectomy and drainage for infectious spondylitis. Int Orthop. 2007;31:367-73.
79. Shin JH, Ha KY, Kim KW, Lee JS, Joo MW. Surgical treatment for delayed pyogenic spondylitis after percutaneous vertebroplasty and kyphoplasty. Report of 4 cases. J Neurosurg. 2008;9:265-72.
80. Tamai K, Kawate K, Kawahara I, Takakura Y, Sakaki K. Inorganic antimicrobial coating for titanium alloy and its effect on bacteria. J Orthop Sci. 2009;14:204-9.
81. Richards BS. Delayed infections following posterior spinal instrumentation for the treatment of idiopathic scoliosis. J Bone Joint Surg. 1995;77A:524-9.
82. Dekel S, Lenthal G, Francis MJ. Release of prostaglandins from the bone and muscle after tibial fracture. An experimental study in rabbit. J Bone Joint Surg. 1981;63B:185-9.
83. Li D, Yhompson DD, Paralkar VM. Prostaglandin E2 receptors in bone formation. Int Orthop. 2007;31:767-72.
84. Robinson Y, Tschoeke SK, Kayser R, Boehm H, Heyde CE. Reconstruction of large defects in vertebral osteomyelitis with expandable titanium cage. Int Orthop. 2009;33:745-9.
85. Sanzen L, Linder L. Infection adjacent to tatanium and bone cement implants: an experimental study in rabbits. Biomaterials. 1995;16:1273-7.
86. Yu SW, Chen WJ, Lin WC, Chen YJ, Tu YK. Serious pyogenic spondylitis following vertebroplasty: a case report. Spine. 2004;29:E209-11.
87. Dunn LT, Javed A, Findlay G, Green ADL. Iatrogenic spinal infection following epidural anesthesia. Case report. Europ Spine J. 1996;5:418-20.
88. Thalgott JS, Cotler HB, Sasso RC, LaRocca H, Gardner V. Postoperative infections in spinal implants. Classification and analysis - a multicenter study. Spine. 1991;16:981-4.
89. Petty W, Spanier S, Shuster JJ, Silverthorne C. The influence of skeletal implants on incidence of infection experiments in a canine model. J Bone Joint Surg. 1985;67A:1236-44.
90. Gagnon RF, Richards GK, Wiesenfeld L. Staphylococcus epidermis biofilms: unexpected outcome of double and triple antibiotic combinations with rifampin. ASAID Trans. 1991;37(3):158-60.
91. Jahansen C, Falholt P, Gram L. Enzymatic removal and disinfection of bacterial biofilms. Appl Environ Microb. 1997;63:3724-8.
92. Koyama A. Transfer of cerotiam into pulmonary tissues and its promotion by serrapeptase. Takeda Bulletin. 1987;6:14-7.
93. Mecikoglu M, Saygi B, Yildirim Y, Karadog-saygi E, Ramadan SS, Esemenli T. The effect of proteolytic enzyme serratiopeptidase in the treatment of experimental implant-related infection. J Bone Joint Surg. 2006;88A:1208-14.
94. Selan L, Berlutti F, Passariello C, Comodi-Ballanti MR, Thaller MC. Proteolytic enzymes: a new treatment therapy strategy for prosthetic infections? Antimicrob Agents Chemothe. 1993;37:2618-2.
95. Takeda News – special issue on Danzen (serratiopeptidase), 1983.
96. Danner RL, Hartman BJ. Update of spinal epidural abscess: 35 cases and review of the literature. Rev Infect Dis. 1987;9:265-74.
97. Mampalam TJ, Rosegay H, Andrews BT, Rosenblum ML, Pitts LH. Nonoperative treatment of spinal epidural infections. J Neurosurg. 1989;71:208-10.
98. Land IM, Hughes JPR, St Clair Forbes W, Makenna F. MRI appearances of cervical epidural abscess. Clin Radiol. 1995;50:446-71.
99. Choi Wt, Choi BY, Lee JW, Moon MS. Pyogenic spinal epidural abscess – A case report. J Korea Orthop Assoc. 2002;37:319-23.

CHAPTER

35

Tuberculosis of Spine—Current Views in Diagnosis and Management and Global Standard

Myung-Sang Moon, Sung-Soo Kim, Jeong-Lim Moon, Jang-Cheol Sihn

Introduction

Tuberculosis still remains an urgent global health problem. Approximately 8 million tuberculosis cases were identified worldwide, resulting in 2 million deaths.[1-5] Ninety-five percent of tuberculosis patients are in the developing world. According to the World Health Organization, tuberculosis causes 1.81 million deaths in Asia each year.[1-5] China has 1.4 million new cases every year.[3] In South Saharan African countries, the number of reported tuberculosis cases has doubled or even tripled because of the spread of HIV/AIDS.[6-12] In HIV-negative patients around 3%-5% of tuberculosis is skeletal, whereas in HIV-positive patients about 60% of the cases involve the bone. The emergence of AIDS has also significantly increased the incidence of disseminated *Mycobacterium avium* complex (MAC) infection, which occurred almost exclusively in patients with a CD4 T-lymphocyte count below 100 cells/mm.[2-5] Apart from the spread of HIV/AIDS, the recent resurgence of chemoresistant variants of *M. tuberculosis* in particular poses further threat, and has raised great concerns worldwide. Taken together, these data indicate a need to prepare for a re-emergence of skeletal tuberculosis in the coming years.[2,5] Tuberculous spondylitis is the most dangerous form of skeletal tuberculosis, although less common.[1-10]

Spine is involved in 50% of osteoarticular tuberculosis patients. Spinal tuberculosis is the most dangerous form as it may cause bone destruction of the vertebral body, spinal deformity and/or paraplegia, and pulmonary insufficiency secondary to deformity of the thoracic cage.[1,2,4,5] When the body of the spine and the neural arch are involved, particularly in children, translational instability of the affected spine with anterior or lateral vertebral translation may occur, the resultant kyphoscoliotic deformity posing a risk of cord compression to the patient.[11]

Regardless of the recent advances in the diagnosis and management of spinal tuberculosis, there remains a significant number of issues that have not received much attention up to now in spite of their significant clinical importance.[5]

This chapter seeks to address these issues in diagnosis and management, in particular newer diagnostic technique, including non-culture laboratory methods, hyperbaric oxygen therapy, immunosuppressant drug use, surgical options for the spinal deformity and associated neural involvement, instrumentation and implant removal time, and the fate of the instrumented mobile segments.

Up to now, none clearly defined and differentiated the noncomplicated spinal tuberculosis from the complicated one on basis of the numerical and/or non-numerical and theoretical data. Surgical treatment is indicated only for the complicated one.

Immunity and Tuberculosis

Following exposure to *M. tuberculosis*, some individuals (about 10%) develop active tuberculosis, while the majority do not. It is not clear what factors determine the development of active disease among individuals infected by *M. tuberculosis*.[5,6] It would be interesting to disclose the factors why some develop active disease after exposure and why the others do not. It has been thought that patient's immune state is closely related with then, what other factors.

Macrophage have been reported to play a pivotal role in the immune response against mycobacteria by producing cytokines, such as TNFα, IFNα and IL-1β along with IFNγ produced by T-lymphocytes. Those cytokines can induce the free oxygen radical, "nitric oxide (NO)" in macrophages via the action of inducible form of the enzyme, "nitric oxide synthetase (iNOS)". NO and related reactive nitrogen intermediate (RNI) can kill and/or inhibit intracellular pathogen like mycobacteria. IFNγ "knockout" mice that are not capable of producing NO and RNI in response to tubercle bacilli, experience a fulminant course of tuberculosis suggesting the role of NO and RNI in the defense mechanism against *M. tuberculosis*. There is evidence that the production of NO and related RNI is well correlated with antimycobacterial effect of murine macrophages. There is, however, few report on the antimycobacterial effect of human macrophages and its correlation with the production of cytokines and NO.[6]

It was found that the peripheral T-lymphocyte CD4 subset count is low in the patients with extrapulmonary tuberculosis.[10-15] Therefore, it is important to know the patient's immune state in the aged and HIV/AIDS patients, and drug abusers, because the immunosuppression is closely linked with the infection (Fig. 35.1).[6,10,16-23]

Humoral immunity requires proper functioning, quantity of complement proteins and immunoglobulins in addition to antigen presentation cells (APC),[22] while cellular immunity is delivered by the direct action of B and T lymphocytes and antigen phagocytes, such as macrophages.[23]

To evaluate the patients' pretherapy physical conditions, the predisposing factors of skeletal tuberculosis as first step measure should be searched: elderly people, malnutrition, agammaglobulinemia, Mannose-binding lactin (MBL) deficiency, diabetes mellitus, HIV infection, malignancy, renal failure, substance abuse, long-term use of anti-rheumatic agents (steroids, anti-TNF-α blockers and B-cell depleting therapeutic agents, methotrexate), and anticancer chemotherapeutic agents.[21-23] Because tuberculosis is a potentially fatal complication of immunosuppressive therapy.

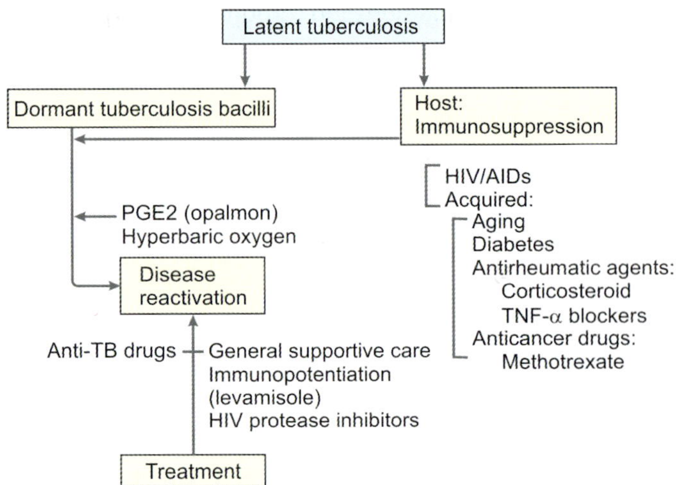

Fig. 35.1 Causes of reactivation of latent tuberculosis and management

Immunity in tuberculosis being a purely cell-mediated defense lymphoproliferative response to antigen or mitogen stimulation has been widely used as *in vitro* correlate of cell-mediated immunity. T-cell-mediated cellular immunity particularly has been suggested as an important factor in mycobacterial infection. Also, it is known that there is an imbalance between helper (H) and suppressor (S) T cells in the pathogenesis of tuberculosis in human. H/S ratio in extrapulmonary tuberculosis is lower than that in pulmonary tuberculosis (1.06 ± 0.44 vs 1.64 ± 0.92).[5]

Immune systems in the elderly patients are generally weakened.[16,19] Therefore, reactivation of the latent tuberculosis is often reported.

In malnourished state immune depression is found at the humoral and cellular levels, and is characterized by altered chemotaxis and phagocytosis, decreased serum albumin levels (<3.5 g/dL) and decreased total lymphocyte counts (<1500–2000 cells/mm^3). Protein malnutrition results in a decreased numbers of circulating T-cells with impaired production of cytokines.[15-17] HIV positive patients' nutritional state in the late stage of the disease becomes worse because of the uncontrollable diarrhea.[5,17,18]

Immune system compromise in diabetic patient has been associated with defects in humoral and cellular immune response. Humoral defects include deficits in complement protein C3 and C4, C1 inhibitor, and alterations in antibody production in reponse to antigen. Cellular deficits have a more complex mechanism and involve alterations in cytokine signaling through TNF, IL-1β, IL-2, IL-6, IL-8, IGF-2, and direct effects on T-cells and their relative populations.[22-24]

HIV/AIDS predispose patients to tuberculous and fungal infections because of defects in the neutrophils, a decrease in cell counts and leukocyte dysfunction. Tuberculous infection when CD4+ lymphocyte (helper-inducer T-cell) counts fall below 200 cells/mm^3, and MAC infection when CD4+ lymphocyte counts fall below 100 cells/mm^3.[2,20,21]

Antirheumatic agents (corticosteroids, methotrexate, anti-TNF-α blockers and chemotherapeutic agents) exert their effects through humoral and cellular levels of immune system and marrow suppression. TNF-α blockers inhibit lymphocyte and macrophage activity.[5,6,18]

Clinical Manifestations

Even at its active stage of the disease symptoms are often insidious. Common symptoms are malaise, loss of appetite, weight loss, and night sweat. The involved spine is stiff and painful on movement with localized hump-back. Back muscle spasms are present. Occasionally patients may have night cries during sleep, because the relaxation of the muscle spasm allows for movement between the inflamed surfaces. Cold abscess and/or sinus may be present. However, during the early stage some of these symptoms and signs may be absent. On palpation a small gibbus may be detected. Rarely neurological deficits may present as the first symptom.

Diagnosis

With the increasing incidence of tuberculosis of all types throughout the world, physicians and surgeons must exercise a high index of suspicion to achieve early diagnosis.

The insidious onset, the lack of early constitutional symptoms and local signs of spinal tuberculosis militate against early diagnosis. Particularly immunosuppressed patients tend to have longer delays to presentation and diagnosis which are almost universal because of less vigorous inflammation and pain generation.[5]

Clinicians typically rely on a battery of means in diagnosing spinal tuberculosis. These include observation and investigation of clinical signs and symptoms, the use of various imaging techniques, smear and/or culture, metabolic product detection (interferon γ test), polymerase chain reaction (PCR) and histological study. Diagnosis may take days to weeks, and involves expensive, invasive and complex procedures.[1,2,4,5]

There is currently no single diagnostic method that can detect all tuberculosis cases.

Tuberculin Skin Test

Tuberculin skin test (TST) has inherent limitations of sensitivity and specificity. Even in high tuberculosis-burden areas abut 20% of individuals are negative to TST throughout life despite the repeated exposure to the tubercle bacilli. Additionally, the sensitivity decreases in immunocompromised patients for whom accurate diagnosis of latent tuberculosis is essential. In terms of specificity, TST is influenced by BCG vaccination and nontuberculous mycobacterial infection.[2,5]

Imaging

Imaging techniques such as simple radiographs, CT, bone scan, and MRI are useful, but not diagnostic. When disk and/or end-plate destruction with surrounding soft tissue swelling is observed on simple radiographs, spine infection should be suspected.

Diffusion-weighted MRI has been found to have limited usefulness for differentiating spinal infection and malignancy.

Laboratory Test

Laboratory aids to diagnosis include complete blood counts, including total lymphocytes and CD4 lymphocyte (helper-inducer T-cell) counts, ESR and CRP, smear and/or culture, histology, detection of specific antigen, metabolic products, patient's antibody response and detection of antibody to *M. tuberculosis*, and DNA sequence polymerase-chain reaction (PCR) of *M. tuberculosis*.[4,5,10,18,21-23]

The diagnostic gold standard has traditionally been the isolation of *M. tuberculosis* by smear and/or culture from clinical samples, such as aspirates (needle or trochar) and tissue specimens (open or percutaneous biopsy), and the typical histology. However, the tubercle bacilli is difficult to culture due to its fastidious growth requirements and slow rate of replication. Hence there are the needs for the development of various laboratory methods.

There are three diagnostic non-culture laboratory tests: (i) immunological tests (antigen and antibody), (ii) metabolic product detection, such as extracorporeal interferon-γ test, and (3) amplification of DNA of *M. tuberculosis* by PCR.[23]

The AMRAD ICT tuberculosis test (an *in vitro* immunological tool for the detection of antibodies to M. tuberculosis in white blood cells) reliably detects tuberculosis in whole blood, enabling rapid and accurate diagnosis at the point of care.[2,5]

When T-lymphocytes are exposed to tubercle bacilli, lymphocytes secrete interferon-γ making extracorporeal interferon γ test particularly for latent tuberculosis noteworthy. Two *ex-vivo* interferon-γ (IFN-γ) assay kits have been marketed; Quanti-FERON* TB Gold [Cellestis limited, Carnegie Victoria, Australia, QFT-G] and T-SPOT, TB [Oxford Immunotec, Oxford, UK, T-SPOT].[2,5] The former uses the ELISA technique and T-SPOT uses enzyme-linked immunosorbent spot (ELISPOT) technique. Both use *M. tuberculosis*-specific antigens, ESAT-6 and CFP-10 as stimulants. As BCG does not contain ESAT-6 and CFP-10, these assays are more specific than TST in the diagnosis of tuberculosis infection. They have variable sensitivity, dependent on host factors and methods used. There are reports that T-SPOT is more sensitive than TST in immunocompromised subjects.

These assays detect tuberculosis infection, but they cannot differentiate between latent tuberculosis from active tuberculosis. Therefore, when the TST and IFN-γ assay results are positive, differentiation of latent infection and active tuberculosis should be carried out on the basis of the clinical history, chest and skeletal imaging, and tissue studies.

The other major nonculture test is the molecular diagnostic test, PCR, which amplifies the DNA of *M. tuberculosis* that provides results within hours. This allows effective and prompt treatment, which in turn, improves prognosis. A primer pair targeting a 123 base pair (bp) segment of the repetitive sequence IS6110 of the *M. tuberculosis* complex is used, and it covers *M. tuberculosis*, *M. africanum*, *M. bovis*, *M. canetti* and *M. microti*. This technique represents an exciting development. It has been used as a marker to monitor response to treatment, and has been shown to provide rapid information on drug resistance and clonality in epidemiological investigation of outbreaks.

Accurate diagnosis should be made at initial presentation to ensure proper treatment.

Classification Based on Staging of Tuberculosis

Disease staging must be practical for the management (Table 35.1). There are no universally accepted staging system, though several staging systems were introduced. Kumar,[7] Moon,[5] Metha and Bhojraj[24] and Oguz et al.[25] proposed their therapeutic classification of the spinal tuberculosis based on the clinical stage of the disease processes. However, they could not satisfy the clinicians in selection of the most appropriate management of the tuberculous lesions of any spinal levels. Because they paid attention only on the aesthetic view points and neurologic state, and did not pay attention on the effect of residual sagittal spinal deformity upon the remaining mobile segments, including the parafusion segments. Thus terms, early and late; early, moderate and advanced; kyphotic and non-kyphotic; and stages I–III have been used in staging the disease. Also vertebral body loss was expressed as percentage and severity of the deformity (Table 35.1). A satisfactory staging system is still awaited.

Table 35.1 Staging of spinal tuberculosis (Moon, 1992)

Disease progress (disease advancement (stages))	*Size of lesion (degree of body destructive loss)*	*Deformity (degree of kyphosis)*
Stage I : minimally (very early)	<20% (2/10)	≤12.2°
Stage II : early	26–50%	12.2–22.25°
Stage III : relatively (moderately)	51–100%	22.26–39.0°
Stage IV : far advanced	101–200%	39.1–72.5°

Note: percentage and degree of kyphosis in cases of conservative treatment is calculated by Rajasekaran's formula (Y=5.5° + 30.5° × degree of body destruction).[11,37]

Management

The treatment goals are primarily not only to save life through eradication of infection, and secondly to provide stability for the affected spine, to meet the patient's aesthetic demand through prevention and/or correction of the spinal deformities, but also to prevent and/or treat paralysis and to reduce the parafusion segment disease. The ideal management would be the one that meets all these goals.

Management decision must be based on the different treatment goals of individual patient.

The management of spinal tuberculosis consists of supportive care, chemotherapy and surgery. Surgical measures include cold abscess drainage, focal debridement of the lesion and/or anterior fusion surgery,[26] decompression surgery, including costotransversectomy, two-stage procedure of posterior instrumentation, and anterior radical surgery,[27] a combined procedure of anterior radical surgery and anterior instrumentation,[28,29] and corrective spinal

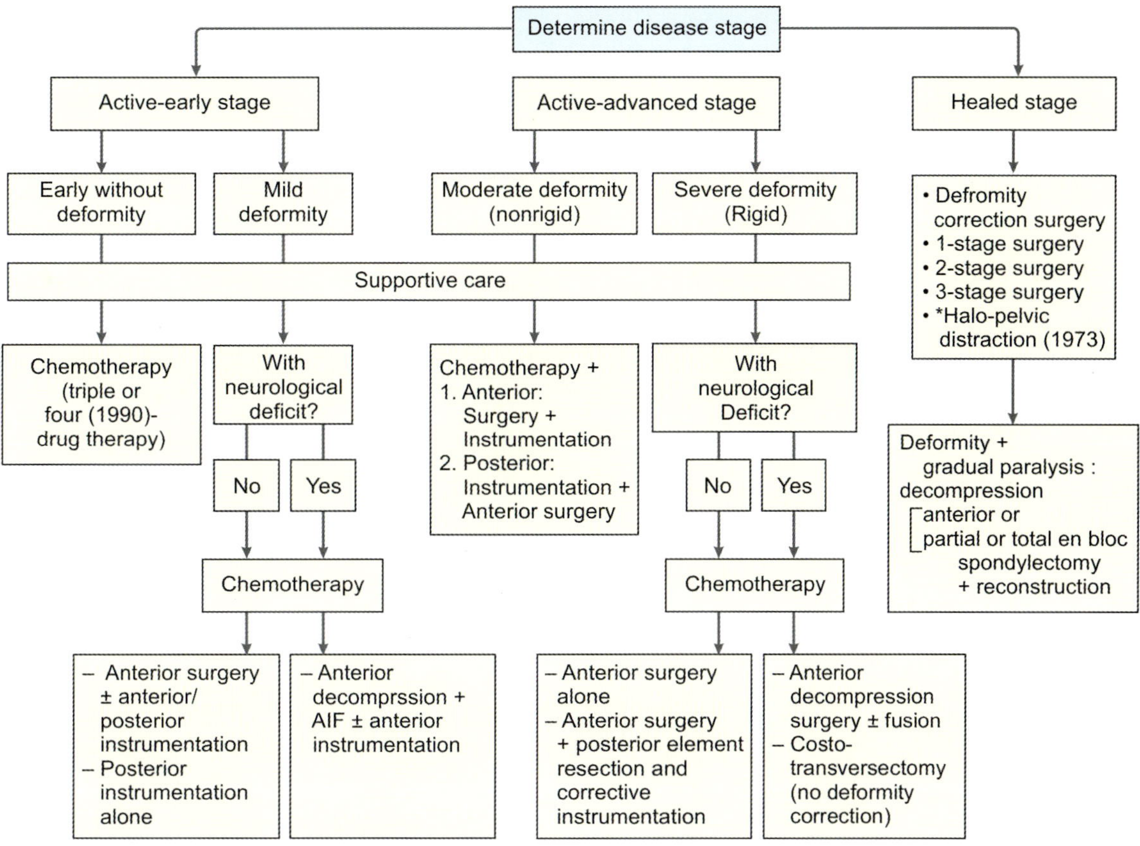

Fig. 35.2 Treatment algorithm for spinal tuberculosis

osteotomy or spondylectomy for healed rigid kyphosis (Fig. 35.2).[2,5] However, without antituberculous chemotherapy surgery alone cannot cure the active disease. Although the final fusion of the affected vertebral segment is an important part of the treatment, it does not necessarily accompany the spontaneous healing process.[29,30]

Recently, the current authors found an important fact that spinal malalignment of the fused segment at the time of the disease cure in adults is a contributing factor in increasing the incidence of parafusion segment disease.[5,30] Therefore, maintenance and/or restoration of normal spinal alignment at the time of the disease cure is strongly recommended.

Myobacterium tuberculosis and its Behavioral Characteristics

Good understanding of the nature of *M. tuberculosis* is vital before initiation of any treatment. Knowledge about the bacterial growth and its response to chemotherapy and biomaterial implants is important.[31,32] Bony tuberculosis has a low bacillary load (i.e. less population). *M. tuberculosis* presents in free floating (planktonic) form, and not in sessile form as seen in pyogenic bacteria. It produces minimal adhesion molecules and slime, and occasionally becomes dormant. Because of the relatively slow replication rate of *M. tuberculosis*, antituberculous chemotherapy given intermittently is as effective as given daily.[1,2,5]

There was a concern that the use of the biomaterials (titanium cage, screws and rods, PVP and stainless steel or ceramic cups) in the tuberculous lesions would hinder the healing of the tuberculosis, or that its use would cause the arrested or quiescent infection to flare up until harmlessness of implants were proven.[34-38] Also, it was found that bacteria adhere less to titanium than stainless steel, because titanium has a less electrochemically active oxide surface compared to stainless steel which has a higher surface free energy (>40 mN/m) and hence more available ligands for binding with cells both bacterial and tissue competing for the biomaterial surface.[30-34] Additionally, to prevent the bacterial adherence to implants surfaces, the implant surfaces were specially treated by polishing and/or cross-linked albumin coating.[33] It follows that stainless steel implants should not be used for spinal stabilization, because it has less resistibility to bacterial adhesion and infections.

In summary, *M. tuberculosis* has little tendency to adhere to implants that the implants can be safely used in tuberculous lesions. However, in HIV positive patients the use of biomaterials in the infected foci is inappropriate, because they are susceptible to a variety of other opportunistic infections.[5, 18,19]

Nutritional Therapy

Hyperalimentation is necessary to recover patients from a physically debilitated pretherapy state to their premorbid nutritional status. The goal should be to achieve a serum albumin level >3 g/dL. An absolute lymphocyte count >800/mm^3, and a 24-hour urine creatinine excretion > 10.5 mg in men and >5.8 mg in women should be restored or maintained.[5,7]

Chemotherapy

When a patient presents early with minimal to moderate bone involvement that does not seem to cause noticeable deformity, conservative chemotherapy alone is indicated. Chemotherapy can be given on an ambulatory basis without bracing.[35,36] Effective institution of chemotherapy and good general supportive care at an early stage of disease are the key to early eradication and minimal sequelae. The advantages and disadvantages of conservative treatment alone are given in Table 35.2.

Studies have shown that conservative treatment at an early stage is beneficial in preventing residual kyphosis.[12] Proper selection of patient for conservative treatment in adults has been used to be based on the predictive residual kyphosis.[11,37]

As yet, there is no standard antituberculosis chemotherapy regimen, though several formulae have been proposed (Tables 35.3 to 35.6). Some clinicians support the use of a 9-month short-term triple chemotherapy,[5,38-41] while others advocate of three-or four-drug regimens for 12 months even for good responders.[2,5,41,42] However, for the slow or doubtful responders chemotherapy for 12–18 months has been prescribed before reformulation.[1,2,4,5] Table 35.4 shows the recommended doses of various chemotherapy agents. First-line chemotherapy for *M. tuberculosis* should include a combination of isoniazid, rifampin, pyrazinamide, and either ethambutol or streptomycin (Table 35.3). Susceptibility testing should be conducted in all isolates, and the regimen adjusted accordingly to include at least two agents the isolate is sensitive to.

For the hepato- and nephropathy patients, the administering dosages of each drug should be adjusted according to the liver and renal function.

Table 35.2 Advantages and disadvantages of chemotherapy alone

Advantages	*Disadvantages*
• Cures tuberculosis effectively • Can be done on an ambulatory basis • Cost-effective • Spontaneous growth correction of the deformed spine in children • Avoids surgical complications and residuals	• Cannot shorten the duration of chemotherapy • Longer time to cure the disease • Cannot always meet esthetic demands • Delayed neurological recovery

Table 35.3 First and second line antituberculous drugs

First-line agents	*Second-line agents*
Isoniazid (H) Rifampicin (rifampin) (R) Pyrazinamide (Z) Ethambutol (E)	Amikacin (AMK) Capreomycin (CPM) Ciprofloxacin Cycloserine (CS) Ethionamide Kanamycin (K) Ofloxacin P-Aminosalicylic acid (PAS) Streptomycin (S) Rifabutin (Rif) } for MAC Clarithromycin (Cla) } for MAC

Table 35.4 Recommended doses for the treatment of tuberculosis

Drug	*Daily dose in mg/kg (maximum dose)*	
	*Children**	*Adults†*
Isoniazid	10–20 (300 mg)	5 (300 mg)
Rifampin	10–20 (600 mg)	19 (600 mg)
Pyrazinamide	15–30 (2 g)	15–30 (2 g)
Ethambutol	15–25	15–25 (1.5 g)
Streptomycin	20–40 (1 g)	15 (1 g)

*Under the age of 12 years.
†Maximum dose depends on body weight

Table 35.5 Antituberculous "standard regimens"

Three-drug regimen

- Davies PC (1996): 2 HRZ 10 HR (12 months)
  - * Drug resistance case: 2S(E) HRZ
- Moon et al. (1987, 1995, 1997, 2004): 12 RHE(Z) (12 months)
- Upadhyay et al. (1999): AIF
  - 3 HPaS, 3HPa (6 months)
  - 3 HPaS 6HPa (9 months)

Four drug regimens:

- Yilmaz C et al. (1999): 2SRHZ 7RH (9 months)
- Metha IS et al. (2001): 2RHEZ 4RHE 6RH (12 months)
- Govender and Kumor (2003): 12 RHZE (12 months)
- Hassan (2003): 12 RHE (at least) (12 months)
- Sundaranaj et al. (2003): 4RHEZ, 14RHE (18 months)

H, INH; R, rifampin; Z, pyrazinamide; E, ethambutol; Pa, PAS; S, streptomycin

Table 35.6 Suggested regimens for the drug-resistant cases

Resistant drug	*Suggested regimen*	*Duration of Therapy*	*Comments*
INH, SM, PZA	RMP, PZA, EMB, AMK	6–9 months	Estimated 100% response rate and <5% relapse rate
INH, EMB (±SM)	RMP, PZA, OFL/CIP, AMK	6–9 months	Efficacy should be comparable to the above regimen
INH, RMP (±SM)	PZA, EMB, OFL/CIP, AMK	18–24 months	Consider surgery
INH, RMP, EMB (±SM)	PZA, OFL/CIP, AMK, plus 2	24 months after conversion	Consider surgery
INH, RMP, PZA (±SM)	EMB, OFL/CIP, AMK, plus 2	24 months after conversion	Consider surgery
INH, RMP, PZA, EMB (±SM)	OFL/CIP, AMK, plus 3	24 months after conversion	Surgery, if possible

INH, isoniazid; SM, streptomycin; PZA, pyrazinamide; EMB, ethambutol; RMP, rifampin; AMK, amikacin; OFL, ofloxacin; CIP, ciprofloxacin

Nonsteroidal anti-inflammatory drugs may be useful in early disease to prevent lesions caused by nonspecific synovial inflammation, and to inhibit or minimize bone resorption caused by prostaglandin-mediated inflammation.[1,2,5,12]

Atypical organisms such as MAC and *M. kansasii* may require additional antibiotics. For the treatment of MAC, a three drug regimen including rifabutin, ethambutol and clarithromycin is the regimen of choice. Multiple-drug therapy is more effective than monotherapy for the treatment of disseminated MAC. Regimens targeting MAC are suppressive rather than curative, thus therapy must be continued indefinitely (Table 35.3).[2,5]

For HIV-negative patients, treatment should be started with at least three agents (isoniazid, rifampicin, pyrazinamide) or, if resistance is suspected, four (the above plus ethambutol) or more (Table 35.6). Despite the diminished cell-mediated immunity, HIV-infected patients usually respond well to standard antituberculous chemotherapy, provided that it is commenced promptly when the patient has compliant, and the organism is not resistant.

Isoniazid chemoprophylaxis is recommended for a HIV-infected individuals with a positive tuberculin skin test, and for those with a history of exposure to an individual with active tuberculosis regardless of tuberculin skin test results.[5]

There are no clear-cut definitions of good (or rapid) and poor (or slow) responses, and nonresponse. The recommended observation period for drug response was differently set between nonparalytics and paralytics: in the nonparalytics a 6-to 8-week assessment (maximum 3 months) is recommended, whereas the assessment for the paralytics is used to be taken at 3–4 weeks after chemotherapy. However, labeling the patient as nonresponder on the basis of an arbitrarily designed assessment guideline may not be justified. That is, exact timing of drug response assessment in patients with or without neurologic deficit remains a matter of debate. The current authors' view is that those different criteria of drug response assessment is rather arbitrary. Our view in interpretation of the different time setting in nonparalytic and paralytic patients is based on the fact that more clinical significance is given to neural condition than the non-neural complications. Because paralysis lasted over a month neurological recovery was less favorable than the one recovered within a months. Also, it is our view that the accurate assessment of the disease activity affected by drugs, is difficult by postchemotherapy 3 months at minimum.[1,5]

Table 35.6 gives recommends for managing resistant tuberculosis. The authors suggest that treatment should last at least 12 months, although others consider chemotherapy of 9 months sufficient to achieve a positive result, and do not recommend long-term suppressive therapy after 9 months of chemotherapy.[36-42]

For rheumatoid arthritis and related disease patients with latent tuberculous infection, antirheumatic agents such as anti-TNF-α treatment should be started at least after 3 weeks of anti-tuberculous chemotherapy, and for rheumatoid patients with active tuberculosis TNF-α agent therapy should be started at least after 2 months of anti-tuberculous chemotherapy.[2,5]

As most of tuberculosis cases after biologic therapy represent reactivation rather than new onset infection, screening before TNF-α blocker therapy is critical to prevent such relapse. However, it is a costly process. It is reminded that if postoperative rigor or fever develops during anti-TNF-α therapy other bacterial infection must be excluded.[5]

The failure of medical treatment is defined in spite of directly observed therapy (DOT), when there is progression of the neurological deficit, lack of improvement of the inflammatory markers after 6–8 weeks of the adequate chemotherapy, and progressive spinal deformity in the following X-rays.[5]

Surgical Treatment

Chemotherapy alone cannot solve the problems arising from bone and joint destruction. Therefore, despite the availability of effective conservative treatments,[42]

surgical procedures still assume an important role in the management of spinal tuberculosis.

Surgery is indicated only for the disease-related complications such as segmental instability, deformity and neurological deficit. To treat the disease and the disease-related complications, the various surgical procedures have been developed and practised with great success. However, the goal of the surgery is only one: the cure of the disease without residual. For each condition, more safe, effective and easy-to-learn procedure have to be selected to meet the each patient's need.[5] It is our view that surgery only for the advanced cases with the severe deformity should be a thing of the past. Therefore, the residuals, such as deformity, neurological deficit, deformity-related late adjacent joint disease must be minimized by our every effort.

Four conditions of spinal tuberculosis, namely cold abscess, tuberculous lesion, paraplegia, and spinal deformity can be managed by various surgical procedures when indicated.

A new classification and guideline for surgical treatment was presented by Oguz et al., which did not deal with the posterior element tuberculosis.[25] Their therapeutic guideline could not meet all the clinicians' complaints. They did not consider the long term outcome related with the patients' aesthetic demands, the adjacent segment disease, the compensatory hyperlordosis over and below the residual kyphotic segment, and also those in children.

The advantages of surgical treatment are given in Table 35.7. Acceptable degree of residual kyphosis is also a topic of great controversy related with aesthetic and biomechanical aspect.

Hither to deformity prevention and/or correction have been based on the predictive value of residual kyphosis.[11,37] The value can be calculated using the following formula: Final kyphosis = 5.5° + 30.5° × degree of vertebral body destruction in 10 grades (0.1–1.0).[11] Its percentile predictive value was initially reported by Rajasekaran et al. to be around 90%[11], while its value assessed by Jain et al. was around 78%.[37] The authors' view was that the discrepancy was caused by the inaccurate estimation of the initial vertebral body loss. Because perfect estimation of the vertebral body loss at prechemotherapy is impossible. The numerical discrepancy of the final kyphosis can reach 6.1° (30.5° x 0.2) because of 10% over- or underestimation of the vertebral body destruction.

Table 35.7 Advantages of surgical treatment

- Early cure by extirpation of the infected focus
- Histological confirmation of diagnosis-active or healed
- Shortening the duration of chemotherapy
- Reduces late-recurrence rates
- Correction and/or prevention of deformity
- Early effective neurological recovery
- Patient satisfaction for esthetic demands through deformity prevention and/or correction

Abscess Drainage

In most cases small and medium-size cold abscesses rapidly resolve spontaneously with chemotherapy alone. In the authors' series, evacuation of abscesses (needle, trochar or open incisional drainage) did not alter patients' general condition, and very often it would result in a draining sinus from which drainage persists for some time. Therefore, surgical drainage is not recommended as a routine practice even for large abscesses. However, as an exception emergency decompression drainage should be carried out for the sudden onset worsening respiratory difficulty by the huge prevertebral cervical abscess compressing the trachea and cord compression above C4.[5,30]

Focal Debridement

Focal debridement is rarely indicated nowadays, because evidence suggests it does not improve healing nor prevent the progressive kyphosis.[29] Radical extirpation of the infected focus may also damage the remaining growth plates in children.[1,2,5,41] Although the procedure is simple, it carries small risks, such as dura tear, cord injury, and injury to nerve roots and autonomous and peripheral nerves.

Anterior Radical Surgery

Bone grafting after anterior radical debridement is safe in the treatment of spinal tuberculosis, even when drainage is present. Anterior radical surgery was once advocated as the treatment of choice for spinal tuberculosis.[25,38] However, it became clear later that the only advantage of anterior fusion is a certain extent of deformity correction and a decreased tendency for deformity progression in adults. The authors' experience suggests that the procedure is not always successful because of frequent graft failure in preventing kyphosis progression and/or correcting pre-existing kyphosis particularly in fusion spanning over two motion segments.

Literature on the treatment of tuberculous kyphoscoliosis and scoliosis is scarce. With non-instrumented anterior radical surgery alone, even nonrigid deformities are difficult to correct, and the corrections, if any, are difficult to be maintained. In rigid deformities, this is even more challenging and the complication rate is relatively high. When anterior surgery is used to treat nonrigid pure tuberculous scoliosis, some overcorrection is recommended to balance the loss of correction during the fusion process. However, if any loss of correction in those overcorrected cases will not occur through some graft absorption or sagging during healing, subsequently iatrogenic scoliosis to the opposite direction can occur. When this type of excessive iatrogenic scoliotic deformity occurs at L4–5 as a result of a rhomboid graft, compensatory pelvic tilt and apparent leg shortening may result.[5] Therefore, utmost care should be taken to avoid inducing excessive coronal deformity iatrogenically by the anterior intercorporal graft. If corrective surgery is indicated in tuberculous scoliosis, combined procedures such as posterior or anterior instrument-aided stabilization is recommended after anterior corrective surgery.[5] It is reminded that spontaneous fusion of adjacent segment happens infrequently after anterior cervical fusion surgery in children.

Cord injury can occur during anterior radical surgery, though the incidence is very low. In two out of 764 anterior procedures in the authors' unit cord was bruised by the misplaced strut graft into the spinal canal. Utmost attention should be paid in placing the graft(s) between the vertebral bodies.[5]

Stabilizing Instrumentation

Corrective and/or stabilizing spinal surgery is most effective in active progressive kyphosis and nonrigid kyphosis.[42-44] However, posterior instrumentation surgery is not recommended in early tuberculosis, because the disease can be cured with conservative chemotherapy alone without significant residual kyphosis.

For kyphosis due to anterior column destruction, posterior instrument-aided correction and stabilization will produce a bone gap in the anterior column, if the posterior column shortening is not combined. This anterior gap should be reconstructed by anterior strut graft surgery. Otherwise, the instrumented spine results in corporal re-collapse and/or instrumentation failure.[5,42-44]

In children with tuberculosis involving both anterior and posterior elements, the affected segment becomes unstable, causing spinal deformity and an increased risk of paraplegia. Prophylactic stabilization particularly in children should be performed if translational instability is suspected at the level of the lesion.[1,2,5,58]

Anterior Radical Surgery and Anterior Instrumentation

Controversies exist regarding the use of biomaterial in the infected focus to reconstruct the gap and/or immobilize the diseased segment(s) internally. Generally, implantation of biomaterial in the infected focus is contraindicated, because the biomaterial may serve as nest for pyogenic bacteria. Bacteria normally produce adhesion molecules to adhere to and survive on the pits of the synthetic surface. However, this is not the case in bone tuberculosis. *M. tuberculosis* divides very slowly with minimal slime production and exists only in a planktonic form, which responds well to chemotherapy. This is thought to be the reason why the fixation or reconstruction biomaterial in the tuberculous focus would not cause biomaterial-centered infections. The use of anterior instrumentation in skeletal tuberculosis is therefore acceptable: it provides effective mechanical stability without hindering the healing process until the disease cure.[1,2,5,44,45,50-54] However, the anterior rods or plate should be well contoured to meet the spinal sagittal alignment, particularly in multisegment long stabilization. Endoscopic instrumentation surgery for the thoracic lesion also has been practiced by some.

Posterior Instrumentation and Anterior Radical Surgery

The authors' clinical experience suggests it is unwise to rely solely on the anterior strut graft to correct the spinal deformity and to maintain the correction without graft collapse. In view of this, since 1981 the senior author (MSM) sought and adopted the combined two-stage procedure–a method of treatment that could prevent major spinal deformity.[1,2,4,5,8,44-49]

Patients presenting late with extensive, multisegment tuberculosis with kyphosis involving more than two vertebral bodies are suitable candidates for the two-stage procedure; posterior corrective and stabilizing instrumentation surgery together with anterior radical surgery under the cover of chemotherapy. Corrective and stabilizing spinal surgery is most effective in active disease with nonrigid spinal deformity.[1,2,4,5,65,66]

Instrument-aided multisegment posterior stabilization of the spine using long rods is more reliable in correcting and stabilizing the flexible spinal deformity without graft failure. Posterior instrument-aided stabilization has several advantages, which include arresting the disease early and bringing about early fusion, correcting the deformity and maintaining the corrected alignment.

With the combined two-stage procedure, the collapsed vertebra can regain its height. Also, the width and/or the extent of anterior interbody fusion can be minimized (Fig. 35.3), and the adjacent unaffected segments can be preserved. The remaining vertebral bodies of the diseased vertebra can be used as graft beds (Fig. 35.4). No graft fracture or absorption has been observed in the authors' series. Furthermore, the procedure can shorten the postoperative bed-rest period.[44]

Multisegment spinal instrumentation immobilizes also the normal mobile segments, and may later cause these segments to be stiffened and degenerated. Therefore, the

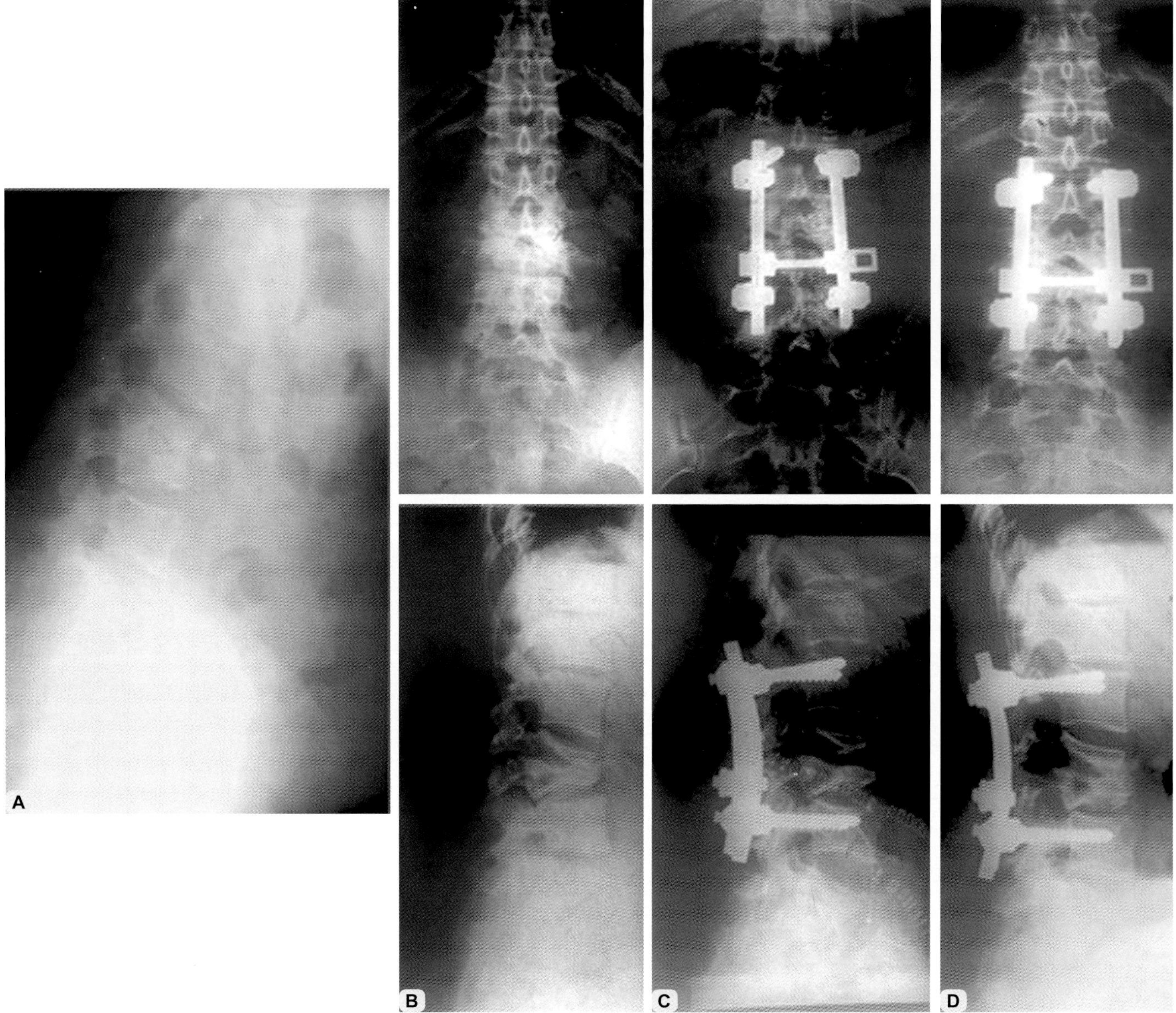

Fig. 35.3 An example of tuberculosis of L3–4 for which short segment posterior instrumentation and anterior interbody fusion between L2 and L5 were performed. (A and B) initial (A) and preoperative (B) radiograms in which progress of kyphosis is seen; (C) After anterior interbody fusion; (D) Final radiograms showing the consolidated a block vertebrae of L3–4

current authors normally remove the rods and screws after solid intercorporal fusion at about 9 months postoperation to remobilize these unaffected fixed segments.

In children, care should be taken not to damage the remaining growth plate during the anterior curettage surgery, and combined posterior instrumentation with or without posterior fusion is recommended to prevent and/or correct kyphosis.[2,5,27,44,48,49]

In summary, the introduced surgical correction procedures up to now for the active spinal tuberculosis with kyphosis are single stage extrapleural anterolateral approach, two-stage anterior and posterior approaches with instrumentation, instrumentation after anterior corpectomy and posterior column shortening, and one stage transpedicular excision, reconstruction and instrumentation.[48,49]

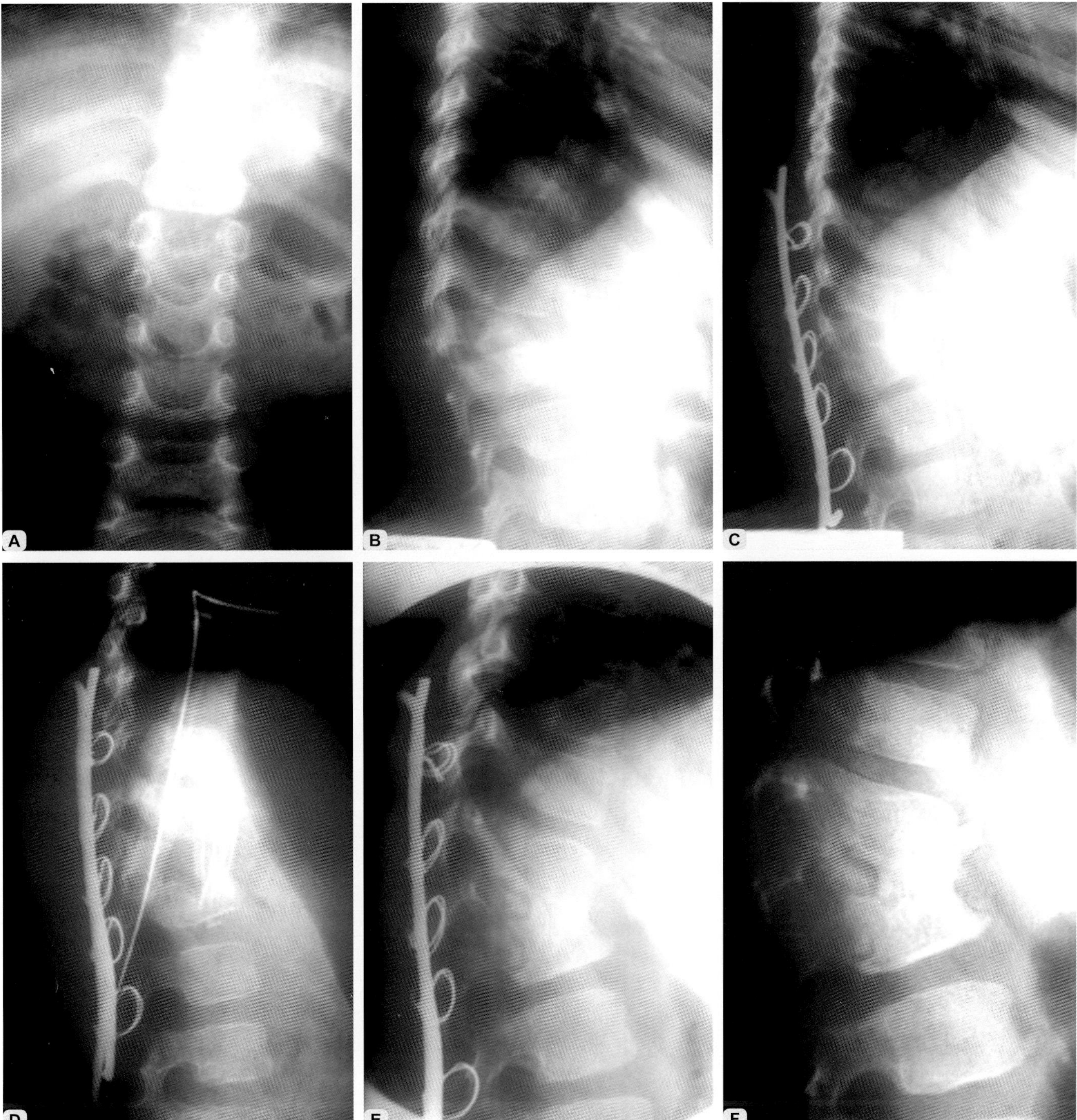

Fig. 35.4 Preoperative radiographs. (A) Anteroposterior view; (B) Lateral view of a 6-year-old boy showing L1 tuberculosis with kyphosis involving neighboring disks; (C) Lateral radiogram immediately after posterior rodding showing a fair amount of correction of kyphosis; (D) Radiograph of immediate postoperative anterior interbody fusion showing three rib grafts, one of which is out of the graft bed; (E) Six-month postoperative radiographs showing good maintenance of corrected kyphosis, although there is some loss of correction; (F) Radiographs 1 year, 3 months after surgery showing complete consolidation of the fused segment, with some natural correction of the kyphosis

Corrective Surgical Procedures for Severe Rigid Kyphosis

In the past, corrective surgery was not recommended for the healed severe kyphotic or kyphoscoliotic spine with normal neurology because of high neurological complication rates, particularly above T11, if it was only for cosmetic reasons. The combined surgery-instrument-aided posterior corrective and stabilizing surgery with anterior reconstruction—is most effective in the management of the active progressive kyphosis and established residual nonrigid kyphosis.[5,31,46,47,50-54]

Recently nonparalytic young patients with severe rigid kyphosis tend to have very high aesthetic demands. This has led to the development of safe and effective corrective surgical procedures for the unsightly kyphosis, but each patient must be considered individually[5] (Fig. 35.5).

In the healed severe tuberculous kyphosis at cord level, the bony anatomy is severely deforme and the cord in this area is ischemic, deformed and less mobile. It is often trapped in the deformed, narrow, hypoplastic canal and is adherent to the dura.[5,52]

There are several possible surgical procedures, ranging from signle-stage to multistage procedures for rigid kyphosis including posterior closing wedge osteotomy, decancellation procedure, and hemi or total spondylectomy as a single stage operative procedure.[1,2,5,45,46]

Recently, some authors reported that the combined procedures of anterior corpectomy, posterior column shortening and posterior instrumentation for the Pott's paraplegics with severe kyphosis brought the favorable results.[5,45-49,52,54]

Long segment stabilization and fusion have been known to be essential in this severe rigid deformity correction surgery. However, it can cause the adjacent joint disease later in life in adults for which none in the past paid attention. So care should be paid for this issue.[5]

Any decision to operate must weigh the high complication and reoperation rates against anticipated improvement. Therefore, an informed consent discussion should include the patient and his or her support group. Risks and complications must be fully understood, and the patient will ultimately choose between those risks and his/her quality of life. The surgeon should offer options and probability, but it is the patient who must bear the consequences of that decision.

The current authors' latest recommendation is to utilize the real-size spinal model to get excellent understanding of the complex spinal pathology in highly selected patient. These models allow complex spinal surgery with or more predictable outcome. By using those models more accurate osteotomy and accurate screwing can be done.[52,53]

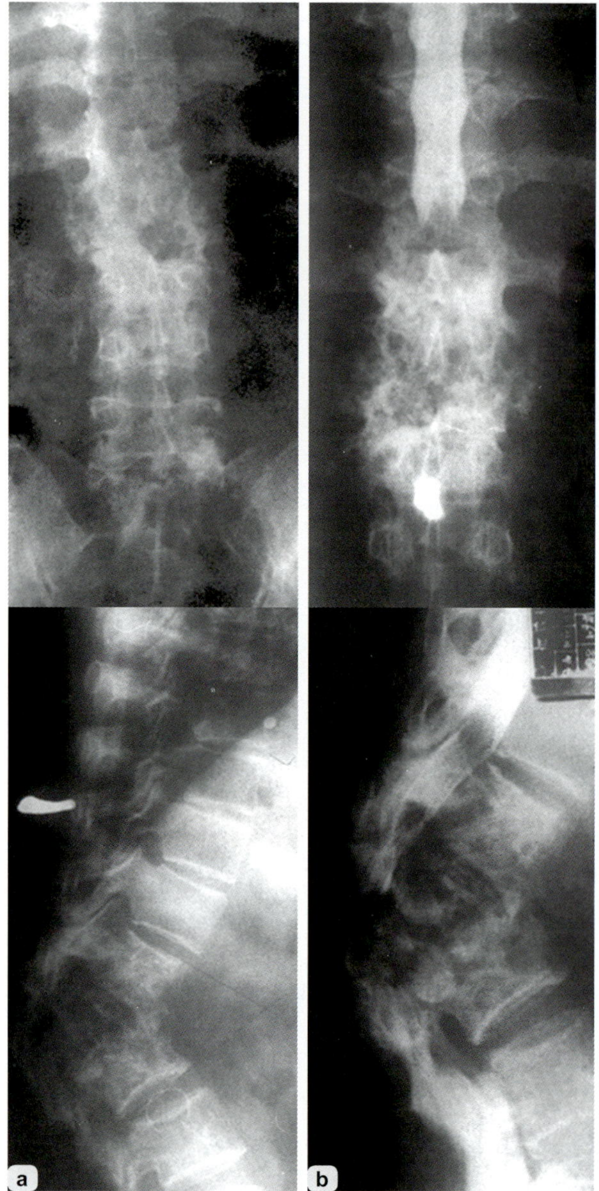

Figs 35.5A Two preoperative radiograms [(a) simple; (b) myelogram)] in a 47 year-old paraparetic woman with tuberculous kyphosis of T12–L2 illustrate 60° of the initial kyphosis. Myelograms show the obliterated spinal canal from T10 level below

Spinal Column Shortening

The ideal size of the longitudinal spondylectomy in the correction of the spinal deformity in relation with the cord function has rarely been discussed, and there is no consensus view in human. In the normal spine, cord length, spinal canal and anterior spinal column length are equal, while in the idiopathic adolescent scoliosis the anterior column is longer than the canal, cord and posterior column. Therefore,

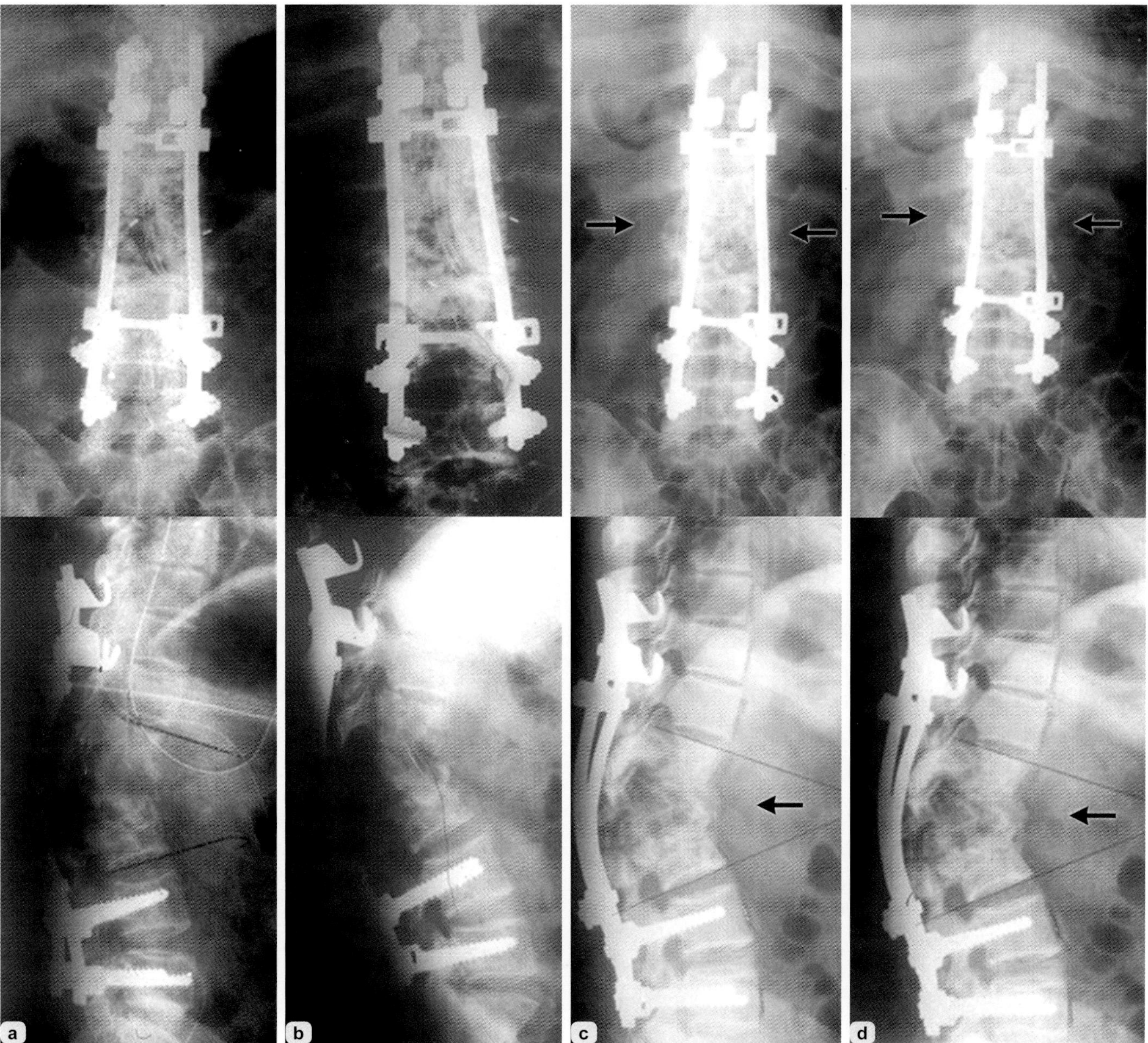

Fig. 35.5B Serial radiograms at postoperative (a) zero month (b) 3 months, (c) 6 months, and (d) 18 months, show 30°, 42°, 43°, and 43° of kyphosis, respectively. Total loss of correction of kyphosis was 13°

if the scoliotic spine is corrected by longitudinal distraction alone, the cord will be stretched which may result in paralysis. Lehemer et al. recommended not to correct over 35° of kyphosis by single level osteotomy. Otherwise, dural buckling can occur which may require dural plasty.

When total *en bloc* spondylectomy is performed for a spine tumor, the preoperative relationship of the cord and spinal column length should be maintained. Sometimes, the spinal column can be lengthened or shortened at the time of anterior column reconstruction and instrumented stabilization; in the former the cord will be stretched and in the latter the cord will be axially compressed which results in cord ischemia leading to paralysis.

Kawahara et al. reported that the dural kinking was not observed in any patients undergoing a column shortening procedure; 22.2% (7 mm ± 4–10 mm) of the corpectomy defect in the 40 patients. Postoperatively neurological degradation was observed in none. They concluded that

20% column shortening in spinal tumor surgery might be safe.[54]

Kobayashi et al. reported the results in dogs of longitudinal column shortening surgery;[55] Up to 7.2 mm shortening produced no morphological change in the dura mater or spinal cord. If the shortening was between 7.2 and 12.5 mm the cord remained straight in spite of 'ruffling' of the dura mater. Above 12.5 mm of shortening, the cord became kinked. Abnormal evoked potentials were recorded with column shortening of 15 mm and 20 mm, causing incomplete paralysis of the hind limbs in 1 of 3 and 3 of 4 dogs, respectively. With column shortening of 5, 10, 15, and 20 mm cord blood flow changed to 146%, 160%, 102%, and 93% of the preoperative blood flow, respectively. Column shortening less than 15 mm significantly increased the diameter of the anterior spinal artery, while shortening over 15mm decreased the anterior flow. They concluded that the safety limit for column shortening was 12.5 mm (62.5%).

Tanaka et al. reported the results of the cranial half shortening spondylectomy (14–23 mm, mean 20 mm) of the L1 body for adult patients with tethered cord syndrome; there were symptomatic improvements after spinal column shortening. The procedure was found safe and effective, but they did not discuss spondylectomy size.[56]

Residual Spinal Deformity and Parafusion Segment Disease

Maintenance of normal spinal alignment of the diseased segment(s) and also the restoration of deformed segment(s) to normal alignment are essential to reduce the ill-effect on the proximal and distal mobile segments (Fig. 35.6 and 35.7). Therefore since 2001 the current authors have strongly recommended to minimize the residual kyphosis at least less than 10° in case of monosegment fusion and less than 5° in case of bisegment fusion.[5,32]

Posterior Fixation Failure (Loosening and/or Fracture of Screws and Rods) and Increase of Deformity

Failure of posterior stabilization because of rod and/or screw loosening and/or fracture is rare, but if it occurs it is a formidable complication, particularly in children with rapidly progressing spinal deformity (Fig. 35.8).

Tuberculous Kyphosis in Children

In children with Pott's disease, the risk of late kyphosis depends on their age (<5 years), level of involvement (thoracic), extent of the disease (>2 vertebrae), endplate damages and the patterns of involvement and vertebral body remnant shape. Dislocation of facets, posterior retropulsion of the diseased fragment and toppling of the cephalad vertebra suggest the worst prognosis for kyphosis.[1,4,5,11] Buckling (invaginating angulatory) collapse of the spine is unique to pediatric spinal tuberculosis at the lower dorsal and dorsolumbar spine. Fortunately, the above risk factors has never been seen in early spinal tuberculosis. However, in adults when the lumbar spine is involved, the pattern of vertebral collapse is telescoping (nonkyphotic vertebral body collapse) in nature which is different from that of the dorsolumbar spine.[11,12] It is strongly advised that kyphosis of more than 45° should not be allowed, because this puts the posterior spinal muscles at a mechanical disadvantage adding to the deforming force. This contributes not only to a progression of kyphosis, but also to the occurrence of paraplegia.[5,13,14] Prophylactic stabilization and/or corrective procedures should, therefore, definitely be considered to prevent further progression of kyphosis in children.[5]

In children spontaneous intercorporeal fusion rarely occurs during chemotherapy. [1,2,5,11,38,43,57] It occurs later after the cure of the disease at lower rates than that in adults. This phenomenon has not been satisfactorily explained. Study of BMP and anti-BMP factors and other inflammatory cytokines in the tissue around the tuberculous lesion may clarify the cause.[12,30]

In children, the deformity can correct spontaneously because of bone reformation from the remaining growth plates. Thus, the growth plates are important because of their capability of bone growth and reformation of the destroyed vertebral body.[5] However, in most children in spite of disease cure there was a gradual increase of spinal deformity in cases of either unfused and fused vertebrae with the growth plate destruction. When the unfused segment was unstable, the deformity progressed more rapidly than that of the fused block vertebrae.[5,11,59]

There are two contradicting views on the effect of wedged-single vertebral remnant and the fused wedge block vertebrae on the development of kyphosis during growth.

According to Upadhyay et al. the children who underwent radical surgery showed an overall correction which was virtually maintained up to final follow-up, and they concluded that there was no disproportionate posterior spinal growth after anterior intercorporal fusion which contributed to the progression of deformity.[38] On the contrary, Schulitz et al. reported that they observed the progressive kyphosis in the children with fused block vertebra,[9] and Rajasekaran reported that in children with unfused tuberculous kyphosis after cure of tuberculosis there was a posterior longitudinal overgrowth that

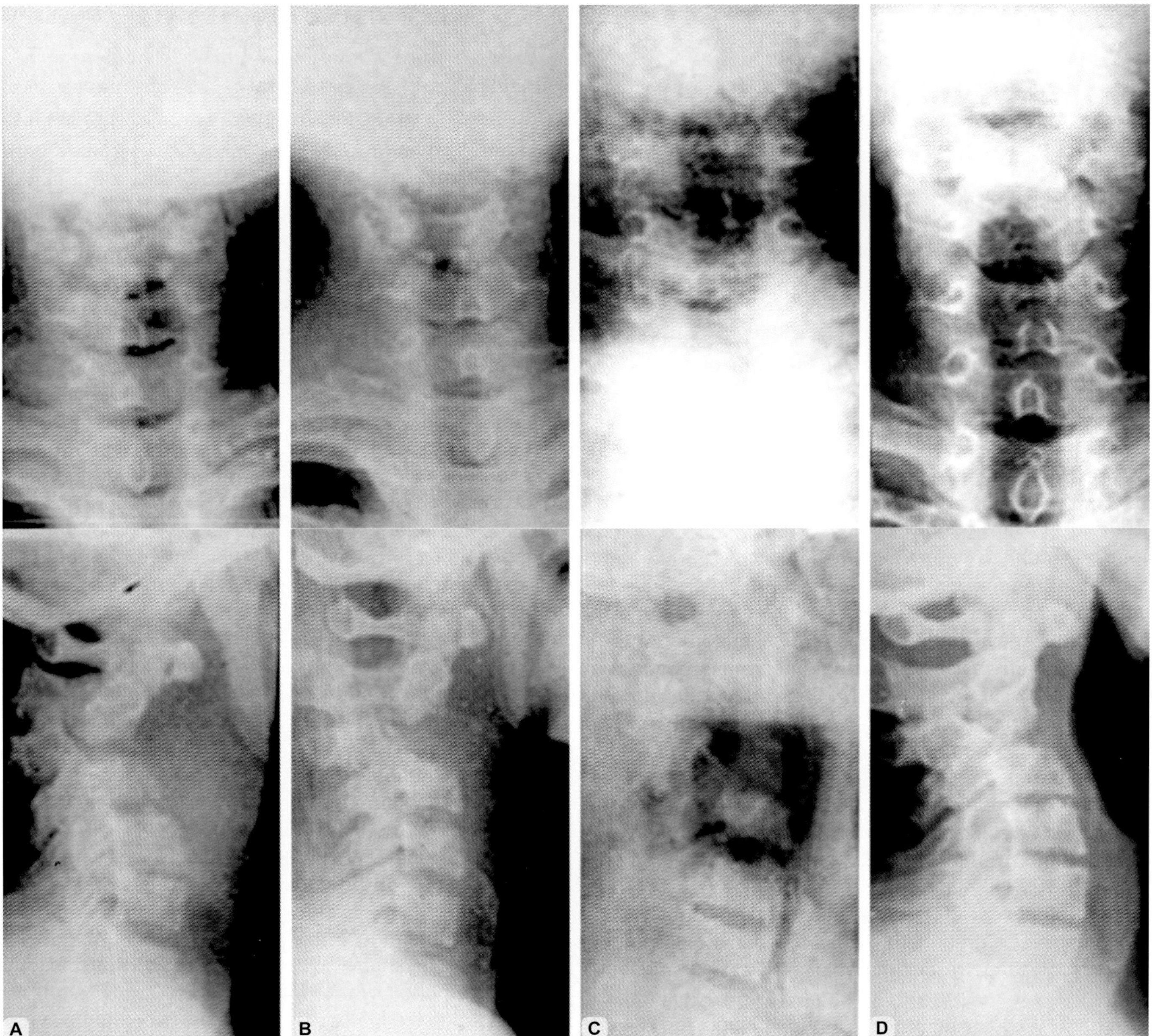

Fig. 35.6 (A) A pretreatment radiograms of a 29 year-old man treated nonoperatively show tuberculous kyphosis at C2–4 with a substantial prevertebral abscess that displaced the trachea and esophagus anteriorly. He received triple chemotherapy for 12 months; (B) The kyphosis was corrected by traction, and the abscess was completely absorbed; (C) A Minerva cast was applied 2 months after traction and chemotherapy; (D) Twelve months after treatment, there was spontaneous anterior fusion without residual kyphosis

eventually caused facet joint subluxation with greatest risk for spinal deformity.[11,57] The current authors support the latter's views.

The unsightly residual hunchback can be distressing to the pediatric patients, their parents and surgeons alike. In the early 1970s initially the authors used posterior interspinous wiring and fusion. This was followed by interspinous wiring and cementation to stabilize the involved segment and to arrest the posterior spinal column growth. Both techniques failed because of loosening of wires and cement, and those procedures were succeeded by the modern posterior instrumentation.[8,42,44,47] Posterior instrumentation in the management of the pediatric tuberculous kyphosis could contribute to gradual correction of the kyphosis by growth arrest of the posterior column when applied before age 10–11 years, though the effect of growth arrest between the

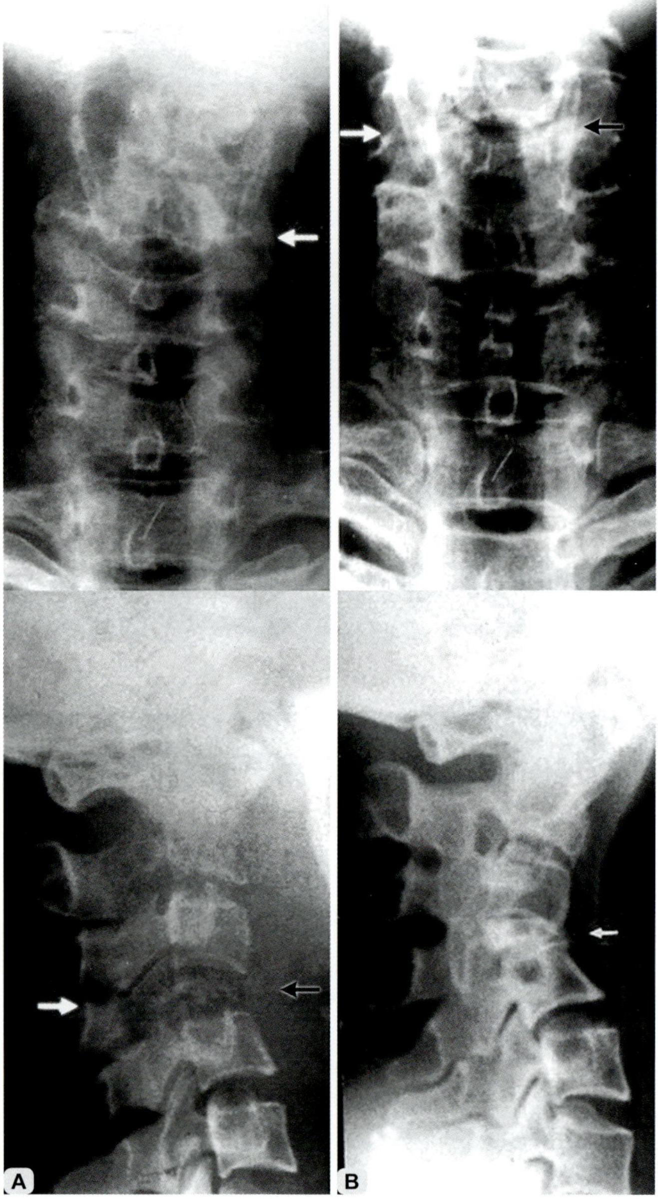

Fig. 35.7 (A) Anterior and lateral pretreatment radiograms of a 32-year-old woman treated nonoperatively demonstrate tuberculous lesion at C3–5. She had multiple lesions T6–7, L1–2, and ribs. Complete destruction of C4 body with a substantial prevertebral abscess and mild kyphosis of 15°; (B) She received triple chemotherapy for 12 months, and anteroposterior and lateral radiograms taken at 4 years demonstrate a solid fusion of C3–5 with an increased kyphosis of 37°. Compensatory hyperlordosis of the caudal mobile segments is seen together with slightly posteriorly slipped and hyperextended C5

Luque's segmental stabilization and pedicle screw fixation system might be different.[5]

In summary, thus, in children posterior instrumentation utilizing several tether devices is thought to be the best procedure with or without posterolateral fusion.

Spinal Tuberculosis in the Elderly

The body's immune system is likely to be weakened through aging. This may contribute to the emergence of tuberculosis in those previously infected individual. It may be that the rapid increase in life expectancy now occurring is resulting in an increase in the incidence of tuberculosis among those elderly people because of both endogenous reactivation and exogenous infection.[18,22] Three- and four-drug regimens are well accepted.

However, the elderly patients frequently have co-morbidity. In general there is an increase in the reported adverse effects of drugs in elderly people. The presence of concomitant diseases such as liver or renal failure may necessitate dosage adjustment of some of the treatment regimens.[5,18,23]

Streptomycin is excreted exclusively, and ethambutol predominantly by the kidney. If either of these 2 drugs is to be given to patients with renal failure, the dosage should be adjusted accordingly. Serum concentration of streptomycin should not exceed 5 mg/mL. If the patient is on dialysis, the dose should be given 5 hours beforehand. Ethambutol should be given in a dose of 25 mg/kg 3 times weekly if the creatinine clearance is between 30 and 50 mL/min. The other main antituberculous medicines are hepatotoxic. For patients with alcoholism or hepatitis B antigen carriers isoniazid and rifampicin, together with one nonhepatotoxic drug should be given to ensure that the duration of treatment will not need to be prolonged.

Pott's Paraplegia

The three main causes of Pott's paraplegia are (i) cord compression by abscess and granulation tissue, (ii) cord compression by sequestrums and the posterior bony edge of the vertebral body at the level of the kyphosis, (iii) bony canal stenosis of the deformed spine above the level of the kyphosis,[5,59] and (iv) tuberculoma in the cord.[63,64]

Many factors affect recovery from Pott's paraplegia. These include as follows:

- The patient's general physical condition and age
- The spinal cord condition
- The involved level and number of vertebrae
- The severity of the spinal deformity (almost no recovery even after effective decompression surgery in patients with kyphosis over 60°)
- The duration and severity of the paraplegia
- The time of initiation of treatment, and
- The type of treatment and drug sensitivity.

In treatment of Pott's paraplegia there are two approaches: conservative medical and radical.[5,59-62] Pott's paraplegia caused by abscess and granulation tissue in the early active stage can be managed effectively by

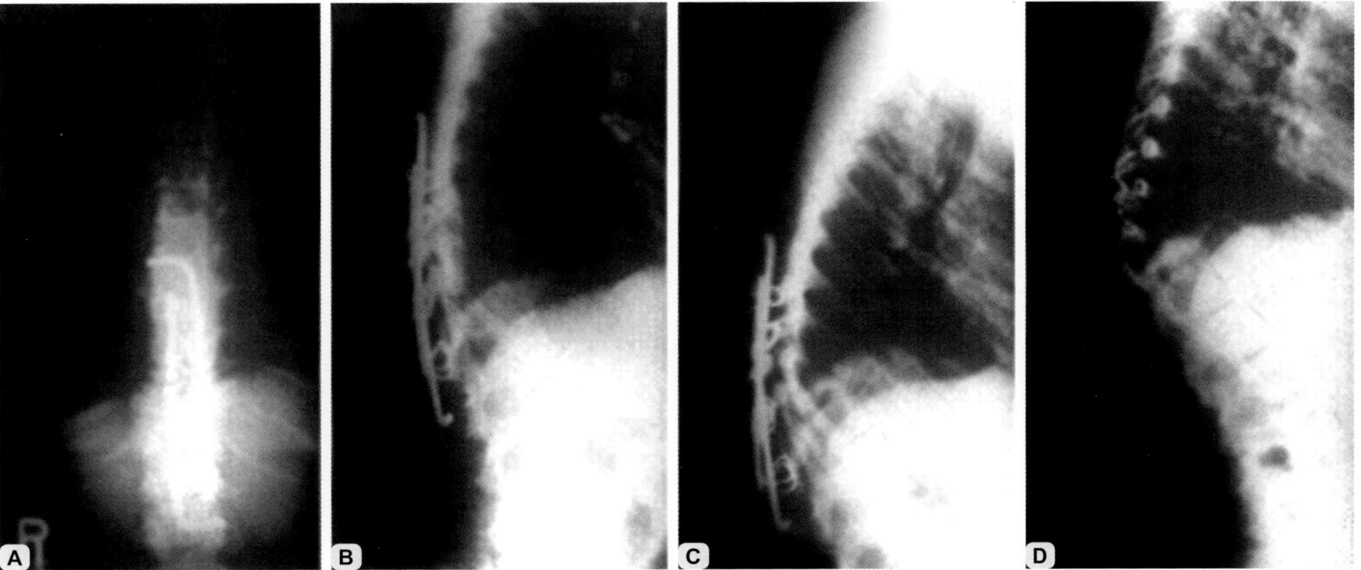

Fig. 35.8 (A to C) An example of modified Luque instrumentation in a 6 year-old boy with tuberculosis of T12–L2; (D) After removal of inferiorly migrated Steinmann's pins and wires, kyphosis developed gradually due to the destroyed vertebral bodies and growth plates

chemotherapy alone, though recovery is slow and gradual. Surgical decompression is indicated when there is acute-onset paralysis with rapidly worsening neurology and respiratory distress in upper cervical tuberculosis, peridural fibrosis and cord compression by bony ridges, and chronic cord compression within the narrow canal.

The time frame for surgery clearly depends on the intensity of the neurologic deficit; dense and progressive deficit needs surgical management much earlier.[5,59-61] Because paraplegia usually resolves rapidly after adequate decompression. Therefore, many surgeons believe that it is unfair to allow a patient to lie paralyzed for some weeks to months awaiting a cure through conservative care, and prefer direct decompression and/or instrumented stabilization.

All types of surgical complications can be encountered during anterior or posterior decompression surgery, though their incidences are low except the cases of rigid severe spinal deformity with distorted neural anatomy.[5]

In one study, the neurological recovery rate in 33 Pott's paraparetics (7 healed, 26 active tuberculosis) with severe spinal deformity was investigated. All seven (2 children and 5 adults) paralytics with healed tuberculosis received surgery. Recovery was relatively good in the two children but poor in the five adults. Among the 26 cases with active disease, 10 (3 children, 7 adults) received chemotherapy alone, and 16 (3 children, 13 adults) underwent surgery. By chemotherapy alone, all three children recovered to a level near normal, and the seven adults also recovered relatively well. In the three surgically treated children, neurological deterioration was observed for a while after surgery, though it later improved by one Frenkel's grade. In the 13 surgically treated adults, less recovery was achieved. Thus, in spite of effective atraumatic decompression surgery, neurological recovery failure rate is rather high in adults. The nonrecovery was thought not to be due to definite surgical trauma but to the preexisting myelopathy secondary to cord ischemia, chronic peridural fibrosis and canal stenosis, especially in cases with kyphosis over 60°. The more severe the kyphosis, the worse the prognosis. Tuli stated that a 60° kyphosis seems to be the watershed for possible neurological recovery after decompression surgery.[14,37]

In summary, neurological recovery was relatively good in children, while it was poor in adults. Although the severity of the paralysis varied between the conservative and surgical groups at the time of treatment, better recovery was achieved in the conservatively treated group and in children.[52,60]

During surgery, there is always a risk of injuring the spinal cord, particularly with extensive anterior decompression at any level of the spine, if the normal landmarks are distorted by the disease. For this reason, meticulous control of hemorrhage is recommended during surgery to identify the dural sac when the anatomical landmarks are severely distorted. In the operative field, one can identify a nerve root and follow it centrally until the dura and the cord are safely identified. An alternative approach is to initiate the decompression over an unaffected area and proceed to the target area following the plane of the dura.[5]

If neurological function worsens in spite of chemotherapy in a Pott's paraplegic patient with severe spinal deformity, only decompressive surgery is recommended to arrest the progression of paralysis and hopefully to restore normal neurology, though in the past some surgeons combined the corrective surgery at the time of decompression.[5] There is only a small chance of neural recovery by surgery, and all patients should be informed of this. The greatest neurological risk is perhaps associated with the correction of a severe fixed kyphosis by osteotomy, and the patients and their family should be advised preoperatively that cord injury may complicate this procedure.

In Moon et al. series of 67 paraplegic patients with minimal to moderate kyphosis, all 13 conservatively treated and 47 (87.0%) of the 54 surgically treated patients recovered. The difference in neurological recovery rates between the two groups was attributed to the difference in the stage of the disease at the time of treatment in addition to surgical complications.[59]

Through the current authors' experiences, it was found that posterior instrument-aided stabilizing surgery alone under the cover of antitubercular chemotherapy regardless of the disease stage and/or severity of deformity can hasten the neurological recovery without direct decompression surgery.[5]

Intramedullary Tuberculoma

There are 4 types of tuberculomas: extra- or intradural and extra- and intramedullary forms. In the past the cord tuberculoma was excised surgically, because there was no other therapeutic choice. Therefore, there has been debate as to whether cord tuberculoma is a medical or surgical condition because of the grave sequellae of surgical excision of the tuberculoma. Recently some recommended the microsurgical resection and antituberculous chemotherapy.[63,64] However, the current authors recommended the combined antitubercular chemotherapy and degranulating agent therapy (anti-TNFα blocker treatment; subcutaneous injection of etanercept, 25 mg twice weekly upto 6–8 weeks) after diagnostic biopsy.[5] This can obviate the need for total excisional surgery for tuberculoma.

Extent of Instrumentation and Timing of Implant Removal

After the instrument-aided corrective surgery of the deformed diseased spine, multisegment stabilization including the 3–4 normal mobile segments is inevitable, while the short segment fixation is more preferred for the monosegment lesion. Multisegment instrumentation immobilizes normal mobile segments and may later cause these segments to be stiffened and degenerated.[64] Therefore, the authors normally removed the instrument to remobilize these instrumented segments at the time of solid intercorporal fusion, about postoperative 9 months, though there was no acceptable standardized regimen for all the surgeons.[2,5,64]

Preservation of proximal and distal normal mobile segments particularly in the cervical and lumbar spine is strongly recommended to restore and/or maintain the near-normal mobile spinal column functions.

In children with unacceptable residual kyphosis, posterior instruments should be left until maturity to maximize gradual growth correction of the deformity due to the tethering effect of the implants.[2,5]

Conclusion

Spinal tuberculosis is a curable disease with the presently available chemotherapeutic agents. With early detection and institution of chemotherapy and improved surgical techniques, patients with kyphosis are rarely seen in daily practice nowadays. Selection of the therapeutic measures to minimize the residual kyphosis in the highly mobile spinal segments after cure of the disease is stressed not only for aesthetic view point but also for reduction of incidence of parafusion segment disease. Paraplegic patients can be well managed with minimal residuals if early diagnosis and effective treatment are achieved. Posterior stabilizing instrumentation alone hastened the neural recovery. Cord tuberculoma could be effectively treated without radical excision by combining the antituberculous medication and anti-TNFα blocker therapy with minimal residual.

Acknowledgment

The authors thank Mr Seog In Moon for his secretariat work.

References

1. Moon MS. Tuberculosis of the spine: controversies and a new challenges: spine update. Spine. 1997;22:1791-7.
2. Moon MS. Managing tuberculosis of spine. Med Progress. 2004;593-602.
3. China Tuberculosis Control Collaboration: The effect of tuberculosis control in China. Lancet. 2004;364:417-22.
4. Moon MS. Development in the management of tuberculosis of the spine. Curr Orthop. 2006;20:132-40.
5. Moon MS. Tuberculosis of spine – Contemporary thoughts on current issues and perspective views. Curr Orthop. 2007;21:364-79.
6. Kwon OJ. The role of nitric oxide in the immune response of tuberculosis. J Korea Med Sci. 1997;12:481-7.

7. Kumar K. Tuberculosis of spine: natural history of disease and its judicious management. J Western Pacific Orthop Assoc. 1988;15(1):1-8.
8. Moon MS. Treatment of spinal infections. Commemoratvie issue. 3rd Spinal Section Congress, WPOA. J Western Pacif Orthop Assoc. 1983;7-11.
9. Schulitz K, Kothe R, Leong J, Wehling P. Growth changes of solidly fused kyphotic bloc after surgery for tuberculosis; comparison of four procedures. Spine. 1997;22:1150-5.
10. Jeong GY, Yang YS, Oh WI. Peripheral lymphocyte subsets in patients with pulmonary and extrapulmonary tuberculosis. Korea J Clin Pathol. 1999;19:696-701.
11. Rajasekaran S, Shammugasundaram TK. Prediction of the angle of gibbus deformity in tuberculosis of the spine. J Bone Joint Surg Am. 1987;69:503-9.
12. Moon MS, Moon YW, Moon JL, Kim SS, Sun DH. Conservative treatment of tuberculosis of the lumbar and lumbosacral spine. Clin Orthop. 2002;398:40-9.
13. Tuli SM: Tuberculosis of the skeletal system (bone, joints, spine and bursal sheath), 3rd Ed. New Delhi; Jaypee Brother Medical publishers pvt. Ltd.; 2004.
14. Tuli SM. Severe kyphotic deformity in tuberculosis of the spine. Internat Orthop (SICOT). 1995;19:327-31.
15. Arora A. Basic science of host immunity in osteoarticular tuberculosis. Indian J Orthop. 2006;40(1):1-5.
16. Maeda Y, Izawa K, Nabeshima T, Yonenobu K. Tuberculous spondylitis in elderly Japanese patients. Internat Orthop. 2008;13:16-20.
17. Cunningham ME, Girardi F, Papadopulos EC, Cammisa FP. Spinal infections in patients with compromised immune systems. Clin Orthop. 2006;444:73-82.
18. Govender S, Parbhoo AH, Kumar KPS, Annamalai K. Anterior spinal decompression in HIV-positive patients with tuberculosis. J Bone Joint Surg. 2001;83-B:864-7.
19. Davies P DO. Tuberculosis in the Elderly: Epidemiology and optimal management. Med Prog. 1996;25-8.
20. Kim HA, Yoo CD, Back HJ, et al. Mycobacterium tuberculosis infection in a corticosteroid-treated rheumatic disease patient. Clin Exp Rheumatol. 1998;16:9-13.
21. Genestier L, Paillet R, Fournel S, Ferrero C, Miossec P, Revillard J. Immunosuppressive properties of methotrexate: apoptosis and clonal deletion of activated peripheral T cells. J Clin Invest. 1998;102:322-8.
22. Cole RA, Lu HM, Shi YZ, et al. Clinical evaluation of a rapid immunochromatographic assay based on the 38 KDa antigen of Mycobacterium tuberculosis on patients with pulmonary tuberculosis in China. Tubercle Lung Dis. 1996;77:363-8.
23. Brisson-Noel A, gicqual B, Lecossier D, et al. Rapid diagnosis of tuberculosis by amplification of mycobacterial DNA in clinical samples. Lancet. 1989;334:1069-71.
24. Mehta JS, Bhojraj SY. Tuberculosis of the thoracic spine. A classification based on the selection of surgical strategies. J Bone Joint Surg. 2001;83-B:859-63.
25. Oguz E, Sehirlioglu A, Altinmakas M, Ozturk C, Komureu M, Solakoglu C, Vaccaro AR. A new classification and guide for surgical treatment of spinal tuberculosis. Internat Orthop. 2008;32:127-33.
26. Hodgson AR, Stock FE: Anterior spine fusion for the treatment of tuberculosis of the spine: the operative findings and results of treatment in the first 100 cases. J Bone Joint Surg. 1960;42A:295-310.
27. Moon MS: Combined posterior instrumentation and anterior interbody fusion for active tuberculous kyphosis of the thoracolumbar spine. Current Orthop. 1991;5:177-9.
28. Zhao J, Lian XF, Hou TS, Ma H, Chen ZM. Anterior debridement and bone grafting of spinal tuberculosis with one-stage instrumentation anteriorly or posteriorly. Internat Orthop. 2007;31:859-63.
29. Nagariya S, Patgaonkar P, Chhabra S, Agrawal V, Franke J. Single stage anterior decompression and instrumentation for spinal tuberculosis. J Spinal Surg. 2010;2(2):373-82.
30. Moon MS, Moon JL, Kim SS, Moon YW. Treatment of tuberculosis of the cervical spine. Clin Orthop. 2007;460:67-77.
31. Oga W, Arizono T, Takasita M, et al. Evaluation of the risk of instrumentation as a foreign body in spinal tuberculosis: clinical and biologic study. Spine. 1993;18:1890-4.
32. Ha KY, Chung YG, Ryoo SJ. Adheaence and biofilm formation of staphylococcus epidermis and mycobacterium tuberculosis on various spinal infections. Spine. 2004;29(24):1-6.
33. An YH, Stuart GW, McDowell CJ, McDaniel SE, Kang O, Friedman RJ. Prevention of bacterial adherence to implant surfaces with a crosslinked albumin coating in vitro. J Orthop Res. 1996;14:846-9.
34. Kim YY, Yoon YS. Replacement arthroplasty using Charnley prosthesis in old tuberculosis of the hip. Intenat Orthop. 1979;3:81.
35. Medical Research Council Working Party on Tuberculosis of Spine: Results at three years of a study in Korea. J Bone Joint Surg. 1993;75B:240-8.
36. Griffith DLI: Short-course chemotherapy in the treatment of spinal tuberculosis. J Bone Joint Surg. 1986;68B:158.
37. Jain AK, Aggarval PK, Arora A, Singh S: Behavior of the kyphotic angle in spinal tuberculosis. Int Orthop. 2004;28(2):110-4.
38. Upadhyay SS, Saji MJ, Yau CMC. Duration of antituberculous chemotherapy in conjunction with radical surgery in the management of spinal tuberculosis. Spine. 1996;21:1898-903.
39. Moulding T, Dutt AK, Reichman LB. Fixed-dose combinations of antituberculous medications to prevent drug resistance. Ann Intern Med. 1995;122(12):951-4.
40. Upadhyay SS, Sell P, Saji MJ, Sell B, Yau ACMC, Leong JCY. 17-year prospective study of surgical management of spinal tuberculosis in children. Spine. 1993;18(12):1704-11.
41. Moon MS, Kim L, Woo YK, et al. Conservative treatment of tuberculosis of the thoracic and lumbar spine in adults and children. Internat Orthop (SICOT). 1987;11:315-22.
42. Moon MS, Rhee SK, Kang YK. Harrington rods in treatment of active spinal tuberculosis with kyphosis. J Western Pacif Orthop Assoc. 1986;23:53-8.
43. Kloeckner C, Valencia R. Sagittal alignment after anterior debridement and fusion with or without additional posterior instrumentation in the treatment of pyogenic and tuberculous spondylodiscitis. Spine. 2003;28:1036-42.

44. Moon MS, Yoo YK, Lee KS, et al. Posterior instrumentation and anterior interbody fusion for tuberculosis kyphosis of dorsal and lumbar spine. Spine. 1995;20:1910-6.
45. Bhojraj S, Patel T, Kalkotwar S, Prasad G. Transpedicular approach: A gateway to the spine. J Spinal Surg. 2010;2(2):420-5.
46. Lee S, Sung J, Park Y. Single stage transpedicular decompression and posterior instrumentation in treatment of thoracic and thoracolumbar spinal tuberculosis. J Spinal Disorder Tech. 2006;19(8):595-602.
47. Benli IT, Maya A, Acaroglu E. Anterior instrumentation in tuberculous spondylitis. Clin. Orthop. 2007;460:108-16.
48. Jain AK, Dhammi IK, Jain S, Mishra P. Kyphosis in spinal tuberculosis - prevention and correction. Indian J Orthop. 2010;44(2):127-36.
49. Jain AK: Tuberculosis of the spine - A fresh look at an old disease. J Bone Joint Surg. 2010;92B:905-13.
50. Yau AMC, Hsu LCS, O'Brien JP, et al. Tuberculous kyphosis: correction with spinal osteotomy, halopelvic distraction, and anterior posterior fusion. J Bone Joint Surg. 1974;56A:1419-34.
51. Lehman SM, Kappler L, Biscup RS, et al. Posterior transvertebral osteotomy for adult thoracolumbar kyphosis. Spine. 1994;19:2060-7.
52. Shimode M, Kojima T, Sowa K: Spinal wedge osteotomy by a single posterior approach for correction of severe and rigid kyphosis or kyphoscoliosis. Spine. 2002;27(20):2260-76.
53. Van Dijk M, Smit TH, Jiya TW, Waisman PI. Polyurethan real-size models used in planning complex spinal surgery. Spine. 2001;26(17):1920-6.
54. Kawahara N, Tomita K, Murakami H, Akameru M, Hata T. Spinal Shortening in total enbloc spondylectomy. Japan Orthop. Congress Book. 2005;3A-P9-4.
55. Kobayashi T, Kawahara N, Murakami H, et al. An experimental study on the influence of spinal shortening on the spinal cord. Japan Orthop. Assoc. Congress Book, 2005;3A-P9-1.
56. Tanaka Y, Kokubun S, Ozawa K, et al. Shortening spinal osteotomy for tethered cord syndrome. Japan Orthop. Assoc Congress Book. 2005;3A-P9-2.
57. Rajasekaran S. The natural history of post-tubercular kyphosis in children: radiological signs which predict late increase in deformity. J. Bone Joint Surg. 2001;83B:954-62.
58. Jain AK, Sinha S: Evaluation of systems of grading of neurological deficit in tuberculosis. Spinal Cord. 2005;43:375-80.
59. Moon MS, Ha KY, Sun DH, et al. Pott's paraplegia: 67 cases. Clin Orthop. 1996;323:122-8.
60. Moon MS, Moon JL, Moon YW, Kim SS, Sun DH. Pott's paraplegia in patients with severely deformed dorsal or dorsolumbar spines: treatment and prognosis. Spinal Cord. 2003;41:164-71.
61. Wong YW, Leong JCY, Luk KDK. Direct intenal kyphectomy for severe angular tuberculous kyphosis. Clin Orthop. 2007;480:124-9.
62. Laheri VJ, Badhe NP, Dewnany GT. Single stage decompression, anterior interbody fusion and posterior instrumentation for tuberculous kyphosis of the dorsolumbar spine. Spinal Cord. 2001;39:429-36.
63. Harsha CKS, Shetty AP, Rajasekaran S. Intradural spinal tuberculosis in the absence of vertebral or meningeal tuberculosis: a case report. J Orthop Surg. 2006;14(1):71-5.
64. Liu YD, Wang FY, Xu JM, Guan Y, Guan H. Intramedullary thoracic tuberculoma (a case report). Spinal Cord. 2010;48:80-2.
65. Kahanovitz N, Arnoczky SP, Levine DB, Otis JP. The effects of internal fixation on the articular cartilage of unfused canine facet joints. Spine. 1984;9:268-72.

CHAPTER

36

Sacropelvic Fixation

Ioannis Avramis, Nicholas Pirnia, Munish Gupta

Introduction

As the terminal segment of the spine, the sacrum is subjected to substantial forces as it transmits axial loads from the lumbar spine to the adjacent ilia via the sacroiliac joints. This relationship leads to several pathologies that are specific to the sacrum, in addition to the extra demands applied as a consequence of surgical treatments. Fixation into the sacrum remains somewhat more challenging than other regions of the caudal spine. The remnant vertebral bodies of the sacrum are relatively small and the cancellous bone quality is often poor. This leaves comparatively little bone for fixation and generally only the S1 and S2 segments are amenable to screw placement. Additionally, the sacral instrumentation may be the most distal fixation for long constructs that span the entire thoracolumbar spine, placing great strain upon these two or four screws. These factors have led to the routine use of supplemental iliac fixation to prevent failure of sacral fixation, sacral insufficiency fractures and decrease the pseudarthrosis rate. In spite of these limitations for fixation across the lumbosacral junction, there are numerous options including pedicle screws, alar screws, posterior sacral plates, S1 screws combined with intrasacral rods, and iliac bolts.

Historical Background

Although internal fixation for lumbosacral fusion has been described as early as the 1940s, effective sacral fixation is relatively new technology. In 1948, King described the use of bilateral facet screws for lumbosacral fusions which allowed early mobilization.[1] These screws were not widely adopted in part because there was a high incidence of early failure and pseudarthrosis.[2] The first commonly used form of spinal internal fixation was the Harrington rod. Harrington rods were used for fusions to the sacrum on many occasions, but fusing to the sacrum proved difficult. The bone of the S1 lamina is thin and often would not support a Harrington hook, plus there were concerns of S2 nerve root irritation from the tip of the laminar hooks.[3] This limited fixation led to the development of the Harrington sacral bar, effectively the first iliac fixation. These Harrington bars were trans-iliac rods that bridged across the posterior superior iliac spine and gave a strong foundation for Harrington constructs to the sacrum.[4] These Harrington bar constructs had much better purchase in bone, but also had many limitations. They were prone to migrating over time and required a separate skin incision that often resulted in wound complications. Furthermore, they could freely rotate in the ilium and did little to resist flexion and extension moments.[5] Additionally, long fusions to the sacrum using this distraction instrumentation system had a pseudarthrosis rate approaching 40%[6] and flattened the patient's lumbar lordosis leading to the now well known "flat-back" syndrome.[7] Because of these limitations, most surgeons strongly avoided long fusions to the sacrum and short lumbosacral fusions were often not instrumented. The Harrington system was later modified to allow some rod contouring as well as angling of the distal hook to allow for lumbar lordosis. This helped, but loss of lumbar lordosis was still the norm and "flat-back" still a common occurrence.[8]

Anterior fixation also proved more challenging than within the lumbar spine. Dwyer instrumentation was developed and implemented in the late1960s followed by Zielke in the 1970s[9] principally for lumbar deformity correction and to aid arthrodesis for long fusions.[10] The system was effective and rapidly grew in popularity for lumbar deformity, although early series showed loss of lumbar lordosis as a common occurrence. However, the shape of the sacrum and the position of the iliac crest precluded extension of these systems past the lumbosacral junction. Some authors attempted hybrid implant systems, using Zielke or Dwyer in the lumbar spine, placing an ALIF at L5-S1, and applying an anterior staple across the lumbosacral junction.[11] These early staples were conceptually similar to modern anterior lumbosacral plating systems, but they lacked threads or tines and easily displaced or migrated. They also were not rigid and, therefore, did not provide much stability. Pseudarthrosis was common in those procedures.

The 1970s saw the first wide spread interest in the treatment of spinal stenosis, first described by Verbiest in 1951. Many spine surgeons appreciated the need for concomitant arthrodesis in addition to multi-level decompressions for stenosis.[12] With few fixation options available, surgeons experimented with both Harrington rods and Knodt rods to stabilize these decompressions and fusions.[13, 14] These implants were not well suited to the task. Firstly, both were distraction systems that typically flattened the normal lumbar lordosis. Secondly, both systems relied on hooks with supplemental use of sublaminar wires, but with loss of the posterior elements for the decompression there was no place to apply these hooks or wires. This meant that surgeons had to instrument an unaffected vertebra above the decompression.[15] Distal fixation often consisted of supralaminar hooks applied to S1 or hooks tamped into the ala. Supplemental wires could be placed around the S1 or S2 lamina via small drill holes or through the dorsal sacral foramens. Again, implant dislodgement, breakage, and pseudarthrosis were very common.

Effective sacral fixation was not available until the advent of pedicle screws. Roy-Camille was among the first to experiment with the concept of screw and plate constructs[16] while Harrington began using L5 lag screws fixed with wire to a Harrington distraction rod for treating severe spondylolisthesis.[17] It would take another two decades before they saw widespread use and were popularized in the US by the work of Arthur Steffee, mostly during the 1980s.[18] Pedicle screws offered the first effective means of capturing the good quality bone of the sacral bodies via posterior instrumentation. These delivered much more robust fixation than prior hook or wire constructs, as well as, allowing for multiaxial control for reduction of deformity and maintenance of normal sagittal contour.[19]

The S1 screw is still the only pedicle screw that is amenable to routine bicortical purchase, which greatly enhances pull-out strength.[20] However, in spite of the benefits of bicortical purchase S1 screws are often a weak link in a lumbosacral construct. Much of this is due to sacral anatomy as the cancellous bone is not dense and the cortex is often rather thin. The S1 pedicles themselves are usually quite large relative to the lumbar pedicles and overall screw purchase is often less than lumbar pedicle screws. These weaknesses have led to several additions to enhance S1 screws. These include sacral plates (Chopin plate/Colorado system), S2 alar screws, Jackson intrasacral rods, and routine use of anterior column support and supplemental iliac screws for long fusions to the sacrum (more than 3 levels).

Iliac bolts or screws were developed originally for neuromuscular scoliosis treatment and have an evolution from Galveston rods. The use of polyaxial screws as the iliac bolt with a rodded connector to the remainder of the spinal instrumentation construct have obviated the need for complex bends of longitudinal rods using the Galveston technique. As the ease of fixation into the ilium has occurred, so too has the indication for use. Iliac bolts are routinely used for high grade spondylolisthesis, long fusions across the lumbosacral junction, and sacral reconstruction for either tumor or trauma.

Sacral and Pelvic Anatomy

The sacrum is a physiologically and anatomically unique component of the axial skeleton. It functions to transmit forces from the mobile spine to adjacent ilia and therefore converts compressive forces from the lumbar spine to shear forces at the sacroiliac joints. Functionally the sacrum serves as a bipod with forces entering at the sacral promontory, bifurcating, and exiting through the alae and sacroiliac joints. This unique function necessitates unique anatomy. As a result, the sacral promontory and alae must withstand significant stress and this drives the bony architecture of the sacrum on both a macro and microanatomical level.

The surface anatomy of the sacrum is unique, but demonstrates the remnants of key vertebral features from the cephalad spine. It is formed by the fusion of five sacral vertebrae that still retain many homologous features of the mobile spine, but also exhibit features that are unique to sacral vertebrae (Fig. 36.1).

The bodies of the sacral vertebrae are highly tapered and rapidly decrease in cross sectional area from cranial to caudal. The average anterior-posterior length of the S1

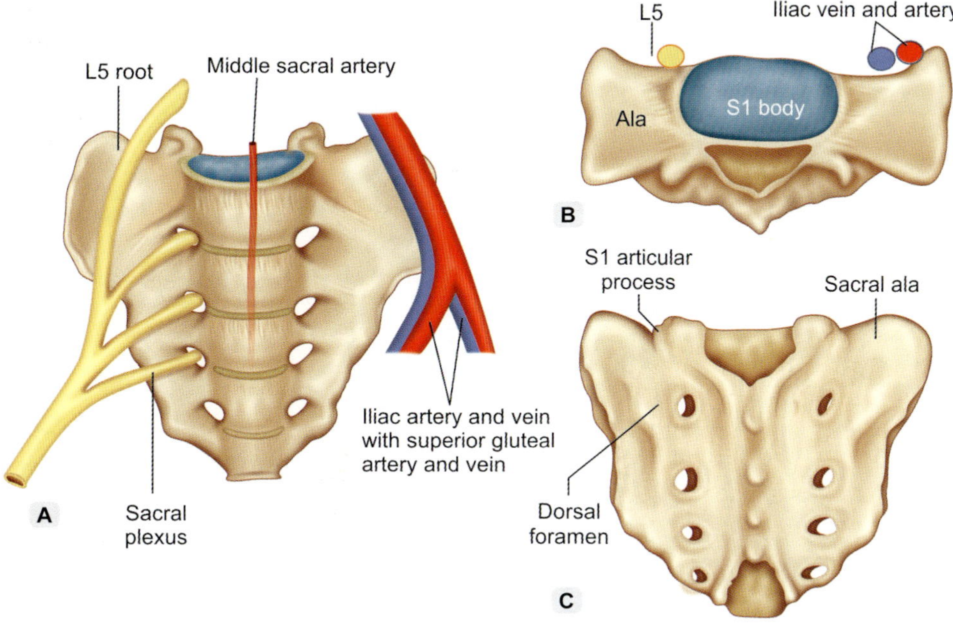

Fig. 36.1 Sacral bony anatomy—landmarks for instrumentation. (A) Anterior sacrum; (B) Posterior sacrum; (C) Axial view of S1 body and ala

body is 50 mm for men and 47 mm for women, this figure dramatically decreases to 31 mm and 28 mm for men and women respectively, at S2.[21] Sacral vertebrae are also larger in the coronal than sagittal plane and have relatively small bodies.

The anterior costal and posterior transverse processes of S1 to S3 are very large and broad, fusing to form the paired alae. The ala contains some of the denser bone found within the sacrum. Because of the fusion of the anterior and transverse processes, each sacral level must contain two foramens to transmit both the ventral and dorsal primary spinal rami. The ventral foramen are much larger as they convey the substantial root contributions of the sciatic nerve. The comparatively small dorsal roots are accompanied by branches of the sinuvertebral artery and can be a source of brisk bleeding during dissection.

In spite of the substantial forces transmitted through the sacrum, much of the sacral cancellous bone is of low density and quality. This is consistent with the bipod like function of the sacrum as the densest bone is found within the sacral promontory and paired alas, but the remainder of the sacrum has poor quality bone as it is functionally stress shielded.

Anterior to the sacrum reside many important visceral structures including the paired common and internal iliac artery and vein, paired L5 nerve roots, sigmoid colon, middle sacral artery, and sympathetic plexus. All of these structures may be subject to risk during surgical instrumentation and approach to the lumbosacral junction. The safest region of the anterior sacrum is the paracentral portion of the S1 body. The vascular structures bifurcate above the S1 body and trace laterally, traversing far from the midline at the level of S1. The L5 nerve roots also course laterally and lie at the junction of the S1 vertebral body and ala. The only midline structure is the middle sacral artery which lies directly on the midline of the anterior sacrum. With this in mind, the safest location for implants that exit the anterior aspect of the sacrum is slightly lateral to the midline within the S1 body. Implants that exit the cortex within the ala place the neurovascular structures at much greater risk. S1 screws are the safest of the bicortical implants as their tips should lie within the medial aspect of the S1 body (Figs 36.1 and 36.2).

The iliac wings are attached to the sacrum through the minimally mobile sacroiliac joints which contain some of the strongest ligaments in the human body. The angle at which the iliac wings are attached to the sacrum is variable, especially between men and women, with men tending to have a more anteriorly directed iliac wing and women more laterally directed. The path of the iliac bolt starts at the PSIS and is directed approximately 30° inferiorly and laterally, the amount lateral trajectory depends on the overall shape of the pelvis as described above (Figs 36.3 and 36.4). The screw path is superior to the greater sciatic notch, violation of which can cause injury to the superior gluteal artery. Perforation of the medial wall of the tract can cause injury to the pelvic vasculature and organs.

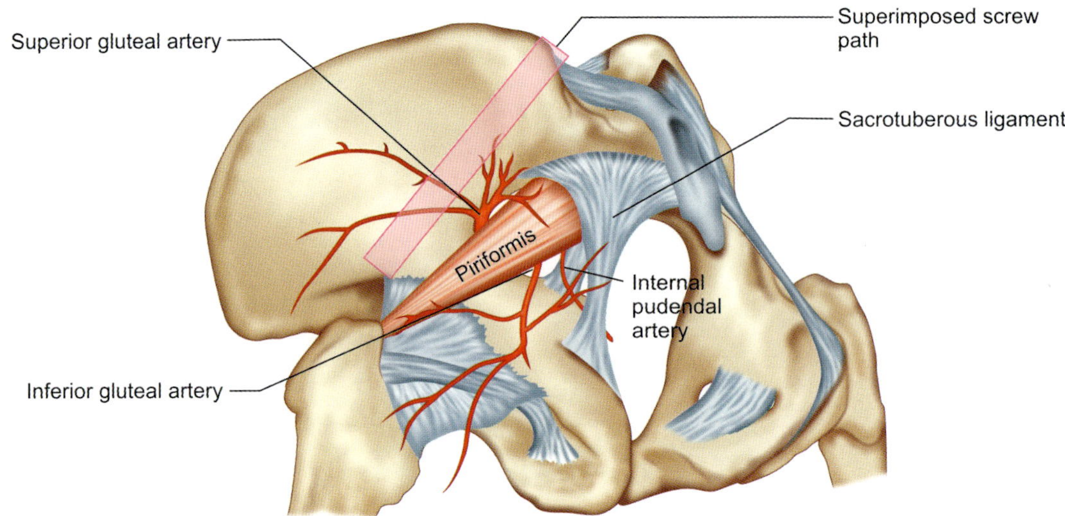

Fig. 36.2 Anterior sacral and pelvic neurovascular anatomy. Greater sciatic notch and the associated neurovascular structures, the path of the iliac bolt is superimposed. For relative position of large blood vessels and nerve roots over the anterior aspect of the sacrum, see Figure 36.1A.

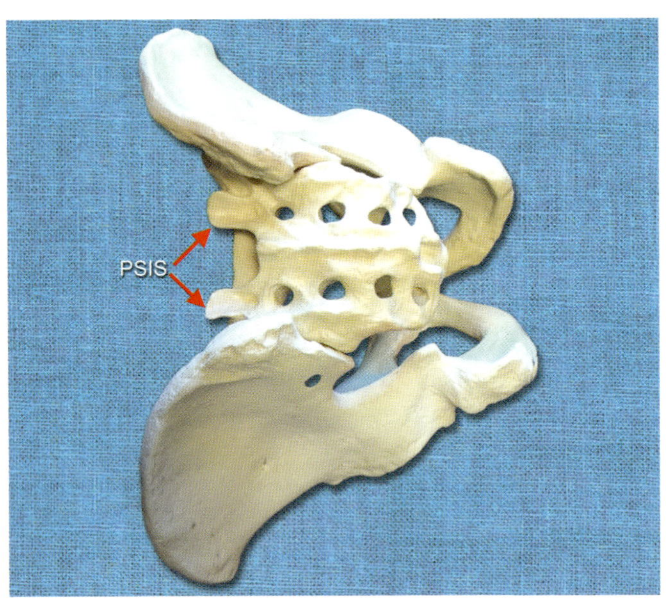

Fig. 36.3 Posterolateral view of the pelvis with the PSIS visible in the orientation viewed by the surgeon

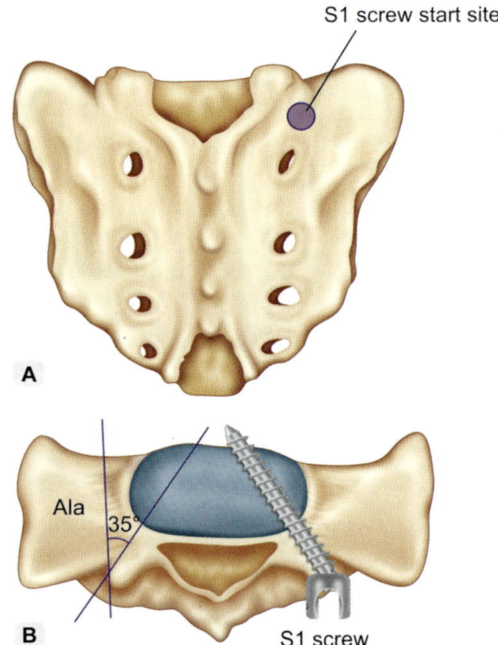

Fig. 36.4 Landmarks for placement of S1 pedicle screws. (A) Dorsal start point at the confluence of the S1 articular process and the superios portion of the sacral ala; (B) Axial view of S1 depicting the appropriate amount of medial trajectory of the S1 pedicle screw

Biomechanics

There are several important biomechanical principles that drive the choice of sacral fixation, especially for long fusions. One of the most important is the concept of the lumbosacral pivot point described by McCord et al.[22] The lumbosacral pivot point is centered within the posterior longitudinal ligament at the level of the L5–S1 disk space and it is a powerful predictor of the efficacy of lumbosacral fixation. As an implant extends further anterior from the lumbosacral pivot point it will provide more construct stiffness and a higher load to failure. Implants that remain posterior to the lumbosacral pivot point impart little additional stability. Implants that extend far anterior, such as iliac bolts, impart substantial biomechanical benefits in resisting flexion moment. Due to the normal pelvic incidence of an ambulatory adult, a typical S2 pedicle screw will not extend anterior to the lumbosacral pivot point, while an S2 alar screw does extend anterior and is biomechanically preferred. Among the common implants and techniques available for sacral fixation, only S1 pedicle screws, S2 alar screws, S2 alar iliac screws and iliac bolts will reach or extend anterior to the lumbosacral pivot point. Triangulation of implants dramatically increases the pullout strength of a construct. Iliac bolts and S2 alar iliac screws have the advantage of being a trajectory that is out of plane from lumbar pedicle screws. A force acting to pull out lumbar pedicle screws would cause a break out force on the pelvic fixation, which is much more resistant to failure leading to overall resilience of the spinal instrumentation construct. Ruland et al. found that medially directed and cross linked S1 pedicle screws outperformed either hooks or stand-alone pedicle screws.[23] This reinforces to the biomechanical benefits of the medially S1 pedicle screw over alar screws or sacral hook constructs.

Sacral Fixation

S1 Pedicle Screws

Pedicle screws placed into the S1 vertebra remain the mainstay of direct sacral fixation in modern spine surgery. The technique for placement is familiar to the majority of spine surgeons, as it is similar to pedicle screw fixation in the lumbar spine and the quality of fixation is relatively good, if placed properly. It harmoniously integrates with posterior instrumentation of the lumbar spine, provides direct sacral fixation, and is relatively safe. S1 pedicle screws work well as the inferior most fixation point in fusions of the lower lumbar spine, up to L3. For longer fusions to L2 and superiorly, S1 screws should be reinforced with fixation into the ilium, the combination of the two is the most biomechanically robust posterior construct.

Placement of S1 screws is much like placement of lumbar pedicle screws but a few anatomic factors can make placing an ideal S1 pedicle screw more difficult than screws at more cranial levels. The wide interpedicular distance at S1, and need to medialize tip of the screw to capture, the dense bone of the promontory require a very medial projection of the S1 screw. The start site for S1 pedicle screws, is at the confluence of the sacral ala and the S1 facet, the trajectory is angled more medial than the lumbar pedicle screws. This is a result of both the more lateral start point and the need to aim the screw, just lateral to midline especially for bicortical screws. However, the iliac crest can block the ideal path for the screw, especially in men with large iliac crests. In these instances, the Steffe probe can be helpful, as it generally has more angle than a Lenke probe, allowing it to be guided medially. Fractures of the sacrum, especially S1, or any other pathology resulting in destruction or weakening of the pedicle represent relative contraindications to placing S1 pedicle screws (Figs 36.4 and 36.5).

Preoperative planning with advanced imaging, such as MRI or CT is encouraged. This imaging allows for evaluation of pedicle size, trajectory, and length of screws. Screw length and trajectory becomes very important if bicortical screws are planned. Bicortical screws have on average 31% more pull out strength than unicortical when using 6.5 mm diameter screws; imaging can visualize the neurovascular structure anterior to the S1 body.[20] As the S1 pedicles tend to be large than lumbar pedicles, imaging can also evaluate the possibility of placing a larger diameter screw into the S1 pedicles, increasing the strength through increased insertional torque by allowing the screw to have fixation

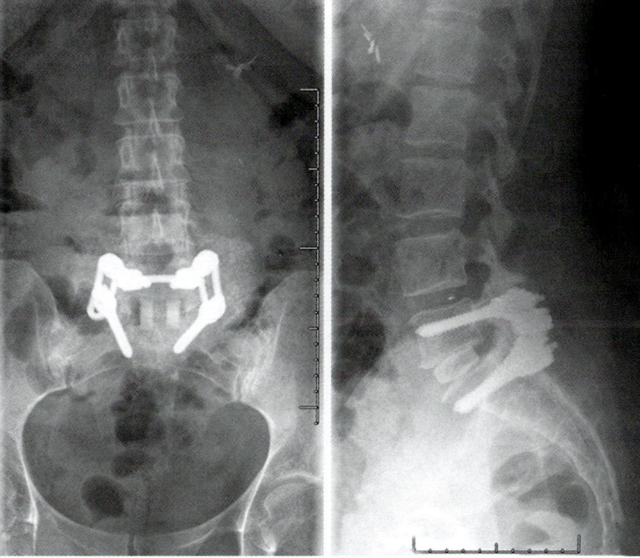

Fig. 36.5 Radiograph of bicortical S1 pedicle screws

into the cortical bone of the pedicle, not just the cancellous bone. Imaging will uncover anatomic variations that may present problems during approach and placement of screws, such as spina bifida occulta, sacralized L5 or lumbarized S1.

S1 pedicle screws can be inserted from several different approaches including midline, Wiltse and minimally invasively, yet the start is always the same at the intersection of the sacral ala and the S1 articular process. If fusion is planned, the need for decortication of the sacral ala should be planned for, and is generally more easily accomplished before screw insertion. The location of the dorsal S1 foramen should be considered during dissection as brisk bleeding can be caused, if the foramen is encountered. Also, the L5-S1 interlaminar window is particularly large and durotomies can occur during dissection if one strays over the window. Midline defects of the S1and S2 lamina also pose a danger of durotomies with electrocautery during exposure.

Once the approach is completed the sacral ala and S1 facet is delineated, removal of osteophytes around the L5–S1 fact joint may be necessary to have clear access to the start site of the S1 pedicle screw. Following creation of a pilot hole using a high speed burr or awl, the pedicle probe is inserted and angled 30°–35° medial and 15°–25° cephalad from the dorsal axis of the sacrum. The probe should advance for 30–40 mm, if significant resistance is encountered early, the probe may need to be redirected more cephalad or medial. If an endpoint is reached after advancing 30 to 40 mm, the anterior cortex should be broached by tapping the probe with a mallet. Dangers during insertion include injury to iliac vessels and L5 nerve root for lateralized trajectories, caudal breaches place the S1 nerve root at risk, cephalad breaches may also occur into the L5–S1 disk space.

Jackson Intrasacral Rod Technique

The Jackson intrasacral rod technique is a powerful adjunctive method of sacral fixation that reduces the strain on S1 screws without fixation into the ilium. It is also very low profile and ideal for patients with thin soft tissues that may breakdown over iliac bolts. It is technically demanding, requiring perfect rod contouring and caudal to cranial rod insertion. Specialized Jackson intrasacral curette and pedicle screw and rod system that contains mono-axial pedicle screws with closed heads is also required. If used for long fusions to the sacrum, the need for caudal to cranial rod placement may be a significant limitation. In these cases the use of separate cranial and caudal rods that are joined by a domino or other rod connector may be very helpful. Biomechanical testing has shown it to provide robust fixation that is more effective for bending resistance than rotation and is very dependent upon sacral bone stock. The technique requires fluoroscopy and closed top S1 screws with a low profile head. This allows for countersinking into the sacrum and assists guiding of the rod into the proper portion of the sacrum.

The approach for using the intrasacral rod technique starts with the preparation of a S1 pedicle screw tract as described above. Next, an appropriate length closed headed pedicle screw is advanced through the screw tract and the head of the screw countersunk into the bone until, the top of the screw is nearly flush with the dorsal surface of the sacrum. A curette is used to expose the cranial aspect of the screw head, including the portion that accepts the rod. The special Jackson intrasacral curette or right angle awl is passed through the screw head and advanced caudally into the sacrum under fluoroscopic guidance. The curette should be directed along the long axis of the sacrum in the sagittal plane and slightly lateral in the coronal plane. The curette is advanced under constant pressure until the inferior cortex is encountered, just medial to the distal portion of the sacroiliac joint. The curette is then advanced through the cortex to create the exit hole. The tract is palpated with a pedicle sound and the length of the tract measured. The rod is then cut to length, incorporating the needs of the rest of the construct, and carefully contoured to match the created rod tract. The rod is inserted into the closed head of the S1 screw and carefully advanced through the screw tract under fluoroscopic guidance. Small rotational movements aid the passage of the rod. Once the rod reaches and passes the exit hole, a set screw is applied to the S1 screw to lockdown the construct (Figs 36.6 to 36.8). The process is then repeated on the contralateral side and the rod reduced down to the cranial portion of the construct. Reduction of the caudal construct to the cranial construct is a powerful maneuver that can greatly aid the creation of lumbosacral lordosis.

S2 Alar Screws

The vertebral body of S2 is much smaller than the body of S1, typically having roughly 60% of the anteroposterior dimensions of S1.[21] The bone quality is also lesser, leaving the surgeon with a dubious combination of short screws with little purchase. With these limitations, most choose to use the S2 screw as more of an alar screw, directing in a superolateral direction to increase length and capture the alar bone stock. A few biomechanical studies have included S2 screws as a mode of fixation and most studies have found them to be inferior to iliac screws if testing was performed

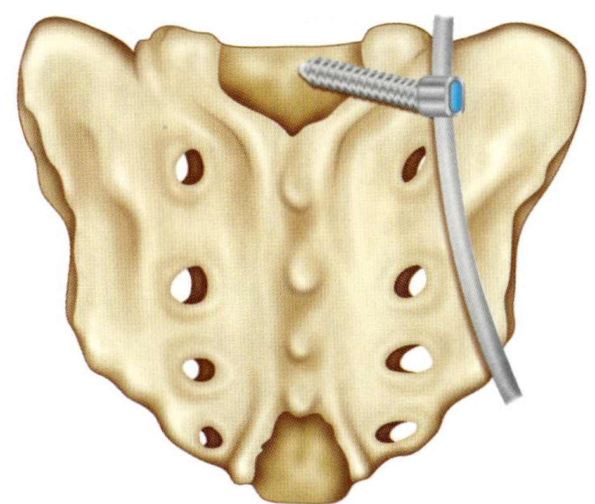

Fig. 36.6 Dorsal view of the Jackson intrasacral rod

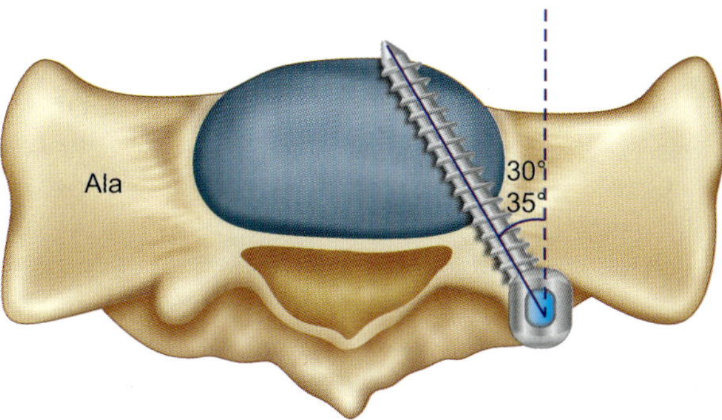

Fig. 36.7 Axial view of Jackson intrasacral rod

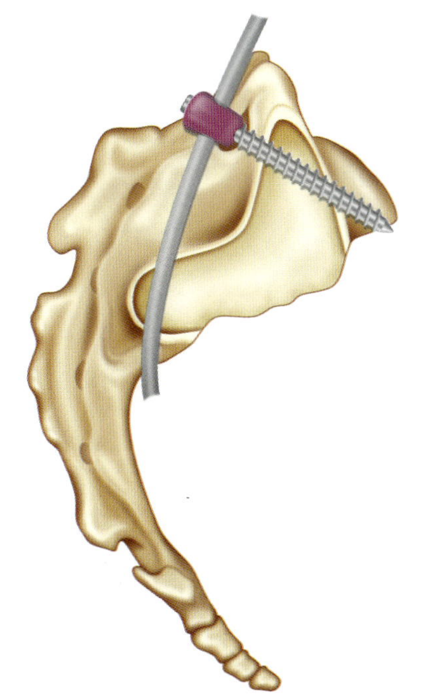

Fig. 36.8 Lateral view of Jackson intrasacral rod

on cadavers.[20-24] However, S2 screws remain an effective technique to supplement S1 pedicle screws, especially as a salvage technique for those who cannot have iliac fixation, such as those who previously had substantial posterior iliac crest harvesting for bone graft. S2 screws are also useful in patients, who have failure of fixation through S1, including S1 screw pullout, traumatic fracture of S1 or insufficiency fracture of S1.[25]

Insertion of S2 alar screws begins with midline exposure inferior to the S2 dorsal foramen. Lateral exposure should extend to the tip of the ala craniolaterally and laterally to the lateral sacral crest. Bony surfaces should be carefully cleaned so that key landmarks can be identified, particularly the dorsal intermediate crest and dorsal foramina. The dorsal foramina of S1 and S2 are identified as key landmarks for screw placement, but care must be taken to avoid brisk bleeding from the accompanying branches of the sinu vertebral arteries. A pilot hole is created using a high speed burr, the starting point is midway between the S1 and S2, dorsal foramina on the lateral edge of the foramina. A pedicle probe is introduced into the pilot hole and directed superolaterally towards the apex of the ala. The proper angle varies between patients, but is typically 50° to 60° cranial and 30° to 40° lateral from the posterior axis of the sacrum. Once far cortex is encountered, the pedicle probe can be gently tapped through with mallet (Figs 36.9 to 36.11). Typical screw lengths are 35–50 mm if bicortical purchase is achieved and should be measured on advanced imaging. Using fluoroscopic guidance is helpful in placing alar screws. Bicortical purchase is biomechanically superior for alar screws, but riskier as injury to neurovascular structures is much more common with bicortical alar screws than bicortical S1 screws. Screw tracts that are too short are usually not aimed cranial or lateral enough.

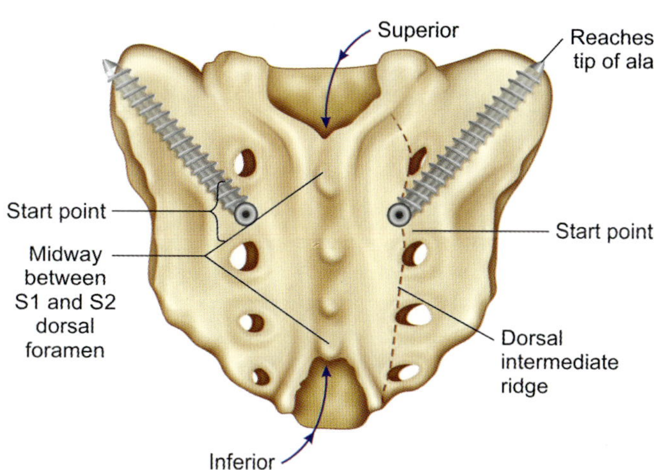

Fig. 36.9 Ideal start point of S2 alar screws between S1 and S2 foramina

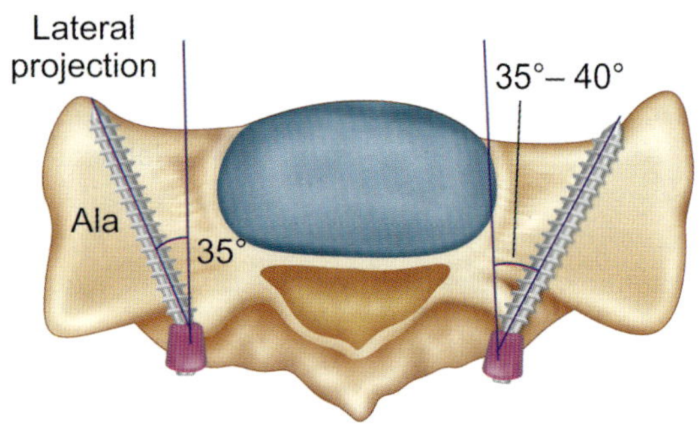

Fig. 36.10 Ideal trajectory on the axial view of S2 alar screws

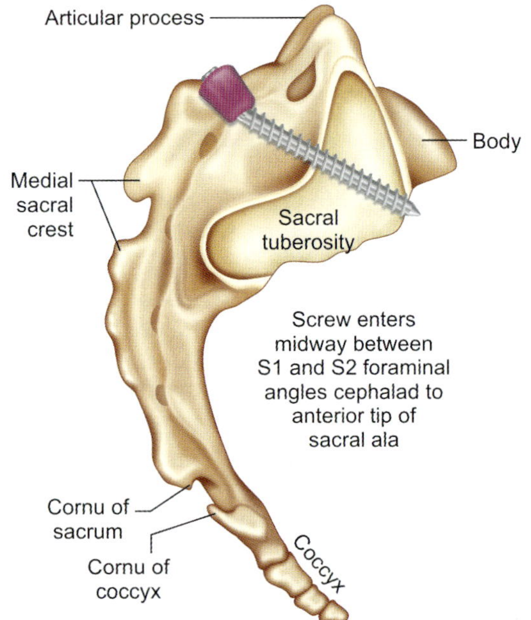

Fig. 36.11 Ideal trajectory on the lateral view of S2 alar screws

Chopin Plate/Colorado II Sacral Plate

The established limitations of stand-alone S1 pedicle screws or alar screws led to a combined fixation system originally termed "the sacral block". This implant was developed and reported by Chopin in 1991 and combines an S1 pedicle screw with an alar screw placed into one sacral plate with one fixation point. The concept of two divergent sacral screws has been biomechanically validated and compared to a single S1 pedicle screw was found to grant superior fixation with greater stiffness and loads to failure.[26] The Chopin plate has been adopted by the Colorado II plate system (Medtronic ™) as an available alternative to S1 pedicle screws and can still be used in conjunction with iliac screws. The disadvantages of the Chopin plate include slightly more dissection for placement of the plate and more constraint for the placement of the S1 pedicle screws and alar screws. Additionally, the screw or plate system is of a conventional design (non-locking) and the potential for sequential screw pull-out and failure exists as it does for independent screws. Nevertheless, this system remains superior to S1 pedicles screws alone or alar screws alone.

Surgical insertion of the Chopin plate begins with the standard exposure for S1 pedicle screws and is then extended to visualize the sacral ala to match the Chopin plate footprint. Overhang of the iliac wing over the sacral ala can increase the difficulty of placing the plate and screws. Once the S1 pedicle screw tract is made the Chopin or Colorado II sacral plate is then applied to the sacrum, oriented longitudinally so that it sits relatively flush on the sacrum. The proximal hole of the plate should directly overly the pilot hole for the S1 screw. The S1 screw is then screwed down through the plate, though it should not be over tightened to avoid tilting the plate. The plate itself assists with orienting the alar screw, a starting awl is used to make the pilot home and a pedicle probe advanced through the plate and into the ala. The pedicle probe should be directed 30° to 35° anterolateral and should not penetrate the SI joint. The length of the screw path is checked and the alar screw placed through the plate and into the ala. The S1 and alar screws are tightened in an alternating fashion to ensure that the plate stays well applied to the bone (Figs 36.12 to 36.14). The sacral plate can then be connected to the remainder of the fixation in the usual fashion.

Complications of Sacral Fixation

Some complications of sacral fixation obviously unique to the previously discussed techniques; however, there are

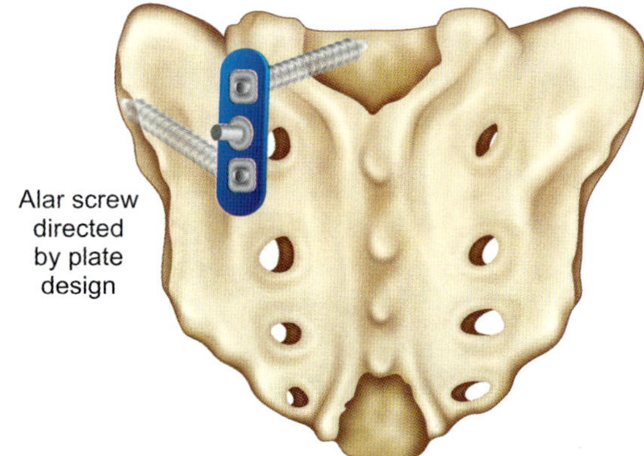

Fig. 36.12 Dorsal view of the Chopin plate system/Colorado II plate system. Note the S1 pedicle screw has standard startpoint and the S2 screw startpoint dictated by design of the plate, overall resulting in divergent screws

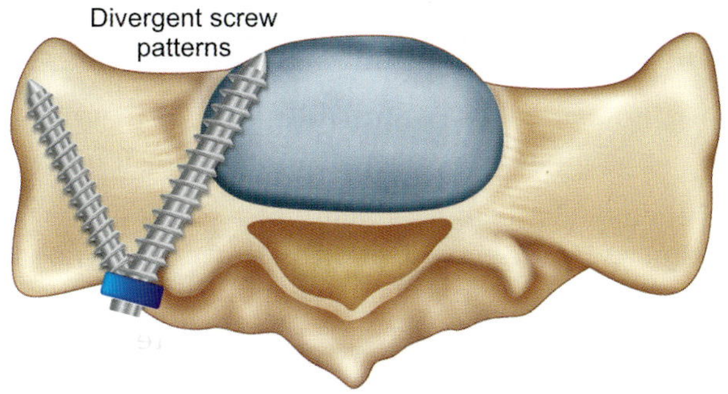

Fig. 36.13 Axial view of the Chopin plate system/Colorado II plate system

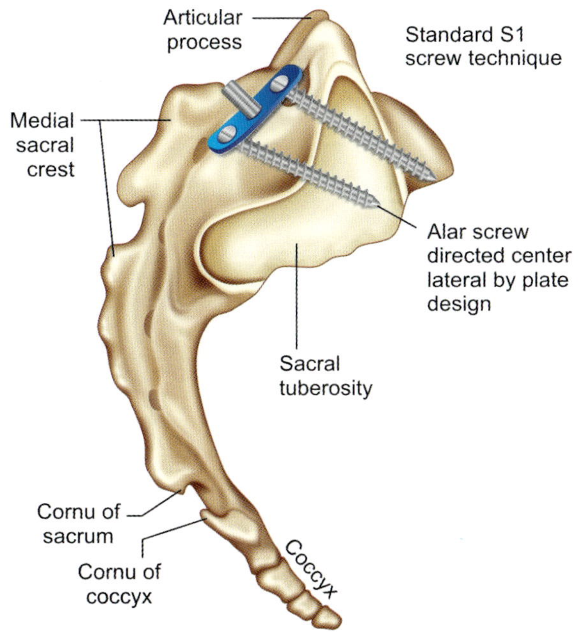

Fig. 36.14 Lateral view of the Chopin plate system/Colorado II plate system, note screws are slightly convergent, with the S2 screw directed towards apex of the ala

some complications shared by all sacral fixation techniques. Most of these complications occur due to violation of the anterior cortex and injury to the structures anterior to the sacrum, with the specific structure injured related to the trajectory of the implant. S1 screws place convergently put the middle sacral artery and vein and the superior hypogastric plexus at risk. S1 screws placed directly anterior can place all anterior structures at risk depending on the start site, particularly the common iliac vein on the left. Diverging S1 screws directed towards the ala risk injury of the common or internal iliac vasculature, namely the arteries. All S1 screws place the sacrum at risk for fracture at the level of the pedicle; this can be prevented by augmenting S1 screws with S2 alar screws, S2 alar iliac screws or iliac bolts, which provides the strongest construct. S2 converging screws can injure the inferior hypogastric plexus or colon with deep perforation of the anterior cortex or excessively long screws.

Pelvic Fixation

Iliac Bolt

Iliac bolts evolved from sacral fixation and the failures seen at the lumbosacral junction, namely pseudarthrosis and sacral fractures. Galveston rods were one of the earliest, widespread techniques to reinforce sacral fixation and anchor longitudinal spinal instrumentation constructs to the pelvis. Galveston rod technique required complicated rod contouring to allow, it to be placed between the inner and outer table of the iliac wing. The use of polyaxial screws inserted into the iliac wing have obviated the need for the complex rod contouring found in the Galveston technique by allowing connection to the longitudinal rod using a rodded connector to the iliac fixation screw.

Indications for the use of iliac bolts include long fusions to the sacrum, L2 and superiorly, as in neuromuscular scoliosis or flat-back deformity requiring corrective osteotomy treatment. Additional indications include grade III or higher spondylolisthesis due to the high stress at the S1 screws,[27-29] sacral fractures with spino-pelvic dissociation, and lumbosacral fusions in patients with osteoporosis as in adult scoliosis.

After standard midline approach to the spine, the incised midline fascia is towel clipped back together using one or two clips. Dissection in the plane superficial to the fascia is carried out from the midline, using palpation of the posterior superior iliac spine (PSIS) to guide the level and amount of dissection which should be as minimal as possible (Fig. 36.15). Using palpation, the fascia is then incised with electrocautery over the PSIS approximately 5 centimeters (cm), and the periosteum is dissected off the PSIS both laterally and medially (Figs 36.16 and 36.17). The medial dissection is carried out until it communicates with the midline dissection. The lateral dissection is carried out to the edge of the outer table at which point a sharp cobb or periosteal elevator can be used to expose the outer table along the trajectory of the iliac bolt. This allows clinical guidance of the broach and screw during placement; there is an arcade of bone that can be palpated and the screw trajectory should follow this arcade (Fig. 36.18).

With the PSIS exposed and the outer table dissected allowing for palpation and visual guidance of the broach and screw trajectory, insertion of the iliac bolt can proceed. A large rounger is used to remove approximately a 1 cm cube of bone from the PSIS, this allows access to the cancellous bone and helps to recess the polyaxial head of the bolt to reduce instrumentation prominence. A T-handle or Lenke probe is then used to dilate a screw path, the trajectory is guided by visualization of the outer table and palpation of the arcade of bone (Fig. 36.19). This arcade of bone represents the thickest bone in this region of the pelvis and placing the bolt

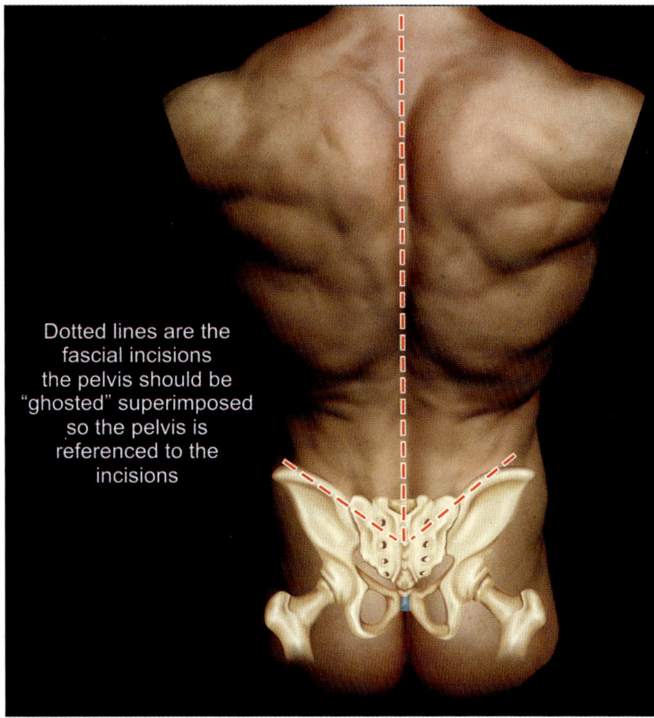

Fig. 36.15 Diagram of prone patient with midline and two lateral fascial incisions for iliac bolt placement

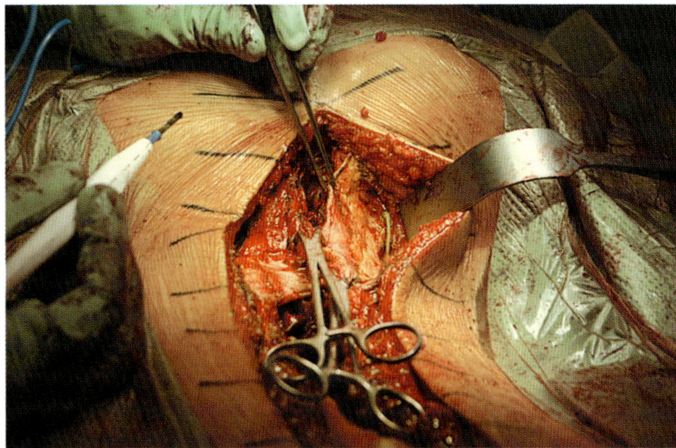

Fig. 36.16 Diagram of incision of midline fascia with towel clip and planned lateral incisions for iliac bolt placement

here decreases the chance of inner or outer table breaches. Using rotation more than a longitudinal force, the broach is advanced to approximately 8 cm and the tract is palpated and measured with the ball tip probe to ensure there is a cylinder of bone with a floor. The tract is then tapped with

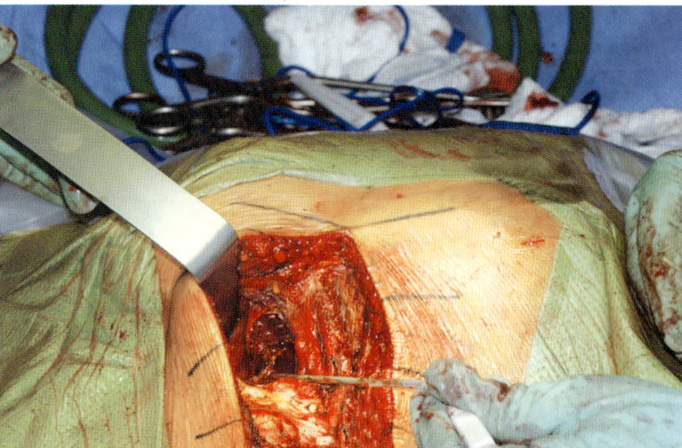

Fig. 36.17 Exposed PSIS is the start site for the iliac bolt and can be easily palpated through the fascia to guide the lateral fascial incision

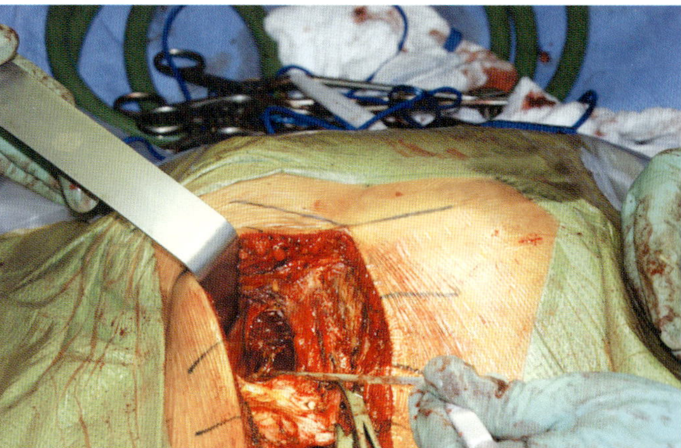

Fig. 36.18 Exposure of lateral iliac wall can visualize the iliac bolt trajectory while palpation of the column of bone superior to the greater sciatic notch can also guide screw placement down this column of bone

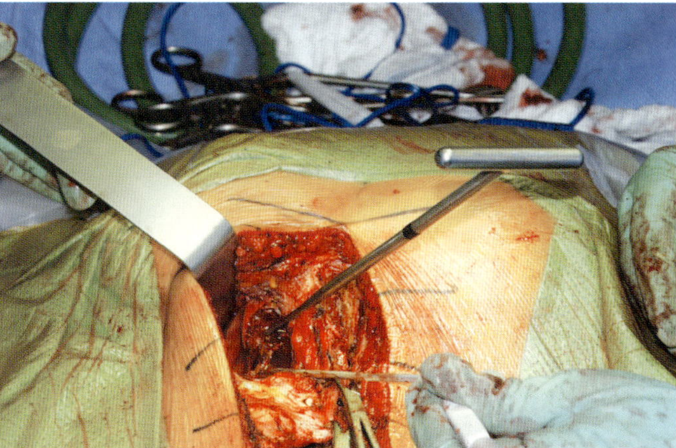

Fig. 36.19 Diagram of insertion of T handle broach

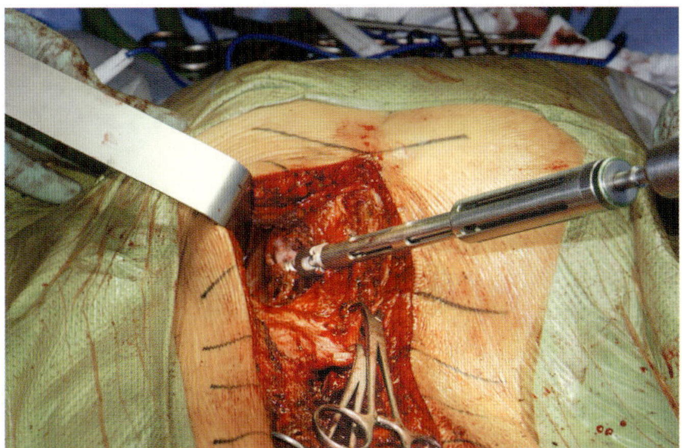

Fig. 36.20 Diagram of insertion of iliac bolt

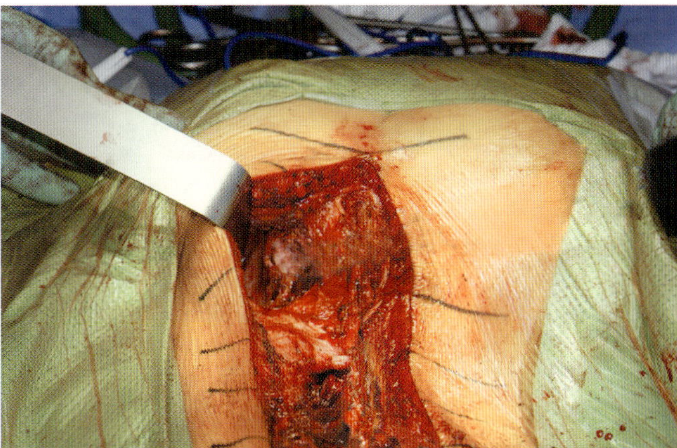

Fig. 36.21 Diagram of lifting fascial slip between the midline and lateral fascial incisions over the iliac bolt polyaxial head to visualize the head in the midline wound

the appropriate size tap and the screw is inserted. The iliac bolt size is usually 8 by 80 millimeters (mm) in average sized adults and adolescents, smaller children tolerate a 6 mm screw and the length should be determined using the ball tip probe and a ruler (Fig. 36.20).

The structures at risk during iliac bolt placement are the acetabulum and the sciatic notch. Within the sciatic notch lie the superior gluteal artery and the sciatic nerve. By exposing the outer table, which allows for visualization and palpation, the sciatic notch can be avoided. The notch can be palpated through the overlying soft tissues and a finger can be placed there during broaching to insure the broach is directed superior to the notch. Violation of the acetabulum can be avoided by using more rotation than longitudinal force when inserting the broach, the thick cortical bone of the dome of the acetabulum can be palpated and differentiated from the cancellous bone with the broach and more easily so with the ball tip probe. In osteoporotic patients where the cortical bone will not be as strong and easy to differentiate, alternating between the ball tip probe and broach is helpful.

There is no fusion across the sacroiliac (SI) joint, hence no decortication is necessary lateral to the sacrum. The sacral ala and lamina of S1 are decorticated using a high speed burr after irrigation and prior to application of bone graft.

Once the screw has been inserted the laterally incised fascia can be placed superior to the iliac bolt and the screw head will be visualized in the midline dissection provided by the medial dissection of the periosteum from the PSIS (Fig. 36.21). The iliac bolts must have a polyaxial head to facilitate connection to the longitudinal rods. A rodded connector, usually of length 40 mm, is used to attach the bolts to the longitudinal rods (Figs 36.22 and 36.23). Although rarely necessary, the rodded connectors themselves can be contoured to allow attachment, for example if the

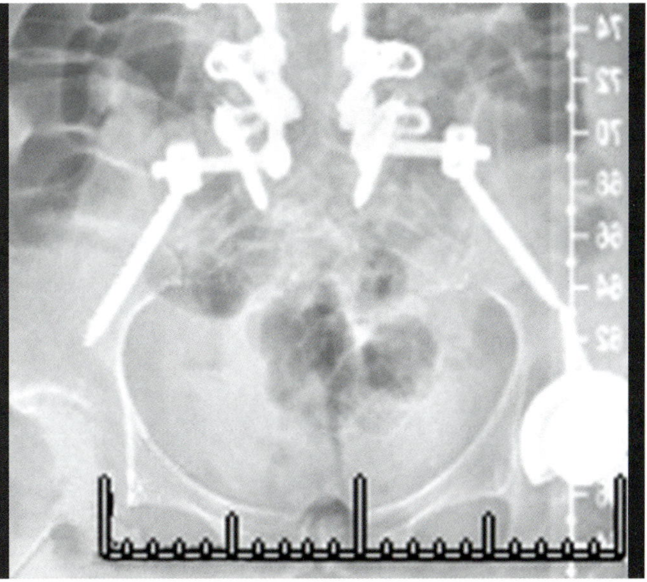

Fig. 36.22 Diagram of the use of a rodded connector from iliac bolt to longitudinal rod with L5 pedicle screws

longitudinal rod is cut too short. The lateral fascial incisions should be closed prior to the midline fascial closure to allow ease of closing the less accessible lateral fascial incisions.

S2 Alar Iliac Screw

The S2 alar iliac screw has been championed by some surgeons as a more advantageous alternative to iliac bolts due to less hardware prominence and positioning the screw head in line with the longitudinal rod of the fusion construct. The screw is placed by starting 2–4 mm lateral and 4–8 mm inferior to the S1 foramen. A 2.5 mm drill is used to

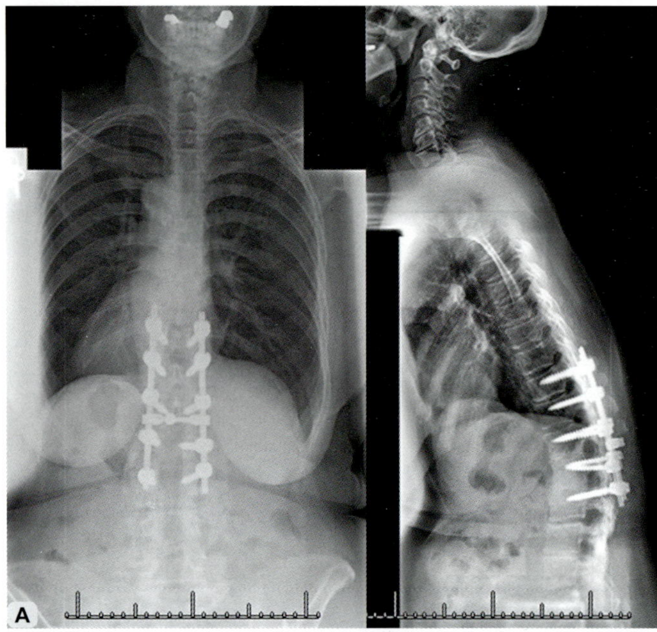

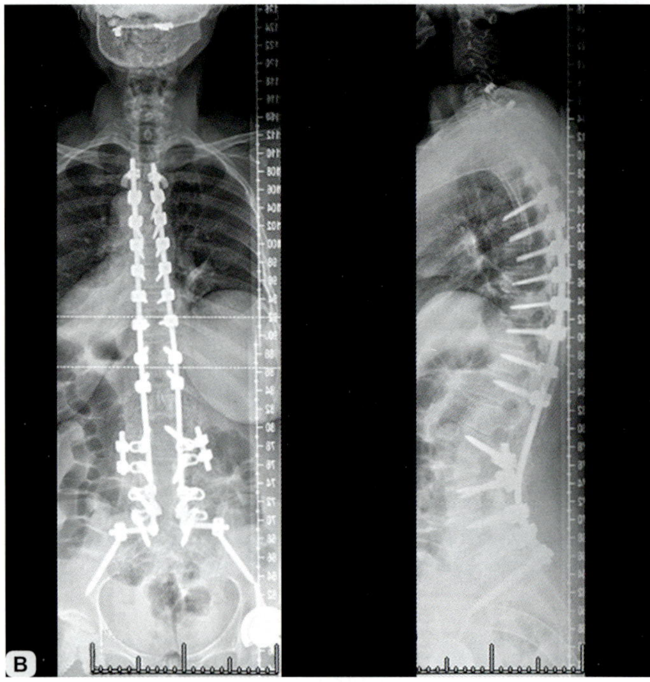

Fig. 36.23 (A) Pre- and (B) postoperative radiographs of flat back deformity correction utilizing iliac bolts

drill through the S2 ala, across the SI joint, in to the ilium. Once the ilium is entered the 2.5 mm drill is exchanged for 3.2 mm to prevent breakage. The trajectory is 40° lateral and 20° to 30° inferior, the path should be 20 mm above the greater sciatic notch[30] (Figs 36.24 and 36.25). Fluoroscopy can be helpful, the teardrop view of the hemi pelvis should be obtained and the screw path should be in the teardrop.

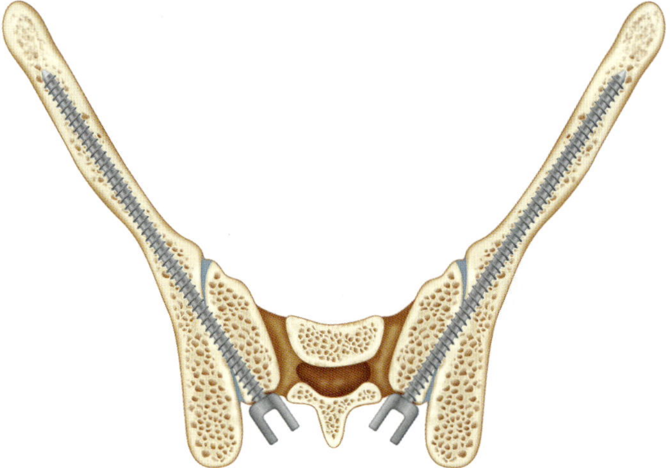

Fig. 36.24 Diagram of the S2 alar iliac screw

Complications of Pelvic Fixation

The structures at risk during iliac bolt placement are the acetabulum and the sciatic notch. Within the sciatic notch lie the superior gluteal artery and the sciatic nerve. The superior portion of the greater sciatic notch can be palpated inferiorly to the column of bone in the ilium that the screw path should be in. Palpation of the notch and column of bone, as well as, visualization of the column of bone should prevent breaching into the sciatic notch. Violation of the medial wall of the iliac bolt can put the internal iliac artery and vein at risk for injury, as well as, lumbar plexus or sciatic nerve. A mild injury from medial wall violation would be an iliacus hematoma.

Instrumentation prominence leading to pain and overlying soft tissue irritation is the most common complication. The iliac bolts can be removed once there is certainty that lumbosacral fusion has occurred. Removal rates of iliac bolts of 22–34% have been reported.[31-33] Removal before fusion can result in kyphosis and breakage of remaining instrumentation of the sacrum.

Implant loosening despite lumbosacral fusion may be symptomatic and require screw removal. Loosening in the ilium may be related to motion at the SI joint. Motion at the SI joint may also cause loosing of the cross connector; however, if lumbosacral fusion is achieved this is not problematic. Loosening or breakage without fusion at the lumbosacral junction can occur as at any level in an instrumented spinal fusion. Some authors recommend anterior column support with interbody fusion at L4–L5 and L5–S1. These interbody grafts are anterior to the lumbosacral pivot point and hence subject to compression, facilitating fusion and decreasing the chance of iliac screw loosening or breakage due to pseudarthrosis and fatigue stress.[34-37] Pseudarthrosis rates

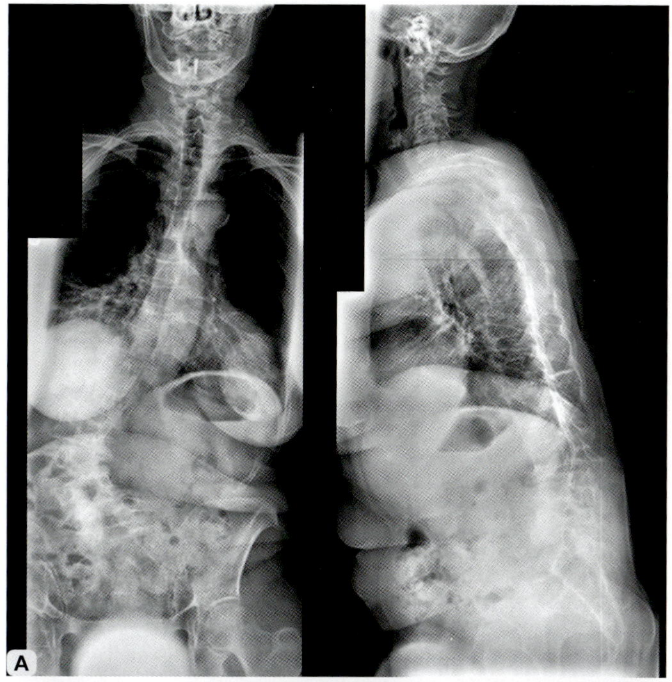

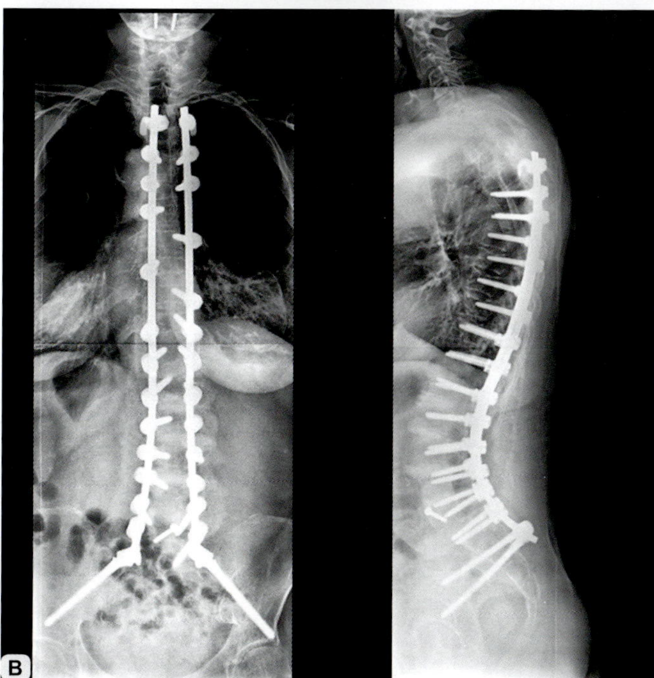

Fig. 36.25 (A) Pre- and (B) postoperative radiographs of flat back deformity correction utilizing S2 alar iliac screws

range from 5% to 17% depending on factors host factors and fusion construct, for example, inclusion of S1 pedicle screws and anterior fusion, both of which decreased the pseudarthrosis rate.[38,39]

Infection rate as high as 4% was seen in one study. This increase may be attributed to the necessary soft tissue dissection as well as the overlying soft tissue coverage.[40]

Conclusion

Instrumentation across the lumbosacral junction has evolved with time and understanding of the biomechanics and stresses across the lumbosacral junction. Of the many techniques described above, currently use S1 pedicle screws and iliac bolts are the most widespread. S1 screws alone for patients requiring fusion and instrumentation of the lower lumbar spine, to L3, have been accepted and declared suitable with biomechanical testing. Longer fusions have required anterior augmentation of L4–5 and L5–S1 or iliac bolts to reduce the stress at the S1 pedicle screws and reduce the risk of pseudarthrosis. With newer techniques like the S2 alar iliac screw, surgeons look to continue to enjoy the benefits of improved sacropelvic fixation with less risk and lower complications in the future.

References

1. King D. Internal fixation for lumbosacral fusion. J Bone Joint Surg Am. 1948 Jul;30A(3):560-5.
2. Thompson WAL, Ralston EL. Pseudarthrosis following spine fusion, J. Bone Joint Surg. 1949;31A:400.
3. White AH, Zucherman JF, Hsu K. Lumbosacral fusions with Harrington rods and intersegmental wiring. Clin Orthop Relat Res. 1986;(203):185-90.
4. Harrington PR. Treatment of scoliosis: correction and internal fixation by spine instrumentation. J Bone Joint Surg Am. 1962;44:591-610.
5. Olsson TH, Selvik G, Willner S. Mobility in the lumbosacral spine after fusion studied with the aid of roentgen stereophotogrammetry. Clin Orthop Relat Res. 1977;(129):181-90.
6. Balderston RA, Winter RB, Moe JH, Bradford DS, Lonstein JE. Fusion to the sacrum for nonparalytic scoliosis in the adult. Spine. 1986;11:824-9.
7. Kostuik JP. Treatment of scoliosis in the adult thoracolumbar spine with special reference to fusion to the sacrum. Orthop Clin North Am. 1988;19:371-81.
8. Casey MP, Asher MA, Jacobs RR, Orrick JM. The effect of Harrington rod contouring on lumbar lordosis. Spine (Phila Pa 1976). 1987;12(8):750-3.
9. Moe JH, Purcell GA, Bradford DS. Zielke instrumentation (VDS) for the correction of spinal curvature. Analysis of results in 66 patients. Clin Orthop Relat Res. 1983;(180):133-53.
10. Kostuik JP. Recent advances in the treatment of painful adult scoliosis. Clin Orthop Relat Res. 1980;(147):238-52.

11. Kostuik JP, Hall BB. Spinal fusions to the sacrum in adults with scoliosis. Spine (Phila Pa 1976). 1983;8(5):489-500.
12. Wiltse LL, Kirkaldy-Willis WH, McIvor GW. The treatment of spinal stenosis. Clin Orthop Relat Res. 1976;(115):83-91.
13. White AH, Wynne G, Taylor LW. Knodt rod distraction lumbar fusion. Spine (Phila Pa 1976). 1983;8(4):434-7.
14. White AH, Zucherman JF, Hsu K. Lumbosacral fusions with Harrington rods and intersegmental wiring. Clin Orthop Relat Res. 1986;(203):185-90.
15. Selby D. Internal fixation with Knodt's rods. Clin Orthop Relat Res. 1986;(203):179-84.
16. Roy-Camille R, Roy-Camille M, Demeulenaere C. Osteosynthesis of dorsal, lumbar, and lumbosacral spine with metallic plates screwed into vertebral pedicles and articular apophyses. Presse Med. 1970;78(32):1447-8.
17. Harrington PR, Dickson JH. Spinal instrumentation in the treatment of severe progressive spondylolisthesis. Clin Orthop Relat Res. 1976;(117):157-63.
18. Steffee AD, Sitkowski DJ, Topham LS. Total vertebral body and pedicle arthroplasty. Clin Orthop Relat Res. 1986;(203):203-8.
19. Krag MH, Beynnon BD, Pope MH, Frymoyer JW, Haugh LD, Weaver DL. An internal fixator for posterior application to short segments of the thoracic, lumbar, or lumbosacral spine. Design and testing. Clin Orthop Relat Res. 1986;(203):75-98.
20. Zindrick MR, Wiltse LL, Widell EH, et al. A biomechanical study of intrapedicular screw fixation in the lumbosacral spine. Clin Orthop. 1986;203:99-112.
21. Asher MA, Strippgen WE. Anthropometric studies of the human sacrum relating to dorsal transsacral implant designs. Clin Orthop Relat Res. 1986;203:58-62.
22. McCord DH, Cunningham BW, Shono Y, Myers JJ, McAfee PC. Biomechanical analysis of lumbosacral fixation. Spine (Phila Pa 1976). 1992;17(8 Suppl):S235-43.
23. Ruland CM, McAfee PC, Warden KE, Cunningham BW. Triangulation of pedicular instrumentation. A biomechanical analysis. Spine (Phila Pa 1976). 1991;16(6 Suppl):S270-6.
24. Nagel DA, Edwards WT, Schneider E. Biomechanics of spinal fixation and fusion. Spine 1991;16(suppl):151-4.
25. Alegre GM, Gupta MC, Bay BK, Smith TS, Laubach JE. S1 screw bending moment with posterior spinal instrumentation across the lumbosacral junction after unilateral iliac crest harvest. Spine (Phila Pa 1976). 2001;26(18):1950-5.
26. Leong JC, Lu WW, Zheng Y, Zhu Q, Zhong S. Comparison of the strengths of lumbosacral fixation achieved with techniques using one and two triangulated sacral screws. Spine (Phila Pa 1976). 1998;23(21):2289-94.
27. Bridwell KH, Kuklo T, Edwards CC II, et al. Sacropelvic Fixation. Memphis, TN. Medtronic Sofamor Danek; 2004.
28. Chewning SJ Jr. Pelvic fixation. Spine State Art Rev. 1992;6:359-68.
29. Potter BK, Kuklo TR, O'Brien MF. Sacro-iliac fixation for treatment of high-grade spondylolisthesis. Semin Spine Surg. 2004;16:119-25.
30. Kebaish KM. Sacropelvic Fixation Techniques and Complications. Spine (Phila Pa 1976). 2010;35:2245-51.
31. Emami A, Deviren V, Berven S, et al. Outcome and complications of long fusions to the sacrum in adult spine deformity: Luque-Galveston, combined iliac and sacral screws, and sacral fixation. Spine (Phila Pa 1976). 2002;27:776-86.
32. Tsuchiya K, Bridwell KH, Kuklo TR, et al. Minimum 5-year analysis of L5–S1 fusion using sacropelvic fixation (bilateral S1 and iliac screws) for spinal deformity. Spine (Phila Pa 1976). 2006;31:303-8.
33. Weistroffer JK Perra, JH, Lonstein JE, Schwender JD, Garvey TA, Transfeldt EE, et al. Complications in long fusions to the sacrum for adult scoliosis minimum five-year analysis of fifty patients. Spine (Phila Pa 1976). 2008;33(13):1478-83.
34. Allen BL Jr, Ferguson RL. The Galveston technique of pelvic fixation with L-rod instrumentation of the spine. Spine (Phila Pa 1976). 1984;9:388-94.
35. Allen BL Jr, Ferguson RL. A pictorial guide to the Galveston LRI pelvic fixation technique. Contemp Orthop. 1983;7:51-61.
36. Allen BL Jr, Ferguson RL. The Galveston experience with L-rod instrumentation for adolescent idiopathic scoliosis. Clin Orthop Relat Res. 1988;229:59-69.
37. Farcy JPC, Margulies JY. Iliosacral screw fixation. In Margulies JY, Floman Y, Farcy JP, et al. (eds): Lumbosacral and Spinopelvic Fixation. Philadelphia, PA: Lippincott-Raven;1996. pp 601-9.
38. Kim YJ, Bridwell KH, Lenke LG, Cho KJ, Edwards II CC, Rinella AS. Spinal deformity following multisegmental instrumentation and arthodesis. JBJS. 2006;88A,4:721-8.
39. Kim YJ, Bridwell KH, Lenke LG, Rinella AS, Edwards II C. Pseudarthrosis in primary fusions for adult idiopathic scoliosis: Incidence, Risk Factors, and Outcome Anaylsis. Spine (Phila Pa 1976). 2005;30:468-74.
40. Kuklo TR, Bridwell KH, Lewis SJ, et al. Minimum 2-year analysis of sacropelvic fixation and L5–S1 fusion using S1 and iliac screws. Spine (Phila Pa 1976). 2001;26:1976-83.

CHAPTER

37

Surgery for Sacrum Tumors

Mehmet Zileli

Primary sacral tumors, although rare, include benign neoplasms, such as osteochondroma, giant cell tumors, and osteoid osteoma, as well as the more common malignant lesions such as chordoma, osteosarcoma, and myeloma.[1,2] Because of their mild symptoms, sacral neoplasms are usually not diagnosed early in their disease course. These tumors are often large by the time they are diagnosed, and they then pose a technically challenging surgical problem. Excision of malignant or benign, aggressive sacral tumors with intralesional margins is rarely curative, because of the high likelihood of local recurrence.[1,3] A radical surgical approach, such as partial or total sacrectomy, with sacrifice of sacral roots, is often warranted to achieve total resection with wide margins.[4] The risk of infection, loss of large amounts of blood, wound complications, and neurological dysfunction are problems associated with sacrectomy. Total sacrectomy also presents the challenge of spinal-pelvic fixation to achieve stabilization after complete dissociation of the spine and pelvis.[5] In this report, we present a surgical series of patients with primary sacral tumors and discuss the challenges associated with sacrectomies.

Radical sacrum surgery and sacrectomy is a long and troublesome approach which a good teamwork is necessary. Problems such as over bleeding, wound problems, appropriate stabilization should be solved and new techniques are necessary for those challenging issues. In spite of these problems, an extramarginal resection aiming an oncologic surgery can be performed and a curative result may be achieved in comparison to mobile spine.

Pathology

The most frequent primary tumor in sacrum is chordomas.[6] They originate from primitive notochord and have a very aggressive behavior. Approximately, one third of chordomas are localized in skull base, and 50% are in sacrococcygeal region. Localization in mobile spine is quite rare (15–20%).[7,8]

Since they cause no symptoms for long periods, sacral chordomas may reach giant dimensions and hence their removal may be quite hard. They can invade sacral roots and a radical surgery may risk the roots. Although rare, they can metastasize to lung and other bones. Local recurrence of chordomas is quite often and although histology is like a benign tumor their behavior is very malignant.[9]

Sacral chordomas are aggressive malignant tumors that can metastasize although their histopathology is benign.

Since the survival time is most affected by tumor free margins of excision material, an aggressive surgery is necessary.

Clinic

The most frequent symptom is the local axial pain. In later stages, sphincter problems, erection disturbance, distal motor paralysis may develope. If they reach giant dimensions, they can cause rectal obstruction and venous edema in lower extremities.

Surgery

In general, surgical decision making in sacrum tumors must start with a biopsy. If the biopsy shows a metastasis or a histology sensitive to chemotherapy, initial therapy must be started with radiotherapy or chemotherapy. If it is a primary tumor such as chordoma, chondrosarcoma or giant cell tumor, the first step must be a radical surgery.

In primary malignant tumors or aggressive benign tumors, an extramarginal resection without entering the tumor mass must be the aim of the surgery.[10-13] However, since such a resection is a major and complicated approach and may result with significant morbidity which may not be accepted by the patients, intralesional surgery and curettage are the type of the surgery in most instances. Chordomas do not respond chemotherapy and resistant to radiation.[4,14,15] For that reason, a radical extramarginal resection aiming intact borders in postoperative histological examination is a well accepted view by many surgeons.[4,14,15] As mentioned before, the amount of resection is associated with functional deficits.[15,16-20] For a better surgical planning, the expected deficits must be discussed with the patient.[20]

For radical excision of primary sacral tumors, three approaches have been described. Radicality against preserving the upper three sacral roots are the biggest concerns in all of them:

1. ***Posterior approach:*** Tumors arising caudal to S2 level may be excised by a posterior only approach. Such a surgery is quite shorter and results with less morbidity. Excessive bleeding, penetration of the pelvic organs are the major risks.
   In tumors localized to distal sacrum and coccyx the dissection may be started with a transperineal or transcoccygeal approach. However, such small tumors are quite rare and only 10% of primary sacral tumors are in this location and dimension. Some surgeons stress that a posterior only surgery is possible in tumors localized at and caudal to S3 level.[21] I believe that posterior approach could be performed in tumors at or caudal to S2 level, although the risk of entering the tumor is potential risk in this condition. Sacrificing the S2 roots bilaterally would cause significant bladder and fecal incontinence.
2. ***Combined anterior-posterior approach:*** Tumors invading S1 cannot be resected without overbleeding if the ventral control major vessels are not provided. Besides, perforation of the pelvic viscera may occur. Before starting posterior osteotomies a ventral dissection and mobilization of rectum, ureters, iliac arteries and veins are necessary. Ligation of internal iliac arteries and central sacral artery would help to decrease the bleeding. Then, a posterior surgery at the same session is performed.
3. ***Single stage abdominosacral approach:*** Some surgeons has preferred a simultaneous approach on lateral position. An oblique incision between iliac crest and lower edge of the ribs is used to enter the abdomen.[22] Colon and rectum are mobilized, left ureter is dissected, and pelvic structures were exposed until levator ani. Median and lateral sacral arteries are ligated. Without changing the position, posterior dissection is performed, muscular and ligamentous connections of the sacrum are cut.
   It is my preference to start the sacrectomy by an anterior retroperitoneal dissection, and posterior osteotomies at the same session.

Radical excision of primary sacral tumors by a so-called sacrectomy is possible,[19,23-30] but poses major problems such as preserving the sacral nerves, vascular and visceral structures, preventing excessive bleeding, wound problems and infection, and providing lumbosacral and sacroiliac stability (Table 37.1).

Radical resection may be the best available treatment for low-grade malignancies and aggressive, benign sacral tumors that are resistant to noninterventional therapies. Because they are technically difficult procedures, however, partial and total sacrectomies pose several complex challenges, and require the expertise of specialists from several fields.

Problems of Radical Sacrum Surgery and Sacrectomy

1. ***Preserving vascular structures:*** A total sacrectomy with a posterior only surgery is not possible because of anteriorly located iliac arteries and veins. Retroperitoneal or transperitoneal dissection of anterior structures, releasing arteries and veins from sacrum is an important part of surgery. This should be done before starting posterior surgery. These structures can be protected using meticulous dissection techniques, aided by a vascular surgeon for handling of the ventral compressed vascular structures. I personally prefer to sacrifice the median sacral artery and vein, internal iliac arteries and veins, and iliolumbar arteries by ligation to cut off the vascular supply to the sacrum and tumor.

Table 37.1 Problems of sacrectomy

Problems of sacrectomy
1. Preserving vascular structures
2. Preserving visceral structures
3. Preserving roots
4. Excessive bleeding
5. Wound problems and infection
6. Lumbosacral and sacroiliac stability

2. ***Preserving visceral structures:*** Care must also be taken to protect the visceral structures, including the ureters, urinary bladder, intestines, and rectum. Because of very anterior location, preserving the ureter and bladder is quite easy. However, rectum wall may be adherent to sacral tumor, even infiltrated. It is recommended to open an elective colostomy before primary surgery, to avoid rectal perforation. Cleaning colon before surgery is also important step for same reasons. An abdominal surgeon or vascular surgeon is necessary for dissections in this phase of surgery.
3. ***Preserving the roots and plexus:*** Neurological deficits resulting from the sacrifice of sacral nerve roots are extensive and permanent. There are two reasons of neurologic deficits after sacrectomy:
   a. Sacrificing sacral roots during sacrectomy. It is well known that the roots from S2 to S4 carry the primary afferent and efferents of sphincters and they are responsible from urinary and fecal continence. The key root in this region is S2. Bilateral preservation of S2 roots mean sphincter problem will not be so severe. Besides, unilateral loss of S2, S3 and S4 roots do not cause significant sphincter dysfunction.[26,31] However, in patients with bilateral section of S2, S3 and S4 roots desire for defecation decreases and, they cannot differentiate feces from gas, neither feel the fullness of bladder.
   b. Injury or stretch to the lumbosacral plexus around superior medial iliac crest or inside the sciatic notch. In this instance, neurological deficits are more like an L5 root involvement resulting with a foot drop.

   Functional results of the loss of sacral roots are as follows:
   a. Urinary incontinence. There happens a false bladder paralysis. Patients should either use drapes or permanent bladder catheters.
   b. Fecal incontinence. The patients describe incontinence in case of diarrhea. However, if the stool is hard, constipation prevents incontinence. They may discharge by increasing intra-abdominal pressure or with fingers.
   c. Loss of erection in male patients. It happens in most of the male patients. It may not occur in case of unilateral sacrifice of the roots.

   In total sacrectomies, most of the sacral roots invaded by the tumor are sacrificed, and this usually results in loss of bladder and sexual function and bowel control.[32,33] In most cases, preservation of the lumbar roots is possible, and they allow the patient to be ambulatory. Sparing the L5 root bilaterally may be adequate for plantar flexion of the foot.[17] Sacrificing the sacral roots in case of no significant sphincter disturbance before surgery are discussed as an ethical problem. The patient must be informed in detail about the disability of such an approach.
4. ***Excessive Bleeding:*** One of the important problems of sacral tumor surgery is excessive bleeding. The reasons are very rich blood supply of presacral area, epidural veins, large osteotomy for sacrectomy, excessive muscle dissection and resection. This may be a life-threatening problem in radical sacral surgery. Considerable blood loss (7–80 L in some series) has been reported.[34,35]

   Different methods to overcome excessive bleeding have been proposed. A meticulous bleeding control and muscle dissection done by monopolar cautery would significantly diminish bleeding, although they cause to increase the operation time. The other cautions recommended to overcome excessive bleeding are the application of bone wax on the osteotomy margins, spongostan, compressive gauzes, the application of polymethylmethacrylate,[36] fluid nitrogen,[37-40] phenol, hydrogen peroxidase, and hot water. Applying substances, such as hemostatic gauze, fibrin glue, or an omentum flap onto the bed of the tumor are also possibilities for preventing blood loss, as is cryosurgery.[41] Cell saver autotransfusion may be used following excessive blood loss, but it cannot be applied to malignant tumors. It must better be used before entering the tumor, since tumor cells will be distributed to the body if used during tumor aspiration.

   To overcome excessive bleeding a balloon dilation catheter may be placed in the distal abdominal aorta via the femoral artery which was also by used by our team.[42,43] Just after the skin incision, the balloon dilatation catheter was inflated with contrast medium and total occlusion of the aorta was achieved. We believe that this method prevents hemodynamical problems caused by massive bleeding and complications secondary to massive transfusion.[43]
5. ***Wound Problems and Infection:*** In many patients, the surgery may result with problems of skin closure, and sometime necrosis of the skin days and weeks after surgery.[29] There are many reasons of that—the skin incision of previous surgery must be resected to overcome recurrence. Excessive muscle and bone excision negatively affect the vascularization of the skin. Pressure to the skin increases with wide bone and muscle excision. These potential complications pose another challenge.[21,44-46]

   For those reasons, contribution of plastic surgeons is necessary by turning flaps to relieve the pressure on skin and also increase the vascularization on the skin. Vascularized flaps are also helpful to diminish the cavity after wide resections. Any tension on the skin must be relieved and soft tissues and muscles below must be reconstructed.

To facilitate wound healing, various types of muscle flaps and incisions were made. In partial sacrectomy, or in the presence of previous incisions, we made a median longitudinal incision. In total sacrectomy, in which the resulting tissue defect was large, we made a downward-based, C-shaped incision with a median longitudinal extension at its apex. We used gluteal muscles as a flap inside the defect, and in some cases a rectus abdominis myocutaneous pure island pedicle flap was used.[47]

Another issue in these cases is the cavity created by sacrectomy. In order to fill out this cavity with a viable tissue and reconstruction of the sacrum there are different maneuvers such as placing meshes to avoid rectum prolapse posteriorly, to fill the space with allograft bones in addition to sacropelvic fixation.

Infection is another problem after such long and bloody surgeries. There are numerous reasons of postoperative infection, some of which are working around rectum, excessive retraction of tissues, diminished vascularization of the remaining tissues and excessive blood transfusion. To avoid infection, surgeons must obey the intraoperative asepsis meticulously. The colon must be empty with preparation before surgery. In case of invasion of rectum, an elective colostomy must be performed before resection. Prophylactic antibiotherapy must always be applied. Some authors have proposed using a Vicryl net bag containing gentamicin beads to fill the defect, to prevent infection and herniation until the granulation tissue develops.[3]

6. ***Lumbosacral and sacroiliac stability:*** Spinal-pelvic stability is one of the most difficult challenges faced in total sacrectomy, partly because of the large loads carried by the lumbosacral junction, and the angular position of the sacrum. This region is a transition zone from the mobile spine to the rigid pelvis.

Distal amputations below sacroiliac joint do not cause instability. Even sacral amputations crossing from S1 foramina may not cause an instability because upper 1/3 of sacroiliac joint is preserved. This joint together with its anterior and posterior interosseous ligaments is a very strong structure and holds the sacrum. Even if a short segment of both sacroiliac joints is preserved, iliolumbar ligaments are very strong and instability would not develope. All sacrectomies rostral to S1 destabilizes the sacrum and pelvic ring, and warrants a fixation surgery. Total destruction of even one sacroiliac joint will cause a significant instability.[32,35,48,49] For patients with an intact sacrum and minimal spinal-pelvic instability, sacral and iliac screws may be sufficient.

If sacrectomy involves S1, stabilization must always be done. The pelvic ring has been cut, the relation between vertebral column and pelvis has been lost. When these patients stand up, pelvic tilt will be spoiled, lumbar vertebrae would sink down to the pelvis and they would feel significant pain and disability when walking. If the sacroiliac joint is spoiled unilaterally, the pelvic balance will be lost unilaterally and the gait of the patient would be similar to after shortening of one lower extremity.

The last stage of surgery must aim to achieve stability. However, if the duration of surgery has significantly increased, if too much blood transfused because of excessive bleeding, and plastic surgery planned flaps for skin protection, stabilization surgery may be delayed to a second stage.

Many different techniques for stabilization have been described. But, the most frequently applied and known technique is spinopelvic stabilization using Galveston rods.[25,27,29,50] In this technique, contoured rods bend with special rod bender are placed inside the iliac bone. Rods are anchored to lumbar vertebrae using pedicle screws.[29,46,51-55] We use a custom made system developed in Turkey for this purpose.[29]

Fixation Systems

Lumbar–iliac L-rod pelvic fixation, known as the Galveston technique, was the first system used for sacroiliac fixation, and was proposed by Allen and Ferguson[56] for the treatment of scoliosis and pelvic obliquity. Use of the sublaminar wiring described by these authors requires intact laminae, however, and does not provide as much rigidity as screws. Shikata et al.[57] described the first lumbar-iliac fixation system for sacrectomy in which a combination of Harrington rods and hooks, sacral bars, and massive bone grafts were used. Iliac bones were joined with the sacral bars, and L5 was lowered 2 cm and shifted anteriorly. This technique does not provide much rotational stability around the horizontal axis of the spine;[58] furthermore, the sacral bars joining the soft posterior iliac wings do not provide firm fixation.[59] Gokaslan et al.[58] modified the procedures described earlier. They replaced the sublaminar wiring used in the Galveston technique, and the Harrington rods, with lumbar pedicle screws. Two L-shaped Galveston rods were used to connect the lumbar pedicles to the iliac wings, one transiliac threaded rod was used to reconstruct the pelvic ring, and a tibial strut allograft was placed between the ilia to augment the instrumentation. Jackson and Gokaslan[24] also proposed rod insertion into the iliac wings. The modified Galveston technique described by Gokaslan et al. provides more rigidity than the wiring technique, but has the disadvantage of requiring rod contouring, which can be time-consuming and difficult.[24]

Custom-made systems have also been used successfully in lumbosacral reconstruction.[3,41,60] Wuisman et al. have used a three-dimensional, real-sized model to design and test a sacral prosthesis.[3] The prosthesis consisted of an L-shaped plate covering the L5 corpus vertebrae and the surface of the L5 endplate. An iliac wing flange covered and connected the remaining external anterior part of the iliac wing. To provide torsional stability, Althausen et al.[41] have used iliac screws and bolts, a reconstruction plate, and cross connectors of varying lengths to connect this system to lumbar pedicle screws and rods. The reconstruction system used by Salehi et al.[60] also included a transverse iliac bar and iliac screws, but the iliac bar traversed a mesh cage resting on the lower end plate of the L5 vertebral body.[60] This system allowed immediate spinal-pelvic stability and early ambulation in patients with metastatic tumors who underwent subtotal resection.

Our first stabilization system was semirigid, consisting of iliac plates fixed with navicular screws.[29] Because a significant amount of contouring was necessary during surgery, we modified the design in the last two cases. In those patients we used two transverse bars connected to lumbar rods with special connectors, and lumbar pedicle screws similar to those used by Gokaslan et al.[58] This modified system does not require rod contouring, and it is more rigid than the previous system of iliac plates and screws.

Surgical Technique

A posterior only surgery is sufficient for tumors at S2 or S3 (Figs 37.1 and 37.3). However, for tumors involving S1 a combined anterior-posterior approach is necessary (Figs 37.2, 37.4 and 37.5).

Our surgical team consisted of a spinal surgeon, an abdominal or vascular surgeon, and in some cases a plastic surgeon. In case of hemipelvectomy and/or if the tumor invades the hip joint, an orthopedic surgeon must also be in the team. Sacrectomy can be performed using either two sequential approaches,[28] which we preferred, or by using a synchronous AP approach in the lateral (right) position.[31,61] We perform sacrectomy in two sessions at the same stage:

I. ***Anterior approach:*** The anterior approach starts with an U-shaped incision by preserving the rectus abdominis muscle. A retroperitoneal dissection of the lower lumbar and pelvic area is then performed. Both the iliac arteries and veins are dissected, and the internal iliac arteries are ligated. We recommend to perform this part of the operation by a general surgeon. Next, the visceral and vascular structures of the pelvis are mobilized away from the tumor. After dissecting the rectum, sacral nerve roots entering the tumor are sacrificed. If we plan a high sacral amputation, we perform an L5–S1 anterior discectomy and partial ventral sacroiliac osteotomies. If not, we preserve the S2 roots and perform an anterior sacral at the junction of S1–S2. A piece of sterile gauze was placed in the abdomen dorsal to the rectum to isolate the rectum from the lumbar vertebrae and sacrum, and the abdominal incision was closed.
II. ***Posterior approach:*** The patient was turned to the prone position and a Y- or inverted C-shaped incision was made. If there had been a previous operation, a vertical midline cut was preferred, and the existing incision lines were resected. After dissecting and retracting the gluteal muscles, the sciatic notch was identified and posterior osteotomies were performed.

An L5 laminectomy was performed, and after identification of the dural sac and the L5 and S1 roots, the dura mater and sacral roots were ligated distal to the L5 roots. After completion of the osteotomies, the tumor mass was completely removed. Closed suction drainage catheters were placed as needed. Myocutaneous flap closure was used in most cases.

When we plan a high sacral amputation, we perform an L5 laminectomy, then a posterior osteotomy through sacral alae as medial as possible. Sometimes, we add partial or total pelvectomy depending on the iliac extension ot the tumor. Now, it is the time for dissection and identification of the dura and roots. If there is any root entering the tumor, it should be sacrificed. If the plan is a high sacral amputation, dura was ligated with its sacral roots just after the exit of S1 roots, and the distal part is cut. Then, depending on the tumor extension, posterior osteotomies were performed medial or lateral to the sacroiliac joints. At this stage, sciatic notch must be explored. The sciatic nerve and gluteal artery and vein must be explored and if possible, protected. Piriform muscle is a good landmark to identify the trace of the sciatic nerve. Then posterior osteotomies are finished by releasing ventral muscles and ligaments and the sacrum is removed.

Posterior lumbopelvic fixation is performed at the same or another stage depending on the duration of surgery and amount of bleeding.

Tables 37.2 to 37.5 gives the characteristics of a series of patients operated between 1991 and 2003 by the author.[29]

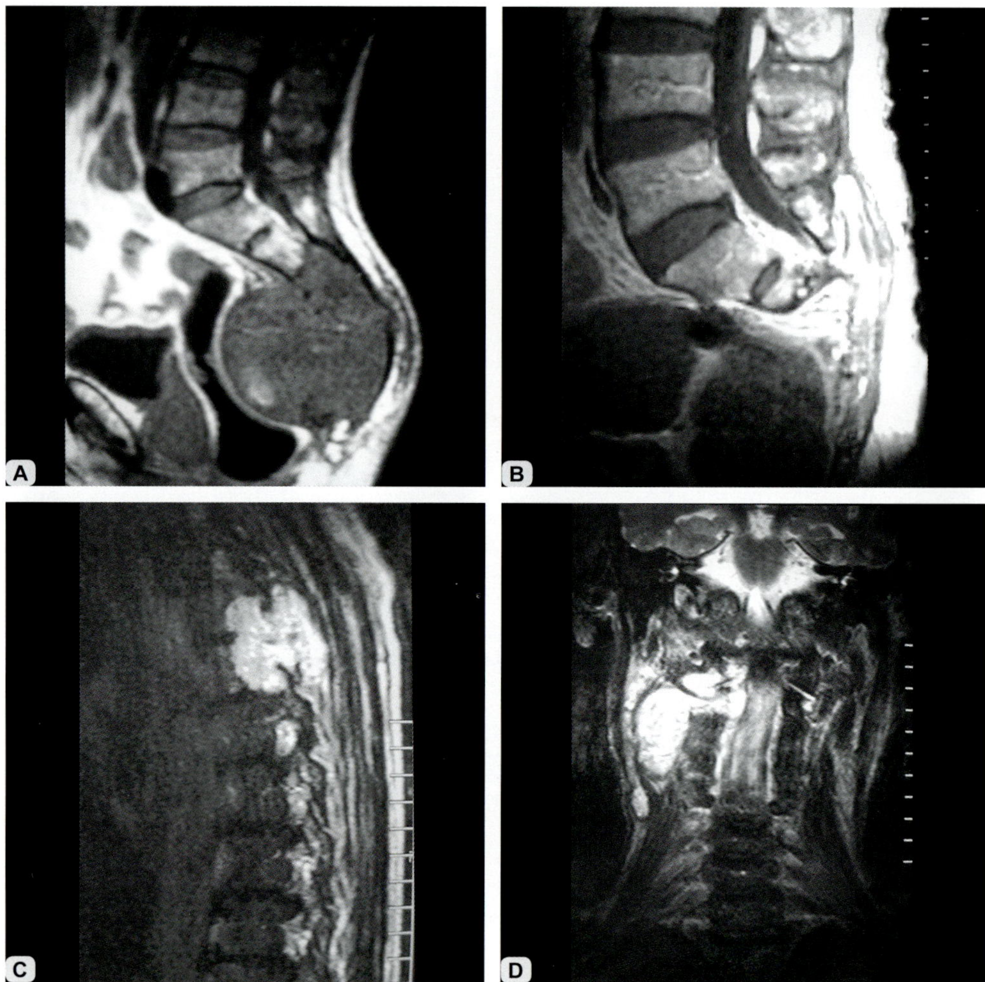

Fig. 37.1 Sacral chordoma, distal sacrectomy, metastasis. A 66-years-old male came with a swelling on his left hip, local pain and weakness of left foot. (A) Tumor below S2 in diameters of 80 × 14 cm has been excised with a posterior distal sacrectomy; (B) Postoperative MR images 6 months after showed no recidive; (C) Three years later he came with a thoracic (T4–5) metastasis and operated for this cord compression; (D) Five years later another metastasis in cervical region from C1–C2 downward to C5 in paraspinal area was revealed and operated again (d). He is alive 10 years after primary surgery with metastatic tumors

Radiotherapy and Chemotherapy

Radiotherapy may be added if the histology shows a radiosensitive tumor and if excision is partial. Some surgeons recommend adjuvant radiotherapy in all cases for possibility of insufficient resections.[62] However, reports showing the significant effect of radiation is quite rare. Although chordomas are resistant to radiotherapy, there are reports that a conventional radiation therapy may prolong the disease-free intervals and diminish symptoms.[4,8,50,63-65] A special type of radiotherapy, proton beam radiation has been shown to provide longer survival rates.[66] For that reason, if the surgery is incomplete or the histologic examination shows borders of a sacrectomy are not tumor free, radiotherapy should be applied. If recurrence occurs, radiation must always be applied. However, the real effect of radiotherapy to outcomes in sacral chordomas are critical.[4,14,44,63,67,68] There is no role of chemotherapy in chordoma patients.

Outcome

The outcomes of sacral tumor surgery are primarily related to tumor biology. The recurrence rates of sacral chordomas are significantly high even in case of sacrectomy and

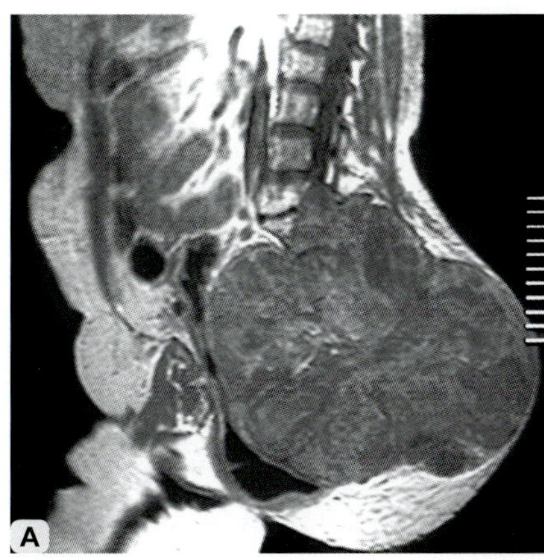
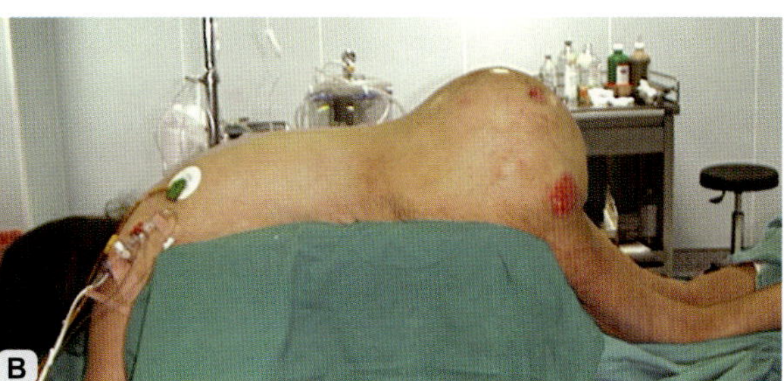

Fig. 37.2 Giant sacral chordoma. Intralesional posterior surgery. A 45-years-old female patient. She has not accepted despite significant swelling on sacrum for 2.5 years. (A) MR images show the dimensions has reached 18 × 32 cm. Significant sphincter problem has caused renal failure and biopsy showed chordoma. She had bilateral foot drop, no anal tonus, and perianal anesthesia; (B) An intralesional surgery with subtotal excision and colostomy at the same session were performed. A postoperative radiotherapy was applied. She had one more surgery 3 years later and she is alive with recurrence 7 years after primary surgery. Renal insufficiency became compensatory

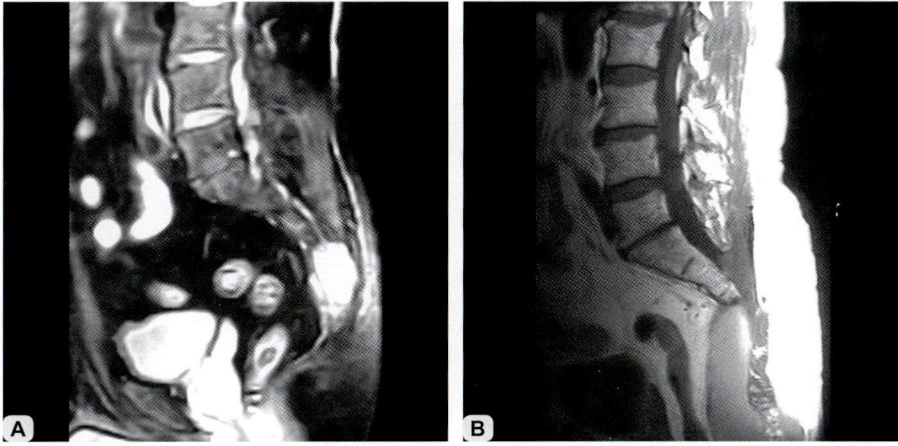

Fig. 37.3 S3 chordoma. Posterior distal sacrectomy. A small chordoma at S3 level was resected by a distal sacrectomy. MR images one year later show no recurrence. He however died 2 years later due to a myocard infarction

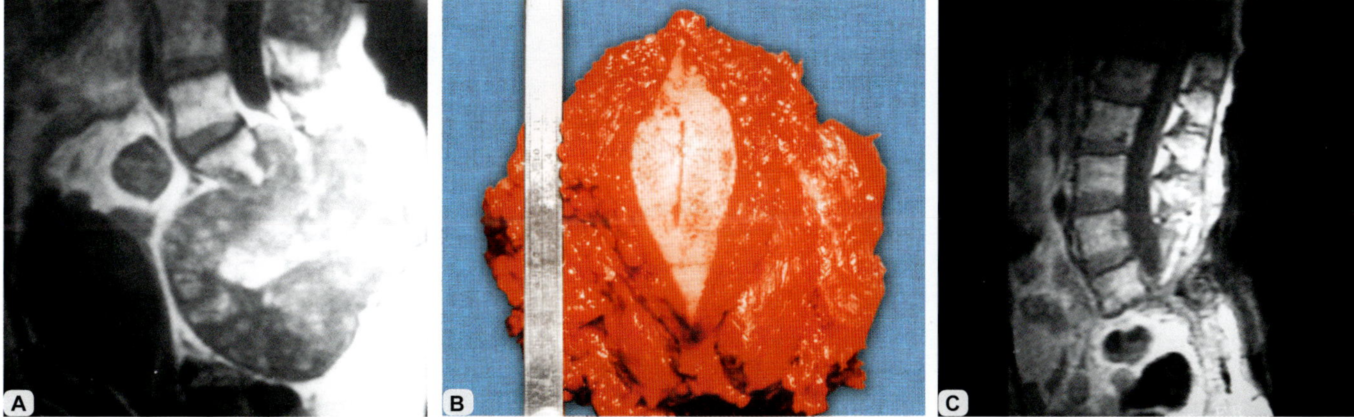

Fig. 37.4 S1 chordoma. Antero-posterior cerrahi, total sacrectomy. (A) A 58-year-old female patient had local pain, perianal anesthesia and sphincter disturbance; (B) An anteroposterior surgery with total sacrectomy was applied. During surgery site of previous biopsy incision was also excised; (C) She received a postoperative radiation. Although there is no tumor at the site of surgery 6 months later she had a recurrence 2 years later and operated again. She died 5 years later because of tumor

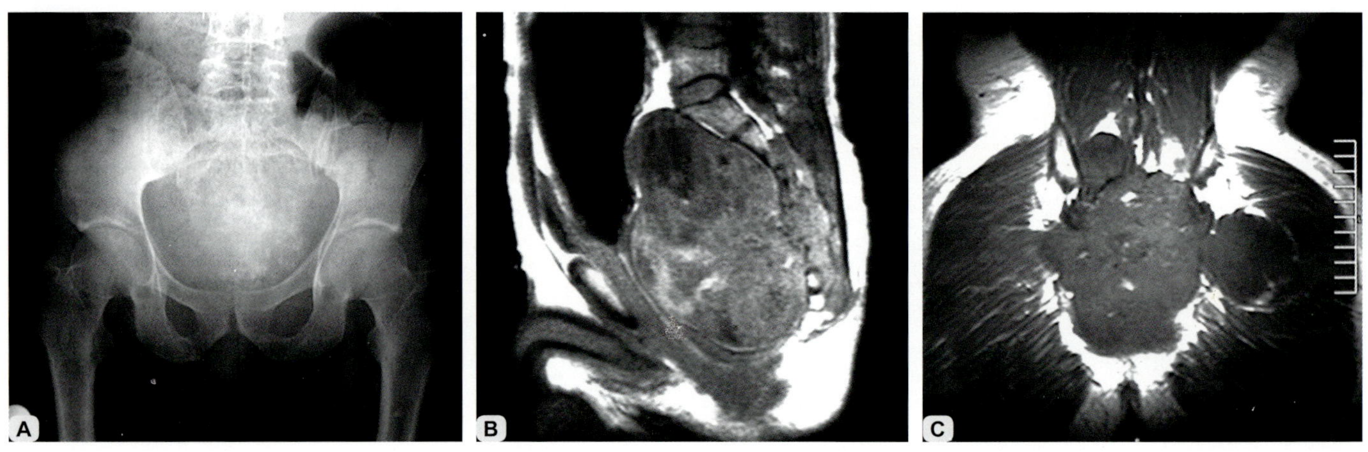

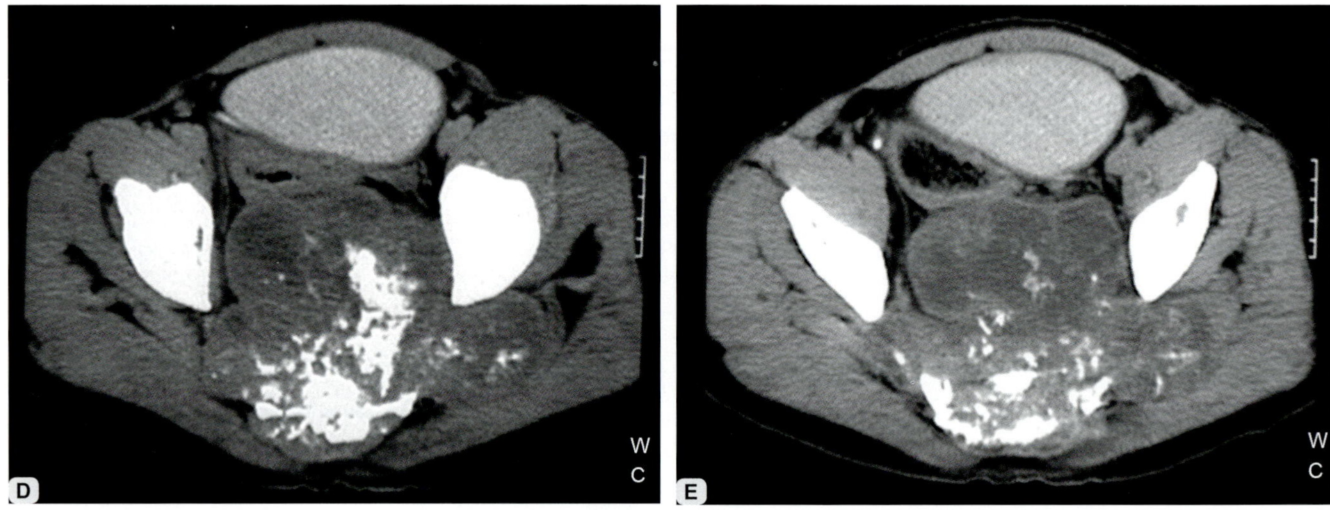
W
C
W
C

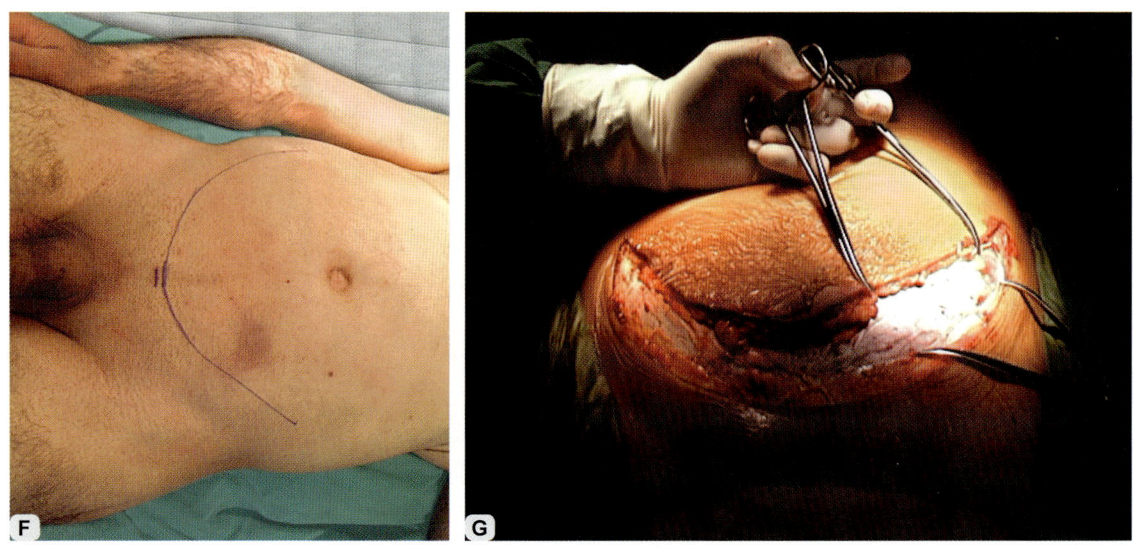

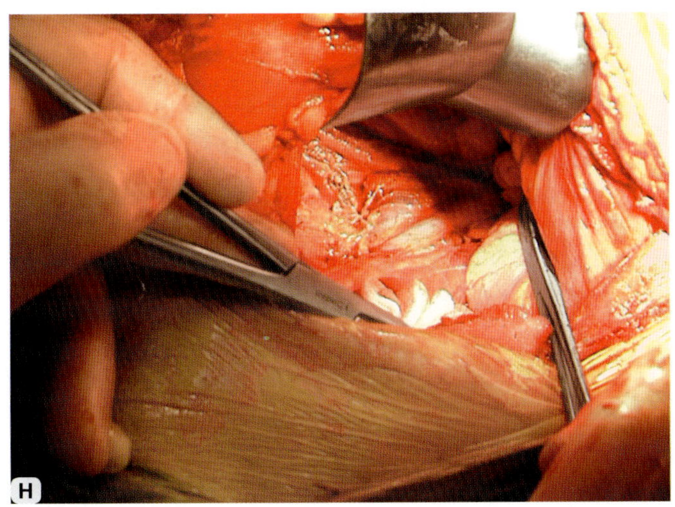
H

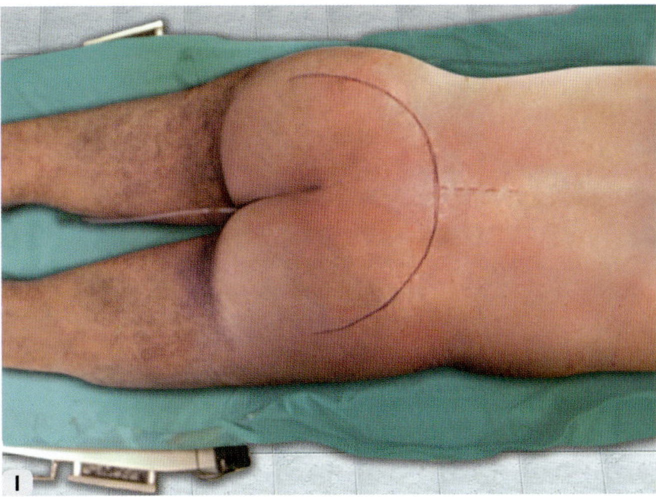
I

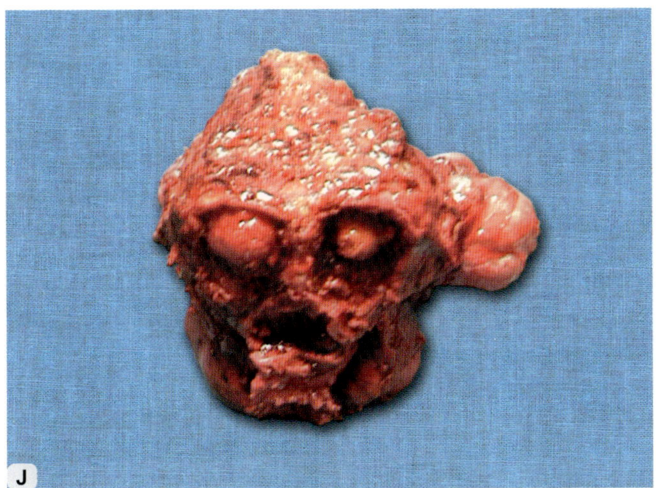
J

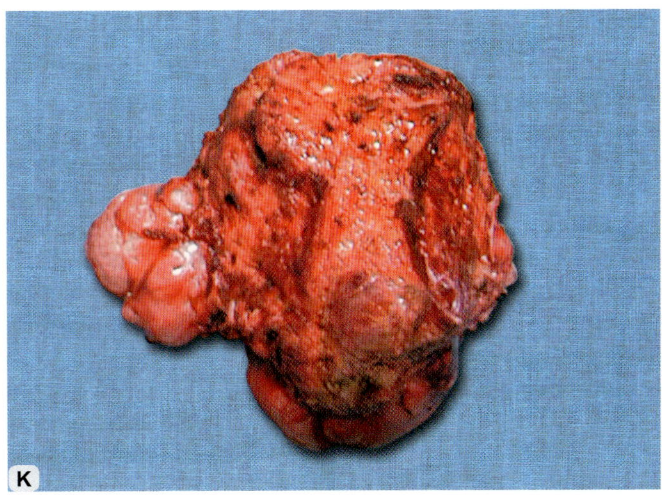
K

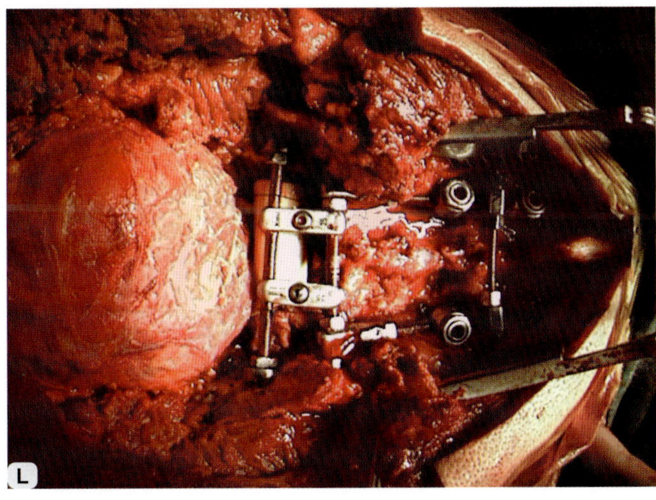
L

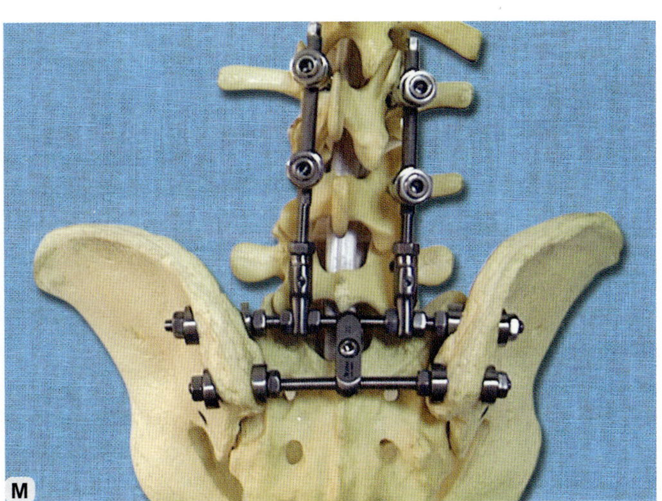
M

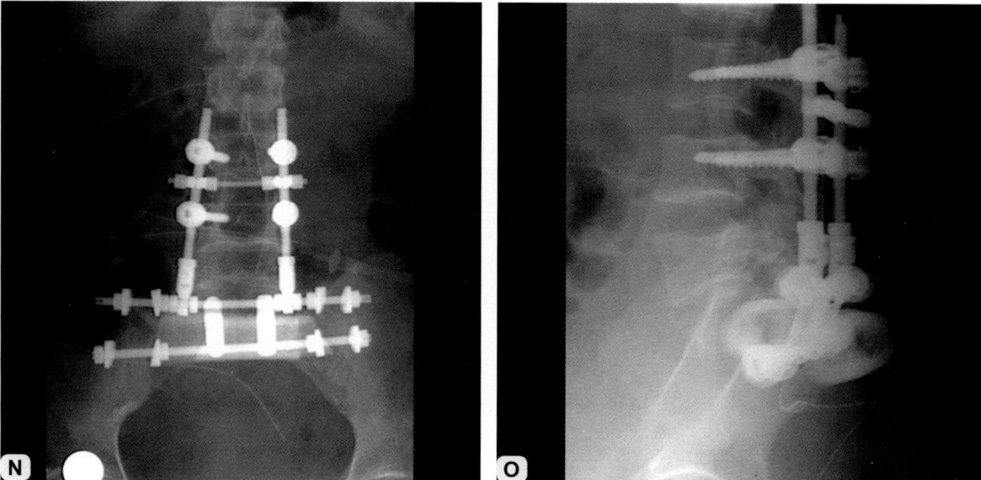

Figs 37.5 Sacral chondrosarcoma. (A) Pelvic radiogram; (B) sagittal MR image; (C) coronal MR image; (D and E) axial CT scans show a huge mass with destruction of the sacrum and extension to the pelvis. The histology was also deliniated with biopsy. On CT scans, there are calcification inside the tumor typical for chondrosarcoma. During the ventral approach, (F) a U-shaped incision was performed with (G and H) bilateral retroperitoneal dissection, mobilization of intestines from the mass, ligation of both internal iliac arteries and veins and median sacral artery were performed. Then, from the dorsal approach, (I) an inverse C-shaped incision was made and (J and K) the sacrum was excised with posterior osteotomies. A posterior lumbopelvic fixation was performed at the same session using (L) a custom-made system during the same operative session. Femoral allograft supported with autografts and a mesh covering for the rectum were placed dorsal to the iliac bars. This custom-made system (TIPSAN Co., Izmir, Turkey) is consisted of two threaded, lateral bars connecting both iliac wings, and (M) sagittal rods connected to transverse rods (N) postoperative AP; and (O) lateral X-ray films obtained after instrumentation. The patient is disease free without any recurrence 8 years after surgery

Table 37.2 Demographic and clinical data obtained in 34 patients who underwent resection of primary sacral tumors

Age: 14–71 years (mean 42)	
Sex: male 14/female 20	
Duration of symptoms: 7 days–10 years, (mean 20 months)	
Pain	
Unilateral sciatic pain	15 patients
Bilateral sciatic pain	6 patients
Local pain only	11 patients
No pain at all	2 patients
Neurological findings	
Monoparesis	4
Cauda equina syndrome	6
Sphincter disturbance	18
No neurology	16

Table 37.3 Histological findings in primary sacral tumors resected in 34 patients

Tumor type	*No. of patients*
Malignant	**20**
Chordoma	8
Chondrosarcoma	3
Osteosarcoma	2
Liposarcoma	1
Solitary plasmocytoma	2
Ependymoma	3
Malignant hemangiopericytoma	1
Benign tumors	**14**
Giant cell tumor	6
Giant schwannoma	6
Aneurysmal bone cyst	1
Hemangioma	1

adjuvant therapies. Although chordomas are low grade tumors survival times are still not too long.[71] Worse outcome are related with two factors: (a) long duration of symptoms and late diagnosis, (b) the large dimeters of tumors.

Five years survival rates are 45–77%, and 10 years survival rates are 28–50% in different series.[44,66,69,70] Mortality in 15 years follow-up are more than 50%.

Local recurrence is the worst factor affecting the prognosis and recurrence rates are 46% in 5 years, and 54% in 10 years.[10,13,71-73]

Metastasis is also a bad sign for prognosis. The rate of metastasis is between 10–40% in different series.[74] Samson et al. have reported 50% metastasis rate in 10 years.[44] Sarsik et al. studies the possibility of recurrence of chordomas.[75]

Table 37.4 Type of surgical treatments for primary sacral tumors in 34 patients

Type of surgery		*No. of patients*
Total sacrectomy (Lesions above S2-Anteroposterior resection)		9
Chordoma	5	
Chondrosarcoma	3	
Osteosarcoma	1	
Distal sacrectomy (Lesions below S2-Posterior resection only)		2
Chordoma	2	
Gross-total resection		12
Intralesional subtotal resection		6
Intralesional partial resection		5
Total		34

Table 37.5 Outcome and complications after surgery

Outcome		
Alive		27
Dead		6
Early postoperative death (1st month) Death at follow up (3 months, 13 months, 5 years)	3 3	
Lost to follow up		1
Recidive-Recurrence		
Residual tumor		17
Metastasis		5
Lyposarcoma Plasmocytoma Chordoma Osteosarcoma	1 2 1 1	
No recidive or recurrence		12
Complications in 11 patients after sacrectomy		
Early postoperative death (1st month) Fat emboli Rectal perforation	 1 2	3
Vascular injury		0
Motor deficits (foot drop)		3
Local infection, wound problems		5
Dural tear, CSF fistula		1

Conclusion

Radical resection can prolong the overall survival time of patients with primary malignant or benign, aggressive neoplasms in the sacrum that are resistant to noninterventional forms of therapy. Although sacrectomies may yield low mortality and acceptable morbidity rates, they remain a challenge for surgeons and oncologists alike because of their complexity, the need for collaboration among specialists from several areas, and the potential for complications, including risks of infection, neurological deficits, and lumbopelvic instability. Although the patient's quality of life largely depends on the extent of sacral root resection and the establishment of sacroiliac stability, this study illustrates that sacrectomy can be performed successfully, and is an important procedure in the treatment of primary sacral tumors.

References

1. Capanna R, Briccoli A, Campanacci LC, et al. Benign and malignant tumors of the sacrum, in Frymoyer JW (ed): The Adult Spine: Principles and Practice, ed 2. Philadelphia: Lippincott-Raven. 1997;pp.2367-405.
2. Raque GH Jr, Vitaz TW, Shields CB: Treatment of neoplastic diseases of the sacrum. J Surg Oncol. 2001;76:301-7.
3. Wuisman P, Lieshout O, van Dijk M, et al. Reconstruction after total en bloc sacrectomy for osteosarcoma using a custom-made prosthesis: a technical note. Spine. 2001;26:431-9.
4. Cheng EY, Ozerdemoglu RA, Transfeldt EE, Thompson RC Jr. Lumbosacral chordoma. Prognostic factors and treatment. Spine. 1999;24:1639-45.
5. Gunterberg B, Petersen I. Sexual function after major resections of the sacrum with bilateral or unilateral sacrifice of sacral nerves. Fertil Steril. 1976;27:1146-53.
6. Pitcher JD, Springfield DS. Benign primary bony lesions of the sacrum. In: Surgical Disorders of the Sacrum. JR Doty, SS Rengachary (eds), Thieme Med Pub, New York. 1994;pp.221-9.
7. Sung MS, Lee GK, Kang HS, Kwon ST, Park JG, Suh JS, et al. Sacrococcygeal chordoma: MR imaging in 30 patients. Skeletal Radiol. 2005;34(2):87-94.
8. Unni KK. Dahlin's bone tumors: general aspects and data on 11,087 cases. 5th ed. Philadelphia: Lippincott-Raven. 1996;pp.291-305.
9. Fan F, Templeton K, Damjanov I. Epithelioid cellular chordoma of the sacrum: a potential diagnostic problem. Ann Diagn Pathol. 2005;9(3):139-42.
10. Bergh P, Kindblom LG, Gunterberg B, Remotti F, Ryd W, Meis-Kindblom JM. Prognostic factors in chordoma of the sacrum and mobile spine: a study of 39 patients. Cancer. 2000;88:2122-34.
11. Kaiser TE, Pritchard DJ, Unni KK. Clinicopathologic study of sacrococcygeal chordoma. Cancer. 1984;53:2574-8.
12. Krol G, Sze G, Arbit E, Marcove R, Sundaresan N. Intradural metastases of chordoma. AJNR Am J Neuroradiol. 1989;10:193-5.
13. Ozaki T, Hillmann A, Winkelmann W. Surgical treatment of sacrococcygeal chordoma. J Surg Oncol. 1997;64:274-9.
14. Chandawarkar RY. Sacrococcygeal chordoma: review of 50 consecutive patients. World J Surg. 1996;20:717-9.

15. Soo MY. Chordoma: review of clinicoradiological features and factors affecting survival. Australas Radiol. 2001;45:427-34.
16. Gunterberg B, Kewenter J, Petersen I, Stener B. Anorectal function after major resections of the sacrum with bilateral or unilateral sacrifice of sacral nerves. Br J Surg. 1976;63:546-54
17. Gunterberg B, Norlen L, Stener B, Sundin T. Neurourologic evaluation after resection of the sacrum. Invest Urol. 1975;13:183-8.
18. Gunterberg B, Romanus B, Stener B. Pelvic strength after major amputation of the sacrum. An experimental study. Acta Orthop Scand. 1976;47:635-42.
19. Stener B. Technique of high sacral amputation. in: Sundaresan N, Schmidek HH, Schiller AL, Rosenthal DI (eds): Tumors of the Spine: Diagnosis and Clinical Management. Philadelphia: WB Saunders. 1990;pp.411-6.
20. Todd LT Jr, Yaszemski MJ, Currier BL, Fuchs B, Kim CW, Sim FH. Bowel and bladder function after major sacral resection. Clin Orthop Relat Res. 2002;397:36-9.
21. Gennari L, Azzarelli A, Quagliuolo V. A posterior approach for the excision of sacral chordoma. J Bone Joint Surg Br. 1987;69:565-8.
22. Huth JF, Dawson EG, Eilber FR. Abdominosacral resection for malignant tumors of the sacrum. Am J Surg. 1984;148:157-61.
23. Harrison SJ, McDonnell DE. Sacrectomy. In: Surgical Disorders of the Sacrum. JR Doty, SS Rengachary (eds), Thieme Med Pub, New York. 1994;pp.279-93.
24. Jackson RJ, Gökaslan ZL. Spinal-pelvic fixation in patients with lumbosacral neoplasms. J Neurosurg (Spine). 2000;92:61-70.
25. McGee AM, Bache CE, Spilsbury J, et al. A simplified Galveston technique for the stabilisation of pathological fractures of the sacrum. Eur Spine J. 2000;9:451-4.
26. Nakai S, Yoshizawa H, Kobayashi S, et al. Anorectal and bladder function after sacrifice of the sacral nerves. Spine. 2000;25:2234-9.
27. Neff JR. Technique of subtotal and total sacral amputation for neoplasm. In: Surgical Disorders of the Sacrum. JR Doty, SS Rengachary (eds). Thieme Med Pub: New York. 1994;pp.266-78.
28. Stener B, Gunterberg B. High amputation of the sacrum for extirpation of tumors. Principles and technique. Spine. 1978;3:351-66.
29. Zileli M, Hoscoskun C, Brastianos P, Sabah D. Surgical treatment of primary sacral tumors: complications associated with sacrectomy. Neurosurg Focus. 2003;15(5):Article 9.
30. Zileli M. Sacral Chordomas. J Surg Medical Sci. 2007;3(51):123-9.
31. Localio SA, Eng K. Sphincter-saving operations for cancer of the rectum. New Engl J Med. 1979;300:1028-30.
32. Gunterberg B. Effects of major resection of the sacrum. Clinical studies on urogenital and anorectal function and a biomechanical study on pelvic strength. Acta Orthop Scand Suppl. 1976;162:1-38.
33. Karakousis CP. Sacral resection with preservation of continence. Surg Gynecol Obstet. 1986;163:270-3.
34. Dahlin DC, Cupps RE, Johnson EW Jr. Giant-cell tumor: a study of 195 cases. Cancer. 1970;25:1061-70.
35. Tomita K, Tsıchiya H. Total sacrectomy and reconstruction for huge sacral tumors. Spine. 1990;15:1223-7.
36. O'Donnell RJ, Springfield DS, Motwani HK, et al. Recurrence of giant-cell tumors of the long bones after curettage and packing with cement. J Bone Joint Surg Am. 1994;76:1827-33.
37. Malawer MM, Bickels J, Meller I, et al. Cryosurgery in the treatment of giant cell tumor. A long-term followup study. Clin Orthop. 1999;359:176-88.
38. Marcove RC, Lyden JP, Huvos AG, et al. Giant-cell tumors treated by cryosurgery. A report of twenty-five cases. J Bone Joint Surg Am. 1973;55:1633-44.
39. Marcove RC, Sheth DS, Brien EW, et al. Conservative surgery for giant cell tumors of the sacrum. The role of cryosurgery as a supplement to curettage and partial excision. Cancer. 1994;74:1253-60.
40. Marcove RC, Weis LD, Vaghaiwalla MR, et al. Cryosurgery in the treatment of giant cell tumors of bone. A report of 52 consecutive cases. Cancer. 1978;41:957-69.
41. Althausen PL, Schneider PD, Bold RJ, et al. Multimodality management of a giant cell tumor arising in the proximal sacrum: case report. Spine. 2002;27:E361-5.
42. Mi C, Lu H, Liu H. Surgical excision of sacral tumors assisted by occluding the abdominal aorta with a balloon dilation catheter: a report of 3 cases. Spine. 2005;30:E614–6.
43. Ozgiray E, Cagli S, Zileli M, Cinar C, Oran I. Occlusion of the Abdominal Aorta by Balloon Dilation Catheter Assisting Surgical Excision of a Sacrum Chordoma: Case Report. Turkish Neurosurgery. 2009;19/3:265-8.
44. Samson IR, Springfield DS, Suit HD, Mankin HJ. Operative treatment of sacrococcygeal chordoma. A review of twenty-one cases. J Bone Joint Surg Am. 1993;75:1476-84.
45. Simpson AH, Porter A, Davis A, et al. Cephalad sacral resection with a combined extended ilioinguinal and posterior approach. J Bone Joint Surg Am. 1995;77:405-11.
46. Sung HW, Shu WP, Wang HM, Yuai SY, Tsai YB. Surgical treatment of primary tumors of the sacrum. Clin Orthop Relat Res. 1987;215:91-8.
47. Alper M, Bilkay U, Keçeci Y, et al. Transsacral usage of a pure island TRAM flap for a large sacral defect: a case report. Ann Plastic Surg. 2000;44:417-21.
48. Bohinski RJ, Mendel E, Rhines LD. Novel use of a threadwire saw for high sacral amputation. Technical note and description of operative technique. J Neurosurg Spine. 2005;3(1):71-8.
49. Doita M, Harada T, Iguchi T, Sumi M, Sha H, Yoshiya S, Kurosaka M. Total sacrectomy and reconstruction for sacral tumors. Spine. 2003;1;28(15):E296-301.
50. Kamada T, Tsujii H, Tsuji H, Yanagi T, Mizoe JE, Miyamoto T, et al. Working Group for the Bone and Soft Tissue Sarcomas. Efficacy and safety of carbon ion radiotherapy in bone and soft tissue sarcomas. J Clin Oncol. 2002;20:4466-71.
51. Fourney DR, Gokaslan ZL. Current management of sacral chordoma. Neurosurg Focus. 2003;15;15(2):E9.
52. Fourney DR, Rhines LD, Hentschel SJ, Skibber JM, Wolinsky JP, Weber KL, et al. En bloc resection of primary sacral tumors: classification of surgical approaches and outcome. J Neurosurg Spine. 2005;3(2):111-22.

53. Fuchs B, Dickey ID, Yaszemski MJ, Inwards CY, Sim FH. Operative management of sacral chordoma. J Bone Joint Surg Am. 2005;87(10):2211-6.
54. Gallia GL, Haque R, Garonzik I, Witham TF, Khavkin YA, Wolinsky JP, et al. Spinal pelvic reconstruction after total sacrectomy for en bloc resection of a giant sacral chordoma. Technical note. J Neurosurg Spine. 2005;3:501-6.
55. Randall RL, Bruckner J, Lloyd C, Pohlman TH, Conrad EU 3rd. Sacral resection and reconstruction for tumors and tumor-like conditions. Orthopedics. 2005;28(3):307-13.
56. Allen BL Jr, Ferguson RL. The Galveston technique for L rod instrumentation of the scoliotic spine. Spine. 1982;7:276-84.
57. Shikata J, Yamamuro T, Kotoura Y, et al. Total sacrectomy and reconstruction for primary tumors. Report of two cases. J Bone Joint Surg Am. 1988;70:122-5.
58. Gokaslan ZL, Romsdahl MM, Kroll SS, et al. Total sacrectomy and Galveston L-rod reconstruction for malignant neoplasms. Technical note. J Neurosurg. 1997;87:781-7.
59. Thomson J, Doty JR. Sacral biomechanics and reconstruction. In Doty JR, Rengachary SS (eds): Surgical Disorders of the Sacrium. New York: Thieme Medical; 1994;pp.253-6.
60. Salehi SA, McCafferty RR, Karahalios D, et al. Neural function preservation and early mobilization after resection of metastatic sacral tumors and lumbosacropelvic junction reconstruction. Report of three cases. J Neurosurg (Spine 1). 2002;97:88-93.
61. Localio SA, Eng K, Ranson JH. Abdominosacral approach for retrorectal tumors. Ann Surg. 1980;191:555-60.
62. Keisch ME, Garcia DM, Shibuya RB. Retrospective long-term follow-up analysis in 21 patients with chordomas of various sites treated at a single institution. J Neurosurg. 1991;75:374-7.
63. Catton C, O'Sullivan B, Bell R, Laperriere N, Cummings B, Fornasier V, et al. Chordoma: long-term follow-up after radical photon irradiation. Radiother Oncol. 1996;41:67-72.
64. Cummings BJ, Hodson DI, Bush RS. Chordoma: the results of megavoltage radiation therapy. Int J Radiat Oncol Biol Phys. 1983;9:633-42.
65. Rich TA, Schiller A, Suit HD, Mankin HJ. Clinical and pathologic review of 48 cases of chordoma. Cancer. 1985;56:182-7.
66. Austin-Seymour M, Munzenrider J, Goitein M, et al. Fractionated proton radiation therapy of chordoma and low-grade chondrosarcoma of the base of the skull. J Neurosurg. 1989;70:13-7.
67. Azzarelli A, Quagliuolo V, Cerasoli S, Zucali R, Bignami P, Mazzaferro V, et al. Chordoma: Natural history and treatment results in 33 cases. J Surg Oncol. 1988;37:185-91.
68. Breteau N, Demasure M, Favre A, Leloup R, Lescrainier J, Sabattier R. Fast neutron therapy for inoperable or recurrent sacrococcygeal chordomas. Bull Cancer Radiother. 1996;83(suppl.)142s-5s.
69. Smith J, Ludwig RL, Marcove RC. Sacrococcygeal chordoma. A clinicoradiological study of 60 patients. Skeletal Radiol. 1987;16:37-44.
70. Sundaresan N. Chordomas. Clin Orthop Relat Res. 1986;204:135-42.
71. Ishii K, Chiba K, Watanabe M, Yabe H, Fujimura Y, Toyama Y. Local recurrence after S2-3 sacrectomy in sacral chordoma. Report of four cases. J Neurosurg. 2002;97(1 Suppl):98-101.
72. Sar C, Eralp L. Surgical treatment of primary tumors of the sacrum. Arch Orthop Trauma Surg. 2002;122:148-55.
73. York JE, Kaczaraj A, Abi-Said D, Fuller GN, Skibber JM, Janjan NA, et al. Sacral chordoma: 40-year experience at a major cancer center. Neurosurgery. 1999;44:74-80.
74. Torelli T, Campo B, Ordesi G, Pirovano C, Azzarelli A, Zanolla R. Sacral chordoma and rehabilitative treatment of urinary disorders. Tumori. 1988;74:475-8.
75. Sarsik B, Doganavsargil B, Basdemir G, Zileli M, Sabah D, Oztop F. Chordomas: Is it possible to predict recurrence? Skull base, vertebral and sacral chordomas. Turkish J Pathology www.logos.com.tr/pataloji.asp 2009.

CHAPTER

38

Novel Interlaminar Dynamic Stabilization Concept and Device (IntraSPINE) for the Treatment of Early and Late Degenerative Problems in the Lumbar Spine

Darwono A Bambang

Degenerative Cascade of the Lumbar Spine

Degenerative cascade as described by Kirkaldy-Willis, et al. is starting from anterior column—the disk and middle column—the facet (Fig. 38.1).[1]

Baastrup CI[2-4] describes a degenerative changes at the spinous process. The spinous process enlarges by age in width and height, breaking down the interspinous ligament, developing a neoarthrosis between the adjacent spinous process, causing kissing of spinous process and/ or lamina and resulting the loss of lumbar lordosis toward a flat back (Fig. 38.2).

The Auckland study (Aylott, et al.)[2] shows that spinous processes increase 50% in width, increase 30% in height from the age 20–80, and the result is loss of the lumbar lordosis (Fig. 38.3).

The loss of lordosis is not merely due to the decrease of the disk height (Kirkaldy-Willis) but also by the enlargement of the spinous process (Baastrup) (Fig. 38.4).[1-4]

The Anatomical Trilogy of the degenerative cascade may start from any part of the three columns of the spine: Anterior the disk, middle—the facet, and posterior—the spinous processes, even though the end stage will be the same involving all three columns. It can suffer the three columns alone or together, from inflammatory to compressive reaction.[2-4]

Treatment of Lumbar Degenerative Cascade

Since the degeneration may involve the three columns of the spine, the treatment has a very wide range of justification, from conservative to various types of surgeries related to the encountered pathologies. The degenerative cascade changes the biomechanic property of the spinal motion segment (SMS) and the conservative treatment has a disadvantage of being unable to recover the changes.[1,4,5-17]

Various types of surgeries were designed to solve the variable stages of degenerative cascade from minimal invasive until open surgery, but cannot stop the degeneration itself. The stabilization and fusion is designed to solve the early and late degenerative cascade. At the end stage of degeneration involving three columns (*de novo* scoliosis, listhesis, spinal canal and lateral recess stenosis) decompression and fusion stabilization is the gold standard. Even though this technique may solve the static and dynamic component of the SMS, but it may induce the degenerative cascade of the adjacent levels.[12,18-28] The long fusion in some way may solve the deformity, but in another way may disturb the dynamic mobility of some population, i.e. squatting, sitting on the floor.

The dynamic stabilization[10,16,29-38] is designed to solve the static component of SMS and preserving the dynamic component, but the degenerative cascade will come to

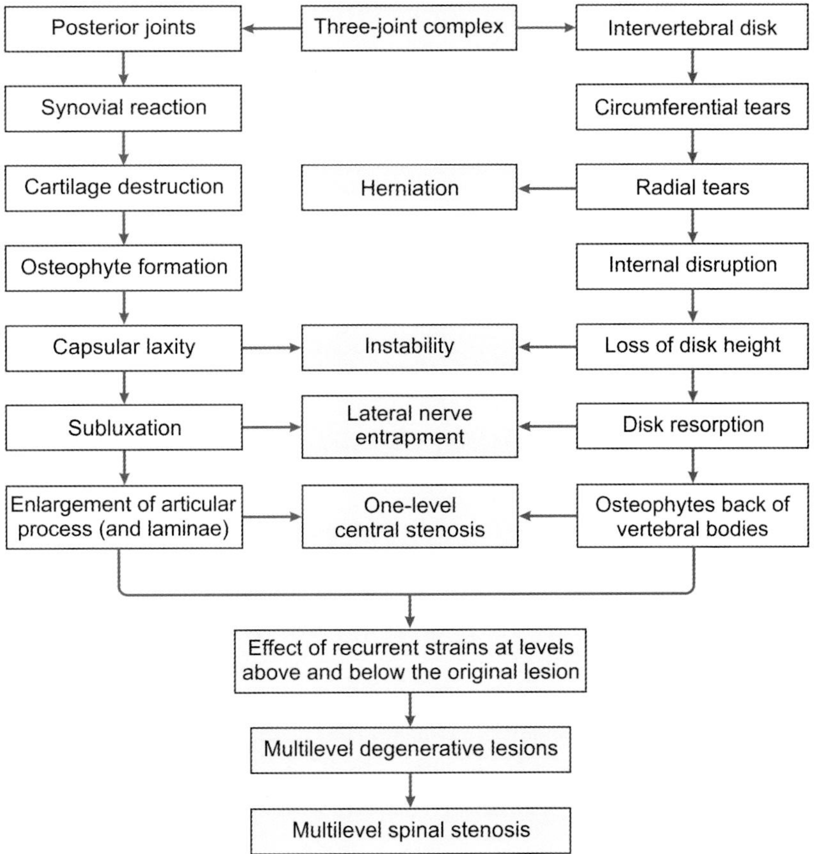

Fig. 38.1 Pathophysiology of multilevel degenerative lumbar spine
Source: Kirkaldy-Willis, et al. Spine. 1978;3(4):319.

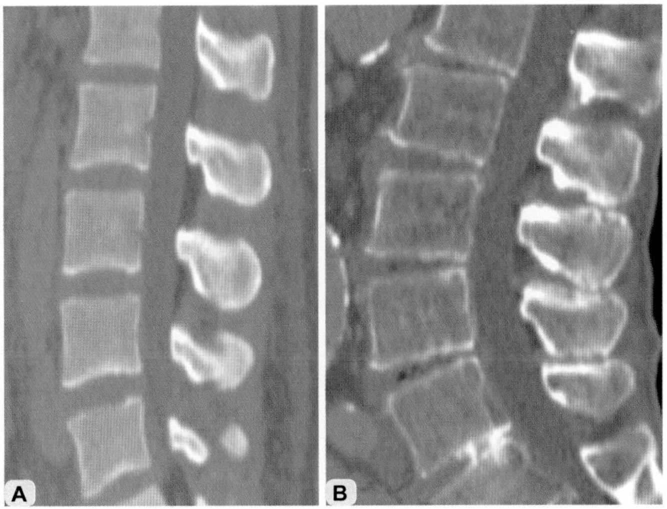

Fig. 38.2 Spinous processes. (A) Young age; (B) Old age

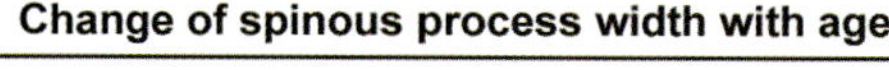
Change of spinous process width with age

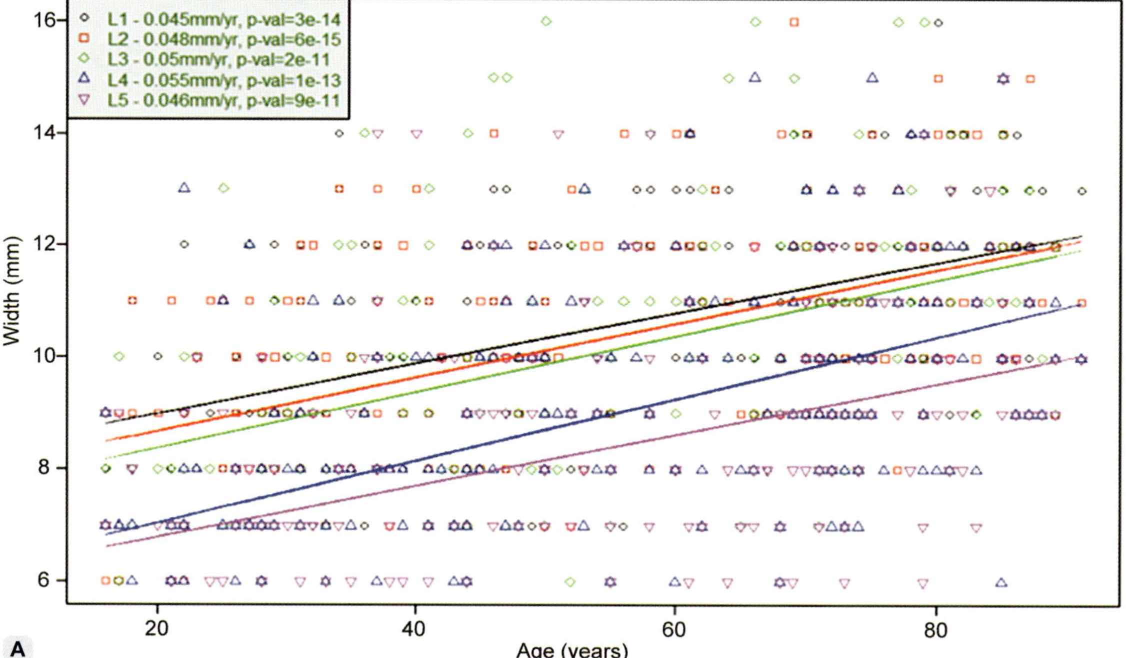
L1 - 0.045mm/yr, p-val=3e-14
L2 - 0.048mm/yr, p-val=6e-15
L3 - 0.05mm/yr, p-val=2e-11
L4 - 0.055mm/yr, p-val=1e-13
L5 - 0.046mm/yr, p-val=9e-11
Width (mm)
6
8
10
12
14
16
20
40
60
80
Age (years)
A

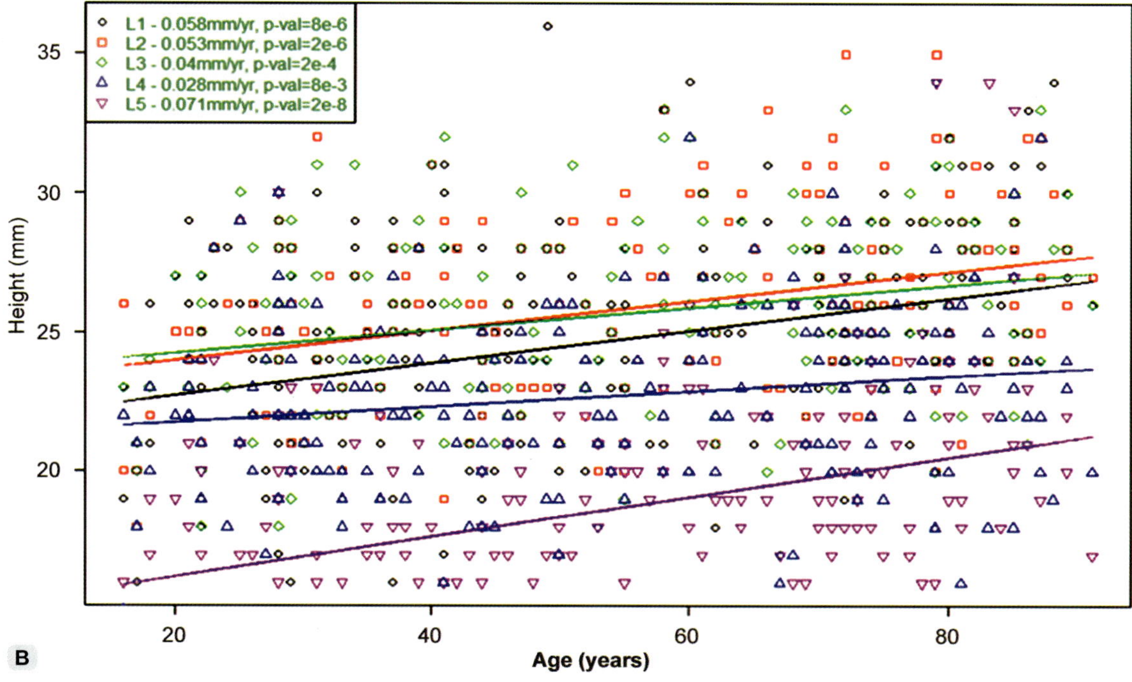
Change of spinous process height and age
L1 - 0.058mm/yr, p-val=8e-6
L2 - 0.053mm/yr, p-val=2e-6
L3 - 0.04mm/yr, p-val=2e-4
L4 - 0.028mm/yr, p-val=8e-3
L5 - 0.071mm/yr, p-val=2e-8
Height (mm)
20
25
30
35
20
40
60
80
Age (years)
B

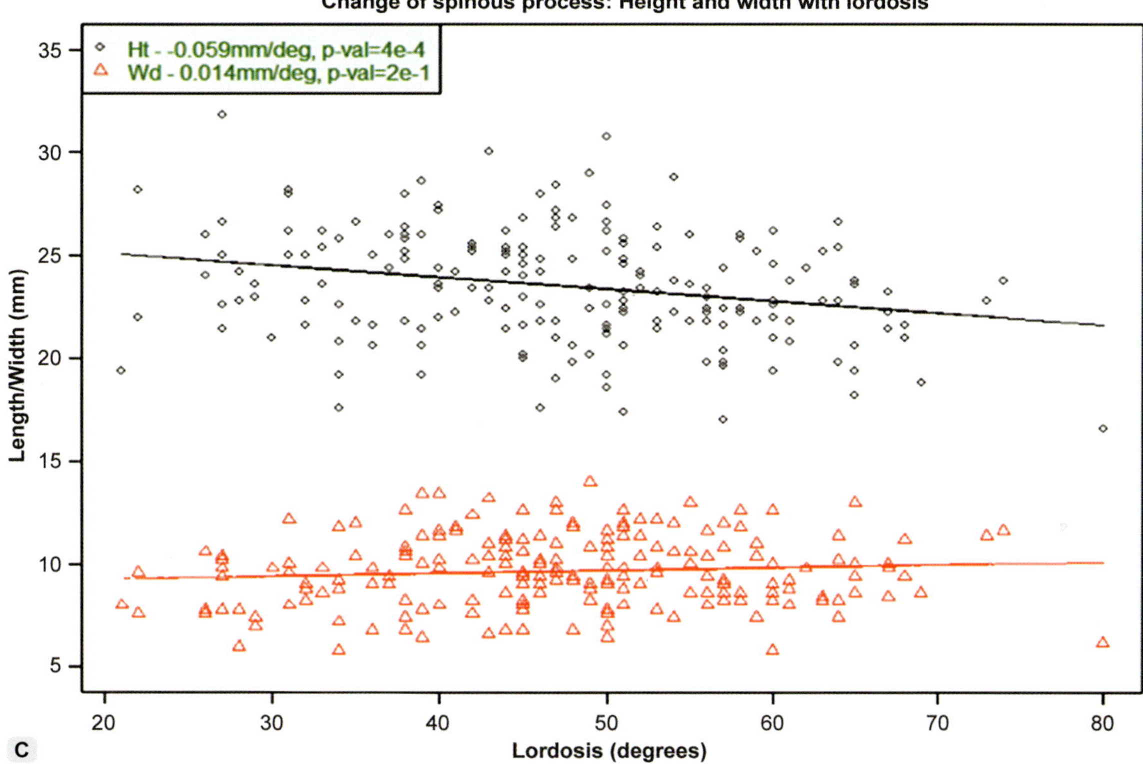

Fig. 38.3 (A) Width increases 50%, p = 0.0004 (Aylott, et al.); (B) Height increases 30%, p = 0.2 (Aylott, et al.); (C) Loss of Lordosis (Aylott, et al.)

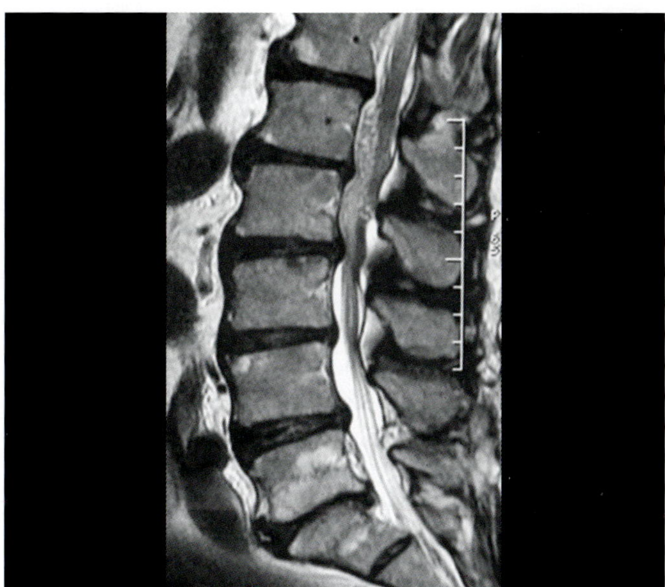

Fig. 38.4 The loss of lordosis: Disk degeneration and enlargement of spinous processes

the same level. The total disk replacement and various interspinous devices are designed to solve a single column degeneration and have a limitation in the amount level. An alternative treatment for the end stage of degeneration is decompression and stabilization using dynamic rod like Dynesis with unlimited amount level. The stabilization is located at the middle column-pedicle and use rod as connector of the pedicle devices.

Middle Column of the Spine

The anterior column-disk[39] is the largest component of the spine with its function as shock absorber since 80% of the burden falls in the front. The posterior column[39] consists of spinous processes, interspinous ligament, muscles and a complex fascia supraspinatus. Its function is the primary limiters in flexion and muscles contraction in extension. Rauschning[40] describes that supraspinatus is not a ligament but a multiple tendon insertion called the complex fascia supraspinatus (CFS) (Fig. 38.5). The CFS in the posterior column is acting as a natural connector like ALL and PLL. Theoretically, preserving the integrity of all natural connectors is very important to gain the stability of the spine.

The middle column[39] consist of pedicles, lamina, transverse processes, and the ganglion which control the back muscles contraction, is located in the middle column as well. The middle column control the load distribution between the anterior column and posterior column,

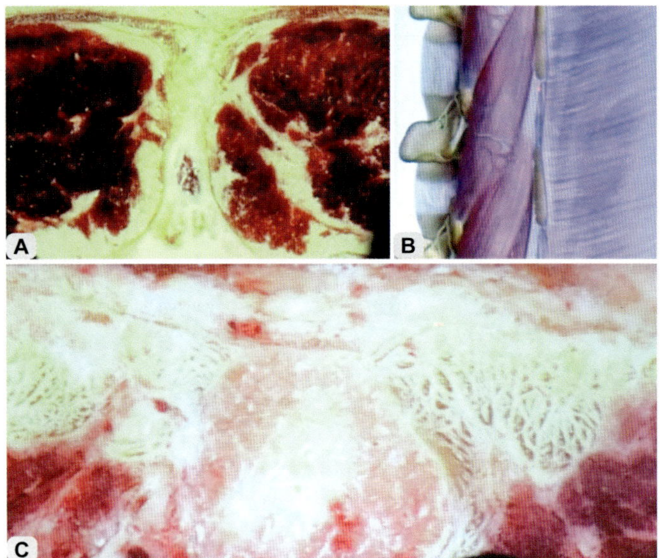

Fig. 38.5 Complex fascia supraspinatus: A multiple tendon insertions. *Courtesy* by Professor Rauschning

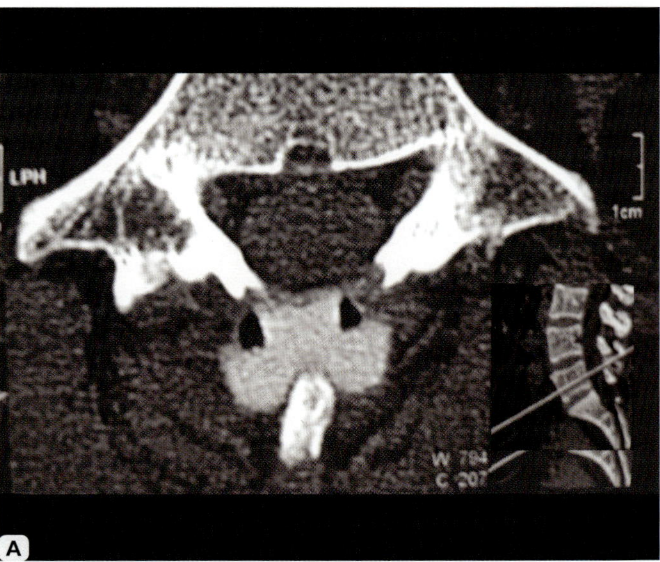

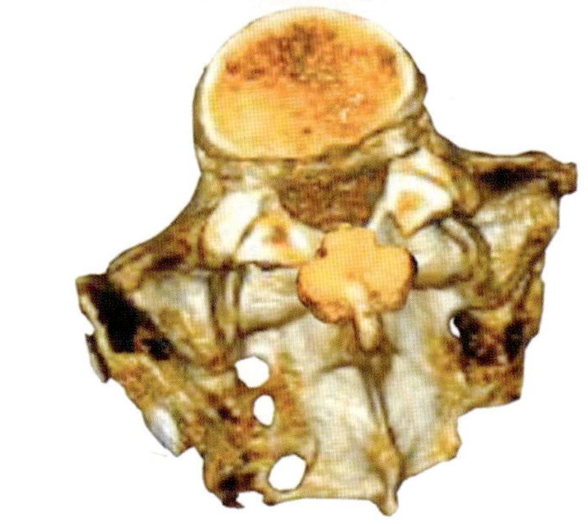

Fig. 38.7 Device is located at the interlamina

similar to crane—mechanically the middle control the load of anterior and posterior part (Fig. 38.6) The middle column with the help of the muscles drives the movement of the mobile segment and are used to control the loads, that changes dynamically in the different position of the spine.[41-49]

The bony neural arch is the only rigid area in the middle column where the device can be placed to control the loads distribution, and the lamina is located close to the axis of instantaneous rotation at the back of the disk (Fig. 38.7).[42-46]

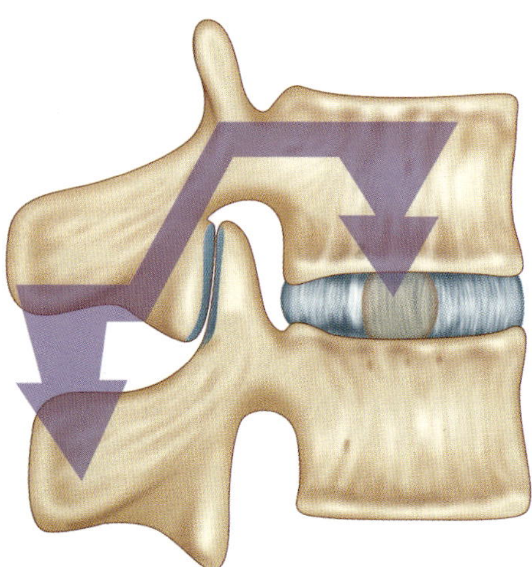

Fig. 38.6 The middle column similar to crane control the loads distribution

Dynamic Interlaminar Device

The device IntraSPINE (Cousin Biotech) is made of Silicone 65 coated by Polyethylene Terephthalate (PET) sleeve. A semi-rigid ligament is also available and can be used to reinforce the CFS in case of insufficiency or laxity (Fig. 38.8).[41-49]

The design of IntraSPINE device (Fig. 38.9):

1. The anterior part = the nose is located at the interlamina (middle column) and the size is related to the interlaminar distance. This part is unloading the disk and facet joints, while controlling the loads distribution between anterior and posterior column.
2. The posterior part = the wing is located at the posterior column to stabilize the device, since the cranial horn is located on the cranial lamina and the caudal horn is located on the caudal lamina.
3. The device do not limit the range of motion of SMS, because the posterior part has a cushion effect created by the holes.

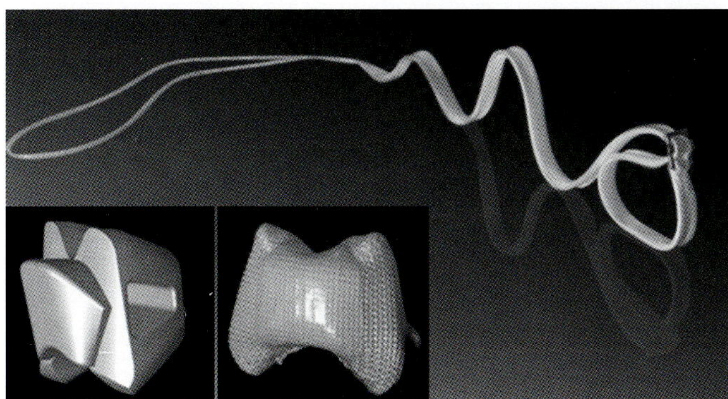

Fig. 38.8 IntraSPINE: Device and semi-rigid ligament (Cousin Biotech)

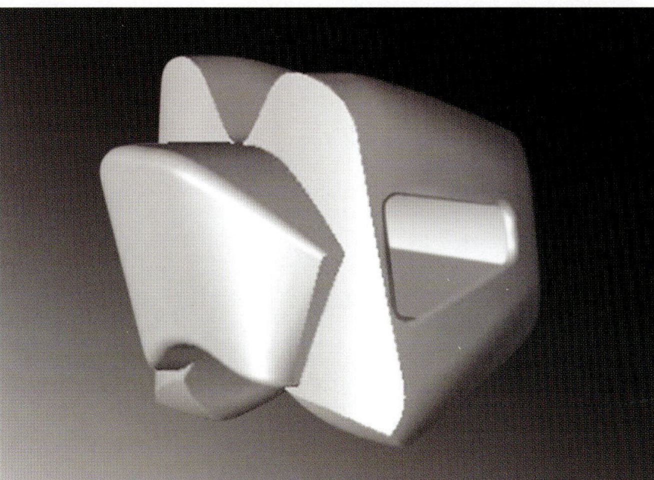

Fig. 38.9 The nose, wing and the hole of the Device (Cousin Biotech)

The interlaminar device can be used as dynamic stabilization for the treatment of the late degenerative cascade after decompression as well as the early degeneration without decompression (Fig. 38.10).[42-46]

The complex fascia supraspinatus is the natural connector in the posterior column and is critically important to preserve it rather to sacrifice as a trick in surgery. In case of an insufficiency or laxity of the CFS due to late degenerative cascade, the semi-rigid ligament can be used to reinforce either at the upper arc and/or the lower arc of the lumbar lordosis as well (Fig. 38.11).[40,42-46]

The Goals of Interlaminar Dynamic Stabilization are:[42-46]

1. Stabilize the segmental instability.
2. Maintain the sagittal balance of the spine.
3. Allow physiologic movement and loads distribution of mobile segment.

Indications[41-49]

1. Early degenerative cascade
   - Large expelled herniated disk in young patients with instability (naturally after removing the hernia)
   - Soft stenosis and/or foraminal stenosis with instability (naturally without decompression)
   - Black disk desease with facet disorder with instability (after a facet joint block test with positive result).
2. Late degenerative cascade:
   - Multilevels degeneration with instability:
     - Canal stenosis, lateral recess stenosis
     - Listhesis (lateral, anterior, retro) grade 1 or less
     - Facet hypertrophy

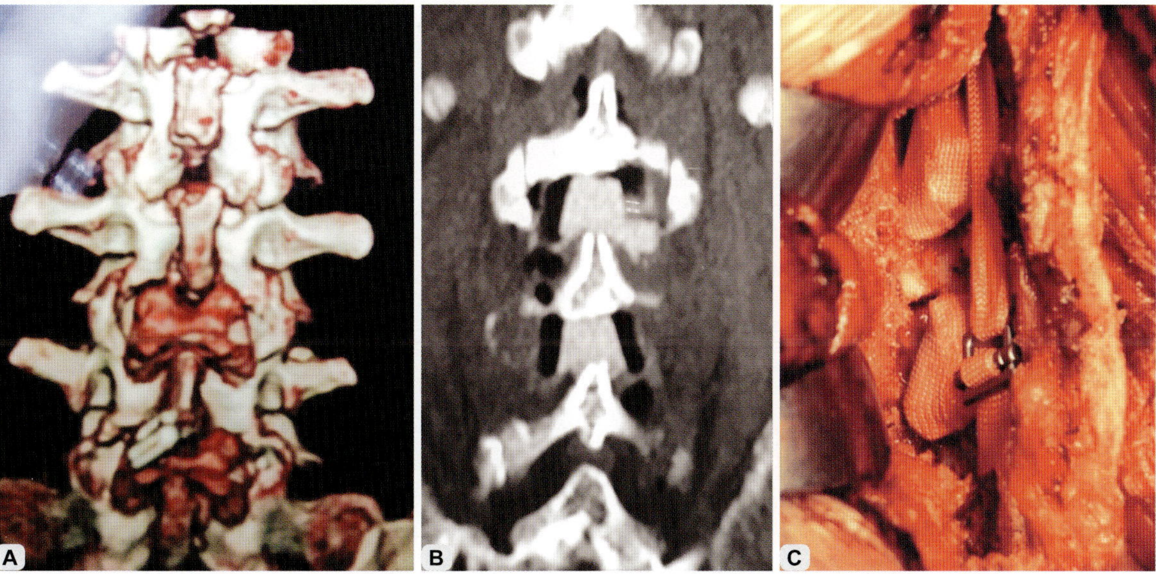

Fig. 38.10 Final position of the interlaminar device

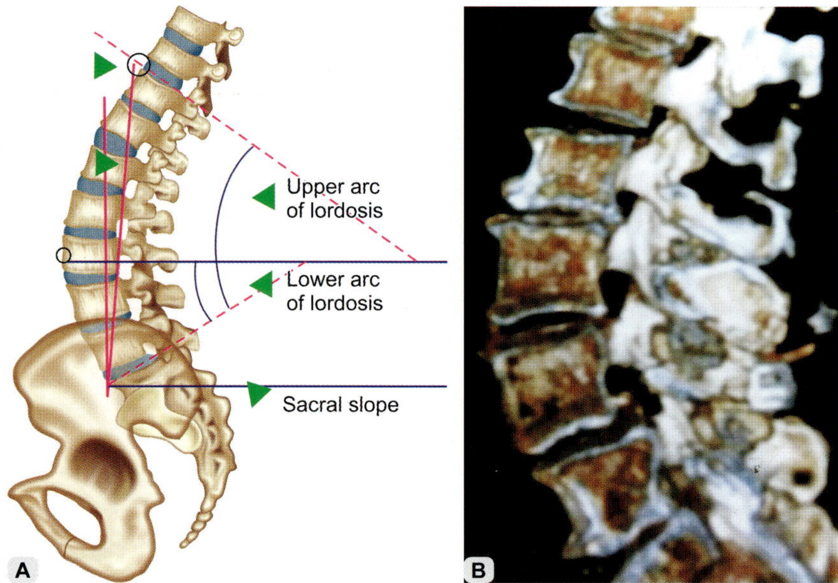

Fig. 38.11 Upper (L1–3) and lower (L3–5) arc of lumbar lordosis

- Disk bulging, resorption
- Flavum ligament buckling, in-folding
- *De novo* scoliosis.

Contraindications[41-49]

- Grade II or III spondylolisthesis
- Fractures at the level now affected
- Spinal tumors
- Congenital bone anomaly at the level now affected
- Significant osteomalacia
- Infection
- Allergic to one of the components
- Dependency of drug and/or alcohol, or psychological problems
- Kissing spine and/or kissing lamina.

Surgical Technique

The basic instrument set for IntraSPINE (Fig. 38.12):[41-46]

- Spinous processes distractor
- Probe sizing device
- IntraSpine grasper and inserter
- Foot pusher
- Semi-rigid ligament inserter
- Semi-rigid ligament tightener
  - Patient position is prone and flexion at the affected level
  - General anesthesia
  - C- Arm/Image intensifier
  - Use needle at the tip of the spinous processes of the affected levels and draw the skin landmark (Fig. 38.13)

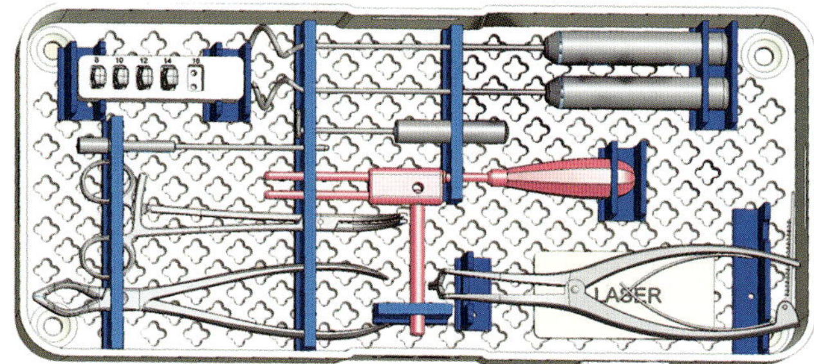

Fig. 38.12 Basic instrument set (Cousin Biotech)

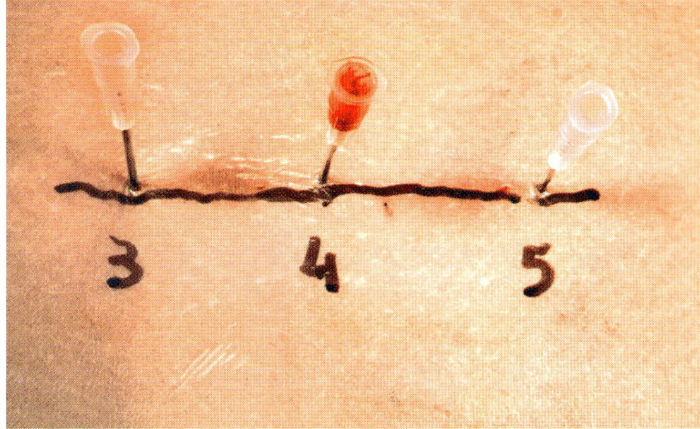

Fig. 38.13 Needle for marking at the tip of spinous process VL3–5

  - Dissecting subcutaneously to the lateral exposing thoracolumbar fascia (Fig. 38.14)
  - Incision of the fascia 1 cm away from midline to preserve the CFS (Fig. 38.15)

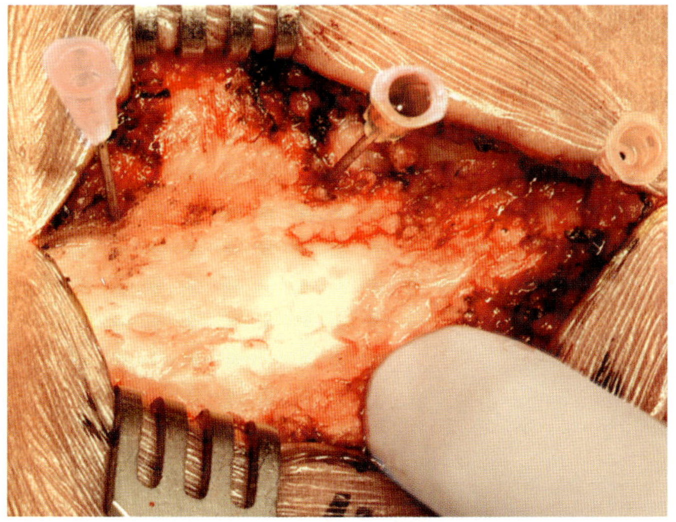

Fig. 38.14 Midline skin incision, and reflecting skin and subcutaneous tissue to lateral

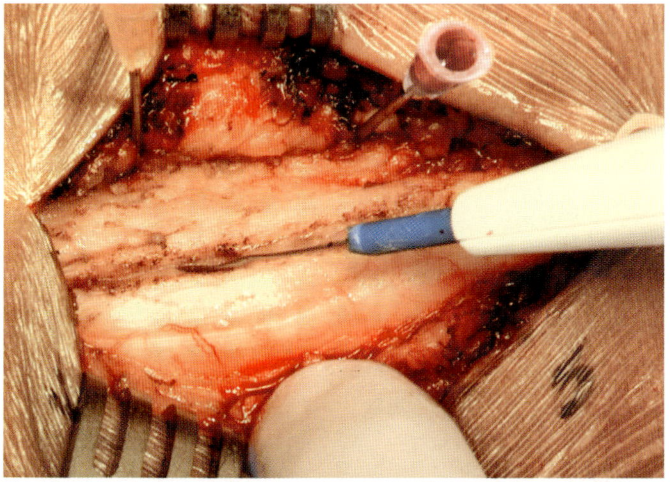

Fig. 38.15 Thoracolumbar fascia incision 1 cm away from midline to preserve CFS

- Reflecting the CFS (Fig. 38.16)
- Separating CFS from muscles (Fig. 38.17)
- Expose the anatomical landmark: spinous process, lamina, facet, interspinous ligament, flavum, CFS (Fig. 38.18)
- Use the interspinous distractor to widen the space for decompression and also to create the maximum tension of the CFS and the ligaments: ALL, PLL, outermost annulus fibrosus of the disk (Fig. 38.19)
- Decompression: Partial facetectomy of the hypertrophied inferior facet using osteotome (Fig. 38.20)
- Flavumectomy of the infolding flavum using no 11 knife and special curve rongeur (Fig. 38.21)
- Partial facet-ectomy of hypertrophied superior facet using osteotome (Fig. 38.22)

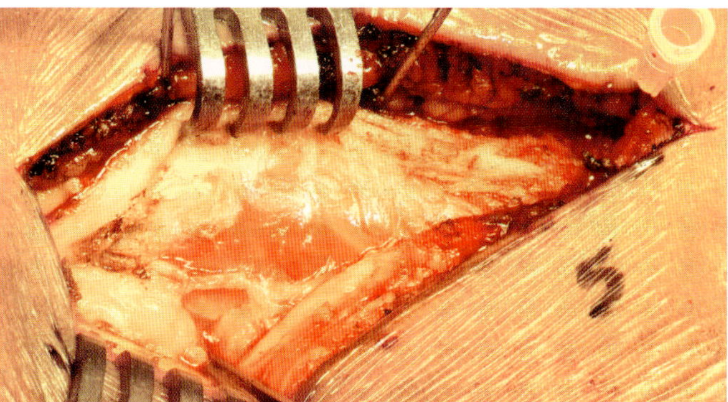

Fig. 38.16 Reflecting the CFS using retractor

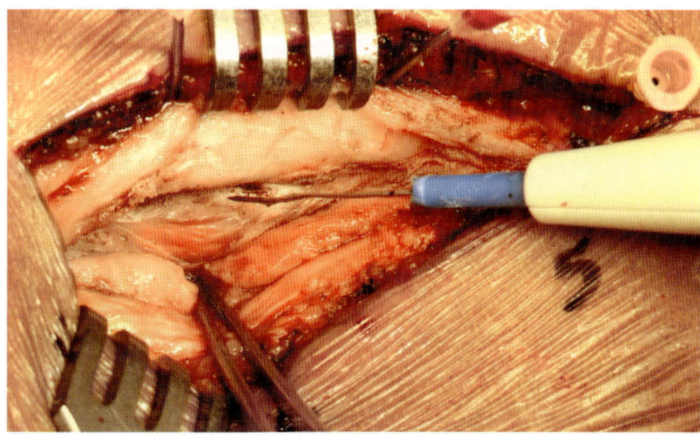

Fig. 38.17 Separate multifidus muscle from CFS

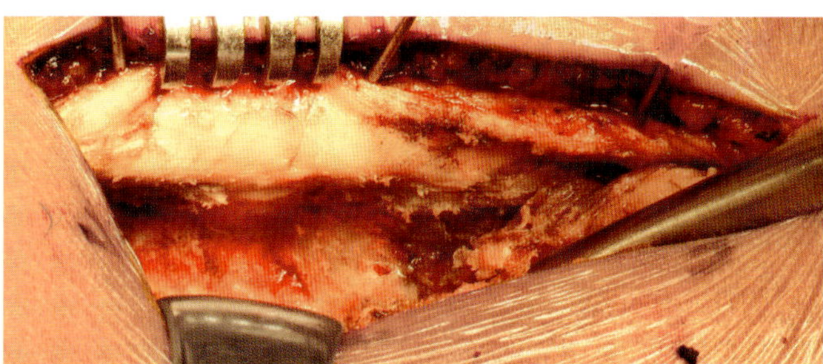

Fig. 38.18 View of spinous process, lamina, facet, ligament flavum after relecting muscles to the lateral

- Sizing the inter lamina space using probe (Fig. 38.23)
- Inserting the IntraSPINE using inserter and foot pusher (Fig. 38.24)
- In any insufficiency or laxity of CFS use the semi-rigid ligament and tightened. Important step before tightening—operation table should be changed from flexion to flat or slight extension (Figs 38.25 and 38.26)
- Closing the CFS and the skin: 3 cm for 1 level, 5 cm for 2 levels, 7 cm for 4 levels, and 10 cm for 4–5 levels (Fig. 38.27).

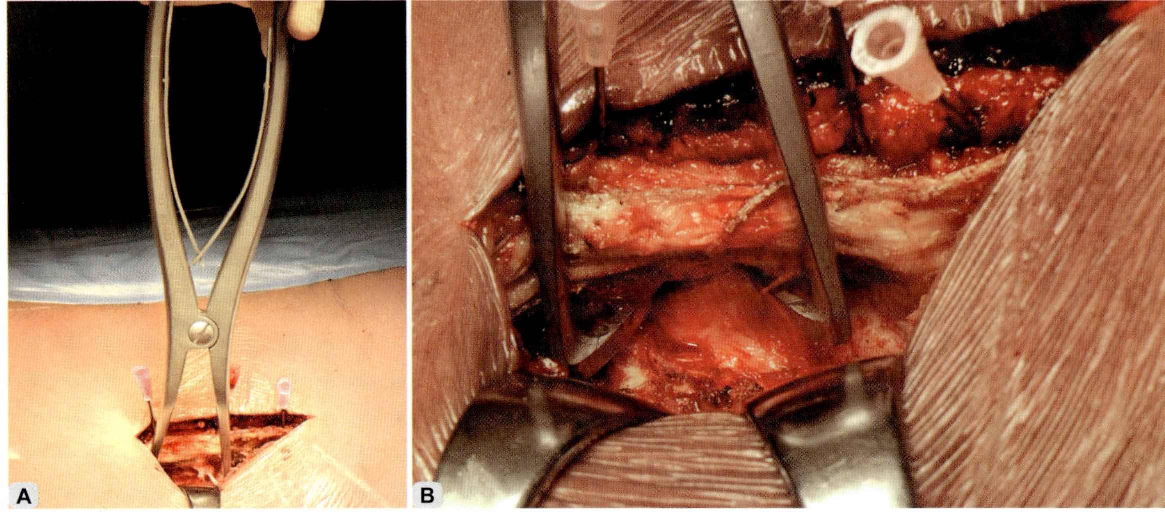

Fig. 38.19 (A) Distraction to widen the interspinous space, and to provide optimum tension of CFS; (B) posterior longitudinal ligament, outermost annulus fibrosus

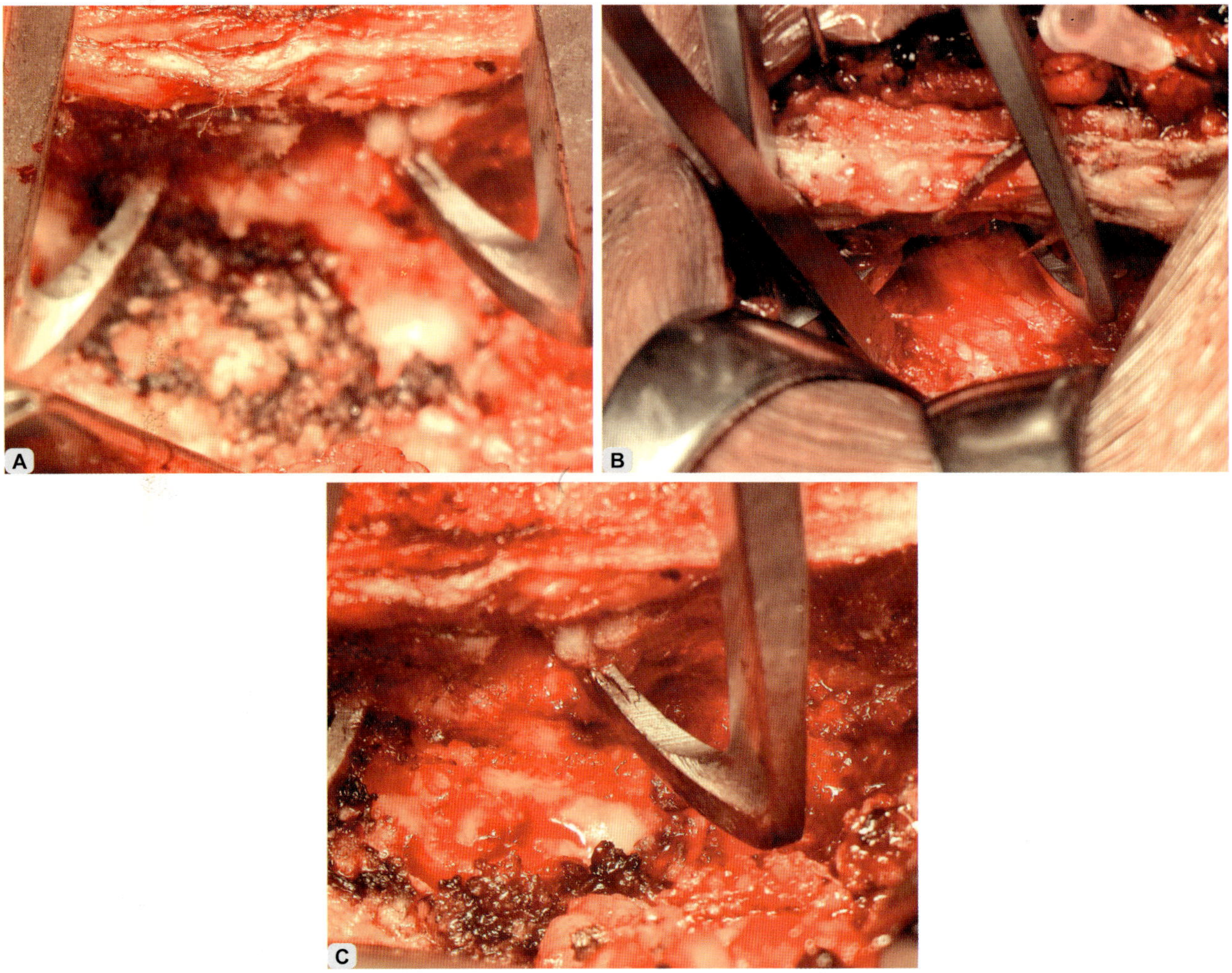

Fig. 38.20 Partial facetectomy of inferior facet using osteotome

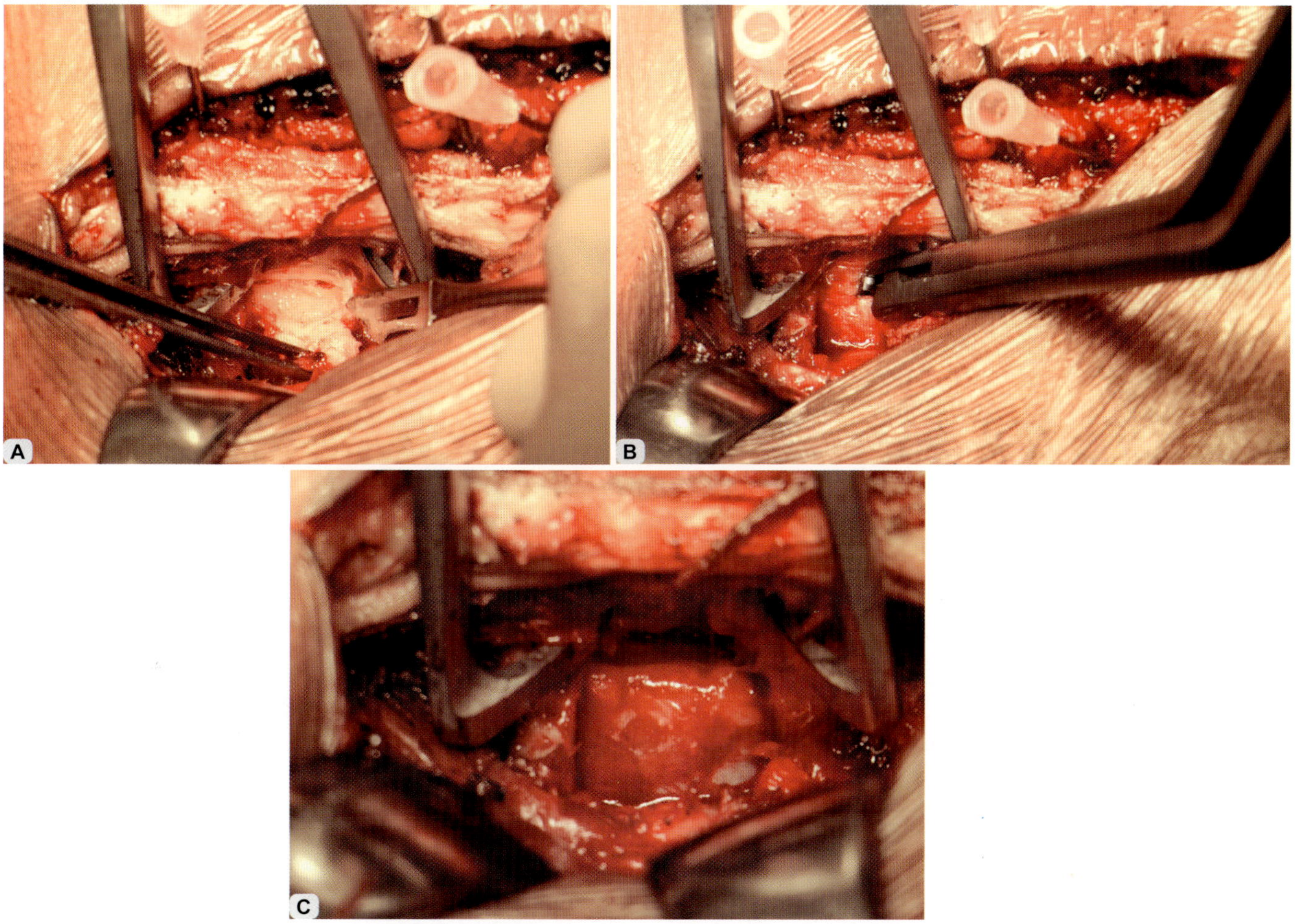

Fig. 38.21 Flavectomy using no. 11 knife and Kerison rongeur

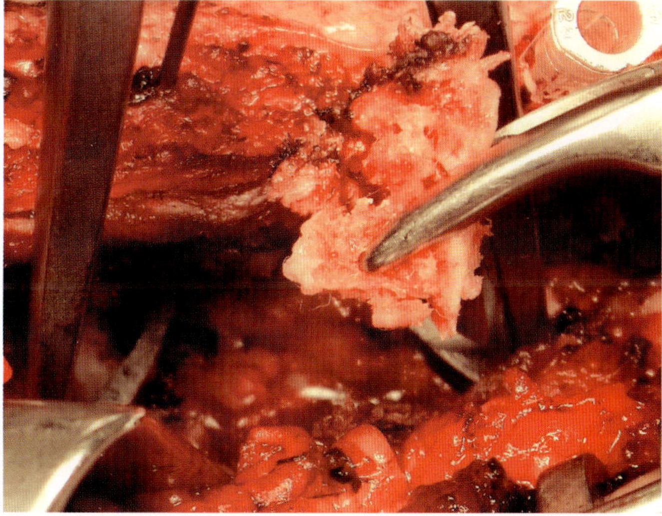

Fig. 38.22 Partial facetectomy of superior facet using osteotome

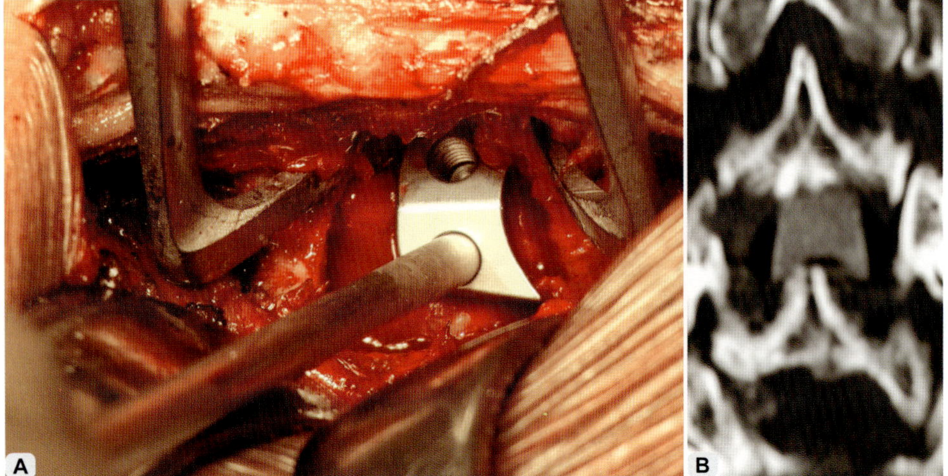

Fig. 38.23 Probe sizing

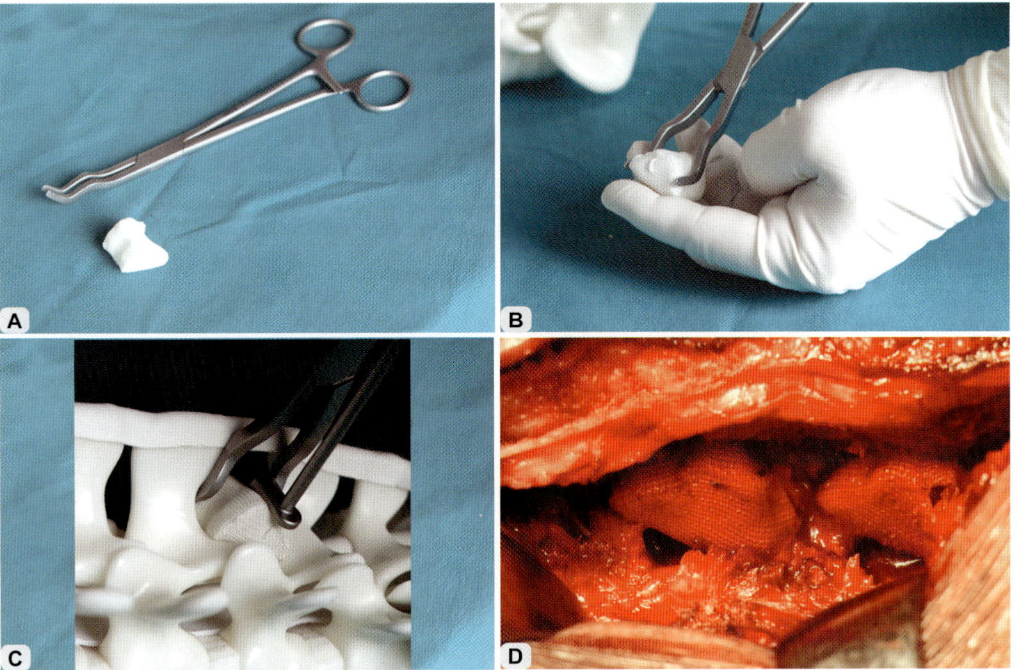

Fig. 38.24 Insert the implant using implant inserter

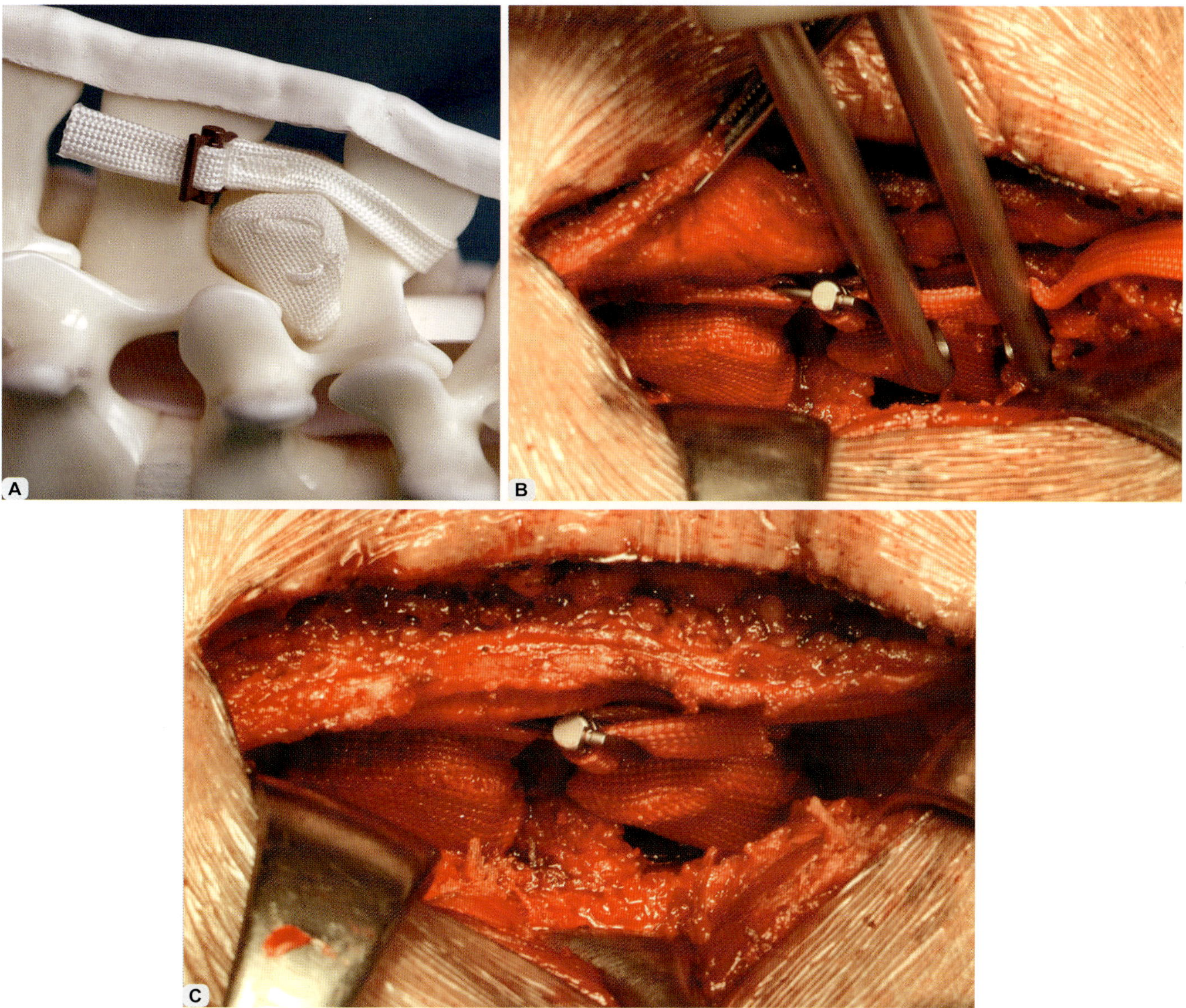

Fig. 38.25 (A and B) Insertion and tightening the semirigid ligament to reinforce the CFS; (C) Final position of the implant with ligament

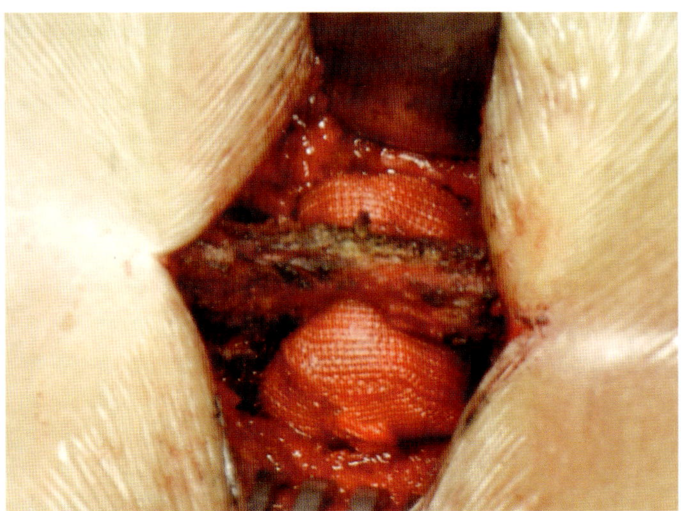

Fig. 38.26 Final position of the implant without ligament

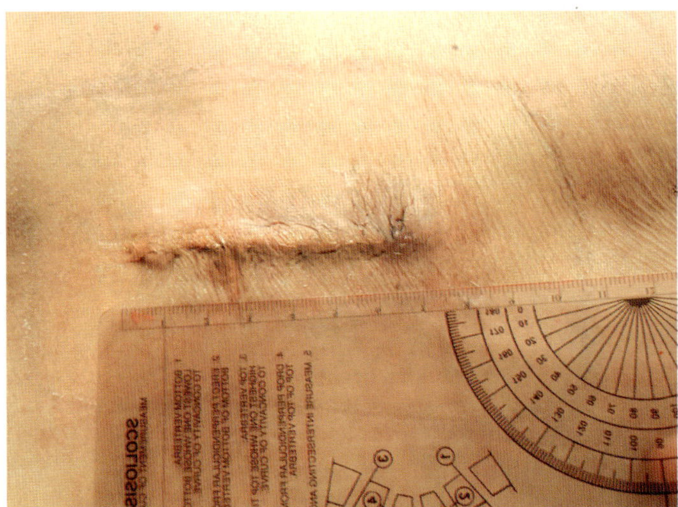

Fig. 38.27 7 cm of skin incision for surgery of 3 levels

Case Studies

Three years non-randomized prospective follow-up study of 60 cases have been treated using IntraSPINE dynamic stabilization for early and late degenerative problems of the lumbar spine. Follow-up made 2 weeks, 1, 2, 3, and 6 months after surgery. The dynamic stabilization using IntraSPINE was performed by a single surgeon. Assessment by dynamic X-ray, MRI, CT-scan, and VAS before and after surgery.

A total of 22 males and 38 females with average age 56.9 (27 – 85 years) were treated with IntraSPINE. The variation level of dynamic stabilization is related to the degenerative level from 1 to 5 levels and from L1–2 until L5–S1. The skin incision is from 3–10 cm, the surgical time for 1 level with decompression is 45′ to 4 hours for 4–5 levels. After 6 months the result is excellent: VAS from average 8.3 to 1.2, dynamic X-ray stable, patient can do normal activity of daily living.[7-11]

Case 1

A female aged 50 years with complaint of low back pain at certain movement. MRI shows an early degeneration on L3–4, L4–5, and L5–S1: bulging disk (Fig. 38.28). 2 years previously she already treated with IDET in another hospital but the complaint still exists. PELD was done for the L5–S1 and IntraSPINE for L3–4, L 4–5 without decompression. Three months after surgery she gain normal ROM of the spine, no complaint of LBP, and a good MRI result (Fig. 38.29).

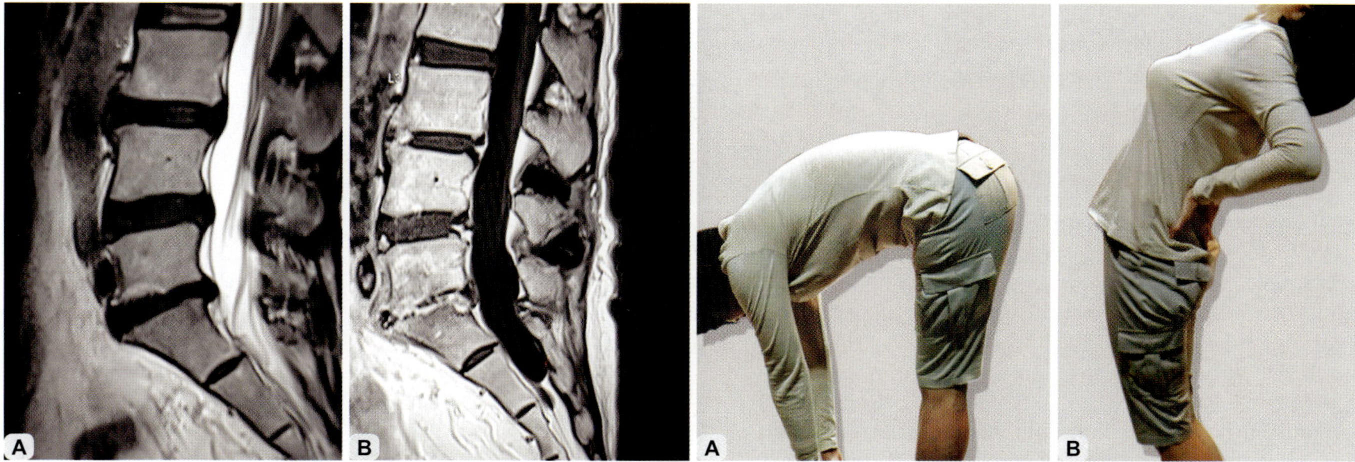

Fig. 38.28 Pretreatment MRI

Fig. 38.29 After treatment: normal ROM of spine

Case 2

A female aged 70 years with complaint of severe low back pain and claudication. Dynamic X-ray shows a grade I listhesis and lateral listhesis at L4–5. MRI shows a huge bulging and stenosis at L4–5. IntraSPINE with decompression and diskectomy was performed at L4–5. Three months later she gains a good quality of life and no complaint in any movement (Fig. 38.30).

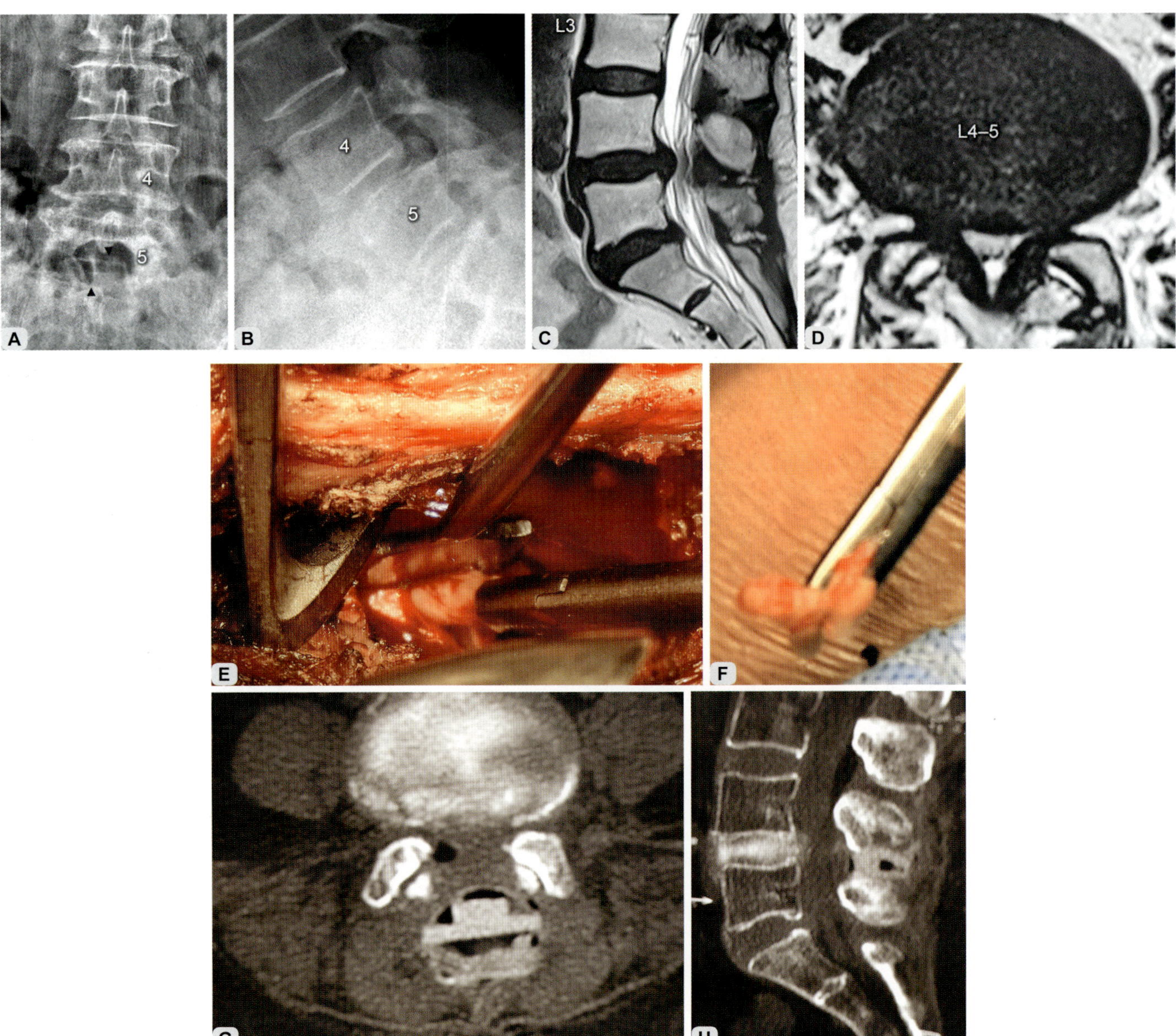

Fig. 38.30 (A and B) Radiographs showing grade I listhesis at L4–5; (C and D) MRI showing a huge bulging of L4–5; (E and F) Decompression and diskectomy performed; (G and H) Postoperative MRI showing no complaint

Case 3

A man aged 53 years with complain of low back pain and sciatica bilateral. Claudication and the pain increase with sitting and flexion. Dynamic X-ray shows instability at L3–4 and L4–5. Two years previously he experienced two levels of operation using interspinous device, but the complaint still exist. The interspinous device were removed and replaced with two levels IntraSPINE and 1 ligament. After 3 months he gains a good ROM and no complain of LBP and sciatica (Fig. 38.31).

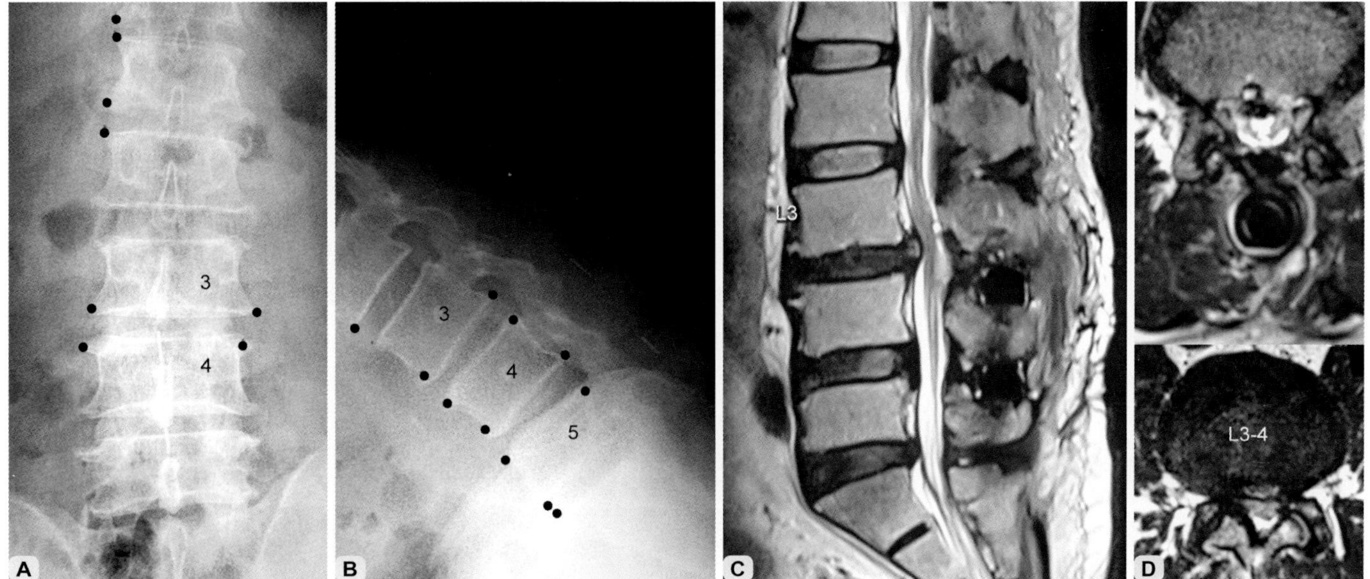

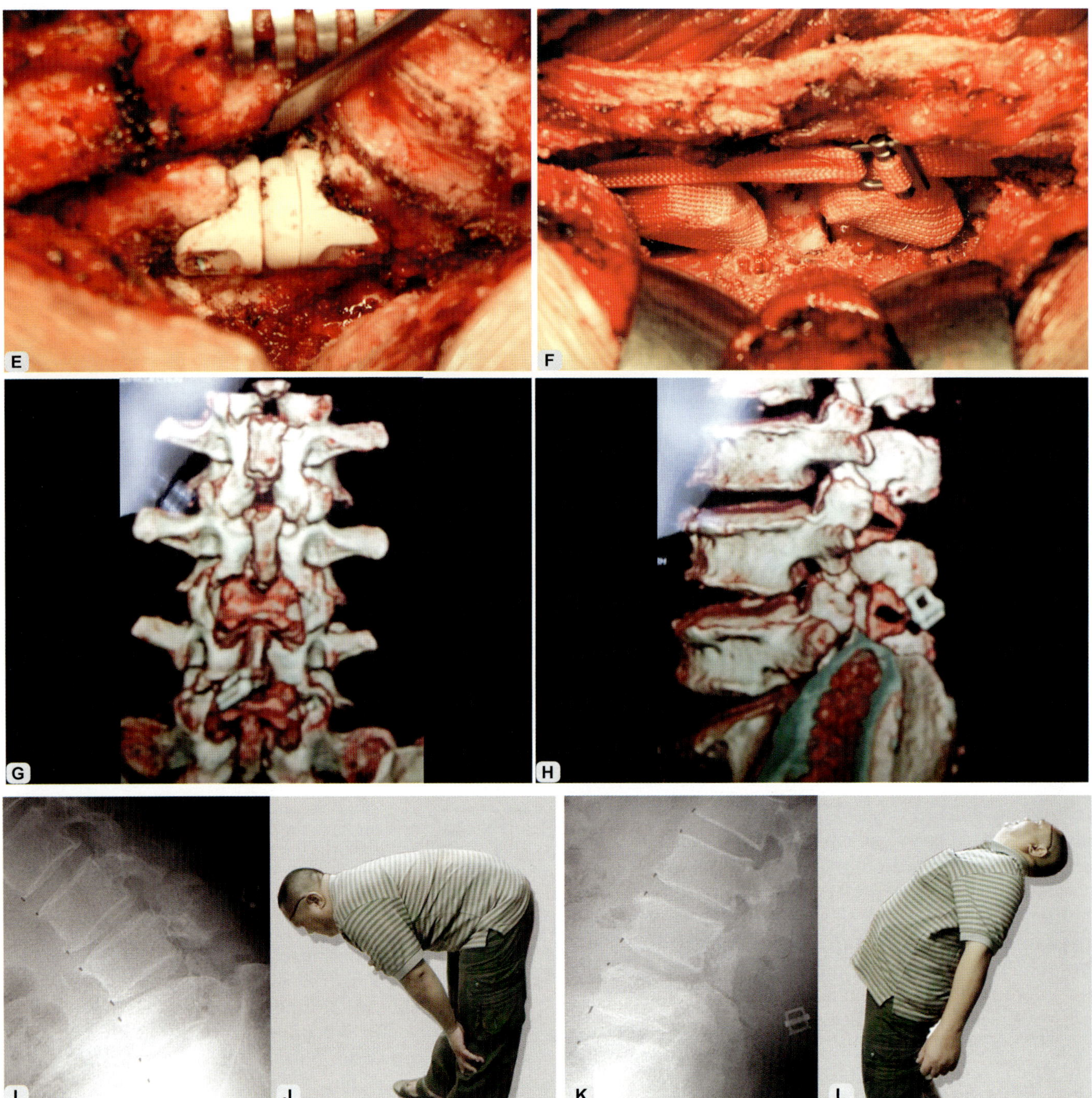

Fig. 38.31 (A to D) Preoperative X-ray and MRI; (E and F) Insertion of intraspine ligaments; (G and H) Postoperative photographs; (I and J) No problem in forward bending; (K and L) No problem in backward bending

Case 4

A woman aged 85 years with complain of low back pain, sciatica bilateral and claudication. She is wheelchair case with sagittal imbalance, pain increase at night and in body movement. Dynamic X-ray shows a scoliosis and *de novo* scoliosis, instability at L2–3, L3–4, L4–5, L5–S1. MRI shows multilevels stenosis, bulging disk and flavum buckling. Four levels IntraSPINE was performed with decompression and 3 months later she can do a good activity of daily living with no complain (Fig. 38.32).

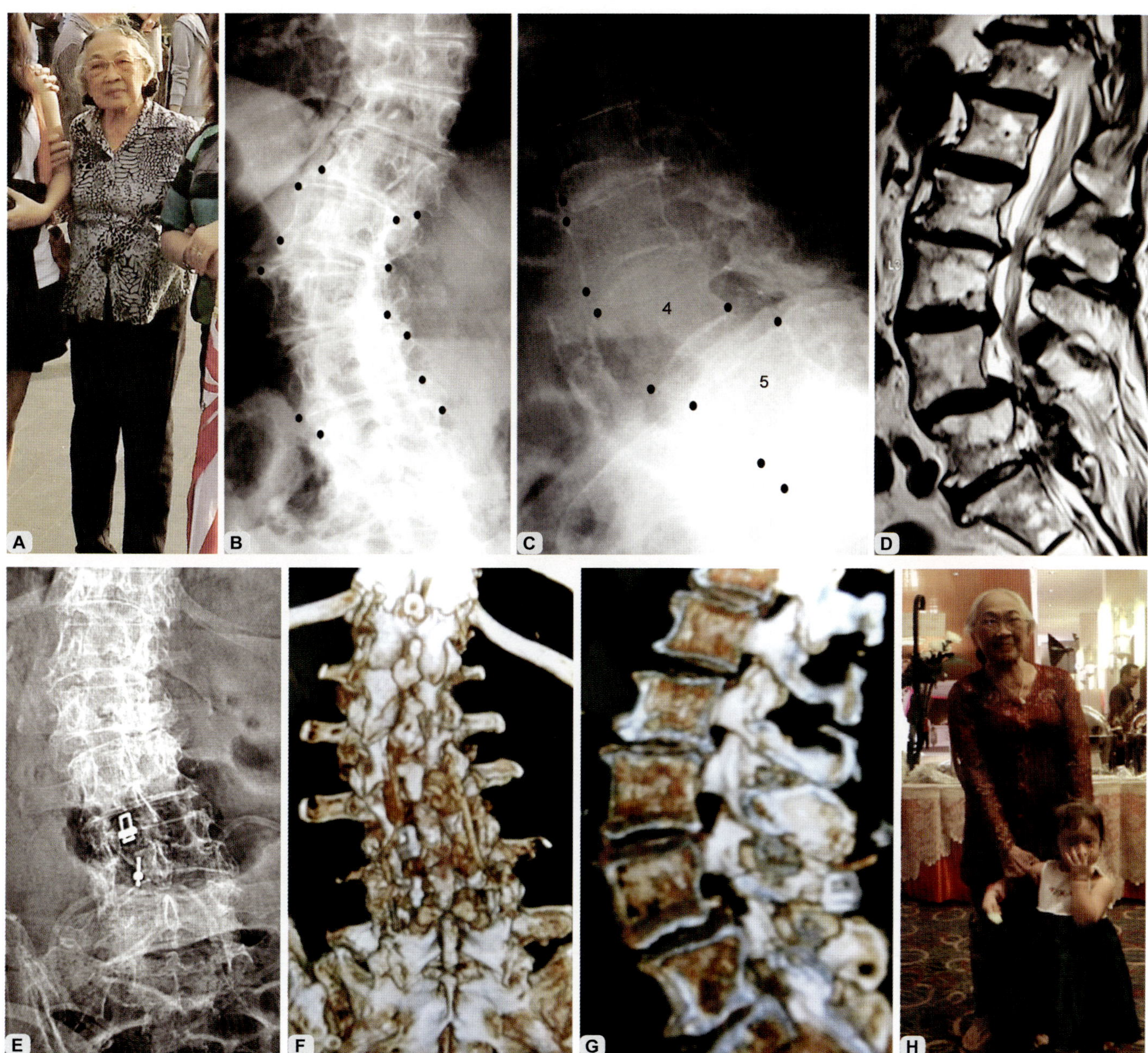

Fig. 38.32 (A) The patient; (B to G) Clinical radiographs of pre- and post-treatment; (H) Patient with no complaints

Conclusion

The fundamental feature in the design of the new device IntraSPINE is related to the anatomical reconstruction of the SMS and regarding the overturned anvil, the anterior part (nose) should be placed in between the lamina (Middle column) to control the load distribution and to achieve the sagittal balance. The interlaminar area is closer to the axis of instantaneous rotation of SMS. The complex fascia supraspinatus (CFS) is being used as Natural connector for this system, which is completely different with metal connector being used in pedicle screw system. In any laxity or insufficiency of the CFS, a semi-rigid ligament can be used to reinforce it either in upper and/or lower arc of lumbar lordosis. The IntraSPINE is made of medical grade silicone 65 shore coated by a pure PET sleeve and do not limit the ROM due to the cushion effect of the hole in the wing.

This system match the goals of dynamic stabilization: 1. Stabilize the segmental instability, 2. Maintain the sagittal balance, 3. Restore the physiologic movement of SMS.[6-11,19-21]

References

1. Kirkaldy-Willis WH, Wedge JH, Yong-Hing K, et al. Pathology and pathogenesis of lumbar spondylosis and stenosis. Spine. 1978;3:319-28.
2. Aylott CEW, Puna R, Robertson PA, et al. Spinous process morphology: the effect of ageing through adulthood on spinous process size and relationship to sagittal alignment. Eur Spine J 2012;21:1007-12.
3. Baastrup C. On the spinous processes of the lumbar vertebrae and the soft tissues between them, and on pathological changes in that region. Acta Radiol. 1933;14:52-4.
4. Kwong Y, Roan N, Latief K. MDCT findings in Baastrup disease: Disease or normal features of the aging spine ? Am Journal of Roentgenology. 2011;196(5).
5. Frymoyer JW, Krag MH. Spinal stability and instability: Definitions, classification, and general priciples of management. In Kahn A (ed): The Unstable Spine. New York: Grune & Stratton; 1986.
6. Frymoyer JW, Selby DK. Segmental instability: Rationale for treatment. Spine. 1985;10:280-6.
7. Fujiwara A, Lim TH, An HS, et al. The effect of disc degeneration and facet joint osteoarthritis on the segmental flexibility of the lumbar spine. Spine. 2000;25:3036-44.
8. Fujiwara A, Tamai K, An HS, et al. The relationship between disc degeneration, facet joint osteoarthritis, and stability of the degenerative lumbar spine. J Spinal Disord. 2000;13:444-50.
9. Jinkins JR. Acquired degenerative changes of the intervertebral segments at and suprajacent to the lumbosacral junction. A Radioanatomic analysis of the nondiskal structures of the spinal column and perispinal soft tissues. Radiol Clin N Am. 2001;39(1).
10. KCE Reports, Spinal Dynamic Stabilization Implants, Bruxelles, 29 october, 2009.
11. Keller TS, Hanson TH, Abram AC, et al. Regional variations in the compressive properties of lumbar vertebral trabeculae. Effect of disc degeneration. Spine. 1989;14:1012-9.
12. Lee CK. Accelerated degeneration of the segment adjacent to a lumbar fusion. Spine. 1988;13:375-7.
13. Moore RJ, Vernon-Roberts B, Fraser RD, et al. The origin and fate of herniated lumbarintervertebral disc tissue. Spine. 1996;21:2149-55.
14. Paajanen H, Tertti M. Association of incipient disc degeneration and instabilityin spondylolisthesis. A magnetic resonance and flexion-extension radiographic study of 20-year-old low back pain patients. Arch Orthop Trauma Surg. 1991;111:16-9.
15. Pearcy MD, Tibrewal SB. Lumbar intervertebral disc and ligament deformations measured in vivo. Clin Orthop. 1984;191:281-6.
16. Seligman JV, Gertzbein SD, Tile M, et al. Computer analysis of spinal segment motion in degenerative disc with and without axial loading. Spine. 1984;9:566-73.
17. Simpson EK, Parkinson IH, Manthey B, et al. Intervertebral disc disorganization is related to trabecular bone architecture in the lumbar spine. J Bone Miner Res. 2001;16:681-7.
18. Barrick WT, Schofferman JA, Reynolds JB, et al. Anterior lumbar fusion improves discogenic pain at levels of prior posterolateral fusion, Spine. 2000;25:853-7.
19. Bono CM, Bawa M, White K, et al. How much radiographic motion is present after solid fusion. Presented at the Annual Meeting of the International Society for the Study of the Lumbar Spine, Vancouver, BC, 2003.
20. Brantigan JW, Stefee AD, Lewis ML, et al. Lumbar interbody fusion using the Brantigan I/F cage for posterior lumbar interbody fusion and the variable pedicle screw placement system. Spine. 2000;25:1437-46.
21. DePalma AF, Rothman RH. Surgery of the lumbar spine. Clin Orthop. 1969;63:162-70.
22. Eck JC, Humphreys SC, Hodges SD. Adjacent-segment degenerationafter lumbar fusion. A review of clinical, biomechanical, and radiologic studies. Am J Orthop. 1999;28:336-40.
23. Etebar S, Cahill DW. Risk factors for adjacent-segment failure following lumbar fixation with rigid instrumentation for degenerative instability. J Neurosurg. 1999;90:163-9.
24. Molz F, Partin J, Kirkpatrick J. The acute effect of L3/L4 fusion on the motion of vertebrae in a whole lumbar cadaveric spine. Presented at the Annual Meeting of the International Society for the Study of the Lumbar Spine, Vancouver, BC, 2003.
25. Parker LM, Murrell SE, Boden SD, et al. The outcome of posterolateral fusion in highly selected patients with discogenic low back pain. Spine. 1997;21:1909-16.

26. Patel C, Truumees E, Gittlin J, et al. Symptomatic spinal stenosis adjacent to a previous lumbar fusion. Spine J. 2002;2(Suppl):54S-55S.
27. Schecter NA, France MP, Lee CK. Painful internal disc derangements of the lumbosacral spine: Discographic diagnosis and treatment by posterior lumbal interbody fusion. Orthopaedics. 1991;14:447-51.
28. Weinhoffer SL, Guyer RD, Herbert M, et al. Intradiscal pressure measuments above an instrumented fusion. A cadaver study. Spine. 1995;20:526-31.
29. Kanayama M, Hasshimoto T, Shigenubu K, et al. Adjacent-segment morbidity after Graft ligamentoplasty compared with posteroleteral lumbar fusion. J Neurosurg. 2001;95:5-10.
30. Kanayama M, Hashimoto M, Shigenobu K, et al. Non-fusion surgery for degenerative spondylolisthesis using artificial ligament stabilization: Surgical indication and clinical results. Spine. 2005;30:588-92.
31. Lindsey DP, Swanson KE, Fuchs P, et al. The effects of an intrespinous implant on the kinematics of the instrumented and adjacent levels in the lumbar spine. Spine. 2003;28:2192-7.
32. McAfee PC, Cunningham BW, Devine J, et al. Classification of heterotopic ossification (HO) in the artificial disk replacement. J Spinal Disord Tech. 2003;16:384-9.
33. Mulholland RC, Sengupta DK. Rationale, principles and experimental evaluation of the concept of soft stabilization. Eur Spine J. 2002;11(Suppl 2):S198-205.
34. Okawa A, Shinomiya K, Komori H, et al. Dynamic motion study of the whole lumbar spine by videofluoroscopy. Spine. 1998;23:1743-9.
35. Putzier M, Schneider SV, Funk JF, et al. The surgical treatment of the lumbar disc prolapse nucleotomy with additional transpedicular dynamic stabilization versus nucleotomy alone. Eur Spine J. 2003;12:108-16.
36. Sengupta DK, Demetropoulos CK, Herkowitz HN, et al. Instant centre of rotation and intradiscal pressure study to identify load-sharing property of dynamic stabilization devices in the lumbar spine without fusion—a biomechanical study in cadaver spine. Presented at World Spine II, Chicago, Aug 2003.
37. Stoll TM, Dubois G, Schwarzenbach O. The dynamic neutralization system for the spine : A multi-center sudy of a novel non-fusion system. Eur Spine J. 2002;11:170-8.
38. Swanson KE, Lindsey DP, Hsu KY, et al. The effects of an interspinous implant on intervertebral disc pressure. Spine. 2003;28:26-32.
39. Roy-Camille R, Massin P. Traitement des fractures du rachis dorsolombaire par la method de Bohler. Rev Chir Orthop. 1989;75:479-89.
40. Rauschning W. Department of Orthopaedic Surgery Academic University Hospital, SE-75185 UPPSALA, Sweden, Personal Communication, 2013.
41. Brochure IntraSpine, Cousin Biotech, France.
42. Darwono B. The role of IntraSpine in the treatment of late degenerative problems, COA 2012 Meeting, Beijing, 15-17 October, 2012.
43. Darwono B. The role of Interlaminar (IntraSpine) in the treatment of early and late degenerative problems, IntraSpine Users Meeting, Nice, France, 21-23 February, 2013.
44. Darwono B. The role of interlaminar (IntraSpine) device in the treatment of early & late degenerative problems, ISMISS, Turkey, 11-14 April, 2013.
45. Darwono B. The role of new interlaminar device (IntraSPINE) in the treatment of early & late degenerative problems, Indonesian Spine Society Meeting, Palembang, Indonesia, 28-30 June, 2013.
46. Darwono B. The role of interlaminar stabilization device (IntraSPINE) in the treatment of early & late degenerative problems, 13th Annual Meeting PASMISS, Miyazaki, Japan, 1-3 August, 2013.
47. Guizzardi G, Petrini P. DIAM Spinal Stabilization Systeem, Chapter 68 in Motion Preservation Surgery of the Spine, Advanced Technique and Controversies, Saunders Elsevier. 2007;519-22.
48. Guizzardi G, Morichi R, Mattioli CM, et al. Italian Multicentre study on the use of A New Interlaminar Prosthesis (INTRASPINE) in DDD of The Lumbar Spine. Preliminary Report, Deutscher Wierbelsaulenkongress, Congress Centrum, Ulm, 27-29 November, 2008.
49. Guizzardi G, Petrini P. Interspinous versus Interlaminar devices in DDD : Biomechanic Tests, Deutscher Wierbelsaulenkongress, Internationales Congress Centrum, Munchen, 10-12 December, 2009.

Index

Page numbers followed by *f* refer to figure and *t* refer to table.

R

S

T